2023-24 GUIDE TO

MEDICATIONS FOR THE TREATMENT OF DIABETES MELLITUS

Edited by
JOHN R. WHITE, JR., PA-C, PharmD

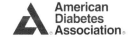

American
Diabetes
Association.

Director, Book Operations, Victor Van Beuren; *Managing Editor, Books*, John Clark; *Director, Book Marketing*, Annette Reape; *Project Manager, Editor, and Composition*, Jeska Horgan-Kobelski; *Printer*, Lightning Source.

Printed in the United States of America
1 3 5 7 9 10 8 6 4 2

The suggestions and information contained in this publication are generally consistent with the *Standards of Care in Diabetes* and other policies of the American Diabetes Association, but they do not represent the policy or position of the Association or any of its boards or committees. Reasonable steps have been taken to ensure the accuracy of the information presented. However, the American Diabetes Association cannot ensure the safety or efficacy of any product or service described in this publication. Individuals are advised to consult a physician or other appropriate health care professional before undertaking any diet or exercise program or taking any medication referred to in this publication. Professionals must use and apply their own professional judgment, experience, and training and should not rely solely on the information contained in this publication before prescribing any diet, exercise, or medication. The American Diabetes Association—its officers, directors, employees, volunteers, and members—assumes no responsibility or liability for personal or other injury, loss, or damage that may result from the suggestions or information in this publication.

♾ The paper in this publication meets the requirements of the ANSI Standard Z39.48-1992 (permanence of paper).

American Diabetes Association titles may be purchased for business or promotional use or for special sales. To purchase more than 50 copies of this book at a discount, or for custom editions of this book with your logo, contact the American Diabetes Association at the bulk book sales address below, at booksales@diabetes.org, or by calling 703-299-2046.

American Diabetes Association
Bulk Book Sales
PO Box 7023
Merrifield, Virginia 22116-7023

American Diabetes Association
2451 Crystal Drive, Suite 900
Arlington, VA 22202

DOI: 10.2337/9781580407649

Library of Congress Control Number: 2023939129

This book is dedicated to the memory of R. Keith Campbell.

Keith was a close friend, a mentor, and an inspiration to me as well as to innumerable other healthcare providers, patients, students, and other people. This book was originally his brainchild. He co-edited each of the previous editions/permutations of this book.

Keith was diagnosed with type 1 diabetes when he was 8 years old. He lived with diabetes for more than 68 years, all the while remaining positive and helping myriad others with diabetes. He was always firmly at the forefront of knowledge in the diabetes arena. He published more than 600 manuscripts, 14 books, 55 book chapters, and made over 1,500 professional presentations. His multifaceted career at Washington State University as an academic spanned 45 years and included many roles and titles. He received numerous awards including the American College of Clinical Pharmacy's Paul F. Parker Medal, the National Community Pharmacists Association's Outstanding Pharmacy Administration Professor in the U.S., the American Diabetes Association's Outstanding Health Care Educator in the Field of Diabetes, and the American Association of Diabetes Educator's (AADE's) Distinguished Service Award. He served on the board of directors of the American Diabetes Association, Washington State Pharmacy Association, and AADE. He was beloved by his friends, family, and students, and was known for his outgoing personality. He was a remarkable, one-of-a-kind individual who is greatly missed. He will always be remembered for his indefatigable ability to manage a difficult, complicated, chronic disease with grace, for his larger-than-life personality, and for his ever-present cat-that-caught-the-mouse smile.

—*John R. White, Jr.*

Contents

Contributors

EDITOR

John R. White, Jr., PA-C, PharmD
Professor and Department Chair
Department of Pharmacotherapy
College of Pharmacy and
  Pharmaceutical Sciences
Washington State University
Spokane, WA

CONTRIBUTORS

Damianne Brand-Eubanks, PharmD
Associate Professor, Pharmacotherapy
College of Pharmacy and
  Pharmaceutical Sciences
Washington State University
Yakima, WA

Christina R. Buchman, PharmD, BCACP
Clinical Assistant Professor,
  Pharmacotherapy
College of Pharmacy and
  Pharmaceutical Sciences
Washington State University
Yakima, WA

Kam L. Capoccia, PharmD, BCPS, CDCES
Clinical Professor of Community Care
PGY-1 Community-Based Residency
  Program Director
College of Pharmacy and Health
  Sciences
Western New England University
Springfield, MA

Megan Giruzzi, PharmD, BCPS
Clinical Assistant Professor,
  Pharmacotherapy
College of Pharmacy and
  Pharmaceutical Sciences
Washington State University
Yakima, WA

Nicholas R. Giruzzi, PharmD, BCPS
Clinical Assistant Professor,
  Pharmacotherapy
College of Pharmacy and
  Pharmaceutical Sciences
Washington State University
Yakima, WA

Anne P. Kim, PharmD, MPH, MIT
Associate Professor, Pharmacotherapy
Director, Yakima Campus
College of Pharmacy and
  Pharmaceutical Sciences
Washington State University
Yakima, WA

Lisa Kroon, PharmD
Chair and Professor
Department of Clinical Pharmacy
School of Pharmacy
University of California, San Francisco
San Francisco, CA
Assistant Chief Pharmacy Officer,
  Research, Education and Clinical
  Services
UCSF Health

Kimberly C. McKeirnan, PharmD, BCACP
Clinical Associate Professor
Department of Pharmacotherapy
College of Pharmacy and
  Pharmaceutical Sciences
Washington State University
Spokane, WA

Joshua J. Neumiller, PharmD, CDCES, FADCES, FASCP
Vice Chair and Allen I. White
  Distinguished Associate Professor,
  Pharmacotherapy
Department of Pharmacotherapy
College of Pharmacy and
  Pharmaceutical Sciences
Washington State University
Spokane, WA

Cheyenne Frazier, PharmD, PhC, BCACP
Associate Professor, Pharmacotherapy
College of Pharmacy and
  Pharmaceutical Sciences
Washington State University
Spokane, WA

Peggy Soule Odegard, BSPharm, PharmD, CDCES
Vice Dean, Professional Pharmacy
  Education
Lynn and Geraldine Brady Endowed
  Professor of Pharmacy
School of Pharmacy
University of Washington
Seattle, WA

Nicole M. Rodin, PharmD, MBA
Assistant Professor
Department of Pharmacotherapy
College of Pharmacy and
  Pharmaceutical Sciences
Washington State University
Spokane, WA

Emmeline Tran, PharmD
Assistant Professor
College of Pharmacy
Medical University of South Carolina
Charleston, SC

Jennifer M. Trujillo, PharmD, BCPS, FCCP, CDCES, BC-ADM
Professor
Skaggs School of Pharmacy and
  Pharmaceutical Sciences
University of Colorado Anschutz
  Medical Campus
Aurora, CO

Megan Willson, PharmD, BCPS
Clinical Professor, Pharmacotherapy
College of Pharmacy and
  Pharmaceutical Sciences
Washington State University
Spokane, WA

Crystal Zhou, PharmD
Clinical Associate Professor
Department of Clinical Pharmacy
School of Pharmacy
University of California, San Francisco
San Francisco, CA

Chapter 1
Pharmacologic Therapy for Type 1 Diabetes

9.1 Most individuals with type 1 diabetes should be treated with multiple daily injections of prandial and basal insulin, or continuous subcutaneous insulin infusion. **A**

9.2 Most individuals with type 1 diabetes should use rapid-acting insulin analogs to reduce hypoglycemia risk. **A**

9.3 Individuals with type 1 diabetes should receive education on how to match mealtime insulin doses to carbohydrate intake, fat and protein content, and anticipated physical activity. **B**

INSULIN THERAPY

Because the hallmark of type 1 diabetes is absent or near-absent β-cell function, insulin treatment is essential for individuals with type 1 diabetes. In addition to hyperglycemia, insulinopenia can contribute to other metabolic disturbances like hypertriglyceridemia and ketoacidosis as well as tissue catabolism that can be life threatening. Severe metabolic decompensation can be, and was, mostly prevented with once or twice daily injections for the six or seven decades after the discovery of insulin. However, over the past three decades, evidence has accumulated supporting more intensive insulin replacement, using multiple daily injections of insulin or continuous subcutaneous administration through an insulin pump, as providing the best combination of effectiveness and safety for people with type 1 diabetes. The Diabetes Control and Complications Trial (DCCT) demonstrated that intensive therapy with multiple daily injections or continuous subcutaneous insulin infusion (CSII) reduced A1C and was associated with improved long-term outcomes.[1-3] The study was carried out with short-acting (regular) and intermediate-acting (NPH) human insulins. In this landmark trial, lower A1C with intensive control (7%) led to ~50% reductions in microvascular complications over 6 years of treatment. However, intensive therapy was associated with a higher rate of

---

Chapter 4 is an excerpt from ElSayed NA, Aleppo G, Aroda VR, et al., American Diabetes Association. 9. Pharmacologic approaches to glycemic treatment: Standards of Care in Diabetes—2023. *Diabetes Care* 2023;46(Suppl. 1):S140–S157

* See Table 1.1 (p. 2) for an explanation of the American Diabetes Association evidence-grading system for *Standards of Care in Diabetes*.

severe hypoglycemia than conventional treatment (62 compared with 19 episodes per 100 patient-years of therapy). Follow-up of subjects from the DCCT more than 10 years after the active treatment component of the study demonstrated fewer macrovascular as well as fewer microvascular complications in the group that received intensive treatment.[2,4]

Insulin replacement regimens typically consist of basal insulin, mealtime insulin, and correction insulin.[5] Basal insulin includes NPH insulin, long-acting insulin analogs, and continuous delivery of rapid-acting insulin via an insulin pump. Basal insulin analogs have longer duration of action with flatter, more constant plasma concentrations and activity profiles than NPH insulin; rapidacting analogs (RAA) have a quicker onset and peak and shorter duration of action than regular human insulin. In people with type 1 diabetes, treatment with analog insulins is associated with less hypoglycemia and weight gain as well as lower A1C compared with human insulins.[6–8] More recently, two new injectable insulin formulations with enhanced rapid action profiles have been introduced. Inhaled human insulin has a rapid peak and shortened duration of action compared with RAA and may cause less hypoglycemia and weight gain[9] (see also subsection "Alternative Insulin Routes" in section "Pharmacologic Therapy for Adults with Type 2 Diabetes"), and faster-acting insulin aspart and insulin lispro-aabc may reduce prandial excur-

Table 1.1—American Diabetes Association Evidence-grading System for *Standards of Care in Diabetes*

Level of evidence	Description
A	Clear evidence from well-conducted, generalizable randomized controlled trials that are adequately powered, including ■ Evidence from a well-conducted multicenter trial ■ Evidence from a meta-analysis that incorporated quality ratings in the analysis Compelling nonexperimental evidence, i.e., "all or none" rule developed by the Centre for Evidence-Based Medicine at the University of Oxford Supportive evidence from well-conducted randomized controlled trials that are adequately powered, including ■ Evidence from a well-conducted trial at one or more institutions ■ Evidence from a meta-analysis that incorporated quality ratings in the analysis
B	Supportive evidence from well-conducted cohort studies ■ Evidence from a well-conducted prospective cohort study or registry ■ Evidence from a well-conducted meta-analysis of cohort studies Supportive evidence from a well-conducted case-control study
C	Supportive evidence from poorly controlled or uncontrolled studies ■ Evidence from randomized clinical trials with one or more major or three or more minor methodological flaws that could invalidate the results ■ Evidence from observational studies with high potential for bias (such as case series with comparison with historical controls) ■ Evidence from case series or case reports Conflicting evidence with the weight of evidence supporting the recommendation
E	Expert consensus or clinical experience

sions better than RAA.[10–12] In addition, longer-acting basal analogs (U-300 glargine or degludec) may confer a lower hypoglycemia risk compared with U-100 glargine in individuals with type 1 diabetes.[13,14] Despite the advantages of insulin analogs in individuals with type 1 diabetes, for some individuals the expense and/or intensity of treatment required for their use is prohibitive. There are multiple approaches to insulin treatment, and the central precept in the management of type 1 diabetes is that some form of insulin be given in a planned regimen tailored to the individual to keep them safe and out of diabetic ketoacidosis and to avoid significant hypoglycemia, with every effort made to reach the individual's glycemic targets.

Most studies comparing multiple daily injections with CSII have been relatively small and of short duration. However, a systematic review and metaanalysis concluded that CSII via pump therapy has modest advantages for lowering A1C (0.30% [95% CI 0.58 to 0.02]) and for reducing severe hypoglycemia rates in children and adults.[15] However, there is no consensus to guide the choice of injection or pump therapy in a given individual, and research to guide this decision-making is needed.[16] The arrival of continuous glucose monitors (CGM) to clinical practice has proven beneficial in people using insulin therapy. Its use is now considered standard of care for most people with type 1 diabetes[5] (see Section 7, "Diabetes Technology"). Reduction of nocturnal hypoglycemia in individuals with type 1 diabetes using insulin pumps with CGM is improved by automatic suspension of insulin delivery at a preset glucose level.[16–18] When choosing among insulin delivery systems, individual preferences, cost, insulin type and dosing regimen, and self-management capabilities should be considered (see Section 7, "Diabetes Technology").

The U.S. Food and Drug Administration (FDA) has now approved multiple hybrid closed-loop pump systems (also called automated insulin delivery [AID] systems). The safety and efficacy of hybrid closed-loop systems has been supported in the literature in adolescents and adults with type 1 diabetes,[19,20] and evidence suggests that a closed-loop system is superior to sensor-augmented pump therapy for glycemic control and reduction of hypoglycemia over 3 months of comparison in children and adults with type 1 diabetes.[21] In the International Diabetes Closed Loop (iDCL) trial, a 6-month trial in people with type 1 diabetes at least 14 years of age, the use of a closed-loop system was associated with a greater percentage of time spent in the target glycemic range, reduced mean glucose and A1C levels, and a lower percentage of time spent in hypoglycemia compared with use of a sensor-augmented pump.[22]

Intensive insulin management using a version of CSII and continuous glucose monitoring should be considered in most individuals with type 1 diabetes. AID systems may be considered in individuals with type 1 diabetes who are capable of using the device safely (either by themselves or with a caregiver) in order to improve time in range and reduce A1C and hypoglycemia.[22] See Section 7, "Diabetes Technology," for a full discussion of insulin delivery devices.

In general, individuals with type 1 diabetes require 50% of their daily insulin as basal and 50% as prandial, but this is dependent on a number of factors, including whether the individual consumes lower or higher carbohydrate meals. Total daily insulin requirements can be estimated based on weight, with typical doses ranging from 0.4 to 1.0 units/kg/day. Higher amounts are required during puberty, pregnancy, and medical illness. The *American Diabetes Association/JDRF Type 1*

Diabetes Sourcebook notes 0.5 units/kg/day as a typical starting dose in individuals with type 1 diabetes who are metabolically stable, with half administered as prandial insulin given to control blood glucose after meals and the other half as basal insulin to control glycemia in the periods between meal absorption;[23] this guideline provides detailed information on intensification of therapy to meet individualized needs. In addition, the American Diabetes Association (ADA) position statement "Type 1 Diabetes Management Through the Life Span" provides a thorough overview of type 1 diabetes treatment.[24]

Typical multidose regimens for individuals with type 1 diabetes combine premeal use of shorter-acting insulins with a longer-acting formulation. The long-acting basal dose is titrated to regulate overnight and fasting glucose. Postprandial glucose excursions are best controlled by a well-timed injection of prandial insulin. The optimal time to administer prandial insulin varies, based on the pharmacokinetics of the formulation (regular, RAA, inhaled), the premeal blood glucose level, and carbohydrate consumption. Recommendations for prandial insulin dose administration should therefore be individualized. Physiologic insulin secretion varies with glycemia, meal size, meal composition, and tissue demands for glucose. To approach this variability in people using insulin treatment, strategies have evolved to adjust prandial doses based on predicted needs. Thus, education on how to adjust prandial insulin to account for carbohydrate intake, premeal glucose levels, and anticipated activity can be effective and should be offered to most individuals.[25,26] For individuals in whom carbohydrate counting is effective, estimates of the fat and protein content of meals can be incorporated into their prandial dosing for added benefit[27] (see Section 5, "Facilitating Positive Health Behaviors and Well-being to Improve Health Outcomes").

The 2021 ADA/European Association for the Study of Diabetes (EASD) consensus report on the management of type 1 diabetes in adults summarizes different insulin regimens and glucose monitoring strategies in individuals with type 1 diabetes (Fig. 1.1 and Table 1.2).[5]

INSULIN INJECTION TECHNIQUE

Ensuring that individuals and/or caregivers understand correct insulin injection technique is important to optimize glucose control and insulin use safety. Thus, it is important that insulin be delivered into the proper tissue in the correct way. Recommendations have been published elsewhere outlining best practices for insulin injection.[28] Proper insulin injection technique includes injecting into appropriate body areas, injection site rotation, appropriate care of injection sites to avoid infection or other complications, and avoidance of intramuscular (IM) insulin delivery.

Exogenously delivered insulin should be injected into subcutaneous tissue, not intramuscularly. Recommended sites for insulin injection include the abdomen, thigh, buttock, and upper arm. Insulin absorption from IM sites differs from that in subcutaneous sites and is also influenced by the activity of the muscle. Inadvertent IM injection can lead to unpredictable insulin absorption and variable effects on glucose and is associated with frequent and unexplained hypoglycemia. Risk for IM insulin delivery is increased in younger, leaner individuals when injecting into the limbs rather than truncal sites (abdomen and buttocks) and when using longer needles. Recent evidence supports the use of short needles (e.g., 4-mm pen needles) as effective and well tolerated when compared with longer needles, including a study performed in adults with obesity.[29]

Injection site rotation is additionally necessary to avoid lipohypertrophy, an accumulation of subcutaneous fat in response to the adipogenic actions of insulin at a site of multiple injections.

Lipohypertrophy appears as soft, smooth raised areas several centimeters in breadth and can contribute to erratic insulin absorption, increased glycemic variability, and unexplained hypoglycemic episodes. People treated with insulin and/

Representative relative attributes of insulin delivery approaches in people with type 1 diabetes[1]

Injected insulin regimens	Flexibility	Lower risk of hypoglycemia	Higher costs
MDI with LAA + RAA or URAA	+++	+++	+++

Less-preferred, alternative injected insulin regimens

	Flexibility	Lower risk of hypoglycemia	Higher costs
MDI with NPH + RAA or URAA	++	++	++
MDI with NPH + short-acting (regular) insulin	++	+	+
Two daily injections with NPH + short-acting (regular) insulin or premixed	+	+	+

Continuous insulin infusion regimens	Flexibility	Lower risk of hypoglycemia	Higher costs
Hybrid closed-loop technology	+++++	+++++	++++++
Insulin pump with threshold/predictive low-glucose suspend	++++	++++	+++++
Insulin pump therapy without automation	+++	+++	++++

Figure 1.1—Choices of insulin regimens in people with type 1 diabetes. Continuous glucose monitoring improves outcomes with injected or infused insulin and is superior to blood glucose monitoring. Inhaled insulin may be used in place of injectable prandial insulin in the U.S. [1]The number of plus signs (+) is an estimate of relative association of the regimen with increased flexibility, lower risk of hypoglycemia, and higher costs between the considered regimens. LAA, long-acting insulin analog; MDI, multiple daily injections; RAA, rapid-acting insulin analog; URAA, ultra-rapid-acting insulin analog. Reprinted from Holt et al.[5]

Table 1.2—Examples of Subcutaneous Insulin Regimens

Regimen	Timing and distribution	Advantages	Disadvantages	Adjusting doses
		Regimens that more closely mimic normal insulin secretion		
Insulin pump therapy (hybrid closed-loop, low-glucose suspend, CGM-augmented open-loop, BGM-augmented open-loop)	Basal delivery of URAA or RAA; generally 40–60% of TDD. Mealtime and correction: URAA or RAA by bolus based on ICR and/or ISF and target glucose, with pre-meal insulin ~15 min before eating.	Can adjust basal rates for varying insulin sensitivity by time of day, for exercise and for sick days. Flexibility in meal timing and content. Pump can deliver insulin in increments of fractions of units. Potential for integration with CGM for low-glucose suspend or hybrid closed-loop. TIR % highest and TBR % lowest with: hybrid closed-loop > low- glucose suspend > CGM-augmented open-loop > BGM- augmented open-loop.	Most expensive regimen. Must continuously wear one or more devices. Risk of rapid development of ketosis or DKA with interruption of insulin delivery. Potential reactions to adhesives and site infections. Most technically complex approach (harder for people with lower numeracy or literacy skills).	Mealtime insulin: if carbohydrate counting is accurate, change ICR if glucose after meal consistently out of target. Correction insulin: adjust ISF and/ or target glucose if correction does not consistently bring glucose into range. Basal rates: adjust based on overnight, fasting, or daytime glucose outside of activity of URAA/RAA bolus.
MDI: LAA + flexible doses of URAA or RAA at meal	LAA once daily (insulin detemir or insulin glargine may require twice-daily dosing); generally 50% of TDD. Mealtime and correction: URAA or RAA based on ICR and/or ISF and target glucose.	Can use pens for all components. Flexibility in meal timing and content. Insulin analogs cause less hypoglycemia than human insulins.	At least four daily injections. More costly insulins. Smallest increment of insulin is 1 unit (0.5 unit with some pens). LAAs may not cover strong dawn phenomenon (rise in glucose in early morning hours) as well as pump therapy.	Mealtime insulin: if carbohydrate counting is accurate, change ICR if glucose after meal consistently out of target. Correction insulin: adjust ISF and/ or target glucose if correction does not consistently bring glucose into range. LAA: based on overnight or fasting glucose or daytime glucose outside of activity time course, or URAA or RAA injections.

(continued)

Table 1.2 (continued)

Regimen	Timing and distribution	Advantages	Disadvantages	Adjusting doses
MDI regimens with less flexibility				
Four injections daily with fixed doses of N and RAA	Pre-breakfast: RAA ~20% of TDD. Pre-lunch: RAA ~10% of TDD. Pre-dinner: RAA ~10% of TDD. Bedtime: N ~50% of TDD.	May be feasible if unable to carbohydrate count. All meals have RAA coverage. N less expensive than LAAs.	Shorter duration RAA may lead to basal deficit during day; may need twice-daily N. Greater risk of nocturnal hypoglycemia with N. Requires relatively consistent mealtimes and carbohydrate intake.	Pre-breakfast RAA: based on BGM after breakfast or before lunch. Pre-lunch RAA: based on BGM after lunch or before dinner. Pre-dinner RAA: based on BGM after dinner or at bedtime. Evening N: based on fasting or overnight BGM.
Four injections daily with fixed doses of N and R	Pre-breakfast: R ~20% of TDD. Pre-lunch: R ~10% of TDD. Pre-dinner: R ~10% of TDD. Bedtime: N ~50% of TDD.	May be feasible if unable to carbohydrate count. R can be dosed based on ICR and correction. All meals have R coverage. Least expensive insulins.	Greater risk of nocturnal hypoglycemia with N. Greater risk of delayed post-meal hypoglycemia with R. Requires relatively consistent mealtimes and carbohydrate intake. R must be injected at least 30 min before meal for better effect.	Pre-breakfast R: based on BGM after breakfast or before lunch. Pre-lunch R: based on BGM after lunch or before dinner. Pre-dinner R: based on BGM after dinner or at bedtime. Evening N: based on fasting or overnight BGM.

(continued)

Table 1.2 (continued)

Regimen	Timing and distribution	Advantages	Disadvantages	Adjusting doses
Regimens with fewer daily injections				
Three injections daily: N+R or N+RAA	Pre-breakfast: ~40% N + ~15% R or RAA. Pre-dinner: ~15% R or RAA. Bedtime: 30% N.	Morning insulins can be mixed in one syringe. May be appropriate for those who cannot take injections in middle of day. Morning N covers lunch to some extent. Same advantages of RAAs over R. Least (N + R) or less expensive insulins than MDI with analogs.	Greater risk of nocturnal hypoglycemia with N than LAAs. Greater risk of delayed post-meal hypoglycemia with R than RAAs. Requires relatively consistent mealtimes and carbohydrate intake. Coverage of post-lunch glucose often suboptimal. R must be injected at least 30 min before meal for better effect.	Morning N: based on pre-dinner BGM. Morning R: based on pre-lunch BGM. Morning RAA: based on post-breakfast or pre- lunch BGM. Pre-dinner R: based on bedtime BGM. Pre-dinner RAA: based on post-dinner or bedtime BGM. Evening N: based on fasting BGM.
Twice-daily "split-mixed": N+R or N+RAA	Pre-breakfast: ~40% N + ~15% R or RAA. Pre-dinner: ~30% N + ~15% R or RAA.	Least number of injections for people with strong preference for this. Insulins can be mixed in one syringe. Least (N+R) or less (N+RAA) expensive insulins vs analogs. Eliminates need for doses during the day.	Risk of hypoglycemia in afternoon or middle of night from N. Fixed mealtimes and meal content. Coverage of post-lunch glucose often suboptimal. Difficult to reach targets for blood glucose without hypoglycemia.	Morning N: based on pre-dinner BGM. Morning R: based on pre-lunch BGM. Morning RAA: based on post-breakfast or prelunch BGM. Evening R: based on bedtime BGM. Evening RAA: based on post-dinner or bedtime BGM. Evening N: based on fasting BGM.

BGM, blood glucose monitoring; CGM, continuous glucose monitoring; ICR, insulin:carbohydrate ratio; ISF, insulin sensitivity factor; LAA, long-acting analog; MDI, multiple daily injections; N, NPH insulin; R, short-acting (regular) insulin; RAA, rapid-acting analog; TDD, total daily insulin dose; URAA, ultra-rapid-acting analog. Reprinted from Holt et al.[5]

or caregivers should receive education about proper injection site rotation and how to recognize and avoid areas of lipohypertrophy. As noted in Table 1.2, examination of insulin injection sites for the presence of lipohypertrophy, as well as assessment of injection device use and injection technique, are key components of a comprehensive diabetes medical evaluation and treatment plan. Proper insulin injection technique may lead to more effective use of this therapy and, as such, holds the potential for improved clinical outcomes.

NONINSULIN TREATMENTS FOR TYPE 1 DIABETES

Injectable and oral glucose-lowering drugs have been studied for their efficacy as adjuncts to insulin treatment of type 1 diabetes. Pramlintide is based on the naturally occurring β-cell peptide amylin and is approved for use in adults with type 1 diabetes. Clinical trials have demonstrated a modest reduction in A1C (0.3–0.4%) and modest weight loss (~1 kg) with pramlintide.[30-33] Similarly, results have been reported for several agents currently approved only for the treatment of type 2 diabetes. The addition of metformin in adults with type 1 diabetes caused small reductions in body weight and lipid levels but did not improve A1C.[34,35] The largest clinical trials of glucagon-like peptide 1 receptor agonists (GLP-1 RAs) in type 1 diabetes have been conducted with liraglutide 1.8 mg daily, showing modest A1C reductions (~0.4%), decreases in weight (~5 kg), and reductions in insulin doses.[36,37] Similarly, sodium–glucose cotransporter 2 (SGLT2) inhibitors have been studied in clinical trials in people with type 1 diabetes, showing improvements in A1C, reduced body weight, and improved blood pressure;[38-40] however, SGLT2 inhibitor use in type 1 diabetes is associated with an increased rate of diabetic ketoacidosis. The risks and benefits of adjunctive agents continue to be evaluated, with consensus statements providing guidance on patient selection and precautions.[41]

SURGICAL TREATMENT FOR TYPE 1 DIABETES

Pancreas and Islet Transplantation

Successful pancreas and islet transplantation can normalize glucose levels and mitigate microvascular complications of type 1 diabetes. However, people receiving these treatments require lifelong immunosuppression to prevent graft rejection and/or recurrence of autoimmune islet destruction. Given the potential adverse effects of immunosuppressive therapy, pancreas transplantation should be reserved for people with type 1 diabetes undergoing simultaneous renal transplantation, following renal transplantation, or for those with recurrent ketoacidosis or severe hypoglycemia despite intensive glycemic management.[42]

The 2021 ADA/EASD consensus report on the management of type 1 diabetes in adults offers a simplified overview of indications for β-cell replacement therapy in people with type 1 diabetes (Fig. 1.2).[5]

Simplified overview of indications for β-cell replacement therapy in people with type 1 diabetes

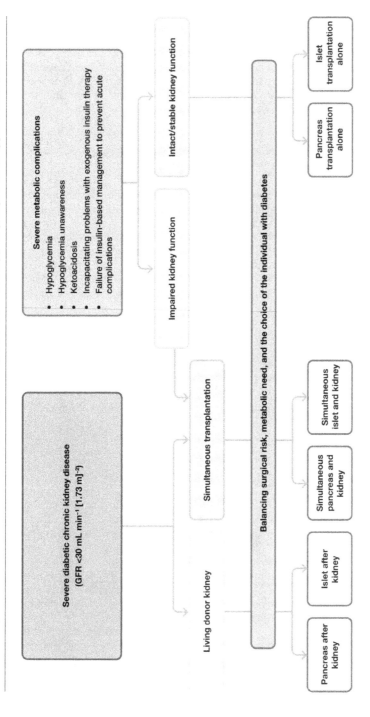

Figure 1.2—Simplified overview of indications for β-cell replacement therapy in people with type 1 diabetes. The two main forms of β-cell replacement therapy are whole-pancreas transplantation or islet cell transplantation. β-Cell replacement therapy can be combined with kidney transplantation if the individual has end-stage renal disease, which may be performed simultaneously or after kidney transplantation. All decisions about transplantation must balance the surgical risk, metabolic need, and the choice of the individual with diabetes. GFR, glomerular filtration rate. Reprinted from Holt et al.[5]

REFERENCES

1. Cleary PA, Orchard TJ, Genuth S, et al.; DCCT/EDIC Research Group. The effect of intensive glycemic treatment on coronary artery calcification in type 1 diabetic participants of the Diabetes Control and Complications Trial/Epidemiology of Diabetes Interventions and Complications (DCCT/EDIC) Study. *Diabetes* 2006;55:3556–3565

2. Nathan DM, Cleary PA, Backlund JYC, et al.; Diabetes Control and Complications Trial/Epidemiology of Diabetes Interventions and Complications (DCCT/EDIC) Study Research Group. Intensive diabetes treatment and cardiovascular disease in patients with type 1 diabetes. *N Engl J Med* 2005;353:2643–2653

3. Diabetes Control and Complications Trial (DCCT)/Epidemiology of Diabetes Interventions and Complications (EDIC) Study Research Group. Mortality in type 1 diabetes in the DCCT/EDIC versus the general population. *Diabetes Care* 2016;39:1378–1383

4. Writing Team for the Diabetes Control and Complications Trial/Epidemiology of Diabetes Interventions and Complications Research Group. Effect of intensive therapy on the microvascular complications of type 1 diabetes mellitus. *JAMA* 2002;287:2563–2569

5. Holt RIG, DeVries JH, Hess-Fischl A, et al. The management of type 1 diabetes in adults. A consensus report by the American Diabetes Association (ADA) and the European Association for the Study of Diabetes (EASD). *Diabetes Care* 2021;44:2589–2625

6. Tricco AC, Ashoor HM, Antony J, et al. Safety, effectiveness, and cost effectiveness of long acting versus intermediate acting insulin for patients with type 1 diabetes: systematic review and network meta-analysis. *BMJ* 2014;349:g5459

7. Bartley PC, Bogoev M, Larsen J, Philotheou A. Long-term efficacy and safety of insulin detemir compared to neutral protamine Hagedorn insulin in patients with type 1 diabetes using a treat-to-target basal-bolus regimen with insulin aspart at meals: a 2-year, randomized, controlled trial. *Diabet Med* 2008;25:442–449

8. DeWitt DE, Hirsch IB. Outpatient insulin therapy in type 1 and type 2 diabetes mellitus: scientific review. *JAMA* 2003;289:2254–2264

9. Bode BW, McGill JB, Lorber DL, Gross JL, Chang PC; Affinity 1 Study Group. Inhaled technosphere insulin compared with injected prandial insulin in type 1 diabetes: a randomized 24-week trial. *Diabetes Care* 2015;38:2266–2273

10. Russell-Jones D, Bode BW, De Block C, et al. Fast-acting insulin aspart improves glycemic control in basal-bolus treatment for type 1 diabetes: results of a 26-week multicenter, active-controlled, treat-to-target, randomized, parallel-group trial (onset 1). *Diabetes Care* 2017;40:943–950

11. Klaff L, Cao D, Dellva MA, et al. Ultra rapid lispro improves postprandial glucose control compared with lispro in patients with type 1 diabetes: Results from the 26-week PRONTO-T1D study. *Diabetes Obes Metab* 2020;22:1799–1807

12. Blevins T, Zhang Q, Frias JP, Jinnouchi H; PRONTO-T2D Investigators. Randomized double blind clinical trial comparing ultra rapid lispro with lispro in a basal-bolus regimen in patients with type 2 diabetes: PRONTO-T2D. *Diabetes Care* 2020;43:2991–2998

13. Lane W, Bailey TS, Gerety G, et al.; Group Information; SWITCH 1. Effect of insulin degludec vs insulin glargine U100 on hypoglycemia in patients with type 1 diabetes: the SWITCH 1 randomized clinical trial. *JAMA* 2017;318:33–44

14. Home PD, Bergenstal RM, Bolli GB, et al. New insulin glargine 300 units/mL versus glargine 100 units/mL in people with type 1 diabetes: a randomized, phase 3a, open-label clinical trial (EDITION 4). *Diabetes Care* 2015;38:2217–2225

15. Yeh HC, Brown TT, Maruthur N, et al. Comparative effectiveness and safety of methods of insulin delivery and glucose monitoring for diabetes mellitus: a systematic review and meta-analysis. *Ann Intern Med* 2012;157:336–347

16. Pickup JC. The evidence base for diabetes technology: appropriate and inappropriate meta-analysis. *J Diabetes Sci Technol* 2013;7:1567–1574

17. Bergenstal RM, Klonoff DC, Garg SK, et al.; ASPIRE In-Home Study Group. Threshold-based insulin-pump interruption for reduction of hypoglycemia. *N Engl J Med* 2013;369:224–232

18. Buckingham BA, Raghinaru D, Cameron F, et al.; In Home Closed Loop Study Group. Predictive low-glucose insulin suspension reduces duration of nocturnal hypoglycemia in children without increasing ketosis. *Diabetes Care* 2015;38:1197–1204

19. Bergenstal RM, Garg S, Weinzimer SA, et al. Safety of a hybrid closed-loop insulin delivery system in patients with type 1 diabetes. *JAMA* 2016;316:1407–1408

20. Garg SK, Weinzimer SA, Tamborlane WV, et al. Glucose outcomes with the in-home use of a hybrid closed-loop insulin delivery system in adolescents and adults with type 1 diabetes. *Diabetes Technol Ther* 2017;19:155–163

21. Tauschmann M, Thabit H, Bally L, et al.; APCam11 Consortium. Closed-loop insulin delivery in suboptimally controlled type 1 diabetes: a multicentre, 12-week randomised trial. *Lancet* 2018;392:1321–1329

22. Brown SA, Kovatchev BP, Raghinaru D, et al.; iDCL Trial Research Group. Six-month randomized, multicenter trial of closed-loop control in type 1 diabetes. *N Engl J Med* 2019;381:1707–1717

23. Peters AL, Laffel L (Eds.). American Diabetes Association/JDRF Type 1 Diabetes Sourcebook. Alexandria, VA, American Diabetes Association, 2013

24. Chiang JL, Kirkman MS, Laffel LMB; Type 1 Diabetes Sourcebook Authors. Type 1 diabetes through the life span: a position statement of the American Diabetes Association. *Diabetes Care* 2014;37:2034–2054

25. Bell KJ, Barclay AW, Petocz P, Colagiuri S, Brand-Miller JC. Efficacy of carbohydrate counting in type 1 diabetes: a systematic review and meta-analysis. *Lancet Diabetes Endocrinol* 2014;2:133–140

26. Vaz EC, Porfírio GJM, Nunes HRC, Nunes-Nogueira VDS. Effectiveness and safety of carbohydrate counting in the management of adult patients with type 1 diabetes mellitus: a systematic review and meta-analysis. *Arch Endocrinol Metab* 2018;62:337–345

27. Bell KJ, Smart CE, Steil GM, Brand-Miller JC, King B, Wolpert HA. Impact of fat, protein, and glycemic index on postprandial glucose control in type 1 diabetes: implications for intensive diabetes management in the continuous glucose monitoring era. *Diabetes Care* 2015;38:1008–1015

28. Frid AH, Kreugel G, Grassi G, et al. New insulin delivery recommendations. *Mayo Clin Proc* 2016;91:1231–1255

29. Bergenstal RM, Strock ES, Peremislov D, Gibney MA, Parvu V, Hirsch LJ. Safety and efficacy of insulin therapy delivered via a 4mm pen needle in obese patients with diabetes. *Mayo Clin Proc* 2015;90:329–338

30. Whitehouse F, Kruger DF, Fineman M, et al. A randomized study and open-label extension evaluating the long-term efficacy of pramlintide as an adjunct to insulin therapy in type 1 diabetes. *Diabetes Care* 2002;25:724–730

31. Ratner RE, Want LL, Fineman MS, et al. Adjunctive therapy with the amylin analogue pramlintide leads to a combined improvement in glycemic and weight control in insulin-treated subjects with type 2 diabetes. *Diabetes Technol Ther* 2002;4:51–61

32. Hollander PA, Levy P, Fineman MS, et al. Pramlintide as an adjunct to insulin therapy improves long-term glycemic and weight control in patients with type 2 diabetes: a 1-year randomized controlled trial. *Diabetes Care* 2003;26:784–790

33. Ratner RE, Dickey R, Fineman M, et al. Amylin replacement with pramlintide as an adjunct to insulin therapy improves long-term glycaemic and weight control in type 1 diabetes mellitus: a 1-year, randomized controlled trial. *Diabet Med* 2004;21:1204–1212

34. Meng H, Zhang A, Liang Y, Hao J, Zhang X, Lu J. Effect of metformin on glycaemic control in patients with type 1 diabetes: a meta-analysis of randomized controlled trials. *Diabetes Metab Res Rev* 2018;34:e2983

35. Petrie JR, Chaturvedi N, Ford I, et al.; REMOVAL Study Group. Cardiovascular and metabolic effects of metformin in patients with type 1 diabetes

(REMOVAL): a double-blind, randomised, placebo-controlled trial. *Lancet Diabetes Endocrinol* 2017;5:597–609

36. Mathieu C, Zinman B, Hemmingsson JU, et al.; ADJUNCT ONE Investigators. Efficacy and safety of liraglutide added to insulin treatment in type 1 diabetes: the ADJUNCT ONE treat-to-target randomized trial. *Diabetes Care* 2016;39:1702–1710

37. Ahrén B, Hirsch IB, Pieber TR, et al.; ADJUNCT TWO Investigators. Efficacy and safety of liraglutide added to capped insulin treatment in subjects with type 1 diabetes: the ADJUNCT TWO randomized trial. *Diabetes Care* 2016;39:1693–1701

38. Dandona P, Mathieu C, Phillip M, et al.; DEPICT-1 Investigators. Efficacy and safety of dapagliflozin in patients with inadequately controlled type 1 diabetes (DEPICT-1): 24 week results from a multicentre, double-blind, phase 3, randomised controlled trial. *Lancet Diabetes Endocrinol* 2017;5:864–876

39. Rosenstock J, Marquard J, Laffel LM, et al. Empagliflozin as adjunctive to insulin therapy in type 1 diabetes: the EASE trials. *Diabetes Care* 2018;41:2560–2569

40. Snaith JR, Holmes-Walker DJ, Greenfield JR. Reducing type 1 diabetes mortality: role for adjunctive therapies? *Trends Endocrinol Metab* 2020;31:150–164

41. Danne T, Garg S, Peters AL, et al. International consensus on risk management of diabetic ketoacidosis in patients with type 1 diabetes treated with sodium-glucose cotransporter (SGLT) inhibitors. *Diabetes Care* 2019;42:1147–1154

42. Dean PG, Kukla A, Stegall MD, Kudva YC. Pancreas transplantation. *BMJ* 2017;357:j1321. Accessed 18 October 2022. Available from https://www.bmj.com/content/357/bmj.j1321

Chapter 2
Management of Hyperglycemia in Type 1 Diabetes Mellitus

Joshua J. Neumiller, PharmD, CDCES, FADCES, FASCP

According to the Centers for Disease Control and Prevention (CDC) estimates, 37.3 million people currently live with diabetes in the U.S.[1] It is estimated that 5–10% of those living with diabetes have type 1 diabetes (T1D).[2] T1D is the major form of diabetes seen in youth, with the majority of cases of diabetes being T1D in children under the age of 10 years.[2] T1D is classically associated with childhood and adolescents and was formerly known as "juvenile diabetes," but T1D (sometimes referred to as "immune-mediated diabetes") can be diagnosed at any age.[2] For people living with T1D, optimization of glycemic control is one of several key treatment approaches central to avoiding or delaying the microvascular and macrovascular complications of diabetes. Although lifestyle interventions (such as consuming a healthy diet and engaging in regular physical activity) are integral to any T1D management plan, this chapter will focus primarily on the pharmacological management of hyperglycemia in people with T1D.

PATHOPHYSIOLOGY

T1D is classically considered an autoimmune disorder leading to the destruction of pancreatic β-cells and a subsequent lack of endogenous insulin production.[3] While mediated by a complex interplay of environmental and genetic factors,[2] as many as 80–90% of people diagnosed with T1D do not have a positive family history of the disorder.[4] Figure 2.1 provides an overview of a classic model of T1D pathophysiology.[2] The model suggests that autoimmunity ensues when people with a genetic predisposition are exposed to an environmental trigger (such as an infection). Once the process is triggered, autoimmunity and β-cell loss progress at a variable rate, but typically proceed until symptoms of diabetes present.[2] The rate of progression and onset of symptoms can be quite variable from one individual to the next. Some people may present at the time of diagnosis in severe diabetic ketoacidosis (DKA), while others may be diagnosed with relatively mild symptoms and residual β-cell function.[2] Ultimately, the lack of insulin secretion that is associated with T1D results in the classic symptoms of hyperglycemia: polyuria, polydipsia, and polyphagia. Owing to the hallmark autoimmune destruction of pancreatic β-cells that occurs in T1D, supplementation with exogenous insulin therapy is absolutely required to manage hyperglycemia.

GLYCEMIC MANAGEMENT IN PEOPLE WITH T1D

Exogenous insulin therapy is a requirement for people with T1D due to a lack of endogenous insulin secretion from pancreatic β-cells. As such, all people with T1D should be managed with an intensive insulin regimen designed to cover both basal and prandial (mealtime) insulin needs, with the ultimate goal of achieving individualized glycemic goals.[5] Indeed, the Diabetes Control and Complications Trial (DCCT) showed that intensive therapy with multiple daily injections or continuous subcutaneous insulin infusion (CSII) resulted in improved glycemic control and better long-term outcomes in people with T1D.[6-8] The American Diabetes Association makes the following specific recommendations pertaining to insulin therapy in people with T1D:[9]

- Most people with T1D should be treated with multiple daily injections of prandial insulin and basal insulin or CSII.
- Most individuals with T1D should use rapid-acting insulin analogs to reduce hypoglycemia risk.
- Patients with T1D should receive education on how to match prandial insulin doses to carbohydrate intake, fat and protein content, and anticipated physical activity.

Although there are multiple important interventions to consider in decreasing microvascular and macrovascular risk in people with T1D, the following sections will focus specifically on glycemic goal setting and use of pharmacologic interventions to meet individualized glycemic goals.

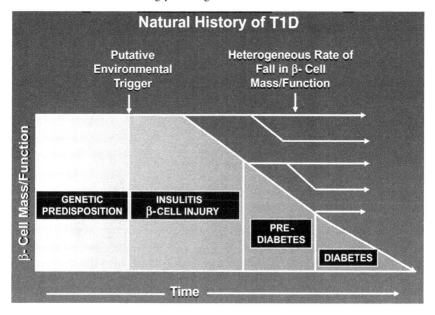

Figure 2.1—Natural history of T1D. *Source:* Reprinted with permission from American Diabetes Association.[2]

Table 2.1 — Glycemic Recommendations for Many Nonpregnant Adults with Diabetes

A1C	<7.0%*
Fasting (Preprandial) Glucose	80–130 mg/dL*
Postprandial Glucose	<180 mg/dL*

*More or less stringent goals may be appropriate for individuals. *Source:* Adapted from American Diabetes Association.[10]

GLYCEMIC TREATMENT GOALS IN PEOPLE WITH T1D

As is the case for all people with diabetes, treatment goals and expectations should be individualized for people with T1D. Aside from the importance of individualization, major organizations such as the American Diabetes Association recommend different general treatment targets for children and adolescents when compared to adults with T1D. Table 2.1 provides a summary of general glycemic recommendations for nonpregnant adults with diabetes. It should be noted that while general recommendations for glycated hemoglobin A_{1c} (A1C) and blood glucose levels are provided, all glycemic goals should be individualized based on person-specific considerations.[9] Factors that may inform glycemic goals in an individual may include risk of hypoglycemia and other adverse drug events, diabetes disease duration, life expectancy, comorbidity burden, presence of vascular complications, attitudes and treatment expectations of the individual, and resources and support available to implement a given treatment plan.[9] As pertaining to glycemic goal setting in children and adolescents with T1D, the American Diabetes Association outlines the following key concepts to consider:[10]

- A1C goals must be individualized and reassessed over time. An A1C of <7% is appropriate for many children and adolescents.
- Less-stringent A1C goals (such as <7.5%) may be appropriate for youth who cannot articulate symptoms of hypoglycemia; have hypoglycemia unawareness; lack access to analog insulins, advanced insulin delivery technology, and/or continuous glucose monitoring; cannot check blood glucose regularly; or have nonglycemic factors that increase A1C.
- Healthcare professionals may reasonably suggest more-stringent A1C goals (such as <6.5%) for selected individual patients if they can be achieved without significant hypoglycemia, negative impacts on well-being, or undue burden of care, or in those who have nonglycemic factors that decrease A1C. Lower targets may also be appropriate during the honeymoon phase.

Ultimately, the American Diabetes Association recommends that treatment decisions and glycemic goal setting should be made in collaboration with the individual, whenever possible, to incorporate his or her needs, preferences, and values.[11]

ANTIHYPERGLYCEMIC DRUG THERAPY IN T1D: INSULIN THERAPY

Insulin both increases glucose uptake by adipose and muscle tissues and suppresses hepatic glucose release. The primary limitation to the usefulness of insulin as a glucose-lowering agent is the occurrence of hypoglycemia. In addition, insulin use often leads to weight gain. There are many common challenges involved in prescribing insulin as well—from choosing insulin regimens to minimizing the hypoglycemia and weight gain that often accompany improved glycemic control. While all insulin products work via stimulation of insulin receptors, their pharmacokinetic and pharmacodynamic profiles can vary significantly. The insulin primarily in use today is manufactured via recombinant DNA technology as either human insulin or as rapid- or longer-acting human insulin analogs. Analog insulins are structurally modified such that the amino acid sequence is intentionally altered to achieve the desired pharmacokinetic characteristics, as detailed in the following sections.[5]

Pharmacokinetics

Several factors impact the pharmacokinetic properties of insulin, regardless of insulin type. The site of injection, thickness of the subcutaneous tissue, amount of total body adipose tissue, subcutaneous blood flow, and amount of insulin administered can all impact the pharmacokinetics of exogenous insulin.[5,12,13] Temperature variation can also have a major influence on insulin absorption. Elevated skin temperature can lead to increased subcutaneous vasodilation and blood flow to the injection site, thus causing insulin to be more rapidly absorbed.[14,15] Additionally, subcutaneous injections can be administered at multiple anatomical sites, such as the abdominal wall area, thigh, or upper arm. Many practitioners recommend use of the abdomen for consistency of absorption. Although most insulin manufacturers recommend rotating injection sites, changing the anatomical site of injection can affect insulin absorption.[5,16] People using insulin should be educated about factors that may influence insulin absorption when initiating insulin therapy and periodically thereafter.

Table 2.2 provides a summary of individual insulin products currently available in the U.S.[2,17–28] Because U-500 regular human insulin is used primarily in people with significant insulin resistance and rarely in T1D, it will not be discussed in this chapter. The following sections discuss individual insulin products, as grouped by their pharmacokinetic and pharmacodynamic profiles, and their relative effects on glucose control.

Short-Acting Insulin

Regular human insulin (RHI) is generally classified as a short-acting insulin product. RHI is a prandial (mealtime) insulin product used to cover carbohydrate intake with meals.[5] When compared to rapid-acting insulin analogs, RHI has a slower onset and a longer duration of action (see Table 2.2). The glucose-lowering effect of RHI starts approximately 30 min after subcutaneous administration, thus RHI is typically injected 30–45 min before a meal to best match the expected postprandial rise in blood glucose.[5,17,18] Although rapid-acting insulin analogs have possible advantages related to their faster onset and shorter durations of action, RHI costs considerably less and can be used effectively in patients unable to afford newer analog insulin products.

Rapid-Acting Insulin Analogs

Currently available injectable rapid-acting analogs (RAAs) include insulin lispro, insulin aspart, and insulin glulisine.[22–25] As noted previously, RAAs are pre-

Table 2.2—Summary of Insulin Products*

Generic name	Brand name(s)	Time to onset of action (h)	Time to peak action (h)	Duration of action (h)
Regular Human Insulin (U-100)	Humulin R; Novolin R	0.5	1.5–2.5	8
Lispro† (U-100, U-200)	Humalog; Lyumjev; Admelog	within 0.25	0.5–1.5	4–6
Aspart†	Novolog, Fiasp	within 0.25	0.5–1.5	4–6
Glulisine	Apidra	within 0.25	0.5–1.5	4–6
Inhaled Human Insulin Powder	Afrezza	within 0.25	0.5–1	1.5–4.5
NPH Insulin	Humulin N; Novolin N	2–4	4–10	12–18
Detemir	Levemir	2–4	flat	14–24
Glargine (U-100)	Lantus; Basaglar; Semglee	2–4	flat	20–24
Glargine (U-300)	Toujeo	6	flat	up to 36
Degludec (U-100, U-200)	Tresiba	1	flat	>42
Regular Human Insulin (U-500)	Humulin R U-500	0.5	4–8	13–24

* Person-specific onset, peak, and duration may vary from times listed in table. Peak and duration are dose-dependent with shorter durations of action seen for smaller doses and longer durations of action with larger doses; † Insulin aspart and insulin lispro are available as multiple branded products: Fiasp, Lyumjev, and Afrezza have a relatively fast onset of action when compared to other rapid-acting insulin products. *Source*: refs. 2,17–28.

ferred for use in people with T1D over RHI.[9] Injectable RAAs are structurally engineered to dissociate and be absorbed more rapidly than RHI,[2] resulting in a faster onset and shorter duration of action.[2,29] The faster onset of action allows for RAAs to be administered closer to the time of meal ingestion (typically from 15 min prior to just before a meal), and the shorter duration of action leads to a reduction in postabsorptive hypoglycemic events.[2] Insulin lispro is commercially available in both U-100 and U-200 strengths, with a follow-on U-100 insulin lispro product approved under the brand name Admelog.[22,26] Insulin aspart is likewise available as two different branded products: Novolog and Fiasp.[23,24] The faster-acting insulin aspart product (Fiasp) is formulated with niacinamide, which is believed to promote formation of insulin monomers after subcutaneous injection, leading to more rapid absorption.[30] Clinical trials comparing Fiasp to Novolog in people with T1D showed a statistically significant improvement in lowering of 1 h postprandial glucose (PPG) levels with Fiasp.[31] Similarly, a faster-acting version of insulin lispro is now available under the brand name Lyumjev.[27] It is generally recommended that RAAs be administered no more than 15 min before a meal; however, it is acceptable for people to inject after a meal if carbohydrate intake is difficult to predict or their rate of carbohydrate absorption is variable due to gastroparesis.[5] It is possible that the faster-acting insulin aspart (Fiasp) and insulin lispro (Lyumjev) products may have an advantage in this scenario due to their relatively rapid absorption profiles.

The mechanism of action of inhaled human insulin powder (brand name Afrezza), also classified as an RAA, differs from the injectable rapid-acting insulins. The product is composed of insulin formulated in "microspheres" with a carrier molecule that allows for the insulin to be delivered into the deep lung for rapid absorption following inhalation.[32] Following oral inhalation of 4, 12, and 48 units, the time to maximum serum concentration ranged from 10–20 min in people with T1D.[19]

Intermediate-Acting Insulin

Neutral protamine Hagedorn (NPH) insulin, also known as isophane insulin, is generally classified as "intermediate-acting" in terms of its pharmacokinetic profile. NPH insulin contains an absorption-inhibiting substance called protamine, which prolongs the action and contributes to the cloudy appearance of NPH insulin.[5] For this reason, NPH and NPH-type insulins should be agitated/mixed prior to injection to resuspend the insulin mixture. NPH insulin may be used to cover basal insulin needs, in which case NPH is typically administered twice daily. NPH reaches peak plasma levels anywhere from 4–10 h after subcutaneous administration.[2,33,34] Because of the notable peak with NPH insulin, its use is associated with higher rates of hypoglycemia when compared to long-acting insulin analogs.[2] Although NPH does carry a higher hypoglycemia risk, it is considerably less expensive than long- and ultra-long-acting insulin analogs and can be used effectively in people who have difficulty obtaining more expensive insulin products.

Long-Acting Insulin

Long-acting insulin products are basal insulin analogs that provide basal insulin coverage for up to 24 h. The two medications within this group include insulin glargine (U-100) and insulin detemir. Some people can realize a full 24 h of basal coverage with these insulin products; others can experience end-of-dose "wearing off," as noted by the duration of action ranges presented in Table 2.2.

Insulin Glargine (U-100)

Insulin glargine (U-100) was approved by the FDA in the year 2000, and differs structurally from human insulin by the addition of two arginines after position B30 and the replacement of asparagine with glycine at position A21.[35] Unlike NPH insulin, insulin glargine is soluble at a pH of 4.0.[35,36] Following subcutaneous injection, the acidic insulin solution is neutralized leading to the formation of insulin microprecipitates from which small amounts of insulin are gradually released over time.[35] U-100 insulin glargine exhibits a duration of action generally ranging from 20–24 h, with a relatively flat pharmacokinetic profile.[2] In clinical trials, U-100 insulin glargine demonstrated similar effects on glycemic control when compared to once- or twice-daily NPH, with the advantage of a decreased rate of hypoglycemic events, particularly nocturnal hypoglycemic events.[35] In addition to the product Lantus, several follow-on U-100 insulin glargine products are available in the U.S., marketed as Basaglar and Semglee.[28,37] Although some people can realize a full 24 h of basal coverage with a single injection of U-100 insulin glargine, some people require twice-daily administration for a full day of basal coverage. This can be especially true in people with T1D on relatively low doses of basal insulin (e.g., 20 units/day).

Insulin Detemir

Insulin detemir is another long-acting basal insulin analog. Insulin detemir has a prolonged duration of action (14–24 h) due to the insulin's ability to reversibly bind to albumin at the injection site and within the bloodstream.[2,38] Unlike insulin glargine, insulin detemir is soluble at a neutral pH. Structurally, insulin detemir differs from human insulin by the omission of threonine at position B30 and the attachment of myristic acid to lysine at position B29.[38] The presence of myristic acid contributes to delayed dissociation and absorption of insulin detemir hexamers and also facilitates a >98% binding of insulin detemir to albumin molecules in the plasma and interstitial fluid.[38] Because only free, non-albumin-bound insulin can be absorbed and bind to insulin receptors, albumin binding contributes to the prolonged duration of action seen with this insulin product. Since the duration of action of insulin detemir can range from 14–24 h, many people with T1D require twice-daily dosing with insulin detemir.

Insulin Glargine (U-300)

U-300 insulin glargine is a concentrated version of insulin glargine. U-300 insulin glargine is similar to the U-100 product in terms of structure and solubility at an acidic pH of 4.0. The longer duration of action realized with the concentrated U-300 product is attributable to the smaller injection volume, which results in a smaller precipitate surface area.[39] The smaller surface area is associated with a slower dissolution rate and a resultant longer duration of action.[39] Please refer to Table 2.2 for specifics related to the pharmacokinetic properties of U-300 insulin glargine. Due to the long half-life of U-300 insulin glargine, time is needed for this insulin product to accumulate and reach steady-state levels, which are generally achieved after 5 days of once-daily administration.[20] The manufacturer recommends titrating the dose no more frequently than every 3–4 days to minimize the risk of hypoglycemia.[20]

Potential advantages of U-300 insulin glargine over the U-100 insulin glargine product include a longer duration of action, the potential for delivery of large insulin doses in a smaller injection volume, and a lower incidence of nocturnal hypoglycemia. Of note, when converting someone from the U-100 insulin glargine product to the U-300 product, larger doses (on a unit per unit basis) are typically needed to achieve the same glucose-lowering effect.[20] Therefore, it can be expected that higher unit doses of U-300 insulin glargine will be required to maintain glycemic control when compared to the previous U-100 insulin glargine dose.

Insulin Degludec (U-100; U-200)

Insulin degludec is another ultra-long-acting basal insulin analog with a duration of action in excess of 42 h at steady state.[21] Steady-state insulin concentrations are achieved by 3–4 days of once-daily subcutaneous administration.[21] When stored in solution with phenol and zinc, insulin degludec forms small, soluble, and stable dihexamers. Upon injection, the phenol component slowly dissipates allowing for self-association of the insulin molecules into large multihexameric chains consisting of thousands of dihexamers connected to one another.[40] Over time, these chains slowly begin to dissolve as the zinc component diffuses, resulting in the release of insulin from the terminal ends of the chain to be absorbed.[40] Insulin degludec is commercially available in U-100 and U-200 concentrations. Similar to U-300 insulin glargine, the manufacturer recommends titrating the dose no more frequently than every 3–4 days to minimize the risk of hypoglycemia.[21] Potential advantages of insulin degludec include its long duration of action, the potential for delivery of large insulin doses in a smaller injection volume (U-200 product), and a lower incidence of nocturnal hypoglycemia when compared to U-100 insulin glargine.

Insulin Adverse Effects

While insulin therapy has been associated with a variety of adverse effects in clinical trials, the more salient adverse effects and monitoring recommendations for insulin products are provided in this section.

Hypoglycemia

Hypoglycemia is the most common and serious adverse event associated with insulin use. Hypoglycemia is defined generally as a blood glucose value ≤70 mg/dL, with lower blood glucose levels associated with worsening hypoglycemic symptoms.[11] Although not an exhaustive list, Table 2.3 provides a list of potential hypoglycemic symptoms.[5] People with hypoglycemia unawareness may not have recognizable symptoms and are at particular risk for severe hypoglycemic events. In people with hypoglycemia unawareness less stringent glycemic targets may be warranted to reduce hypoglycemia risk, especially during the night.[5]

All people who use insulin should be counseled regarding the signs, symptoms, and proper treatment of hypoglycemia. Mild hypoglycemia can be treated by following the "rule of 15": treat with 15 g carbohydrate, wait 15 min, and then check the blood glucose level.[5] If after 15 min blood glucose remains below 70 mg/dL, another 15 g carbohydrate should be consumed. Once the blood

Table 2.3   Symptoms of Hypoglycemia

Shakiness	Blurred/impaired vision
Nervousness or anxiety	Tingling or numbness in the lips or tongue
Sweating, chills, or clamminess	Headache
Irritability or impatience	Anger, stubbornness, or sadness
Confusion	Lack of coordination
Rapid/fast heartbeat	Nightmares
Lightheadedness or dizziness	Seizures
Hunger	Unconsciousness
Sleepiness/fatigue	

Source: Adapted from American Diabetes Association.[5]

glucose is normalized, a snack or meal that includes complex carbohydrates and protein should be consumed to prevent a secondary hypoglycemic episode. When a severe hypoglycemic event occurs and glucose cannot be delivered orally, glucagon use is indicated.[5] The American Diabetes Association *Standards of Care in Diabetes* recommends that glucagon be prescribed to individuals at significant risk of severe hypoglycemia,[11] which would include people who use prandial insulin products, or all people with T1D.

Weight Gain

Weight gain is associated with insulin use and is observed as improvements in glycemic control are achieved. Weight gain can additionally be seen in people with T1D due to increased caloric intake to treat hypoglycemia. As glycemic control improves, glucose is used by the tissues instead of being lost in the urine, thus resulting in weight gain. People starting insulin therapy should be informed of the potential for weight gain and encouraged to implement healthy lifestyle measures to minimize insulin-induced weight gain.[5] In people with T1D, pramlintide can be used as an adjunct therapy with the goal of lowering insulin doses and inducing weight loss.[5] Please see additional information about pramlintide in the section "Other Adjunctive Drug Therapies" presented later in this chapter.

Injection Site Reactions

Long-term use of insulin can lead to lipoatrophy or lipohypertrophy, which can adversely affect insulin absorption. Injection site rotation is important to avoid lipoatrophy and lipohypertrophy. If either occurs, injection into the affected area(s) should be avoided. Lipoatrophy and lipohypertrophy are particularly problematic in people with T1D and can impair long-term glycemic management as the number of viable injection sites decreases over time.

Modes of Insulin Delivery

The method of insulin delivery can include multiple daily injections (with vial and syringe or insulin pens) or use of CSII. The choice of which delivery method to use should be tailored to the individualized needs and preferences of the person with T1D.[5] Figure 2.2 provides a summary of relative attributes of insulin delivery approaches in people with T1D.[9]

Insulin Vials and Syringes

Vials of insulin are typically less expensive than prefilled insulin pens or durable pens that use insulin cartridges. Many people can do quite well with vials and syringes, but use may be difficult for people with vision or dexterity issues. People should be instructed to use a new, clean needle for every dose to prevent injection site infections.

Insulin Pens

Insulin pens provide a mode of delivery that is more convenient, and often more accurate, than insulin administration via vial and syringe. These devices can be very beneficial for people who have vision or dexterity issues that make drawing insulin into a syringe difficult. A new disposable pen needle should be tightened onto the insulin pen before each use to prevent infection. Patients should also be counseled to never share insulin pens. Some of the pens also require priming the pen needle before each use and holding the needle in the injection site for a specific number of seconds (typically 10 seconds), so manufacturer's instructions should be explained to the patient prior to initiation.

Representative relative attributes of insulin delivery approaches in people with type 1 diabetes[1]

Injected insulin regimens	Flexibility	Lower risk of hypoglycemia	Higher costs
MDI with LAA + RAA or URAA	+++	+++	+++

Less-preferred, alternative injected insulin regimens

	Flexibility	Lower risk of hypoglycemia	Higher costs
MDI with NPH + RAA or URAA	++	++	++
MDI with NPH + short-acting (regular) insulin	++	+	+
Two daily injections with NPH + short-acting (regular) insulin or premixed	+	+	+

Continuous insulin infusion regimens	Flexibility	Lower risk of hypoglycemia	Higher costs
Hybrid closed-loop technology	+++++	+++++	++++++
Insulin pump with threshold/predictive low-glucose suspend	++++	++++	+++++
Insulin pump therapy without automation	+++	+++	++++

Figure 2.1—Choices of insulin regimens in people with type 1 diabetes. Continuous glucose monitoring improves outcomes with injected or infused insulin and is superior to blood glucose monitoring. Inhaled insulin may be used in place of injectable prandial insulin in the U.S. 1The number of plus signs (+) is an estimate of relative association of the regimen with increased flexibility, lower risk of hypoglycemia, and higher costs between the considered regimens. LAA, long-acting insulin analog; MDI, multiple daily injections; RAA, rapid-acting insulin analog; URAA, ultra-rapid-acting insulin analog. *Source:* Reprinted with permission from American Diabetes Association.[2]

Continuous Subcutaneous Insulin Infusion

CSII via an insulin pump or patch allows for precise insulin delivery. CSII requires considerable patient education and support until the individual becomes familiar with the use of the device. Insulin pumps use rapid-acting insulin (insulin lispro, insulin aspart, or insulin glulisine) to cover both basal and bolus insulin needs.[5] Insulin pump and patch technology advances very quickly, with new-generation devices entering the market regularly. Examples of recent technological advancements with insulin pump therapies are the incorporation of threshold suspend features and the introduction of the first hybrid closed-loop system that is able to automatically adjust basal insulin delivery in response to continuous glucose monitoring (CGM) input. The American Diabetes Association publishes consumer guides, inclusive of an insulin pump consumer guide, that are readily accessible via the American Diabetes Association's Consumer Guide website (consumerguide.diabetes.org).

Insulin Inhalation

As discussed previously, inhaled human insulin is currently available in the U.S. for prandial use in T1D.[19] The product is available in single-use cartridges for use in the corresponding inhalation device. The product is available in 4-unit, 8-unit, and 12-unit single-use cartridges, which are color-coded to prevent medication errors.[19]. Individual cartridges can be used in combination to customize the dose or if higher doses are needed.

INSULIN DOSING IN T1D

Ideally the exogenous insulin regimen used in people with T1D mimics physiologic insulin secretory patterns to the extent possible. Such an approach involves either initiation of an intensive multiple daily injection (MDI) insulin regimen or use of CSII.[5] An intensive basal/bolus regimen in someone with T1D is generally inclusive of a long- or ultra-long-acting insulin that mimics the normal basal insulin release seen in people without diabetes, where approximately 1 unit of insulin is secreted every hour to handle the fasting insulin needs of the liver and muscle. A short- or rapid-acting insulin is also administered in conjunction with the ingestion of carbohydrates at mealtimes, which simulates the rapid release of insulin from the pancreas that typically occurs in the fed state. Similarly, CSII allows for the infusion of rapid-acting insulin to cover both basal and prandial insulin needs.

Insulin Initiation and Titration

When initiating insulin therapy in someone newly diagnosed with T1D, the starting insulin dose is generally calculated based on weight, with starting doses typically ranging from 0.4–1.0 units/kg/day of total insulin.[2] Many clinicians will begin at 0.5 units/kg/day when the person is metabolically stable, with subsequent titration of the insulin per glycemic response. After calculating the total daily insulin dose, approximately half of the calculated total daily dose is administered as basal insulin, with the other half distributed across meals as prandial insulin (for example, 20% of the total daily dose injected at breakfast, 10% at lunch, and 20% at dinner)[2] It is important to note that this weight-based total daily dose calculation and allocation is a starting point only and should be subsequently adjusted according to individualized insulin needs. The following provides an example total daily insulin dose calculation in a person recently diagnosed with T1D:

Example: RJ is a 60-kg female recently diagnosed with T1D. It is decided that a total daily dose of 0.5 units/kg/day is an appropriate starting point.

- Total Daily Dose = 60 kg x 0.5 units/kg/day = 30 units/day
- Basal Dose = 30 units/2 = 15 units of basal insulin daily
- Prandial Insulin = Remaining 15 units/3 meals = 5 units of prandial insulin per meal

Of note, there is no one gold standard method for initiating insulin in people with T1D. While the example provided above provides a starting point for initiating an intensive insulin regimen, the weight-based dose calculation is an estimation of insulin needs only. The basal and prandial insulin doses will inevitably require adjustment to meet individualized glycemic goals. Blood glucose monitoring data and continuous glucose monitoring (CGM) are important tools to evaluate an insulin regimen and inform insulin titration decisions. Ideally, people with T1D will promptly learn to count carbohydrates and adjust insulin doses based on carbohydrate intake, and also use insulin correction doses to account for residual hyperglycemia before meals and at bedtime.

Insulin:Carbohydrate (I:C) Ratios

Ideally, prandial (mealtime) insulin doses are calculated in people with T1D to cover the amount of carbohydrate to be consumed. A typical ballpark insulin-to-carbohydrate ratio (I:C ratio) in someone with T1D is 1:10 (1 unit of prandial insulin to cover 10 g carbohydrate) or 1:15.[5] These are estimates, however, and each individual's needs vary. For people taking rapid-acting analogs to cover meals, the "500 Rule" provides a reasonable initial estimate for determining a person's I:C ratio.[41] To use the 500 Rule, the current total daily dose of insulin is simply divided into 500 to determine an estimated I:C ratio.

Example: SR, a person with T1D, is currently taking 30 units of U-100 insulin glargine once daily and a total of 20 units of insulin aspart divided among breakfast, lunch, and dinner. His total daily insulin dose is 50 units. SR would like to begin adjusting his mealtime insulin doses using an I:C ratio.

- The 500 Rule = 500/total daily insulin dose = 500/50 = 10
- Interpretation: 1 unit of insulin aspart will cover approximately 10 g carbohydrate consumed with meals
- Application: SR is planning to consume 40 g carbohydrate at lunch. Using his estimated I:C ratio, he will inject 4 units of insulin aspart prior to the meal. RJ was advised to check his blood glucose before the meal and 2 h after the meal to assess and reevaluate the appropriateness of his I:C ratio estimate.

Correction Doses

Correction doses are important when blood glucose levels are unexpectedly elevated. A correction factor is ultimately used to correct for a blood glucose reading in the hyperglycemic range before meals or at bedtime, as examples.[41] The "1800 Rule" is another simple estimating calculation that can be used in people using rapid-acting analogs at meals. The calculation estimates how far 1 unit of rapid-acting insulin will drop an individual's blood glucose in mg/dL. To use the 1800 Rule, the number 1800 is divided by the total daily dose of insulin to determine the individual's correction factor. The following is an example of how to use the 1800 Rule to estimate a correction factor:

Example: RJ is currently taking 30 units of U-100 insulin glargine once daily and an average total of 30 units of insulin aspart divided among breakfast, lunch, and dinner after recently implementing an I:C ratio of 1:10. His total daily insulin dose is approximately 60 units. RJ would now like to determine his correction factor to better control his blood glucose throughout the day.

- The 1,800 Rule = 1,800/total daily insulin dose = 1,800/60 = 30
- Interpretation: 1 unit of insulin aspart will drop RJ's blood glucose by an estimated 30 mg/dL
- Application: RJ is about to consume 40 g carbohydrate at lunch. His premeal blood glucose reading is 160 mg/dL (his goal premeal blood glucose is 100 mg/dL). Using his I:C ratio he will administer 4 units to cover carbohydrates, and using his correction factor he will administer an additional 2 units of insulin to account for the 60 mg/dL he is above his target premeal blood glucose. In total, RJ will administer 6 units of insulin aspart prior to lunch.

Ongoing Insulin Adjustment in T1D

Although there are a variety of tools and estimates that can be used to initiate and titrate insulin in people with T1D, the job of optimizing insulin therapy in the individual with T1D is an ongoing and iterative process. Insulin needs can and will change based on numerous factors. Illness, stress, diet, physical activity, and even the changing of the seasons can have drastic effects on glycemic control and insulin needs in people with T1D. Using information obtained from blood glucose monitoring and CGM can be extremely valuable in pinpointing glycemic trends and making adjustments to diet, physical activity, or insulin doses to improve glucose control. People with T1D should be encouraged and empowered to take an active role in identifying trends and factors that impact their blood glucose to improve their glucose control and quality of life. For additional information and recommendations related to the overall management of people with T1D, please refer to the American Diabetes Association Position Statement "Type 1 Diabetes Through the Life Span."[42]

ADJUNCTIVE DRUG THERAPIES IN T1D

Insulin is the foundation of all pharmacotherapeutic regimens in T1D, but there are several other antihyperglycemic classes of medication that are used on- and off-label for the management of hyperglycemia. A brief discussion of the use of adjunctive antihyperglycemic therapies in T1D follows.

Pramlintide

Amylin is a 37-amino-acid hormone co-secreted with insulin from pancreatic β-cells.[2] Because people with T1D do not have functioning β-cells, they have an absolute deficiency of both insulin and amylin. As a neuroendocrine hormone, amylin acts to slow the appearance of glucose into the bloodstream through three primary mechanisms: suppression of glucagon secretion from pancreatic α-cells, slowing of gastric emptying, and promotion of satiety.[43] Taken together, these actions work in concert with the physiologic actions of insulin to maintain glucose homeostasis.[44]

Pramlintide is an amylinomimetic agent indicated as an adjunctive treatment for people with T1D (and type 2 diabetes [T2D]) receiving mealtime insulin therapy who have failed to achieve desired glucose control despite optimal insulin therapy.[45] Pramlintide is an injectable agent that is administered in addition (as a separate injection) to mealtime insulin prior to meals. In people with T1DM, the starting dose is 15 micrograms (µg) injected subcutaneously before each meal.[45] Because pramlintide slows gastric emptying, some of the most common adverse reactions experienced with use include nausea and vomiting, which are dose related. As such, the dose of pramlintide is gradually increased in 15-µg increments to a target premeal dose of 30 or 60 µg, as tolerated.[45] It is recommended that dose increases not be made any more frequently than every 3 days to minimize nausea.[45] The labeling for pramlintide includes a black box warning for severe hypoglycemia,[45] and mealtime insulin doses should be decreased by approximately 50% upon the initiation of pramlintide to minimize the risk of severe hypoglycemia. The mealtime insulin dose can subsequently be titrated based on individualized response.

The potential advantages of pramlintide use in people with T1D include improved overall glycemic control and potential weight loss. Potential disadvantages, however, include the need for additional injections, severe hypoglycemia risk, and the possible occurrence of common adverse events such as nausea and vomiting.

Other Adjunctive Drug Therapies

Although not approved by the FDA, several other antihyperglycemic classes of medications have been studied and used off-label in people with T1D. Immunotherapies (e.g., teplizumab) for the treatment and/or prevention of T1D and β-cell transplant will not be covered in this chapter. Please refer to the American Diabetes Association's *Standards of Care in Diabetes* for additional information about β-cell replacement therapy in T1D.[9]

Metformin

The addition of metformin to insulin therapy in people with T1D may have benefits.[9] One report found that the addition of metformin led to reduced insulin requirements and modest reductions in weight and total and LDL cholesterol levels.[46] A randomized clinical trial additionally found that among overweight adolescents with T1D, the addition of metformin to insulin did not improve glycemic control, but did increase the risk for gastrointestinal adverse events when compared to placebo.[47] When studied in adults with T1D and increased risk of cardiovascular disease, the addition of metformin to insulin did not significantly improve glycemic control beyond the initial 3 months of treatment, and the progression of atherosclerosis was not significantly improved.[48] Other cardiovascular risk factors such as weight and LDL cholesterol were, however, improved with metformin treatment.[48]

Incretin-Based Therapies

Interest exists for the use of glucagon-like peptide 1 (GLP-1) receptor agonists and dipeptidyl peptidase-4 (DPP-4) inhibitors in T1D, owing to their potential effects on preservation of β-cell mass and suppression of glucagon release.[9] No GLP-1 receptor agonists or DPP-4 inhibitors are currently approved for use in people with T1D. GLP-1 receptor agonists are currently being investigated (and used off-label) in people with T1D due to their insulin-sparing and weight loss effects.[2] The safety and efficacy of incretin-based therapy in people with T1D remains to be fully defined.

Sodium-Glucose Cotransporter 2 (SGLT2) Inhibitors

SGLT2 inhibitors, via inhibition of glucose reabsorption in the proximal renal tubule, decrease glucose levels in an insulin-independent fashion. Because SGLT2 inhibitors lower glucose independent of β-cell function, there is great interest in the potential adjunctive use of these agents in people with T1D. Limited evidence published to date shows potential glycemic benefits in people with diabetes receiving insulin therapy, inclusive of people with T1D.[49] Despite these potential benefits, SGLT2 inhibitor use has been associated with cases of euglycemic diabetic ketoacidosis (eDKA) in people with both T1D and T2D,[9] thus calling into question the safety of using these agents in people with T1D.

MONOGRAPHS

INSULIN PRODUCTS

Insulin Aspart (Fiasp): https://dailymed.nlm.nih.gov/dailymed/drugInfo.cfm?setid=834e7efc-393f-4c55-9125-628562a8a5cf

Insulin Aspart (Novolog): https://dailymed.nlm.nih.gov/dailymed/drugInfo.cfm?setid=e172b4f8-9b25-4019-8e09-afc10b2f30c9

Insulin Degludec [U-100, U-200] (Tresiba): https://dailymed.nlm.nih.gov/dailymed/drugInfo.cfm?setid=456c5e87-3dfd-46fa-8ac0-c6128d4c97c6

Insulin Detemir (Levemir): https://dailymed.nlm.nih.gov/dailymed/drugInfo.cfm?setid=d38d65c1-25bf-401d-9c7e-a2c3222da8af

Insulin Glargine [U-100] (Lantus, Basaglar): https://dailymed.nlm.nih.gov/dailymed/drugInfo.cfm?setid=6328c99d-d75f-43ef-b19e-7e71f91e57f6

Insulin Glargine [U-300] (Toujeo): https://dailymed.nlm.nih.gov/dailymed/drugInfo.cfm?setid=c9561d96-124d-48ca-982f-0aa1575bff36

Insulin Glulisine (Apidra): https://dailymed.nlm.nih.gov/dailymed/drugInfo.cfm?setid=e7af6a7a-8046-4fb4-9979-4ec4230b23aa

Inhaled Human Insulin (Afrezza): https://dailymed.nlm.nih.gov/dailymed/drugInfo.cfm?setid=29f4637b-e204-425b-b89c-7238008d8c10

Insulin Lispro [U-100, U-200] (Humalog, Admelog): https://dailymed.nlm.nih.gov/dailymed/drugInfo.cfm?setid=c8ecbd7a-0e22-4fc7-a503-faa58c1b6f3f

NPH Insulin (Humulin N, Novolin N): https://dailymed.nlm.nih.gov/dailymed/drugInfo.cfm?setid=82f1445c-b2c6-445a-82cf-ba8825fac776

Regular Human Insulin [U-100] (Humulin R, Novolin R): https://dailymed.nlm.nih.gov/dailymed/drugInfo.cfm?setid=b519bd83-038c-4ec5-a231-a51ec5cc291f

Regular Human Insulin [U-500] (Humulin R U-500): https://dailymed.nlm.nih.gov/dailymed/drugInfo.cfm?setid=b60e8dd0-1d48-4dc9-87fd-e14675255e8c

NONINSULIN PRODUCTS (FDA APPROVED FOR USE IN T1D)

Pramlintide (Symlin): https://dailymed.nlm.nih.gov/dailymed/drugInfo.
cfm?setid=4aea30ff-eb0d-45c1-b114-3127966328ff

REFERENCES

1. Centers for Disease Control and Prevention. National Diabetes Statistics Report website. Estimates of Diabetes and Its Burden in the United States. Available from https://www.cdc.gov/diabetes/data/statistics-report/index.html. Accessed 7 March 2023

2. American Diabetes Association/JDRF. *Type 1 Diabetes Sourcebook*. Peters A, Laffel L, Eds. Alexandria, American Diabetes Association, 2013

3. ElSayed NA, Aleppo G, Aroda VR, et al., American Diabetes Association. 2. Classification and diagnosis of diabetes: Standards of Care in Diabetes – 2023. *Diabetes Care* 2023;46(Suppl. 1):S19-S40

4. Haller MJ, Atkinson MA, Schatz DA. Efforts to prevent and halt autoimmune beta cell destruction. *Endocrinol Metab Clin North Am* 2010;39:527–539

5. American Diabetes Association. *Practical Insulin: A Handbook for Prescribing Providers*. 5th ed. Alexandria, American Diabetes Association, 2019

6. Nathan DM, Genuth S, Lachin J, et al.; Diabetes Control and Complications Trial Research Group. The effect of intensive treatment of diabetes on the development and progression of long-term complications in insulin-dependent diabetes mellitus. *N Engl J Med* 1993;329:977–986

7. Nathan DM, Cleary PA, Backlund J-YC, et al.; Diabetes Control and Complications Trial/Epidemiology of Diabetes Interventions and Complications (DCCT/EDIC) Study Research Group. Intensive diabetes treatment and cardiovascular disease in patients with type 1 diabetes. *N Engl J Med* 2005;353:2643–2653

8. DCCTEDIC Study Research Group. Mortality in type 1 diabetes in the DCCT/EDIC versus the general population. *Diabetes Care* 2016;39:1378–1383

9. ElSayed NA, Aleppo G, Aroda VR, et al., American Diabetes Association. 9. Pharmacologic approaches to glycemic treatment: Standards of Care in Diabetes – 2023. *Diabetes Care* 2023;46(Suppl. 1):S140–S157

10. ElSayed NA, Aleppo G, Aroda VR, et al., American Diabetes Association. 14. Children and adolescents: Standards of Care in Diabetes – 2023. *Diabetes Care* 2023;46(Suppl. 1):S230–S253

11. ElSayed NA, Aleppo G, Aroda VR, et al., American Diabetes Association. 6. Glycemic targets: Standards of Care in Diabetes – 2023. *Diabetes Care* 2023;46(Suppl. 1):S97–S110

12. Evans M, Schumm-Draeger PM, Vora J, King AB. A review of modern insulin analogue pharmacokinetic and pharmacodynamics profiles in type 2 diabetes: improvements and limitations. *Diabetes Obes Metab* 2011;13:677–684

13. Ryysy L, Häkkinen AM, Goto T, et al. Hepatic fat content and insulin action on free fatty acids and glucose metabolism rather than insulin absorption are associated with insulin requirements during insulin therapy in type 2 diabetic patients. *Diabetes* 2000;49:749–758

14. Koivisto VA. Sauna-induced acceleration in insulin absorption from subcutaneous injection site. *Br Med J* 1980;280:1411–1413

15. Berger M, Cuppers HJ, Hegner H, Jorgens V, Berchtold P. Absorption kinetics and biologic effects of subcutaneously injected insulin preparations. *Diabetes Care* 1982;5:77–91

16. ter Braak EW, Woodworth JR, Bianchi R, et al. Injection site effects on the pharmacokinetics and glucodynamics of insulin lispro and regular insulin. *Diabetes Care* 1996;19:1437–1440

17. Humulin R (insulin human injection) [package insert]. Indianapolis, IN, Lilly USA, LLC, 2022

18. Novolin R (insulin human injection) [package insert]. Plainsboro, NJ, Novo Nordisk Inc., 2022

19. Afrezza (insulin human inhalation powder) [package insert]. Danbury, CT, MannKind Corporation, 2023

20. Toujeo (insulin glargine injection) [package insert]. Bridgewater, NJ, Sanofi-aventis U.S. LLC, 2022

21. Tresiba (insulin degludec injection) [package insert]. Plainsboro, NJ, Novo Nordisk Inc., 2022

22. Humalog (insulin lispro injection) [package insert]. Indianapolis, IN, Lilly USA, LLC, 2019

23. Novolog (insulin aspart injection) [package insert]. Plainsboro, NJ, Novo Nordisk Inc., 2023

24. Fiasp (insulin aspart injection) [package insert]. Plainsboro, NJ, Novo Nordisk Inc., 2022

25. Apidra (insulin glulisine injection) [package insert]. Bridgewater, NJ, Sanofi-aventis U.S. LLC, 2020

26. Admelog (insulin lispro injection) [package insert]. Bridgewater, NJ, Sanofi-aventis U.S. LLC, 2020

27. Lyumjev (insulin lispro-aabc injection) [package insert]. Indianapolis, IN, Lilly USA, LLC, 2022

28. Semglee (insulin glargine injection) [package insert]. Morgantown, WV, Mylan Specialty L.P., 2022

29. Tibaldi JM. Evolution of insulin: From human to analog. *Am J Med* 2014;127:S25–S38

30. Mathieu C, Bode BW, Franek E, et al. Efficacy and safety of fast-acting insulin aspart in comparison with insulin aspart in type 1 diabetes (onset 1): a 52-week, randomized, treat-to-target, phase III trial. *Diabetes Obes Metab* 2018;20:1148–1155

31. Russell-Jones D, Bode BW, De Block C, et al. Fast-acting insulin aspart improves glycemic control in basal-bolus treatment for type 1 diabetes: results of a 26-week multicenter, active-controlled, treat-to-target, randomized, parallel-group trial (onset 1). *Diabetes Care* 2017;40:943–950

32. Neumiller JJ, Campbell RK. Technosphere insulin: an inhaled prandial insulin product. *Biodrugs* 2010;24:165–172

33. Humulin N (human insulin isophane suspension) [package insert]. Indianapolis, IN, Lilly USA, LLC, 2022

34. Novolin N (isophane insulin human suspension) [package insert]. Plainsboro, NJ, Novo Nordisk Inc., 2022

35. Campbell RK, White JR, Levien T, Baker D. Insulin glargine. *Clin Ther* 2001;23:1938–1957

36. Lantus (insulin glargine injection) [package insert]. Bridgewater, NJ, Sanofi-aventis U.S. LLC, 2022

37. Basaglar (insulin glargine injection) [package insert]. Indianapolis, IN, Lilly USA, LLC, 2021

38. Soran H, Younis N. Insulin detemir: a new basal insulin analogue. *Diabetes Obes Metab* 2006;8:26–30

39. Blair HA, Keating GM. Insulin glargine 300 U/mL: a review in diabetes mellitus. *Drugs* 2016;76:363–374

40. Robinson JD, Neumiller JJ, Campbell RK. Can a new ultra-long-acting insulin analogue improve patient care? Investigating the potential role of insulin degludec. *Drugs* 2012;72:2319–2325

41. Walsh J, Roberts R, Varma C, Bailey T. *Using Insulin*. San Diego, Torrey Pines Press, 2003

42. Chiang JL, Kirkman MS, Laffel LM, et al. Type 1 diabetes through the life span: a position statement of the American Diabetes Association. *Diabetes Care* 2014;37:2034–2054

43. Younk LM, Mikeladze M, Davis SN. Pramlintide and the treatment of diabetes: a review of the data since its introduction. *Expert Opin Pharmacother* 2011;12:1439–1451

44. Edelman SV, Weyer C. Unresolved challenges with insulin therapy in type 1 and type 2 diabetes: potential benefit of replacing amylin, a second beta-cell hormone. *Diabetes Technol Ther* 2002;4:175–189

45. Symlin (pramlintide acetate) [package insert]. Wilmington, DE, AstraZeneca Pharmaceuticals LP, 2019

46. Vella S, Buetow L, Royle P, et al. The use of metformin in type 1 diabetes: a systematic review of efficacy. *Diabetologia* 2010;53:809–820

47. Libman IM, Miller KM, DiMeglio LA, et al.; T1D Exchange Clinic Network Metformin RCT Study Group. Effect of metformin added to insulin on glycemic control among overweight/obese adolescents with type 1 diabetes: a randomized clinical trial. *JAMA* 2015;314:2241–2250

48. Petrie JR, Chaturvedi N, Ford I, et al.; REMOVAL Study group. Cardiovascular and metabolic effects of metformin in patients with type 1 diabetes (REMOVAL): a double-blind, randomised, placebo-controlled trial. *Lancet Diabetes Endocrinol* 2017;5:597–609

49. Yang Y, Chen S, Pan H, et al. Safety and efficiency of SGLT2 inhibitor combining with insulin in subjects with diabetes: systematic review and meta-analysis of randomized controlled trials. *Medicine (Baltimore)* 2017;96:e6944

Chapter 3
Insulin

Joshua J. Neumiller, PharmD, CDCES, FADCES, FASCP
Kimberly C. McKeirnan, PharmD, BCACP

INTRODUCTION

Since the introduction of commercially available insulin (Iletin) in the U.S. in 1923, insulin has remained a cornerstone of diabetes management.[1] Prior to the availability of exogenous insulin, a diagnosis of T1D was essentially a death sentence. While insulin products and delivery systems have dramatically improved since the introduction of Iletin in the 1920s, a century later, insulin remains a medical necessity for all people with T1D.[2,3] The use of insulin is not reserved only for those with T1D, however; insulin is often used in people with T2D to meet individualized glycemic goals.[4]

This chapter will provide an overview of insulin products currently available for use in the U.S. Additional topics covered in this chapter include safety considerations when using insulin therapy, general approaches to insulin use in T1D and T2D, and a brief overview of insulin delivery devices.

PHARMACOLOGY

MECHANISM OF ACTION

Insulin action involves a complex series of responses that affect carbohydrate, lipid, and protein metabolism.[5] Insulin carries out its metabolic and growth-promoting effects via binding to insulin receptors on cell plasma membranes.[5] A key metabolic effect of insulin receptor activation is the stimulation of glucose transport and metabolism. In the context of T1D, patients have an absolute insulin deficiency and are unable to effectively transport and metabolize glucose.[2] In T2D, the tissues are resistant to the effects of insulin leading to a relative insulin deficiency.[6] Over time, pancreatic β-cells begin to fail as they continually work to produce more insulin to counterbalance the persistent insulin resistance within the tissues. Eventually, β-cell function can decline to a level that requires exogenous insulin administration to adequately control blood glucose.[7] While all insulin products work via stimulation of insulin receptors, their pharmacokinetic and pharmacodynamic profiles can vary significantly. The insulin primarily in use today is manufactured via recombinant DNA technology as either human insulin (Figure 3.1) or as rapid- or longer-acting human insulin analogs. Analog insulins are structurally modified to achieve the desired pharmacokinetic characteristics, as detailed in the next section.[7]

PHARMACOKINETICS

Several factors impact the pharmacokinetic properties of insulin, regardless of insulin type. The site of injection, thickness of the subcutaneous tissue, amount of total body adipose tissue, subcutaneous blood flow, and amount of insulin administered can all impact the pharmacokinetics of exogenous insulin.[7–9] Factors such as level of endogenous insulin secretion (T1D vs. T2D) and obesity may additionally contribute to pharmacokinetic differences observed among individual patients.[8] Temperature variation can also have a major influence on insulin absorption. Elevated skin temperature can lead to increased subcutaneous vasodilation, increasing blood flow to the injection site, thus causing insulin to be more rapidly absorbed.[10,11] Additionally, subcutaneous injections can be administered at multiple anatomical sites, such as the abdominal wall area, thigh, or upper arm. While most insulin manufacturers recommend rotating injection sites, changing the anatomical site of injection can affect insulin absorption.[7,12] People using insulin should be educated about factors that may influence insulin absorption when initiating insulin therapy and periodically thereafter.

Table 3.1 provides a summary of key pharmacokinetic properties of individual insulin products currently available in the U.S.[2,13–17] The following sections discuss individual insulin products, as grouped by their pharmacokinetic profiles, and their relative effects on glucose control.

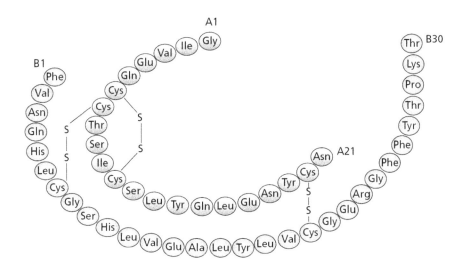

Figure 3.1—Structure of human insulin. Reprinted with permission from American Diabetes Association.[7]

Table 3.1—Summary of Insulin Pharmacokinetics*

Generic name	Brand name(s)	Time to onset of action (h)	Time to peak action (h)	Duration of action (h)
Regular Human Insulin (U-100)	Humulin R; Novolin R	0.5	1.5–2.5	8
Lispro† (U-100, U-200)	Humalog; Lyumjev; Admelog	within 0.25	0.5–1.5	4–6
Aspart†	Novolog; Fiasp	within 0.25	0.5–1.5	4–6
Glulisine	Apidra	within 0.25	0.5–1.5	4–6
Inhaled Human Insulin Powder	Afrezza	within 0.25	0.5–1	1.5–4.5
NPH Insulin	Humulin N; Novolin N	2–4	4–10	12–18
Detemir	Levemir	2–4	flat	14–24
Glargine (U-100)	Lantus; Basaglar; Semglee	2–4	flat	20–24
Glargine (U-300)	Toujeo	6	flat	up to 36
Degludec (U-100, U-200)	Tresiba	1	flat	>42
Regular Human Insulin (U-500)	Humulin R U-500	0.5	4–8	13–24

* Person-specific onset, peak, and duration may vary from times listed in table. Peak and duration are dose-dependent with shorter durations of action seen for smaller doses and longer durations of action with larger doses. † Insulin aspart and insulin lispro are available as multiple branded products—Fiasp, Lyumjev, and Afrezza have a relatively fast onset of action when compared to other rapid-acting insulin products. Source: refs. 2,13–17,19–22,24,29,30,32,33,40,47,55,56.

SHORT-ACTING INSULIN

Regular human insulin (RHI) is generally classified as a short-acting insulin product. RHI is a prandial (mealtime) insulin product used to cover carbohydrate intake with meals.[7] When compared to rapid-acting insulin analogs, RHI has a slower onset and a longer duration of action (see Table 3.1). Following a single subcutaneous injection of 0.1 unit/kg of RHI to healthy subjects, peak insulin concentrations occurred between 1.5–2.5 h post dose, with insulin concentrations returning to baseline after approximately 5 h.[13,14] The glucose-lowering effect of RHI starts approximately 30 min after subcutaneous administration; thus RHI is typically injected 30–45 min before a meal to best match the expected postprandial rise in blood glucose.[7,13,14] RHI administration via continuous intravenous infusion is typically the treatment of choice for managing hyperglycemia in the critical care setting.[18] Although rapid-acting insulin analogs have possible advantages related to their faster onset and shorter durations of action, RHI costs considerably less and can be used effectively in patients unable to afford newer analog insulin products.

RAPID-ACTING INSULIN ANALOGS

Currently available injectable rapid-acting insulin analogs (RAAs) include insulin lispro, insulin aspart, and insulin glulisine.[19–22] Injectable RAAs are structurally engineered to dissociate and be absorbed more rapidly than RHI,[2] resulting in a faster onset and shorter duration of action.[2,23] The faster onset of action allows for RAAs to be administered closer to the time of meal ingestion (typically from 15 min prior to just before a meal), and the shorter duration of action lends to a reduction in postabsorptive hypoglycemic events.[2] As an example, following subcutaneous administration of insulin lispro at doses ranging from 0.1–0.4 unit/kg, peak serum levels were seen within 30–90 min, compared to 50–120 min with RHI.[19] Similar observations have been noted in studies with insulin aspart and insulin glulisine.[20,22] Insulin lispro is commercially available in both U-100 and U-200 strengths, with a follow-on U-100 insulin lispro product approved under the brand name Admelog[19,24] Insulin aspart is likewise available as two different branded products: Novolog and Fiasp.[20,21] The faster-acting insulin aspart product (Fiasp) is formulated with niacinamide, which is believed to promote the formation of insulin monomers after subcutaneous injection leading to more rapid absorption.[25] Clinical trials comparing Fiasp with Novolog in people with T1D and T2D showed a statistically significant improvement in lowering of 1-h PPG levels with Fiasp.[26,27] Similarly, a faster-acting version of insulin lispro is now available under the brand name Lyumjev.[57] It is generally recommended that RAAs be administered no more than 15 min before a meal; however, it is acceptable for people to inject after a meal if carbohydrate intake is difficult to predict or their rate of carbohydrate absorption is variable due to gastroparesis.[7] It is possible that the faster-acting insulin aspart (Fiasp) and insulin lispro (Lyumjev) products may have an advantage in this scenario due to their relatively rapid absorption profiles.

The mechanism of action of inhaled human insulin powder (brand name Afrezza), also classified as an RAA, differs from the injectable rapid-acting insulins. The product is composed of insulin formulated in "microspheres" with a carrier molecule that allows for the insulin to be delivered into the deep lung for rapid absorption following inhalation.[28] Following oral inhalation of 4, 12, and 48 units, the time to maximum serum concentration ranged from 10–20 min in people with T1D.[15] Serum concentrations declined to baseline 60–240 min after inhalation, with a half-life of the inhaled insulin product ranging from 120–206 min.[15] Inhaled human insulin is approved for use in T1D and T2D and is a viable option for people who are unwilling to initiate subcutaneous self-injection and can benefit from prandial insulin administration.[28]

INTERMEDIATE-ACTING INSULIN

NPH insulin, also known as isophane insulin, is generally classified as "intermediate-acting" in terms of its pharmacokinetic profile. NPH insulin contains an absorption-inhibiting substance called protamine, which prolongs the action and contributes to the cloudy appearance of NPH insulin.[7] For this reason, NPH and NPH-type insulins should be agitated/mixed prior to injection to resuspend the insulin mixture. NPH insulin may be used to cover basal insulin needs, in which case NPH is typically administered twice daily. NPH reaches peak plasma levels anywhere from 4–10 h after subcutaneous administration.[2,29,30] Because of the notable peak with NPH insulin, its use is associated with higher rates of hypoglycemia than that of long-acting insulin analogs.[2] Although NPH does carry a higher hypoglycemia risk, it is considerably less expensive than long- and ultra-long-acting insulin analogs and can be used effectively in people who have difficulty obtaining more expensive insulin products.

LONG-ACTING INSULIN

Long-acting insulin products are basal insulin analogs that provide basal insulin coverage for up to 24 h. The two medications within this group include insulin glargine (U-100) and insulin detemir. Some people can realize a full 24 h of basal coverage with these insulin products, but others can experience end-of-dose "wearing off," as noted by the duration of action ranges presented in Table 3.1.

Insulin Glargine (U-100)

Insulin glargine (U-100) was approved by the FDA in the year 2000, and differs structurally from human insulin by the addition of two arginines after position B30 and the replacement of asparagine with glycine at position A21.[31] Unlike NPH insulin, insulin glargine is soluble at a pH of 4.0.[31,32] Following subcutaneous injection, the acidic insulin solution is neutralized leading to the formation of insulin microprecipitates from which small amounts of insulin are gradually released over time.[31] As noted in Table 3.1, U-100 insulin glargine exhibits a duration of action generally ranging from 20–24 h with a relatively flat pharmacokinetic profile.[2] In clinical trials, U-100 insulin glargine demonstrated effects on glycemic control similar to once- or twice-daily NPH, with the advantage of a decreased rate of hypoglycemic events, particularly nocturnal hypoglycemic events.[31] In addition to the product Lantus, several follow-on U-100 insulin glargine products are available in the U.S., marketed as Basaglar and Semglee.[33,56] Although some people can realize a full 24 h of basal coverage with a single injection of U-100 insulin glargine, some people require twice-daily administration for a full day of basal coverage.

Insulin Detemir

Insulin detemir is another long-acting basal insulin analog. Insulin detemir has a prolonged duration of action (14–24 h) due to the insulin's ability to reversibly bind to albumin at the injection site and within the bloodstream.[2,34] Unlike insulin glargine, insulin detemir is soluble at a neutral pH. Structurally, insulin detemir differs from human insulin by the omission of threonine at position B30 and the attachment of myristic acid to lysine at position B29.[34] The presence of myristic acid contributes to delayed dissociation and absorption of insulin detemir hexamers and also facilitates a >98% binding of insulin detemir to albumin molecules in the plasma and interstitial fluid.[34] Because only free, non-albumin-bound insulin can be absorbed and bind to insulin receptors, albumin binding contributes to the prolonged duration of action seen with this insulin product. Since the duration of action of insulin detemir can range from 14–24 h, not everyone can realize a full 24 h of basal insulin coverage with once-daily administration, and twice-daily administration may be required.

ULTRA-LONG-ACTING INSULIN ANALOGS

"Ultra-long-acting" basal insulin products are those that have a duration of action in excess of 24 h. These insulin products will provide a full 24 h of basal coverage with a single daily injection, and may be beneficial in people who do not realize a full 24 h of coverage with U-100 insulin glargine or insulin detemir.

Insulin Glargine (U-300)

U-300 insulin glargine is a concentrated version of insulin glargine. U-300 insulin glargine is similar to the U-100 product in terms of structure and solubility at an acidic pH of 4.0. The longer duration of action realized with the concentrated U-300 product is attributable to the smaller injection volume, which results in a smaller precipitate surface area.[35] The smaller surface area is associated with a slower dissolution rate and a resultant longer duration of action.[35] In terms of its pharmacokinetic profile, the median time to maximum serum concentration following doses of 0.4, 0.6, and 0.9 U/kg of insulin glargine U-300 was 12,[8–14] 12,[12–18] and 16[12–20] h, respectively, and the mean concentrations declined to the lower limit of quantitation by 16, 28, and beyond 36 h, respectively.[16] Please refer to Table 3.1 for general pharmacokinetic properties of U-300 insulin glargine. Due to the pharmacokinetic properties of U-300 insulin glargine, time is needed for this insulin product to accumulate and reach steady-state levels, which are generally achieved after 5 days of once-daily administration.[16] The manufacturer recommends titrating the dose no more frequently than every 3–4 days to minimize the risk of hypoglycemia.[16]

Potential advantages of U-300 insulin glargine over the U-100 insulin glargine product include a longer duration of action, the potential for delivery of large insulin doses in a smaller injection volume, and a lower incidence of nocturnal hypoglycemia. Of note, when converting someone from the U-100 insulin glargine product to the U-300 product, larger doses (on a unit per unit basis) are typically needed to achieve the same glucose-lowering effect.[16] Therefore, it can be expected that higher unit doses of U-300 insulin glargine will be required to maintain glycemic control when compared to the previous U-100 insulin glargine dose.

Insulin Degludec (U-100; U-200)

Insulin degludec is another ultra-long-acting basal insulin analog with a duration of action of action in excess of 42 h at steady state.[17] Steady-state insulin concentrations are achieved by 3–4 days of once-daily subcutaneous administration.[17] To achieve this prolonged glycemic effect, insulin degludec is modified such that the amino acid at B30 is deleted and the lysine at position B29 is conjugated to hexadecanoic acid via a γ-L-glutamyl spacer.[36] When stored in solution with phenol and zinc, insulin degludec forms small, soluble and stable dihexamers. Upon injection, the phenol component slowly dissipates, allowing for self-association of the insulin molecules into large multihexameric chains consisting of thousands of dihexamers connected to one another.[36] Over time, these chains slowly begin to dissolve as the zinc component diffuses, resulting in the release of insulin from the terminal ends of the chain to be absorbed.[36] Insulin degludec is commercially available in U-100 and U-200 concentrations. Similar to U-300 insulin glargine, the manufacturer recommends titrating the dose no more frequently than every 3–4 days to minimize the risk of hypoglycemia.[17] Potential advantages of insulin degludec include its long duration of action, the potential for delivery of large insulin doses in a smaller injection volume (U-200 product), and a lower incidence of nocturnal hypoglycemia when compared to U-100 insulin glargine.

U-500 Regular Insulin

U-500 regular insulin was first introduced in the U.S. in 1952 for use in people with extreme insulin resistance caused by antibody formation against animal-derived insulin products.[37] Although it is a 5-times concentrated RHI product, the pharmacokinetics of U-500 insulin are considerably different than U-100 RHI. U-500 insulin peaks around 30 min after subcutaneous injection and has a duration of action that can range widely (see Table 3.1)[38,39] Historically, U-500 insulin use was associated with a high risk of insulin overdose errors due to injection of U-500 with U-100 insulin syringes. In recent years, however, the availability of U-500 insulin pens and dedicated U-500 insulin syringes has improved the safety of this insulin product. Given the unique pharmacokinetics of U-500 insulin, its use is generally reserved for people with T2D and significant insulin resistance who take in excess of 200 units of insulin daily.[40] Following publication of a U-500 clinical trial that used two dosing algorithms for the initiation and titration of U-500 in T2D patients not achieving adequate glycemic control with high-dose U-100 insulin therapy,[41] dosing algorithms are now readily available to help guide clinicians in the use of U-500 insulin in appropriate patients.

TREATMENT ADVANTAGES/DISADVANTAGES

Insulin therapy has the greatest potential for lowering A1C and improving glycemic control among all available glucose-lowering therapies. The degree to which glycemia can be reduced with insulin is limited only by hypoglycemia. Unlike many other antihyperglycemic options that target either fasting plasma glucose (FPG) or PPG, insulin can be used to target FPG, PPG, or both depending on the needs of the individual. Although insulin is unmatched in terms of glucose-lowering potential, its use comes with risks of hypoglycemia, weight gain, and injection site reactions (please see the section below, "Adverse Effects and Monitoring"). In addition, with the exception of inhaled insulin, insulin administration requires subcutaneous self-injection. Initiation of insulin therapy inherently comes with a requirement of more intensive medical oversight and training related to proper insulin use and administration. These considerations can lead to hesitancy to initiate insulin on the part of both people with diabetes and healthcare providers. The following sections provide a general description of the approaches to insulin use in people with T1D and T2D. The information below may be helpful in understanding the generally recommended approaches to insulin use in these patient populations, but the information provided is by no means the only approach to successfully manage people with insulin.

APPROACH TO THE USE OF INSULIN IN T1D

As noted at the beginning of this chapter, exogenous insulin therapy is a requirement for people with T1D due to an absolute lack of endogenous insulin secretion from pancreatic β-cells. As such, all people with T1D should use an intensive insulin regimen designed to cover both basal and prandial (mealtime) insulin needs with the ultimate goal of achieving individualized glycemic targets.[7] Regarding insulin therapy in T1D, the American Diabetes Association *Standards of Care in Diabetes* make the following recommendations:[4]

- Most people with T1D should be treated with multiple daily injections of prandial insulin and basal insulin or CSII.
- Most individuals with T1D should use rapid-acting insulin analogs to reduce hypoglycemia risk.
- Patients with T1D should receive education on how to match prandial insulin doses to carbohydrate intake, fat and protein content, and anticipated physical activity.

When initiating insulin therapy in someone newly diagnosed with T1D, the starting insulin dose is generally calculated based on weight, with starting doses ranging from 0.4–1.0 units/kg/day of total insulin.[2] Many clinicians will begin at 0.5 units/kg/day when the person is metabolically stable, with titration of the insulin per glycemic response. After calculating the total daily insulin dose, approximately half of the calculated total daily dose is administered as basal insulin, with the other half distributed across meals as prandial insulin (such as 20% of the total daily dose injected at breakfast, 10% at lunch, and 20% at dinner).[2] The insulin is thereafter titrated based on blood glucose monitoring data, with the individual ideally learning to count carbohydrates and dose their prandial insulin based on carbohydrate intake at each meal and snack.

The method of insulin delivery can include multiple daily injections (with vial and syringe or insulin pens) or use of CSII. The choice of which delivery method to use should be tailored to the individualized needs and preferences of the person with T1D. For a more detailed discussion of insulin use and glycemic management in people with T1D please refer to "Chapter 2: Management of Hyperglycemia in Type 1 Diabetes Mellitus."

APPROACH TO THE USE OF INSULIN IN T2D

The approach to insulin use in T2D is quite different than the approach taken in people with T1D.[4,42] People with T1D initiate an intensive insulin regimen shortly after diagnosis; people with T2D can often be managed with noninsulin therapies for years before the addition of insulin is required to meet individualized glycemic goals. That said, many people with T2D can benefit from early basal insulin initiation, depending on individualized needs and preferences. Once people with T2D reach a point where they are not achieving individualized glycemic goals despite the use of multiple noninsulin therapies, people may need to progress to the use of injectable therapies. Figure 3.2 provides recommendations from the 2023 American Diabetes Association *Standards of Care in Diabetes* regarding treatment intensification to injectable therapies.[4] As noted in Figure 3.2, for people with T2D who require injectable therapy to reduce A1C, it is recommended that a GLP-1 receptor agonist be considered as the first injectable agent in most patients. Insulin is recommended as the first injectable in those with very high A1C (>10%), those with symptoms or evidence of catabolism (weight loss, polyuria, polydipsia, etc.), or if a diagnosis of T1D is a possibility.[4] The figure provides some guidance on the initiation and titration of basal insulin, inclusive of a recommended starting dose (10 units/day or 0.1–0.2 units/kg/day) and guidance on titration of the basal insulin to achieve an individualized FPG target.[4] If goal A1C is not met following basal insulin optimization and achieving the target FPG level, the addition of prandial insulin is recommended (or the addition of a second NPH dose in those patients managed on a single NPH injection at bedtime). Alternatively, a GLP-1 receptor agonist can be added to target PPG excursions if the patient is not already receiving one. If prandial insulin is chosen, it is recommended to be started at 4 units/day, or 10% of the basal dose, typically initiated once daily with the largest meal (or meal with the largest PPG excursion). The dose can be up-titrated by 1–2 units or 10–15% twice weekly, with dose reductions of 10–20% recommended in the presence of hypoglycemia. Depending on response, additional injections of prandial insulin, or conversion to a self-mixed/split insulin or twice-daily premixed insulin regimen, can be considered to intensify therapy and meet individualized glycemic targets.[4] While Figure 3.2 provides a framework for insulin initiation and titration in people with T2D, individual patient needs will differ, and strategies should be tailored to meet glycemic goals and minimize hypoglycemia risk.

THERAPEUTIC CONSIDERATIONS

SIGNIFICANT WARNINGS/PRECAUTIONS

The following are warnings and precautions to be considered for use of insulin products.

Hypoglycemia

Hypoglycemia is the most common adverse reaction for all insulin therapies. Extra caution is warranted in people who have recently begun treatment with insulin and those with hypoglycemia unawareness who may not readily recognize hypoglycemic symptoms. Individuals experiencing a hypoglycemic event may experience impaired concentration and/or reaction time, thus hypoglycemia may present risk during activities such as driving or operating machinery.

Hypokalemia

Insulin stimulates potassium movement intracellularly, potentially causing hypokalemia. The risk of hypokalemia is particularly high when administering

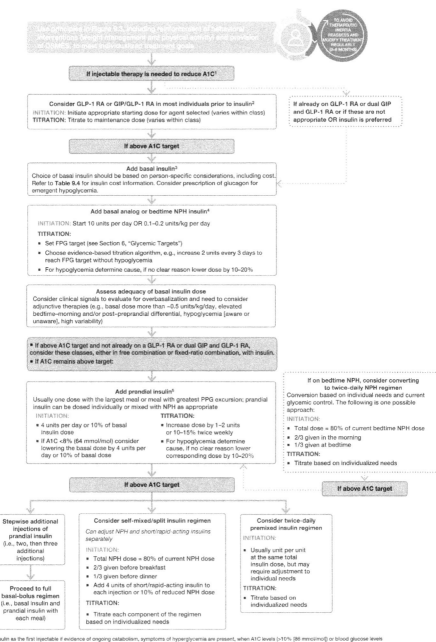

Figure 3.2—Intensifying to injectable therapies in T2D. Reprinted with permission from the American Diabetes Association.[42]

Table 3.2—Symptoms of Hypoglycemia

Shakiness	Tingling or numbness in the lips or tongue
Nervousness or anxiety	Headache
Sweating, chills, or clamminess	Anger, stubbornness, or sadness
Irritability or impatience	Lack of coordination
Confusion	Nightmares
Rapid/fast heartbeat	Seizures
Lightheadedness or dizziness	Unconsciousness
Hunger	
Sleepiness/fatigue	
Blurred/impaired vision	

Source: Adapted from American Diabetes Association.[7]

insulin intravenously.[13,14] Potassium levels should be monitored closely when administering insulin intravenously.

Hypersensitivity and Allergic Reactions

Severe, life-threatening hypersensitivity and allergic reactions can occur with insulin products. If hypersensitivity reactions occur, the offending insulin product should be discontinued until the person is medically treated and evaluated.

SPECIAL POPULATIONS

Although all people with T1D require insulin therapy, and many people with T2D will eventually require insulin to meet glycemic goals there are some considerations with insulin use in special populations as outlined below.

Pregnancy

According to the American Diabetes Association *Standards of Care in Diabetes,* insulin is the preferred medication for treating hyperglycemia during gestational diabetes as well as during pregnancy in women with T1D or T2D.[43] In people with diabetes or gestational diabetes, insulin requirements may decrease during the first trimester, generally increase during the second and third trimesters, and rapidly decline after delivery.[43]

Kidney Impairment

In contrast to endogenously secreted insulin, which undergoes substantial degradation in the liver, exogenous insulin is to a larger degree eliminated by the kidneys.[44] Insulin is filtered by the glomerulus followed by reabsorption in the proximal tubule of the kidney. Insulin clearance decreases in parallel with a decrease in glomerular filtration rate (GFR), leading to an overall decrease in exogenous insulin requirements.[44] Because individual insulin preparations have not been well studied in the context of chronic kidney disease (CKD) and considering individual needs vary considerably, no definitive recommendations exist for insulin dose adjustment based on estimated GFR. Many noninsulin therapies are contraindicated in CKD, so insulin therapy is a mainstay of hyperglycemia management in people with CKD. To mitigate hypoglycemia risk, blood glucose levels should be monitored closely to inform insulin dose adjustments.[44]

Hepatic Impairment

As with kidney disease, individual insulin products have not been well studied in people with hepatic impairment. In general, more frequent glucose monitoring and insulin dose adjustment may be warranted to prevent possible hypoglycemia in people with liver disease.

ADVERSE EFFECTS AND MONITORING

Insulin therapy has been associated with a variety of adverse effects in clinical trials, and the more salient adverse effects and monitoring recommendations for insulin products are provided below.

Hypoglycemia

As noted in the "Significant Warnings/Precautions" section above, hypoglycemia is the most common and serious adverse event associated with insulin use. Hypoglycemia is defined generally as a blood glucose value ≤70 mg/dL, with lower blood glucose levels associated with worsening hypoglycemic symptoms.[45] Hypoglycemia is much more common with the use of prandial insulin products. Careful and methodical titration of basal insulin products can minimize hypoglycemia risk. As such, people with T1D are generally at greater risk for hypoglycemia, as intensive insulin therapy is required for adequate glycemic control. That said, some people with T2D also receive intensive insulin therapy and should be considered high risk for hypoglycemic events, particularly when used in combination with sulfonylureas or other insulin secretagogue medications. Although not an exhaustive list, Table 3.2 provides a list of potential hypoglycemic symptoms.[7] People with hypoglycemia unawareness may not have recognizable symptoms and are at particular risk for severe hypoglycemic events. In people with hypoglycemia unawareness, less stringent glycemic targets may be warranted to reduce hypoglycemia risk, especially during the night.[7]

All people who use insulin should be counseled regarding the signs, symptoms, and proper treatment of hypoglycemia. Mild hypoglycemia can be treated by following the "rule of 15": treat with 15 g carbohydrate, wait 15 min, and then check the blood glucose level.[7] If after 15 min the blood glucose remains below 70 mg/dL, another 15 g carbohydrate should be consumed. Once the blood glucose is normalized, a snack or meal that includes complex carbohydrates and protein should be consumed to prevent a secondary hypoglycemic episode. When a severe hypoglycemic event occurs and glucose cannot be delivered orally, glucagon use (injectable or intranasal) is indicated.[7] The American Diabetes Association *Standards of Care in Diabetes* recommend that glucagon be prescribed to individuals at significant risk of severe hypoglycemia,[45] which would include people who use prandial insulin products.

Weight Gain

Weight gain is associated with insulin use and is observed as improvements in glycemic control are achieved. As glycemic control improves, glucose is used by the tissues instead of being lost in the urine, thus resulting in weight gain. Although weight gain is initially viewed as desirable in people with T1D due to weight loss experienced due to glucosuria and catabolism that is frequently present at the time of diagnosis, intensive insulin therapy can result in undesirable weight gain over time.[46] Indeed, some patients with T1D may even underdose insulin in an effort to avoid weight gain.[46] For those with T2D, who often struggle with overweight and obesity, insulin therapy can further contribute to weight gain. Use of prandial insulin in people with T2D generally contributes to more weight gain than does the use of basal insulin products alone, with both hypoglycemia treatment and possibly increased caloric intake in defense against hypoglycemia.[46] People starting insulin therapy should be informed of the potential for weight gain and encouraged to implement healthy lifestyle measures to minimize insulin-induced weight gain.[7] In people with T2D, adjunctive antihyperglycemic agents such as GLP-1 receptor agonists, SGLT2 inhibitors, and pramlintide can also be used for their insulin-sparing and weight-mitigating effects.[7] Medications approved by the FDA for weight loss can also be considered.

Injection Site Reactions

Long-term use of insulin can lead to lipoatrophy or lipohypertrophy, which can adversely affect insulin absorption. Injection site rotation is important to avoid lipoatrophy and lipohypertrophy. If either occurs, injection into the affected area(s) should be avoided.

Pulmonary Adverse Events (Inhaled Insulin)

Due to its route of administration, inhaled human insulin carries unique adverse-event considerations related to pulmonary function. In clinical trials, the most common reason for discontinuation of inhaled insulin was cough.[15] In addition, participants using the product in clinical trials experienced a greater decline from baseline in forced expiratory volume in 1 second (FEV_1) compared to people treated with other antihyperglycemic therapies.[15] For these reasons, at least in part, inhaled insulin is contraindicated for use in people with chronic lung disease, such as asthma or chronic obstructive pulmonary disease (COPD), due to the risk of acute bronchospasm.[15] For people using the product, pulmonary function testing is recommended at baseline, after the first 6 months of therapy, and annually thereafter, even in the absence of pulmonary symptoms.[15] It is recommended that the product be considered for discontinuation if a $\geq 20\%$ decline in FEV_1 from baseline is observed.

DRUG INTERACTIONS

Drugs affecting glucose metabolism have the potential to interact with insulin and impact overall glycemic control. Some examples of commonly used medications that may lower blood glucose and potentially increase the effect of insulin include oral antihyperglycemic agents, angiotensin converting enzymes inhibitors, angiotensin II receptor blocking agents, disopyramide, pramlintide, fibrates, monoamine oxidase inhibitors, salicylates, sulfonamide antibiotics, and fluoxetine.[13–17,19–22,24,29,30,32,33,40,47] Conversely, examples of medications that may reduce the effect of insulin by increasing blood glucose include corticosteroids, niacin, diuretics, sympathomimetic agents (such as epinephrine or albuterol), isoniazid, thyroid hormones, estrogens, progestin, protease inhibitors, and antipsychotics.[13–17,19–22,24,29,30,32,33,40,47] More specific to the inhaled human insulin product, when coadministered with albuterol, the area under the curve for inhaled human insulin increased by 25%.[15] For patients taking albuterol and inhaled human insulin, dose adjustment of the insulin may be necessary with more frequent blood glucose monitoring recommended.[15] Medications, such as β-blockers, clonidine, lithium salts, and alcohol have been associated with both increasing and decreasing blood glucose levels.[13–17,19–22,24,29,30,32,33,40,47] Signs of hypoglycemia may also be reduced or absent in patients taking antiadrenergic medications, such as β-blockers, clonidine, guanethidine, and reserpine.[13–17,19–22,24,29,30,32,33,40,47] People taking any of these medications in combination with insulin should monitor their blood glucose more closely during use and be counseled on the signs, symptoms, and proper management of hypoglycemic events. Of note, while some antihyperglycemic agents have a low risk of hypoglycemia when used as monotherapy, the risk of hypoglycemia is always increased when additional antihyperglycemic agents are added to background insulin therapy. More diligent blood glucose monitoring with a potential decrease in insulin dose may be warranted when adding additional antihyperglycemic therapies.

DOSAGE AND ADMINISTRATION

The dose of insulin required varies considerably and is dependent on the type of insulin used and the needs of the individual. Although guidelines provide recommendations for insulin initiation and titration for basal and prandial insulin products, these are merely starting points from which to individualize the insulin dose and schedule.

A variety of insulin delivery options are also available, including vials and syringes, pens with disposable cartridges (penfills), prefilled disposable pens with disposable pen needles, and insulin pumps.[7] Table 3.3 provides a summary of individual insulin products available in the U.S., and how the products are supplied, storage recommendations, and pen dosing capabilities (if applicable).[13–17,19–22,24,29,30,32,33,40,47]

Insulin Vials and Syringes

Vials of insulin are typically less expensive than prefilled insulin pens or insulin cartridges. Many people can do quite well with vials and syringes, but use may be difficult for people with vision or dexterity issues. People should be instructed to use a new, clean needle for every dose to prevent injection site infections.

Insulin Pens

Insulin pens provide a mode of delivery that is more convenient, and often more accurate, than insulin administration via vial and syringe. These devices can be beneficial for people who have vision or dexterity issues that make drawing

Table 3.3—Insulin Product Availability and Storage Information

Generic name	Brand name(s)	Product availability	Units per pen (if applicable)	Dose range per injection (pens only)	Recommended pen storage at room temperature (days)
\multicolumn{6}{c}{Prandial (Mealtime) Insulin Products}
Regular Human Insulin	Humulin R, Novolin R	Vial, Prefilled pen	300 units	1–60 units	28
	Humulin R U-500	Vial, Prefilled pen	1,500 units	5–300 units	28
Insulin Lispro	Humalog (U-100)	Vial, Prefilled pen, Pen Cartridges	300 units	1–60 units 0.5–30 units†	28
	Admelog (U-100)	Vial, Prefilled pen	300 units	1–80 units	28
	Humalog (U-200)	Prefilled pen	600 units	1–60 units	28
	Lyumjev (U-100)	Vial, Prefilled pen, Pen Cartridges	300 units	1–60 units 0.5–30 units†	28
	Lyumjev (U-200)	Prefilled pen	600 units	1–60 units	28
Insulin Aspart	Novolog	Vial, Prefilled pen, Pen Cartridges	300 units	1–60 units (FlexPen) 1–80 units (FlexTouch)	28
	Fiasp	Vial, Prefilled pen	300 units	1–80 units	28
Insulin Glulisine	Apidra	Vial, Prefilled pen	300 units	1–80 units	28
Inhaled Human Insulin	Afrezza	Inhalation cartridges	N/A	N/A	N/A
\multicolumn{6}{c}{Basal Insulin Products}
Human Insulin Isophane (NPH)	Humulin N Novolin N	Vial, Prefilled pen	300 units	1–60 units	14
Insulin Detemir	Levemir	Vial, Prefilled pen	300 units	1–60 units	42
Insulin Glargine (U-100)	Lantus	Vial, Prefilled pen	300 units	1–80 units	28
	Basaglar	Prefilled pen	300 units	1–80 units	28
	Semglee	Vial, Prefilled pen	300 units	1–80 units	28

(continued)

Table 3.3 (continued)

Generic name	Brand name(s)	Product availability	Units per pen (if applicable)	Dose range per injection (pens only)	Recommended pen storage at room temperature (days)
Insulin Glargine (U-300)	Toujeo	Prefilled pen	450 units (SoloStar) 900 units (Max SoloStar)	1–80 units (SoloStar) 2–160 units (Max SoloStar)	56
Insulin Degludec (U-100, U-200)	Tresiba	Vial (U-100) Prefilled pen	300 units (U-100) 600 units (U-200)	1–80 units (U-100) 2–160 (U-200)	56

N/A, not applicable. † KwikPen Junior. *Source:* refs. 13–17,19–22,24,29,30,32,33,40,47, 55,57.

insulin into a syringe difficult. A new disposable pen needle should be tightened onto the insulin pen before each use to prevent infection. Some of the pens also require priming the pen needle before each use and holding the needle in the injection site for a specific number of seconds, so manufacturer's instructions should be explained to the patient prior to initiation.

Continuous Subcutaneous Insulin Infusion

CSII via use of an insulin pump or patch allows for precise insulin delivery. CSII is most commonly used by people with T1D at the current time. CSII requires considerable patient education and support until the individual becomes familiar with use of the device. Insulin pumps use rapid-acting insulin (insulin lispro, insulin aspart, or insulin glulisine) to cover both basal and bolus insulin needs.[7] Insulin pump and patch technology advances very quickly with new-generation devices entering the market regularly. The American Diabetes Association publishes consumer guides, inclusive of an insulin pump consumer guide, on a regular basis that are readily accessible via the American Diabetes Association's Consumer Guide website (consumerguide.diabetes.org).

Insulin Inhalation

As discussed previously, inhaled human insulin is currently available in the U.S. for prandial use in T1D and T2D.[15] The product is available in single-use cartridges for use in the corresponding inhalation device. The product is available in 4-unit, 8-unit, and 12-unit single-use cartridges, which are color-coded to prevent medication errors.[15]

COMBINATION THERAPY

Insulin combination therapy is commonly needed in people with T1D (unless they use an insulin pump) and in many people with longstanding T2D. Please refer back to the sections "Approach to the Use of Insulin in Type 1 Diabetes" and "Approach to the Use of Insulin in Type 2 Diabetes" for specific information on approaches to insulin use in these patient groups. When using multiple insulin products, they can be injected individually, mixed in a single syringe (if compatible), or purchased in fixed-ratio combination (FRC) insulin pens.

MIXING INSULIN

Some insulin products can be combined, or "mixed," in the same syringe to reduce the number of required daily injections. NPH or NPH-type insulin can be mixed with either regular human insulin or rapid-acting insulin analogs.[7] By mixing NPH-type insulins with regular insulin or a rapid-acting insulin analog, a biphasic action profile is created, providing both basal and prandial coverage with a single injection. When mixing insulins in a single syringe, the rapid- or short-acting insulin should be drawn up first.[7] It should be noted that long-acting insulins such as insulin glargine, insulin detemir, and insulin degludec should not be mixed with other insulin products.

PREMIXED INSULIN PRODUCTS

Commercially available premixed insulin products contain set percentages of two types of insulin in the same solution. These include mixtures of NPH and RHI (70/30), mixtures of protamine suspensions of rapid-acting analogs with the respective rapid-acting analog (75/25 lispro protamine/insulin lispro, 50/50 lispro protamine/insulin lispro, and 70/30 aspart protamine/aspart), and a combination of insulin degludec with insulin aspart (70/30).[48-52] The primary advantages of these insulin products are convenience and accuracy of administration, particularly for people with vision or dexterity limitations for whom mixing insulin would be difficult or unreliable.[7]

In addition to fixed-dose insulin combination products, there are currently two products available that combine a basal insulin analog with a GLP-1 receptor agonist.[53,54] As discussed in the section "Approach to the Use of Insulin in Type 2 Diabetes," combination therapy with basal insulin and a GLP-1 receptor agonist can effectively target both FPG and PPG values and thus improve A1C and overall glycemic control, while also mitigating insulin-associated weight gain. Table 3.4 provides a summary of fixed-dose combination products currently available in the U.S.[48-54]

Table 3.4—Fixed-Dose Combination (FDC) Insulin Products

Generic name	Brand name(s)	Product availability	Units per pen	Dose range per injection (pens only)	Recommended pen storage at room temperature (days)
Fixed-Dose Combination Insulin Products					
Regular/NPH 70/30	Humulin 70/30 Novolin 70/30	Vial, Prefilled pen	300 units	1–60	10
Lispro mix 50/50	Humalog Mix 50/50	Vial, Prefilled pen	300 units	1–60 units	10
Lispro mix 75/25	Humalog Mix 75/25	Vial, Prefilled pen	300 units	1–60 units	10
Aspart mix 70/30	Novolog Mix 70/30	Vial, Prefilled pen	300 units	1–60 units	14
Fixed-Dose Insulin/GLP-1 Receptor Agonist Products					
Insulin Glargine/ Lixisenatide	Soliqua	Prefilled pen	300 units (insulin glargine)	15–60 units (insulin glargine)	28
Insulin Degludec/ Liraglutide	Xultophy	Prefilled pen	300 units (insulin degludec)	10–50 units (insulin degludec)	21

Source: refs. 48–54.

MONOGRAPHS

SINGLE INSULIN PRODUCTS

Insulin Aspart (Fiasp): https://dailymed.nlm.nih.gov/dailymed/drugInfo.cfm?setid=834e7efc-393f-4c55-9125-628562a8a5cf

Insulin Aspart (Novolog): https://dailymed.nlm.nih.gov/dailymed/drugInfo.cfm?setid=e172b4f8-9b25-4019-8e09-afc10b2f30c9

Insulin Degludec [U-100, U-200] (Tresiba): https://dailymed.nlm.nih.gov/dailymed/drugInfo.cfm?setid=456c5e87-3dfd-46fa-8ac0-c6128d4c97c6

Insulin Detemir (Levemir): https://dailymed.nlm.nih.gov/dailymed/drugInfo.cfm?setid=d38d65c1-25bf-401d-9c7e-a2c3222da8af

Insulin Glargine [U-100] (Lantus, Basaglar, Semglee): https://dailymed.nlm.nih.gov/dailymed/drugInfo.cfm?setid=6328c99d-d75f-43ef-b19e-7e71f91e57f6

Insulin Glargine [U-300] (Toujeo): https://dailymed.nlm.nih.gov/dailymed/drugInfo.cfm?setid=c9561d96-124d-48ca-982f-0aa1575bff36

Insulin Glulisine (Apidra): https://dailymed.nlm.nih.gov/dailymed/drugInfo.cfm?setid=e7af6a7a-8046-4fb4-9979-4ec4230b23aa

Inhaled Human Insulin (Afrezza): https://dailymed.nlm.nih.gov/dailymed/drugInfo.cfm?setid=29f4637b-e204-425b-b89c-7238008d8c10

Insulin Lispro [U-100, U-200] (Humalog, Admelog): https://dailymed.nlm.nih.gov/dailymed/drugInfo.cfm?setid=c8ecbd7a-0e22-4fc7-a503-faa58c1b6f3f

NPH Insulin (Humulin N, Novolin N): https://dailymed.nlm.nih.gov/dailymed/drugInfo.cfm?setid=82f1445c-b2c6-445a-82cf-ba8825fac776

Regular Human Insulin [U-100] (Humulin R, Novolin R): https://dailymed.nlm.nih.gov/dailymed/drugInfo.cfm?setid=b519bd83-038c-4ec5-a231-a51ec5cc291f

Regular Human Insulin [U-500] (Humulin R U-500): https://dailymed.nlm.nih.gov/dailymed/drugInfo.cfm?setid=b60e8dd0-1d48-4dc9-87fd-e14675255e8c

REFERENCES

1. White JR. A brief history of the development of diabetes medications. *Diabetes Spectr* 2014;27:82–86

2. American Diabetes Association/JDRF. *Type 1 Diabetes Sourcebook*. Peters A, Laffel L, Eds. Alexandria, American Diabetes Association, 2013

3. Chiang JL, Kirkman MS, Laffel LMB, Peters AL. Type 1 diabetes through the life span: a position statement of the American Diabetes Association. *Diabetes Care* 2014;37:2034–2054

4. American Diabetes Association. 9. Pharmacologic approaches to glycemic treatment: Standards of Medical Care in Diabetes—2022. *Diabetes Care* 2022;45(Suppl. 1):S125–S143

5. Kahn CR, Baird KL, Flier JS, et al. Insulin receptors, receptor antibodies and the mechanism of insulin action. *Recent Prog Horm Res* 1981;37:477–538

6. Skyler JS, Bakris GL, Bonifacio E, et al. Differentiation of diabetes by pathophysiology, natural history, and prognosis. *Diabetes* 2017;66:241–255

7. American Diabetes Association. *Practical Insulin: A Handbook for Prescribing Providers*. 5th ed. Alexandria, American Diabetes Association, 2019

8. Evans M, Schumm-Draeger PM, Vora J, King AB. A review of modern insulin analogue pharmacokinetic and pharmacodynamics profiles in type 2 diabetes: improvements and limitations. *Diabetes Obes Metab* 2011;13:677–684

9. Ryysy L, Häkkinen AM, Goto T, et al. Hepatic fat content and insulin action on free fatty acids and glucose metabolism rather than insulin absorption are associated with insulin requirements during insulin therapy in type 2 diabetic patients. *Diabetes* 2000;49:749–758

10. Koivisto VA. Sauna-induced acceleration in insulin absorption from subcutaneous injection site. *Br Med J* 1980;280:1411–1413

11. Berger M, Cuppers HJ, Hegner H, Jorgens V, Berchtold P. Absorption kinetics and biologic effects of subcutaneously injected insulin preparations. *Diabetes Care* 1982;5:77-91

12. ter Braak EW, Woodworth JR, Bianchi R, et al. Injection site effects on the pharmacokinetics and glucodynamics of insulin lispro and regular insulin. *Diabetes Care* 1996;19:1437–1440

13. Humulin R (insulin human injection) [package insert]. Indianapolis, IN, Lilly USA, LLC, 2022

14. Novolin R (insulin human injection) [package insert]. Plainsboro, NJ, Novo Nordisk Inc., 2022

15. Afrezza (insulin human inhalation powder) [package insert]. Danbury, CT, MannKind Corporation, 2023

16. Toujeo (insulin glargine injection) [package insert]. Bridgewater, NJ, Sanofi-aventis U.S. LLC, 2022

17. Tresiba (insulin degludec injection) [package insert]. Plainsboro, NJ, Novo Nordisk Inc., 2022

18. ElSayed NA, Aleppo G, Aroda VR,e t al., American Diabetes Association. 16. Diabetes care in the hospital: Standards of Care in Diabetes – 2023. *Diabetes Care* 2023;46(Suppl. 1):S267–S278

19. Humalog (insulin lispro injection) [package insert]. Indianapolis, IN, Lilly USA, LLC, 2019

20. Novolog (insulin aspart injection) [package insert]. Plainsboro, NJ, Novo Nordisk Inc., 2023

21. Fiasp (insulin aspart injection) [package insert]. Plainsboro, NJ, Novo Nordisk Inc., 2022

22. Apidra (insulin glulisine injection) [package insert]. Bridgewater, NJ, Sanofi-aventis U.S. LLC, 2020

23. Tibaldi JM. Evolution of insulin: from human to analog. *Am J Med* 2014;127:S25–S38

24. Admelog (insulin lispro injection) [package insert]. Bridgewater, NJ, Sanofi-aventis U.S. LLC, 2020

25. Mathieu C, Bode BW, Franek E, et al. Efficacy and safety of fast-acting insulin aspart in comparison with insulin aspart in type 1 diabetes (onset 1): a 52-week, randomized, treat-to-target, phase III trial. *Diabetes Obes Metab* 2018;20:1148–1155

26. Russell-Jones D, Bode BW, De Block C, et al. Fast-acting insulin aspart improves glycemic control in basal-bolus treatment for type 1 diabetes: results of a 26-week multicenter, active-controlled, treat-to-target, randomized, parallel-group trial (onset 1). *Diabetes Care* 2017;40:943–950

27. Bowering K, Case C, Harvey J, et al. Faster aspart versus insulin aspart as part of a basal-bolus regimen in inadequately controlled type 2 diabetes: the onset 2 trial. *Diabetes Care* 2017;40:951–957

28. Neumiller JJ, Campbell RK. Technosphere insulin: an inhaled prandial insulin product. *Biodrugs* 2010;24:165–172

29. Humulin N (human insulin isophane suspension) [package insert]. Indianapolis, IN, Lilly USA, LLC, 2022

30. Novolin N (isophane insulin human suspension) [package insert]. Plainsboro, NJ, Novo Nordisk Inc., 2022

31. Campbell RK, White JR, Levien T, Baker D. Insulin glargine. *Clin Ther* 2001;23:1938–1957

32. Lantus (insulin glargine injection) [package insert]. Bridgewater, NJ, Sanofi-aventis U.S. LLC, 2022

33. Basaglar (insulin glargine injection) [package insert]. Indianapolis, IN, Lilly USA, LLC, 2021

34. Soran H, Younis N. Insulin detemir: a new basal insulin analogue. *Diabetes Obes Metab* 2006;8:26–30

35. Blair HA, Keating GM. Insulin glargine 300 U/mL: a review in diabetes mellitus. *Drugs* 2016;76:363–374

36. Robinson JD, Neumiller JJ, Campbell RK. Can a new ultra-long-acting insulin analogue improve patient care? Investigating the potential role of insulin degludec. *Drugs* 2012;72:2319–2325

37. Kahn CR, Flier JS, Bar RS, et al. The syndromes of insulin resistance and acanthosis nigricans: insulin-receptor disorders in man. *N Engl J Med* 1976;294:739–745

38. Lamos EM, Younk LM, Davis SN. Concentrated insulins: the new basal insulins. *Ther Clin Risk Manag* 2016;12:389–400

39. de la Peña A, Riddle M, Morrow LA, et al. Pharmacokinetics and pharmacodynamics of high-dose human regular U-500 insulin versus human regular U-100 insulin in healthy obese subjects. *Diabetes Care* 2011;34:2496–2501

40. Humulin R U-500 (insulin human injection) [package insert]. Indianapolis, IN, Lilly USA, LLC, 2022

41. Hood RC, Arakaki RF, Wysham C, et al. Two treatment approaches for human regular U-500 insulin in patients with type 2 diabetes not achieving adequate glycemic control on high-dose U-100 insulin therapy with or without oral agents: a randomized, titration-to-target clinical trial. *Endocr Pract* 2015;21:782–793

42. Davies MJ, D'Alessio DA, Fradkin J, et al. Management of hyperglycemia in type 2 diabetes, 2018. A consensus report by the American Diabetes Association (ADA) and the European Association for the Study of Diabetes (EASD). *Diabetes Care* 2018 Oct 4. DOI:10.2337/dci18-0033. [Epub ahead of print]

43. ElSayed NA, Aleppo G, Aroda VR, et al., American Diabetes Association. 15. Management of diabetes in pregnancy: Standards of Care in Diabetes – 2023. *Diabetes Care* 2023;46(Suppl. 1):S254–S266

44. Neumiller JJ, Alicic RZ, Tuttle KR. Therapeutic considerations for antihyperglycemic agents in diabetic kidney disease. *J Am Soc Nephrol* 2017;28:2263–2274

45. ElSayed NA, Aleppo G, Aroda VR, et al., American Diabetes Association. 6. Glycemic targets: Standards of Care in Diabetes – 2023. *Diabetes Care* 2023;46(Suppl. 1):S97–S110

46. Russell-Jones D, Khan R. Insulin-associated weight gain in diabetes—causes, effects and coping strategies. *Diabetes Obes Metab* 2007;9(6):799–812

47. Levemir (insulin detemir injection) [package insert]. Plainsboro, NJ, Novo Nordisk Inc., 2022

48. Humulin 70/30 (insulin human injection) [package insert]. Indianapolis, IN, Lilly USA, LLC, 2022

49. Novolin 70/30 (human insulin isophane suspension and human insulin injection) [package insert]. Plainsboro, NJ, Novo Nordisk Inc., 2022

50. Humalog Mix50/50 (insulin lispro injection, suspension) [package insert]. Indianapolis, IN, Lilly USA, LLC, 2019

51. Humalog Mix75/25 (insulin lispro injection, suspension) [package insert]. Indianapolis, IN, Lilly USA, LLC, 2019

52. Novolog Mix 70/30 (insulin aspart protamine and insulin aspart injectable suspension) [package insert]. Plainsboro, NJ, Novo Nordisk Inc., 2023

53. Soliqua 100/33 (insulin glargine and lixisenatide injection) [package insert]. Bridgewater, NJ, Sanofi-aventis U.S. LLC, 2022

54. Xultophy 100/3.6 (insulin degludec and liraglutide injection) [package insert]. Plainsboro, NJ, Novo Nordisk Inc., 2022

55. Semglee (insulin glargine injection) [package insert]. Morgantown, WV, Mylan Specialty L.P., 2022

56. Lyumjev (insulin lispro-aabc injection) [package insert]. Indianapolis, IN, Lilly USA, LLC, 2022

Chapter 4
Pharmacologic Therapy for Type 2 Diabetes

9.4a Healthy lifestyle behaviors, diabetes self-management education and support, avoidance of clinical inertia, and social determinants of health should be considered in the glucose-lowering management of type 2 diabetes. Pharmacologic therapy should be guided by person-centered treatment factors, including comorbidities and treatment goals. **A**

9.4b In adults with type 2 diabetes and established/high risk of atherosclerotic cardiovascular disease, heart failure, and/or chronic kidney disease, the treatment regimen should include agents that reduce cardiorenal risk (Fig. 4.1 and Table 4.1). A

9.4c Pharmacologic approaches that provide adequate efficacy to achieve and maintain treatment goals should be considered, such as metformin or other agents, including combination therapy (Fig. 4.1 and Table 4.1). A

9.4d Weight management is an impactful component of glucose-lowering management in type 2 diabetes. The glucose-lowering treatment regimen should consider approaches that support weight management goals (Fig. 4.1 and Table 4.1). A

9.5 Metformin should be continued upon initiation of insulin therapy (unless contraindicated or not tolerated) for ongoing glycemic and metabolic benefits. **A**

9.6 Early combination therapy can be considered in some individuals at treatment initiation to extend the time to treatment failure.**A**

9.7 The early introduction of insulin should be considered if there is evidence of ongoing catabolism (weight loss), if symptoms of hyperglycemia are present, or when A1C levels (>10% [86 mmol/mol]) or blood glucose levels (≥300 mg/dL [16.7 mmol/L]) are very high. **E**

9.8 A person-centered approach should guide the choice of pharmacologic agents. Consider the effects on cardiovascular and renal comorbidities, efficacy, hypo-glycemia risk, impact on weight, cost and access, risk for side effects, and individual preferences (Table 4.1 and Fig. 4.1). **E**

Chapter 4 is an excerpt from ElSayed NA, Aleppo G, Aroda VR, et al., American Diabetes Association. 9. Pharmacologic approaches to glycemic treatment: Standards of Care in Diabetes—2023. *Diabetes Care* 2023;46(Suppl. 1):S140–S157

* See Table 1.1 (p. 2) for an explanation of the American Diabetes Association evidence-grading system for *Standards of Care in Diabetes.*

9.9   Among individuals with type 2 diabetes who have established atherosclerotic cardiovascular disease or indicators of high cardiovascular risk, established kidney disease, or heart failure, a sodium–glucose cotransporter 2 inhibitor and/or glucagon-like peptide 1 receptor agonist with demonstrated cardiovascular disease benefit (Fig. 4.1, Table 4.1, Table 17.3b, and Table 17.3c) is recommended as part of the glucose-lowering regimen and comprehensive cardiovascular risk reduction, independent of A1C and in consideration of person-specific factors (Fig. 4.1) (see Section 10, "Cardiovascular Disease and Risk Management," for details on cardiovascular risk reduction recommendations). **A**

9.10 In adults with type 2 diabetes, a glucagon-like peptide 1 receptor agonist is preferred to insulin when possible. **A**

9.11 If insulin is used, combination therapy with a glucagon-like peptide 1 receptor agonist is recommended for greater efficacy, durability of treatment effect, and weight and hypoglycemia benefit. **A**

9.12 Recommendation for treatment intensification for individuals not meeting treatment goals should not be delayed. **A**

9.13 Medication regimen and medication-taking behavior should be reevaluated at regular intervals (every 3–6 months) and adjusted as needed to incorporate specific factors that impact choice of treatment (Fig. 4.1 and Table 4.1). **E**

9.14 Clinicians should be aware of the potential for overbasalization with insulin therapy. Clinical signals that may prompt evaluation of overbasalization include basal dose more than ~0.5 units/kg/day, high bedtime–morning or postprepandial glucose differential, hypoglycemia (aware or unaware), and high glycemic variability. Indication of overbasalization should prompt reevaluation to further individualize therapy. **E**

The ADA/EASD consensus report "Management of Hyperglycemia in Type 2 Diabetes, 2022"[1–3] recommends a holistic, multifactorial person-centered approach accounting for the lifelong nature of type 2 diabetes. Person-specific factors that affect choice of treatment include individualized glycemic and weight goals, impact on weight, hypoglycemia and cardiorenal protection (see Section 10, "Cardiovascular Disease and Risk Management," and Section 11 "Chronic Kidney Disease and Risk Management"), underlying physiologic factors, side effect profiles of medications, complexity of regimen, regimen choice to optimize medication use and reduce treatment discontinuation, and access, cost, and availability of medication. Lifestyle modifications and health behaviors that improve health (see Section 5, "Facilitating Positive Health Behaviors and Well-being to Improve Health Outcomes") should be emphasized along with any pharmacologic therapy. Section 13, "Older Adults," and Section 14, "Children and Adolescents," have recommendations specific for older adults and for children and adolescents with type 2 diabetes, respectively. Section 10, "Cardiovascular Disease and Risk Management," and Section 11, "Chronic Kidney Disease and Risk Management," have recommendations for the use of glucose-lowering drugs in the management of cardiovascular and renal disease, respectively.

Table 4.1—Medications for lowering glucose, summary of characteristics

	Efficacy[1]	Hypoglycemia	Weight change[2]	CV effects		Progression of DKD	Renal effects	Oral/SQ	Cost	Clinical considerations
				Effect on MACE	HF		Dosing/use considerations[3]			
Metformin	High	No	Neutral (potential for modest loss)	Potential benefit	Neutral	Neutral	• Contraindicated with eGFR <30 mL/min per 1.73 m²	Oral	Low	• GI side effects common; to mitigate GI side effects, consider slow dose titration, extended release formulations, and administration with food • Potential for vitamin B12 deficiency; monitor at regular intervals
SGLT2 inhibitors	Intermediate to high	No	Loss (intermediate)	Benefit: canagliflozin, empagliflozin	Benefit: canagliflozin, dapagliflozin, empagliflozin, ertugliflozin	Benefit: canagliflozin, dapagliflozin, empagliflozin	• See labels for renal dose considerations of individual agents • Glucose-lowering effect is lower for SGLT2 inhibitors at lower eGFR	Oral	High	• DKA risk, rare in T2DM; discontinue, evaluate, and treat promptly if suspected; be aware of predisposing risk factors and clinical presentation (including euglycemic DKA); discontinue before scheduled surgery (e.g., 3–4 days), during critical illness, or during prolonged fasting to mitigate potential risk • Increased risk of genital mycotic infections • Necrotizing fasciitis of the perineum (Fournier gangrene), rare reports; institute prompt treatment if suspected • Attention to volume status, blood pressure; adjust other volume-contracting agents as applicable
GLP-1 RAs	High to very high	No	Loss (intermediate to very high)	Benefit: dulaglutide, liraglutide, semaglutide (SQ) Neutral: exenatide once weekly, lixisenatide	Neutral	Benefit for renal endpoints in CVOTs, driven by albuminuria outcomes: dulaglutide, liraglutide, semaglutide (SQ)	• See labels for renal dose considerations of individual agents • No dose adjustment for dulaglutide, liraglutide, semaglutide • Monitor renal function when initiating or escalating doses in patients with renal impairment reporting severe adverse GI reactions	SQ; oral (semaglutide)	High	• Risk of thyroid C-cell tumors in rodents; human relevance not determined (liraglutide, dulaglutide, exenatide extended release, semaglutide) • Counsel patients on potential for GI side effects and their typically temporary nature; provide guidance on dietary modifications to mitigate GI side effects (reduction in meal size, mindful eating practices [e.g., stop eating once full], decreasing intake of high-fat or spicy food); consider slower dose titration for patients experiencing GI challenges • Pancreatitis has been reported in clinical trials but causality has not been established. • Discontinue if pancreatitis is suspected • Evaluate for gallbladder disease if cholelithiasis or cholecystitis is suspected
GIP and GLP-1 RA	Very high	No	Loss (very high)	Under investigation	Under investigation	Under investigation	• See label for renal dose considerations • No dose adjustment • Monitor renal function when initiating or escalating doses in patients with renal impairment reporting severe adverse GI reactions	SQ	High	• Risk of thyroid C-cell tumors in rodents; human relevance not determined • Counsel patients on potential for GI side effects and their typically temporary nature; provide guidance on dietary modifications to mitigate GI side effects (reduction in meal size, mindful eating practices [e.g., stop eating once full], decreasing intake of high-fat or spicy food); consider slower dose titration for patients experiencing GI challenges • Pancreatitis has been reported in clinical trials but causality has not been established. • Discontinue if pancreatitis is suspected • Evaluate for gallbladder disease if cholelithiasis or cholecystitis is suspected
DPP-4 inhibitors	Intermediate	No	Neutral	Neutral	Neutral (potential risk, saxagliptin)	Neutral	• Renal dose adjustment required (sitagliptin, saxagliptin, alogliptin); can be used in renal impairment • No dose adjustment required for linagliptin	Oral	High	• Pancreatitis has been reported in clinical trials but causality has not been established. • Discontinue if pancreatitis is suspected • Bullous pemphigoid (postmarketing); discontinue if suspected
Thiazolidinediones	High	No	Gain	Potential benefit: pioglitazone	Increased risk	Neutral	• No dose adjustment required • Generally not recommended in renal impairment due to potential for fluid retention	Oral	Low	• Congestive HF (pioglitazone, rosiglitazone) • Fluid retention/edema; heart failure • Benefit in NASH • Joint pain • Risk of bone fractures • Weight gain: consider lower doses to mitigate weight gain and edema

(continued)

Table 4.1 (continued)

	Efficacy[1]	Hypoglycemia	Weight change[2]	CV effects		Renal effects		Oral/SQ	Cost	Clinical considerations
				Effect on MACE	HF	Progression of DKD	Dosing/use considerations[a]			
Sulfonylureas (2nd generation)	High	Yes	Gain	Neutral	Neutral	Neutral	• Glyburide: generally not recommended in chronic kidney disease • Glipizide and glimepiride: initiate conservatively to avoid hypoglycemia	Oral	Low	• FDA Special Warning on increased risk of CV mortality based on studies of an older sulfonylurea (tolbutamide); glimepiride shown to be CV safe (see text) • Use with caution in persons at risk for hypoglycemia
Insulin Human	High to very high	Yes	Gain	Neutral	Neutral	Neutral	• Lower insulin doses required with a decrease in eGFR; titrate per clinical response	SQ; inhaled	Low (SQ)	• Injection site reactions • Higher risk of hypoglycemia with human insulin (NPH or premixed formulations) vs. analogs
Analogs								SQ	High	

CV, cardiovascular; CVOT, cardiovascular outcomes trial; DKA, diabetic ketoacidosis; DKD, diabetic kidney disease; DPP-4, dipeptidyl peptidase 4; eGFR, estimated glomerular filtration rate; FDA, U.S. Food and Drug Administration; GI, gastrointestinal; GIP, gastric inhibitory polypeptide; GLP-1 RA, glucagon-like peptide 1 receptor agonist; HF, heart failure; NASH, non-alcoholic steatohepatitis; MACE, major adverse cardiovascular events; SGLT2, sodium–glucose cotransporter 2; SQ, subcutaneous; T2DM, type 2 diabetes mellitus. [a]For agent-specific dosing recommendations, please refer to manufacturers' prescribing information. [1]Tsapas et al.[62] [2]Tsapas et al.[114] Reprinted from Davies et al.[45].

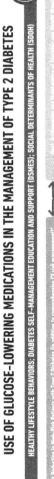

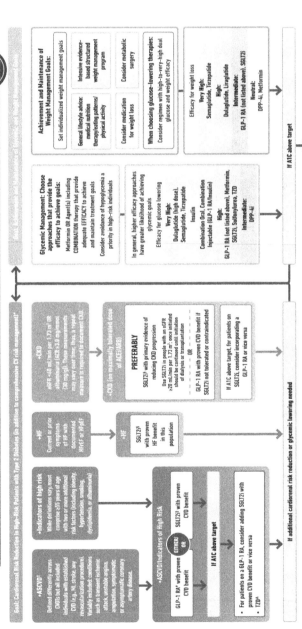

Figure 4.1—Use of glucose-lowering medications in the management of type 2 diabetes. ACEi, angiotensin-converting enzyme inhibitor; ACR, albumin-to-creatinine ratio; ARB, angiotensin receptor blocker; ASCVD, atherosclerotic cardiovascular disease; CGM, continuous glucose monitoring; CKD, chronic kidney disease; CV, cardiovascular; CVD, cardiovascular disease; CVOT, cardiovascular outcomes trial; DPP-4i, dipeptidyl peptidase 4 inhibitor; eGFR, estimated glomerular filtration rate; GLP-1 RA, glucagon-like peptide 1 receptor agonist; HF, heart failure; HFpEF, heart failure with preserved ejection fraction; HFrEF, heart failure with reduced ejection fraction; HHF, hospitalization for heart failure; MACE, major adverse cardiovascular events; MI, myocardial infarction; SDOH, social determinants of health; SGLT2i, sodium-glucose cotransporter 2 inhibitor; T2D, type 2 diabetes; TZD, thiazolidinedione. Adapted from Davies et al.[45]

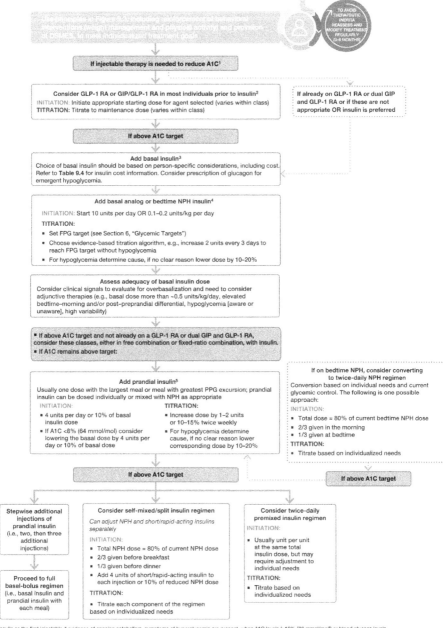

1. Consider insulin as the first injectable if evidence of ongoing catabolism, symptoms of hyperglycemia are present, when A1C levels (>10% [86 mmol/mol]) or blood glucose levels (300 mg/dL [16.7 mmol/L]) are very high, or a diagnosis of type 1 diabetes is a possibility.
2. When selecting GLP-1 RA, consider individual preference, A1C lowering, weight-lowering effect, or frequency of injection. If CVD is present, consider GLP-1 RA with proven CVD benefit. Oral or injectable GLP-1 RA are appropriate.
3. For people on GLP-1 RA and basal insulin combination, consider use of a fixed-ratio combination product (iDegLira or iGlarLixi).
4. Consider switching from evening NPH to a basal analog if the individual develops hypoglycemia and/or frequently forgets to administer NPH in the evening and would be better managed with an A.M. dose of a long-acting basal insulin.
5. If adding prandial insulin to NPH, consider initiation of a self-mixed or premixed insulin regimen to decrease the number of injections required.

Figure 4.2—Intensifying to injectable therapies in type 2 diabetes. DSMES, diabetes self-management education and support; FPG, fasting plasma glucose; GLP-1 RA, glucagon-like peptide 1 receptor agonist; max, maximum; PPG, postprandial glucose. Adapted from Davies et al.[43]

Table 4.2—Median Monthly (30-day) AWP and NADAC of Maximum Approved Daily Dose of Noninsulin Glucose-Lowering Agents in the U.S.

Class	Compound(s)	Dosage strength/ product (if applicable)	Median AWP (min, max)†	Median NADAC (min, max)†	Maximum approved daily dose*
Biguanides	• Metformin	850 mg (IR)	$106 ($5, $189)	$2	2,550 mg
		1,000 mg (IR)	$87 ($3, $144)	$2	2,000 mg
		1,000 mg (ER)	$242 ($242, $7,214)	$32 ($32, $160)	2,000 mg
Sulfonylureas (2nd generation)	• Glimepiride	4 mg	$74 ($71, $198)	$3	8 mg
	• Glipizide	10 mg (IR)	$70 ($67, $91)	$6	40 mg
		10 mg (XL/ER)	$48 ($46, $48)	$11	20 mg
	• Glyburide	6 mg (micronized)	$52 ($48, $71)	$12	12 mg
		5 mg	$79 ($63, $93)	$9	20 mg
Thiazolidinediones	• Pioglitazone	45 mg	$345 ($7, $349)	$4	45 mg
α-Glucosidase inhibitors	• Acarbose	100 mg	$106 ($104, $106)	$29	300 mg
	• Miglitol	100 mg	$241 ($241, $346)	N/A	300 mg
Meglitinides (glinides)	• Nateglinide	120 mg	$155	$27	360 mg
	• Repaglinide	2 mg	$878 ($58, $897)	$31	16 mg
DPP-4 inhibitors	• Alogliptin	25 mg	$234	$154	25 mg
	• Saxagliptin	5 mg	$565	$452	5 mg
	• Linagliptin	5 mg	$606	$485	5 mg
	• Sitagliptin	100 mg	$626	$500	100 mg
SGLT2 inhibitors	• Ertugliflozin	15 mg	$390	$312	15 mg
	• Dapagliflozin	10 mg	$659	$527	10 mg
	• Canagliflozin	300 mg	$684	$548	300 mg
	• Empagliflozin	25 mg	$685	$547	25 mg

(continued)

Table 4.2 (continued)

Class	Compound(s)	Dosage strength/ product (if applicable)	Median AWP (min, max)†	Median NADAC (min, max)†	Maximum approved daily dose*
GLP-1 RAs	• Exenatide (extended release)	2 mg powder for suspension or pen	$936	$726	2 mg**
	• Exenatide	10 µg pen	$961	$770	20 µg
	• Dulaglutide	4.5 mg mL pen	$1,064	$852	4.5 mg**
	• Semaglutide	1 mg pen	$1,070	$858	1 mg**
		14 mg (tablet)	$1,070	$858	14 mg
	• Liraglutide	1.8 mg pen	$1,278	$1,022	1.8 mg
	• Lixisenatide	20 µg pen	$814	N/A	20µg
GLP-1/GIP dual agonist	• Tirzepatide	15 mg pen	$1,169	$935	15 mg**
Bile acid sequestrant	• Colesevelam	625 mg tabs	$711 ($674, $712)	$83	3.75 g
		3.75 g suspension	$674 ($673, $675)	$177	3.75 g
Dopamine-2 agonist	• Bromocriptine	0.8 mg	$1,118	$899	4.8 mg
Amylin mimetic	• Pramlintide	120 µg pen	$2,783	NA	120 µg/injection††

AWP, average wholesale price; DPP-4, dipeptidyl peptidase 4; ER and XL, extended release; GIP, glucose-dependent insulinotropic polypeptide; GLP-1 RA, glucagon-like peptide 1 receptor agonist; IR, immediate release; max, maximum; min, minimum; NA, data not available; NADAC, National Average Drug Acquisition Cost; SGLT2, sodium-glucose cotransporter 2. †Calculated for 30-day supply (AWP [72] or NADAC [73] unit price × number of doses required to provide maximum approved daily dose × 30 days); median AWP or NADAC listed alone when only one product and/or price. *Utilized to calculate median AWP and NADAC (min, max); generic prices used, if available commercially. **Administered once weekly. ††AWP and NADAC calculated based on 120 µg three times daily.

CHOICE OF GLUCOSE-LOWERING THERAPY

Healthy lifestyle behaviors, diabetes self-management, education, and support, avoidance of clinical inertia, and social determinants of health should be considered in the glucose-lowering management of type 2 diabetes. Pharmacologic therapy should be guided by person-centered treatment factors, including comorbidities and treatment goals. Pharmacotherapy should be started at the time type 2 diabetes is diagnosed unless there are contraindications. Pharmacologic approaches that provide the efficacy to achieve treatment goals should be considered, such as metformin or other agents, including combination therapy, that provide adequate efficacy to achieve and maintain treatment goals.[3] In adults with type 2 diabetes and established/high risk of atherosclerotic cardiovascular disease (ASCVD), heart failure (HF), and/or chronic kidney disease (CKD), the treatment regimen should include agents that reduce cardiorenal risk (see Fig. 4.1,

Table 4.1, Section 10, "Cardiovascular Disease and Risk Management," and Section 11, "Chronic Kidney Disease and Risk Management"). Pharmacologic approaches that provide the efficacy to achieve treatment goals should be considered, specified as metformin or agent(s), including combination therapy, that provide adequate efficacy to achieve and maintain treatment goals (Fig. 4.1 and Table 4.1). In general, higher-efficacy approaches have greater likelihood of achieving glycemic goals, with the following considered to have very high efficacy for glucose lowering: the GLP-1 RAs dulaglutide (high dose) and semaglutide, the gastric inhibitory peptide (GIP) and GLP-1 RA tirzepatide, insulin, combination oral therapy, and combination injectable therapy. Weight management is an impactful component of glucose-lowering management in type 2 diabetes.[3,4] The glucose-lowering treatment regimen should consider approaches that support weight management goals, with very high efficacy for weight loss seen with semaglutide and tirzepatide (Fig. 4.1 and Table 4.1).[3]

Metformin is effective and safe, is inexpensive, and may reduce risk of cardiovascular events and death.[5] Metformin is available in an immediate-release form for twice-daily dosing or as an extended-release form that can be given once daily. Compared with sulfonylureas, metformin as first-line therapy has beneficial effects on A1C, weight, and cardiovascular mortality.[6]

The principal side effects of metformin are gastrointestinal intolerance due to bloating, abdominal discomfort, and diarrhea; these can be mitigated by gradual dose titration. The drug is cleared by renal filtration, and very high circulating levels (e.g., as a result of overdose or acute renal failure) have been associated with lactic acidosis. However, the occurrence of this complication is now known to be very rare, and metformin may be safely used in people with reduced estimated glomerular filtration rates (eGFR); the FDA has revised the label for metformin to reflect its safety in people with eGFR ≥30 mL/min/1.73 m2.[7] A randomized trial confirmed previous observations that metformin use is associated with vitamin B12 deficiency and worsening of symptoms of neuropathy.[8] This is compatible with a report from the Diabetes Prevention Program Outcomes Study (DPPOS) suggesting periodic testing of vitamin B12[9] (see Section 3, "Prevention or Delay of Type 2 Diabetes and Associated Comorbidities").

When A1C is ≥1.5% (12.5 mmol/mol) above the glycemic target (see Section 6, "Glycemic Targets," for appropriate targets), many individuals will require dual-combination therapy or a more potent glucose-lowering agent to achieve and maintain their target A1C level[3,10] (Fig. 4.1 and Table 4.1). Insulin has the advantage of being effective where other agents are not and should be considered as part of any combination regimen when hyperglycemia is severe, especially if catabolic features (weight loss, hypertriglyceridemia, ketosis) are present. It is common practice to initiate insulin therapy for people who present with blood glucose levels ≥300 mg/dL (16.7 mmol/L) or A1C >10% (86 mmol/mol) or if the individual has symptoms of hyperglycemia (i.e., polyuria or polydipsia) or evidence of catabolism (weight loss) (Fig. 9.4). As glucose toxicity resolves, simplifying the regimen and/or changing to noninsulin agents is often possible. However, there is evidence that people with uncontrolled hyperglycemia associated with type 2 diabetes can also be effectively treated with a sulfonylurea.[11]

COMBINATION THERAPY

Because type 2 diabetes is a progressive disease in many individuals, maintenance of glycemic targets often requires combination therapy. Traditional recommendations have been to use stepwise addition of medications to metformin to maintain A1C at target. The advantage of this is to provide a clear assessment of the positive and negative effects of new drugs and reduce potential side effects and expense.[12] However, there are data to support initial combination therapy for more rapid attainment of glycemic goals[13,14] and later combination therapy for longer durability of glycemic effect.[15] The VERIFY (Vildagliptin Efficacy in combination with metfoRmln For earlY treatment of type 2 diabetes) trial demonstrated that initial combination therapy is superior to sequential addition of medications for extending primary and secondary failure.[16] In the VERIFY trial, participants receiving the initial combination of metformin and the dipeptidyl peptidase 4 (DPP-4) inhibitor vildagliptin had a slower decline of glycemic control compared with metformin alone and with vildagliptin added sequentially to metformin. These results have not been generalized to oral agents other than vildagliptin, but they suggest that more intensive early treatment has some benefits and should be considered through a shared decision-making process, as appropriate. Initial combination therapy should be considered in people presenting with A1C levels 1.5–2.0% above target. Finally, incorporation of high-glycemic-efficacy therapies or therapies for cardiovascular/renal risk reduction (e.g., GLP-1 RAs, SGLT2 inhibitors) may allow for weaning of the current regimen, particularly of agents that may increase the risk of hypoglycemia. Thus, treatment intensification may not necessarily follow a pure sequential addition of therapy but instead reflect a tailoring of the regimen in alignment with person-centered treatment goals (Fig. 4.1).

Recommendations for treatment intensification for people not meeting treatment goals should not be delayed. Shared decision-making is important in discussions regarding treatment intensification. The choice of medication added to initial therapy is based on the clinical characteristics of the individual and their preferences. Important clinical characteristics include the presence of established ASCVD or indicators of high ASCVD risk, HF, CKD, obesity, nonalcoholic fatty liver disease or nonalcoholic steatohepatitis, and risk for specific adverse drug effects, as well as safety, tolerability, and cost. Results from comparative effectiveness meta-analyses suggest that each new class of noninsulin agents added to initial therapy with metformin generally lowers A1C approximately 0.7–1.0%[17,18] (Fig. 4.1 and Table 4.1).

For people with type 2 diabetes and established ASCVD or indicators of high ASCVD risk, HF, or CKD, an SGLT2 inhibitor and/or GLP-1 RA with demonstrated CVD benefit (see Table 4.1, Table 10.3b, Table 10.3c, and Section 10, "Cardiovascular Disease and Risk Management") is recommended as part of the glucose-lowering regimen independent of A1C, independent of metformin use and in consideration of person-specific factors (Fig. 4.1). For people without established ASCVD, indicators of high ASCVD risk, HF, or CKD, medication choice is guided by efficacy in support of individualized glycemic and weight management goals, avoidance of side effects (particularly hypoglycemia and weight gain), cost/access, and individual preferences.[19] A systematic review and network meta-analysis suggests greatest reductions in A1C level with insulin regimens and specific GLP-1 RAs added to metformin-based background therapy.[20] In all cases, treatment regimens need to be continuously reviewed for efficacy, side effects, and burden (Table 4.1). In some instances, the individual will require medication reduction or discontinuation. Common reasons for this include ineffectiveness, intolerable side effects, expense, or a change in glycemic goals (e.g., in response to development of comorbidities or changes in treatment goals). Section 13, "Older Adults," has a full discussion of treatment considerations in older adults, in whom changes of glycemic goals and de-escalation of therapy are common.

The need for the greater potency of injectable medications is common, particularly in people with a longer duration of diabetes. The addition of basal insulin, either human NPH or one of the long-acting insulin analogs, to oral agent regimens is a well-established approach that is effective for many individuals. In addition, evidence supports the utility of GLP-1 RAs in people not at glycemic goal. While most GLP-1 RAs are injectable, an oral formulation of semaglutide is commercially available.[21] In trials comparing the addition of an injectable GLP-1 RA or insulin in people needing further glucose lowering, glycemic efficacy of injectable GLP-1 RA was similar or greater than that of basal insulin.[22–28] GLP-1 RAs in these trials had a lower risk of hypoglycemia and beneficial effects on body weight compared with insulin, albeit with greater gastrointestinal side effects. Thus, trial results support GLP-1 RAs as the preferred option for individuals requiring the potency of an injectable therapy for glucose control (Fig. 9.4). In individuals who are intensified to insulin therapy, combination therapy with a GLP-1 RA has been shown to have greater efficacy and durability of glycemic treatment effect, as well as weight and hypoglycemia benefit, than treatment intensification with insulin alone.[3] However, cost and tolerability issues are important considerations in GLP-1 RA use.

Costs for diabetes medications have increased dramatically over the past two decades, and an increasing proportion is now passed on to patients and their families.[29] Table 4.2 provides cost information for currently approved noninsulin therapies. Of note, prices listed are average wholesale prices (AWP)[30] and National Average Drug Acquisition Costs (NADAC),[31] separate measures to allow for a comparison of drug prices, but do not account for discounts, rebates, or other price adjustments often involved in prescription sales that affect the actual cost incurred by the patient. Medication costs can be a major source of stress for people with diabetes and contribute to worse medication-taking behavior;[32] cost-reducing strategies may improve medication-taking behavior in some cases.[33]

CARDIOVASCULAR OUTCOMES TRIALS

There are now multiple large randomized controlled trials reporting statistically significant reductions in cardiovascular events in adults with type 2 diabetes treated with an SGLT2 inhibitor or GLP-1 RA; see Section 10, "Cardiovascular Disease and Risk Management" for details. Participants enrolled in many of the cardiovascular outcomes trials had A1C ≥6.5%, with more than 70% taking metformin at baseline, with analyses indicating benefit with or without metformin.[3] Thus, a practical extension of these results to clinical practice is to use these medications preferentially in people with type 2 diabetes and established ASCVD or indicators of high ASCVD risk. For these individuals, incorporating one of the SGLT2 inhibitors and/or GLP-1 RAs that have been demonstrated to have cardiovascular disease benefit is recommended (see Fig. 4.1, Table 4.1, and Section 10, "Cardiovascular Disease and Risk Management"). Emerging data suggest that use of both classes of drugs will provide additional cardiovascular and kidney outcomes benefit; thus, combination therapy with an SGLT2 inhibitor and a GLP-1 RA may be considered to provide the complementary outcomes benefits associated with these classes of medication.[34] In cardiovascular outcomes trials, empagliflozin, canagliflozin, dapagliflozin, liraglutide, semaglutide, and dulaglutide all had beneficial effects on indices of CKD, while dedicated renal outcomes studies have demonstrated benefit of specific SGLT2 inhibitors. See Section 11, "Chronic Kidney Disease and Risk Management," for discussion of how CKD may impact treatment choices. Additional large randomized trials of other agents in these classes are ongoing.

INSULIN THERAPY

Many adults with type 2 diabetes eventually require and benefit from insulin therapy (Fig. 9.4). See the section insulin injection technique, above, for guidance on how to administer insulin safely and effectively. The progressive nature of type 2 diabetes should be regularly and objectively explained to patients, and clinicians should avoid using insulin as a threat or describing it as a sign of personal failure or punishment. Rather, the utility and importance of insulin to maintain glycemic control once progression of the disease overcomes the effect of other agents should be emphasized. Educating and involving patients in insulin management is beneficial. For example, instruction of individuals with type 2 diabetes initiating insulin in self-titration of insulin doses based on glucose monitoring improves glycemic control.[35] Comprehensive education regarding blood glucose monitoring, nutrition, and the avoidance and appropriate treatment of hypoglycemia are critically important in any individual using insulin.

BASAL INSULIN

Basal insulin alone is the most convenient initial insulin treatment and can be added to metformin and other noninsulin injectables. Starting doses can be estimated based on body weight (0.1–0.2 units/kg/day) and the degree of hyperglycemia, with individualized titration over days to weeks as needed. The principal action of basal insulin is to restrain hepatic glucose production and limit hyperglycemia overnight and between meals.[36,37] Control of fasting glucose can be achieved with human NPH insulin or a long-acting insulin analog. In clinical trials, long-acting basal analogs (U-100 glargine or detemir) have been demonstrated to reduce the risk of symptomatic and nocturnal hypoglycemia compared with NPH insulin,[38–43] although these advantages are modest and may not persist.[44] Longer-acting basal analogs (U-300 glargine or degludec) may convey a lower hypoglyce-

Table 4.3—Median cost of insulin products in the U.S. calculated as AWP[30] and NADAC[31] per 1,000 units of specified dosage form/product

Insulins	Compounds	Dosage form/ product	Median AWP (min, max)*	Median NADAC*
Rapid-acting	• Lispro follow-on product	U-100 vial	$118 ($118, $157)	$94
		U-100 prefilled pen	$151	$121
	• Lispro	U-100 vial	$99†	$79†
		U-100 cartridge	$408	$326
		U-100 prefilled pen	$127†	$102†
		U-200 prefilled pen	$424	$339
	• Lispro-aabc	U-100 vial	$330	$261
		U-100 prefilled pen	$424	$339
		U-200 prefilled pen	$424	NA
	• Glulisine	U-100 vial	$341	$272
		U-100 prefilled pen	$439	$351
	• Aspart	U-100 vial	$174†	$140†
		U-100 cartridge	$215†	$172†
		U-100 prefilled pen	$224†	$180†
	• Aspart ("faster acting product")	U-100 vial	$347	$277
		U-100 cartridge	$430	$344
		U-100 prefilled pen	$447	$357
	• Inhaled insulin	Inhalation cartridges	$1,418	NA
Short-acting	• Human regular	U-100 vial	$165††	$132††
		U-100 prefilled pen	$208	$166
Intermediate-acting	• Human NPH	U-100 vial	$165††	$132††
		U-100 prefilled pen	$208	$168
Concentrated human regular insulin	• U-500 human regular insulin	U-500 vial	$178	$142
		U-500 prefilled pen	$230	$184

(continued)

Table 4.3 (continued)

Insulins	Compounds	Dosage form/ product	Median AWP (min, max)*	Median NADAC*
Long-acting	• Glargine follow-on products	U-100 prefilled pen	$261 ($118, $323)	$209 ($209, $258)
		U-100 vial	$118 ($118, $323)	$95
	• Glargine	U-100 vial; U-100 prefilled pen	$136†	$109†
		U-300 prefilled pen	$346	$277
	• Detemir	U-100 vial; U-100 prefilled pen	$370	$296
	• Degludec	U-100 vial; U-100 prefilled pen;	$407	$326
		U-200 prefilled pen		
Premixed insulin products	• NPH/regular 70/30	U-100 vial	$165††	$133††
		U-100 prefilled pen	$208	$167
	• Lispro 50/50	U-100 vial	$342	$274
		U-100 prefilled pen	$424	$339
	• Lispro 75/25	U-100 vial	$342	$273
		U-100 prefilled pen	$127†	$103†
	• Aspart 70/30	U-100 vial	$180†	$146†
		U-100 prefilled pen	$224†	$178†
Premixed insulin/GLP-1 RA products	• Glargine/Lixisenatide	100/33 µg prefilled pen	$646	$517
	• Degludec/ Liraglutide	100/3.6 µg prefilled pen	$944	$760

AWP, average wholesale price; GLP-1 RA, glucagon-like peptide 1 receptor agonist; N/A, not available; NADAC, National Average Drug Acquisition Cost. *AWP or NADAC calculated as in Table 4.2. †Generic prices used when available. ††AWP and NADAC data presented do not include vials of regular human insulin and NPH available at Walmart for approximately $25/vial; median listed alone when only one product and/or price.

mia risk compared with U-100 glargine when used in combination with oral agents.[45-51] Clinicians should be aware of the potential for overbasalization with insulin therapy. Clinical signals that may prompt evaluation of overbasalization include basal dose greater than ~0.5 units/kg, high bedtime-morning or postpreprandial glucose differential (e.g., bedtime–morning glucose differential ≥50 mg/dL), hypoglycemia (aware or unaware), and high variability. Indication of overbasalization should prompt reevaluation to further individualize therapy.[52]

The cost of insulin has been rising steadily over the past two decades, at a pace severalfold that of other medical expenditures.[53] This expense contributes significant burden to patients as insulin has become a growing "out-of-pocket" cost for people with diabetes, and direct patient costs contribute to decrease in medication-taking behavior.[53] Therefore, consideration of cost is an important component of effective management. For many individuals with type 2 diabetes (e.g., individuals with relaxed A1C goals, low rates of hypoglycemia, and prominent insulin resistance, as well as those with cost concerns), human insulin (NPH and regular) may be the appropriate choice of therapy, and clinicians should be familiar with its use.[54] Human regular insulin, NPH, and 70/30 NPH/regular products can be purchased for considerably less than the AWP and NADAC prices listed in Table 4.3 at select pharmacies. Additionally, approval of follow-on biologics for insulin glargine, the first interchangeable insulin glargine product, and generic versions of analog insulins may expand cost-effective options.

PRANDIAL INSULIN

Many individuals with type 2 diabetes require doses of insulin before meals, in addition to basal insulin, to reach glycemic targets. If the individual is not already being treated with a GLP-1 RA, a GLP-1 RA (either in free combination or fixed-ratio combination) should be considered prior to prandial insulin to further address prandial control and to minimize the risks of hypoglycemia and weight gain associated with insulin therapy.[3] For individuals who advance to prandial insulin, a prandial insulin dose of 4 units or 10% of the amount of basal insulin at the largest meal or the meal with the greatest postprandial excursion is a safe estimate for initiating therapy. The prandial insulin regimen can then be intensified based on individual needs (Fig. 9.4). Individuals with type 2 diabetes are generally more insulin resistant than those with type 1 diabetes, require higher daily doses (~1 unit/kg), and have lower rates of hypoglycemia.[55] Titration can be based on home glucose monitoring or A1C. With significant additions to the prandial insulin dose, particularly with the evening meal, consideration should be given to decreasing basal insulin. Meta-analyses of trials comparing rapid-acting insulin analogs with human regular insulin in type 2 diabetes have not reported important differences in A1C or hypoglycemia.[56,57]

CONCENTRATED INSULINS

Several concentrated insulin preparations are currently available. U-500 regular insulin is, by definition, five times more concentrated than U-100 regular insulin. U-500 regular insulin has distinct pharmacokinetics with delayed onset and longer duration of action, has characteristics more like an intermediate-acting (NPH) insulin, and can be used as two or three daily injections.[58] U-300 glargine and U-200 degludec are three and two times as concentrated as their U-100 formulations, respectively, and allow higher doses of basal insulin administration per volume used. U-300 glargine has a longer duration of action than U-100 glargine but modestly lower efficacy per unit administered.[59,60] The FDA has also approved a concentrated formulation of rapid-acting insulin lispro, U-200 (200 units/mL), and insulin lispro-aabc (U-200). These concentrated preparations may be more convenient and comfortable for individuals to inject and may improve treatment plan engagement in those with insulin resistance who require large doses of insulin. While U-500 regular insulin is available in both prefilled pens and vials, other concentrated insulins are available only in pre-filled pens to minimize the risk of dosing errors.

ALTERNATIVE INSULIN ROUTES

Insulins with different routes of administration (inhaled, bolus-only insulin delivery patch pump) are also available.[3] Inhaled insulin is available as a rapid-acting insulin; studies in individuals with type 1 diabetes suggest rapid pharmacokinetics.[61] Studies comparing inhaled insulin with injectable insulin have demonstrated its faster onset and shorter duration compared with rapid-acting insulin lispro as well as clinically meaningful A1C reductions and weight reductions compared with insulin aspart over 24 weeks.[62–64] Use of inhaled insulin may result in a decline in lung function (reduced forced expiratory volume in 1 s [FEV1]). Inhaled insulin is contraindicated in individuals with chronic lung disease, such as asthma and chronic obstructive pulmonary disease, and is not recommended in individuals who smoke or who recently stopped smoking. All individuals require spirometry (FEV1) testing to identify potential lung disease prior to and after starting inhaled insulin therapy.

COMBINATION INJECTABLE THERAPY

If basal insulin has been titrated to an acceptable fasting blood glucose level (or if the dose is >0.5 units/kg/day with indications of need for other therapy) and A1C remains above target, consider advancing to combination injectable therapy (Fig. 9.4). This approach can use a GLP-1 RA or dual GIP and GLP-1 RA added to basal insulin or multiple doses of insulin. The combination of basal insulin and GLP-1 RA has potent glucose-lowering actions and less weight gain and hypoglycemia compared with intensified insulin regimens.[65–70] The DUAL VIII (Durability of Insulin Degludec Plus Liraglutide Versus Insulin Glargine U100 as Initial Injectable Therapy in Type 2 Diabetes) randomized controlled trial demonstrated greater durability of glycemic treatment effect with the combination GLP–1 RA–insulin therapy compared with addition of basal insulin alone.[15] In select individuals, complex insulin regimens can also be simplified with combination GLP-1 RA-insulin therapy in type 2 diabetes.[71] Two different once-daily, fixed dual combination products containing basal insulin plus a GLP-1 RA are available: insulin glargine plus lixisenatide (iGlarLixi) and insulin degludec plus liraglutide (IDegLira).

Intensification of insulin treatment can be done by adding doses of prandial insulin to basal insulin. Starting with a single prandial dose with the largest meal of the day is simple and effective, and it can be advanced to a regimen with multiple prandial doses if necessary.[72] Alternatively, in an individual on basal insulin in whom additional prandial coverage is desired, the regimen can be converted to two doses of a premixed insulin. Each approach has advantages and disadvantages. For example, basal-prandial regimens offer greater flexibility for individuals who eat on irregular schedules. On the other hand, two doses of premixed insulin is a simple, convenient means of spreading insulin across the day. Moreover, human insulins, separately, self-mixed, or as premixed NPH/regular (70/30) formulations, are less costly alternatives to insulin analogs. Figure 9.4 outlines these options as well as recommendations for further intensification, if needed, to achieve glycemic goals. When initiating combination injectable therapy, metformin therapy should be maintained, while sulfonylureas and DPP-4 inhibitors are typically weaned or discontinued. In individuals with suboptimal blood glucose control, especially those requiring large insulin doses, adjunctive use of a thiazolidinedione or an SGLT2 inhibitor may help to improve control and reduce the amount of insulin needed, though potential side effects should be considered. Once a basal-bolus insulin regimen is initiated, dose titration is important, with adjustments made in both mealtime and basal insulins based on the blood glucose levels and an understanding of the pharmacodynamic profile of each formulation (also known as pattern control or pattern management). As people with type 2 diabetes get older, it may become necessary to simplify complex insulin regimens because of a decline in self-management ability (see Section 13, "Older Adults").

REFERENCES

1. Davies MJ, D'Alessio DA, Fradkin J, et al. Management of hyperglycemia in type 2 diabetes, 2018. A consensus report by the American Diabetes Association (ADA) and the European Association for the Study of Diabetes (EASD). Diabetes Care 2018;41:2669–2701

2. Buse JB, Wexler DJ, Tsapas A, et al. 2019 Update to: management of hyperglycemia in type 2 diabetes, 2018. A consensus report by the American Diabetes Association (ADA) and the European Association for the Study of Diabetes (EASD). Diabetes Care 2020;43:487–493

3. Davies MJ, Aroda VR, Collins BS, et al. Management of hyperglycemia in type 2 diabetes, 2022. A consensus report by the American Diabetes Association (ADA) and the European Association for the Study of Diabetes (EASD). Diabetes Care 2022;45:2753–2786

4. Lingvay I, Sumithran P, Cohen RV, le Roux CW. Obesity management as a primary treatment goal for type 2 diabetes: time to reframe the conversation. Lancet 2022;399:394–405

5. Holman RR, Paul SK, Bethel MA, Matthews DR, Neil HAW. 10-year follow-up of intensive glucose control in type 2 diabetes. N Engl J Med 2008;359:1577–1589

6. Maruthur NM, Tseng E, Hutfless S, et al. Diabetes medications as monotherapy or metformin-based combination therapy for type 2 diabetes: a systematic review and meta-analysis. Ann Intern Med 2016;164:740–751

7. U.S. Food and Drug Administration. FDA Drug Safety Communication: FDA revises warnings regarding use of the diabetes medicine metformin in certain patients with reduced kidney function. Accessed 18 October 2022. Available from https://www.fda.gov/drugs/drug-safety-and-availability/fda-drug-safety-communication-fda-revises-warnings-regarding-use-diabetes-medicine-metformin-certain

8. Out M, Kooy A, Lehert P, Schalkwijk CA, Stehouwer CDA. Long-term treatment with metformin in type 2 diabetes and methylmalonic acid: post

hoc analysis of a randomized controlled 4.3-year trial. J Diabetes Complications 2018;32:171–178

9. Aroda VR, Edelstein SL, Goldberg RB, et al.; Diabetes Prevention Program Research Group. Long-term metformin use and vitamin B12 deficiency in the Diabetes Prevention Program Outcomes Study. J Clin Endocrinol Metab 2016;101:1754–1761

10. Henry RR, Murray AV, Marmolejo MH, Hennicken D, Ptaszynska A, List JF. Dapagliflozin, metformin XR, or both: initial pharmacotherapy for type 2 diabetes, a randomised controlled trial. Int J Clin Pract 2012;66:446–456

11. Babu A, Mehta A, Guerrero P, et al. Safe and simple emergency department discharge therapy for patients with type 2 diabetes mellitus and severe hyperglycemia. Endocr Pract 2009;15:696–704

12. Cahn A, Cefalu WT. Clinical considerations for use of initial combination therapy in type 2 diabetes. Diabetes Care 2016;39(Suppl. 2):S137–S145

13. Abdul-Ghani MA, Puckett C, Triplitt C, et al. Initial combination therapy with metformin, pioglitazone and exenatide is more effective than sequential add-on therapy in subjects with new-onset diabetes. Results from the Efficacy and Durability of Initial Combination Therapy for Type 2 Diabetes (EDICT): a randomized trial. Diabetes Obes Metab 2015;17:268–275

14. Phung OJ, Sobieraj DM, Engel SS, Rajpathak SN. Early combination therapy for the treatment of type 2 diabetes mellitus: systematic review and meta-analysis. Diabetes Obes Metab 2014;16:410–417

15. Aroda VR, González-Galvez G, Grøn R, et al. Durability of insulin degludec plus liraglutide versus insulin glargine U100 as initial injectable therapy in type 2 diabetes (DUAL VIII): a multicentre, open-label, phase 3b, randomised controlled trial. Lancet Diabetes Endocrinol 2019;7:596–605

16. Matthews DR, Paldánius PM, Proot P, Chiang Y, Stumvoll M; VERIFY study group. Glycaemic durability of an early combination therapy with vildagliptin and metformin versus sequential metformin monotherapy in newly diagnosed type 2 diabetes (VERIFY): a 5-year, multicentre, randomised, double-blind trial. Lancet 2019;394:1519–1529

17. Bennett WL, Maruthur NM, Singh S, et al. Comparative effectiveness and safety of medications for type 2 diabetes: an update including new drugs and 2-drug combinations. Ann Intern Med 2011;154:602–613

18. Maloney A, Rosenstock J, Fonseca V. A model based meta-analysis of 24 antihyperglycemic drugs for type 2 diabetes: comparison of treatment effects at therapeutic doses. Clin Pharmacol Ther 2019;105:1213–1223

19. Vijan S, Sussman JB, Yudkin JS, Hayward RA. Effect of patients' risks and preferences on health gains with plasma glucose level lowering in type 2 diabetes mellitus. JAMA Intern Med 2014;174:1227–1234

20. Tsapas A, Avgerinos I, Karagiannis T, et al. Comparative effectiveness of glucose-lowering drugs for type 2 diabetes: a systematic review and network meta-analysis. Ann Intern Med 2020;173:278–286

21. Pratley R, Amod A, Hoff ST, et al.; PIONEER 4 investigators. Oral sema-glutide versus subcutaneous liraglutide and placebo in type 2 diabetes (PIO-NEER 4): a randomised, double-blind, phase 3a trial. Lancet 2019;394:39–50

22. Singh S, Wright EE Jr, Kwan AYM, et al. Glucagon-like peptide-1 receptor agonists compared with basal insulins for the treatment of type 2 diabetes mellitus: a systematic review and meta-analysis. Diabetes Obes Metab 2017;19:228–238

23. Levin PA, Nguyen H, Wittbrodt ET, Kim SC. Glucagon-like peptide-1 receptor agonists: a systematic review of comparative effectiveness research. Diabetes Metab Syndr Obes 2017;10:123–139

24. Abd El Aziz MS, Kahle M, Meier JJ, Nauck MA. A meta-analysis comparing clinical effects of short- or long-acting GLP-1 receptor agonists versus insulin treatment from head-to-head studies in type 2 diabetic patients. Diabetes Obes Metab 2017;19:216–227

25. Giorgino F, Benroubi M, Sun JH, Zimmermann AG, Pechtner V. Efficacy and safety of once-weekly dulaglutide versus insulin glargine in patients with type 2 diabetes on metformin and glimepiride (AWARD-2). Diabetes Care 2015;38:2241–2249

26. Aroda VR, Bain SC, Cariou B, et al. Efficacy and safety of once-weekly semaglutide versus once-daily insulin glargine as add-on to metformin (with or without sulfonylureas) in insulin-naive patients with type 2 diabetes (SUSTAIN 4): a randomised, open-label, parallel-group, multicentre, mul-tinational, phase 3a trial. Lancet Diabetes Endocrinol 2017;5:355–366

27. Davies M, Heller S, Sreenan S, et al. Once-weekly exenatide versus once- or twice-daily insulin detemir: randomized, open-label, clinical trial of efficacy and safety in patients with type 2 diabetes treated with metformin alone or in combination with sulfonylureas. Diabetes Care 2013;36:1368–1376

28. Diamant M, Van Gaal L, Stranks S, et al. Once weekly exenatide compared with insulin glargine titrated to target in patients with type 2 diabetes (DURATION-3): an open-label randomised trial. Lancet 2010;375:2234–2243

29. Riddle MC, Herman WH. The cost of diabetes care-an elephant in the room. Diabetes Care 2018;41:929–932

30. IBM. Micromedex Red Book. Accessed 9 November 2022. Available from https://www.ibm.com/products/micromedex-red-book

31. Data.Medicaid.gov. NADAC (National Average Drug Acquisition Cost). Accessed 23 October 2022. Available from https://data.medicaid.gov/data-set/dfa2ab14-06c2-457a-9e36-5cb6d80f8d93

32. Kang H, Lobo JM, Kim S, Sohn MW. Cost-related medication non-adherence among U.S. adults with diabetes. Diabetes Res Clin Pract 2018;143:24–33

33. Patel MR, Piette JD, Resnicow K, Kowalski-Dobson T, HeislerM. Social determinants of health, cost-related nonadherence, and cost-reducing behaviors among adults with diabetes: findings from the National Health interview survey. Med Care 2016;54:796–803

34. Gerstein HC, Sattar N, Rosenstock J, et al.; AMPLITUDE-O Trial Investigators. Cardiovascular and renal outcomes with efpeglenatide in type 2 diabetes. N Engl J Med 2021;385:896–907

35. Blonde L, Merilainen M, Karwe V; TITRATE Study Group. Patient-directed titration for achieving glycaemic goals using a once-daily basal insulin analogue: an assessment of two different fasting plasma glucose targets–the TITRATE study. Diabetes Obes Metab 2009;11:623–631

36. Porcellati F, Lucidi P, Cioli P, et al. Pharmacokinetics and pharmacodynamics of insulin glargine given in the evening as compared with in the morning in type 2 diabetes. Diabetes Care 2015;38:503–512

37. Wang Z, Hedrington MS, Gogitidze Joy N, et al. Dose-response effects of insulin glargine in type 2 diabetes. Diabetes Care 2010;33:1555–1560

38. Singh SR, Ahmad F, Lal A, Yu C, Bai Z, Bennett H. Efficacy and safety of insulin analogues for the management of diabetes mellitus: a meta-analysis. CMAJ 2009;180:385–397

39. Horvath K, Jeitler K, Berghold A, et al. Long-acting insulin analogues versus NPH insulin (human isophane insulin) for type 2 diabetes mellitus. Cochrane Database Syst Rev 2007 2:CD005613

40. Monami M, Marchionni N, Mannucci E. Long-acting insulin analogues versus NPH human insulin in type 2 diabetes: a meta-analysis. Diabetes Res Clin Pract 2008;81:184–189

41. Owens DR, Traylor L, Mullins P, Landgraf W. Patient-level meta-analysis of efficacy and hypoglycaemia in people with type 2 diabetes initiating insulin glargine 100U/mL or neutral protamine Hagedorn insulin analysed according to concomitant oral antidiabetes therapy. Diabetes Res Clin Pract 2017;124(Suppl. C):57–65

42. Riddle MC, Rosenstock J; Insulin Glargine 4002 Study Investigators. The treat-to-target trial: randomized addition of glargine or human NPH insulin to oral therapy of type 2 diabetic patients. Diabetes Care 2003;26:3080–3086

43. Hermansen K, Davies M, Derezinski T, Martinez Ravn G, Clauson P, Home P. A 26-week, randomized, parallel, treat-to-target trial comparing insulin detemir with NPH insulin as add-on therapy to oral glucose-lowering drugs in insulin-naive people with type 2 diabetes. Diabetes Care 2006;29:1269–1274

44. Yki-Järvinen H, Kauppinen-Mäkelin R, Tiikkainen M, et al. Insulin glargine or NPH combined with metformin in type 2 diabetes: the LANMET study. Diabetologia 2006;49:442–451

45. Bolli GB, Riddle MC, Bergenstal RM, et al.; on behalf of the EDITION 3 Study Investigators. New insulin glargine 300 U/ml compared with glargine 100 U/ml in insulin-naïve people with type 2 diabetes on oral glucose-lowering drugs: a randomized controlled trial (EDITION 3). Diabetes Obes Metab 2015;17:386–394

46. Terauchi Y, Koyama M, Cheng X, et al. New insulin glargine 300 U/ml versus glargine 100 U/ml in Japanese people with type 2 diabetes using basal insulin and oral antihyperglycaemic drugs: glucose control and hypoglycaemia in a randomized controlled trial (EDITION JP 2). Diabetes Obes Metab 2016;18:366–374

47. Yki-Järvinen H, Bergenstal RM, Bolli GB, et al. Glycaemic control and hypoglycaemia with new insulin glargine 300 U/ml versus insulin glargine 100 U/ml in people with type 2 diabetes using basal insulin and oral antihyperglycaemic drugs: the EDITION 2 randomized 12-month trial including 6-month extension. Diabetes Obes Metab 2015;17:1142–1149

48. Marso SP, McGuire DK, Zinman B, et al.; DEVOTE Study Group. Efficacy and safety of degludec versus glargine in type 2 diabetes. N Engl J Med 2017;377:723–732

49. Rodbard HW, Cariou B, Zinman B, et al.; BEGIN Once Long Trial Investigators. Comparison of insulin degludec with insulin glargine in insulin-naive subjects with type 2 diabetes: a 2-year randomized, treat-to-target trial. Diabet Med 2013;30:1298–1304

50. Wysham C, Bhargava A, Chaykin L, et al. Effect of insulin degludec vs insulin glargine u100 on hypoglycemia in patients with type 2 diabetes: the SWITCH 2 randomized clinical trial. JAMA 2017;318:45–56

51. Zinman B, Philis-Tsimikas A, Cariou B, et al.; NN1250-3579 (BEGIN Once Long) Trial Investigators. Insulin degludec versus insulin glargine in insulin naive patients with type 2 diabetes: a 1-year, randomized, treat-to-target trial (BEGIN Once Long). Diabetes Care 2012;35:2464–2471

52. Cowart K. Overbasalization: addressing hesitancy in treatment intensification beyond basal insulin. Clin Diabetes 2020;38:304–310

53. Cefalu WT, Dawes DE, Gavlak G, et al.; Insulin Access and Affordability Working Group. Conclusions and recommendations. Diabetes Care 2018;41:1299–1311

54. Lipska KJ, Parker MM, Moffet HH, Huang ES, Karter AJ. Association of initiation of basal insulin analogs vs neutral protamine hagedorn insulin with hypoglycemia-related emergency department visits or hospital admissions and with glycemic control in patients with type 2 diabetes. JAMA 2018;320:53–62

55. McCall AL. Insulin therapy and hypoglycemia. Endocrinol Metab Clin North Am 2012;41:57–87

56. Mannucci E, Monami M, Marchionni N. Short-acting insulin analogues vs. regular human insulin in type 2 diabetes: a meta-analysis. Diabetes Obes Metab 2009;11:53–59

57. Heller S, Bode B, Kozlovski P, Svendsen AL. Meta-analysis of insulin aspart versus regular human insulin used in a basal-bolus regimen for the treatment of diabetes mellitus. J Diabetes 2013;5:482–491

58. Wysham C, Hood RC, Warren ML, Wang T, Morwick TM, Jackson JA. Effect of total daily dose on efficacy, dosing, and safety of 2 dose titration regimens of human regular U500 insulin in severely insulin-resistant patients with type 2 diabetes. Endocr Pract 2016;22:653–665

59. Riddle MC, Yki-Jaärvinen H, Bolli GB, et al. One-year sustained glycaemic control and less hypoglycaemia with new insulin glargine 300 U/ml compared with 100 U/ml in people with type 2 diabetes using basal plus mealtime insulin: the EDITION 1 12-month randomized trial, including 6-month extension. Diabetes Obes Metab 2015;17:835–842

60. Yki-Järvinen H, Bergenstal R, Ziemen M, et al.; EDITION 2 Study Investigators. New insulin glargine 300 units/mL versus glargine 100 units/mL in people with type 2 diabetes using oral agents and basal insulin: glucose control and hypoglycemia in a 6-month randomized controlled trial (EDITION 2). Diabetes Care 2014;37:3235–3243

61. DCCTEDIC Study Research Group. Mortality in type 1 diabetes in the DCCT/EDIC versus the general population. Diabetes Care 2016;39:1378–1383

62. Akturk HK, Snell-Bergeon JK, Rewers A, et al. Improved postprandial glucose with inhaled technosphere insulin compared with insulin aspart in patients with type 1 diabetes on multiple daily injections: the STAT study. Diabetes Technol Ther 2018;20:639–647

63. Hoogwerf BJ, Pantalone KM, Basina M, Jones MC, Grant M, Kendall DM. Results of a 24-week trial of technosphere insulin versus insulin aspart in type 2 diabetes. Endocr Pract 2021;27:38–43

64. Grant M, Heise T, Baughman R. Comparison of pharmacokinetics and pharmacodynamics of inhaled technosphere insulin and subcutaneous insulin lispro in the treatment of type 1 diabetes mellitus. Clin Pharmacokinet 2022;61:413–422

65. Diamant M, Nauck MA, Shaginian R, et al.; 4B Study Group. Glucagon-like peptide 1 receptor agonist or bolus insulin with optimized basal insulin in type 2 diabetes. Diabetes Care 2014;37:2763–2773

66. Eng C, Kramer CK, Zinman B, Retnakaran R. Glucagon-like peptide-1 receptor agonist and basal insulin combination treatment for the manage-

ment of type 2 diabetes: a systematic review and meta-analysis. Lancet 2014;384:2228–2234

67. Maiorino MI, Chiodini P, Bellastella G, Capuano A, Esposito K, Giugliano D. Insulin and glucagon-like peptide 1 receptor agonist combination therapy in type 2 diabetes: a systematic review and meta-analysis of randomized controlled trials. Diabetes Care 2017;40:614–624

68. Aroda VR, Rosenstock J, Wysham C, et al.; LixiLan-L Trial Investigators. Efficacy and safety of LixiLan, a titratable fixed-ratio combination of insulin glargine plus lixisenatide in type 2 diabetes inadequately controlled on basal insulin and metformin: the LixiLan-L randomized trial. Diabetes Care 2016;39:1972–1980

69. Lingvay I, Pérez Manghi F, García-Hernández P, et al.; DUAL V Investigators. Effect of insulin glargine up-titration vs insulin degludec/liraglutide on glycated hemoglobin levels in patients with uncontrolled type 2 diabetes: the DUAL V randomized clinical trial. JAMA 2016;315:898–907

70. Dahl D, Onishi Y, Norwood P, et al. Effect of subcutaneous tirzepatide vs placebo added to titrated insulin glargine on glycemic control in patients with type 2 diabetes: the SURPASS-5 randomized clinical trial. JAMA 2022;327:534–545

71. Taybani Z, Bótyik B, Katkó M, Gyimesi A, Várkonyi T. Simplifying complex insulin regimens while preserving good glycemic control in type 2 diabetes. Diabetes Ther 2019;10:1869–1878

72. Rodbard HW, Visco VE, Andersen H, Hiort LC, Shu DHW. Treatment intensification with stepwise addition of prandial insulin aspart boluses compared with full basal-bolus therapy (FullSTEP Study): a randomised, treat-to-target clinical trial. Lancet Diabetes Endocrinol 2014;2:30–37

73. Tsapas A, Karagiannis T, Kakotrichi P, et al. Comparative efficacy of glucose-lowering medications on body weight and blood pressure in patients with type 2 diabetes: A systematic review and network meta-analysis. Diabetes Obes Metab 2021;23:2116–2124

Chapter 5

Overview of Medications Used to Treat Type 2 Diabetes

John R. White, Jr., PA-C, PharmD

The options available to clinicians in the U.S. for the management of hyperglycemia secondary to T2D have changed dramatically in the past three decades. Currently there are a dozen categories of medications that may be used in the management of diabetes. These include insulins, sulfonylureas, thiazolidinediones (TZDs), glinides, biguanides, amylin derivatives, gliptins (DPP-4 inhibitors), α-glucosidase inhibitors, bile-acid sequestrants, GLP-1 receptor agonists (GLP-1 RAs), dopamine-2 agonists, and SGLT2 inhibitors. The dopamine-2 agonists, amylin derivatives, and bile acid sequestrants will not be mentioned in this chapter, as they are rarely used for the management of hyperglycemia in T2D but are covered in later individual chapters. The glinides and the α-glucosidase inhibitors are mentioned in this chapter but are not widely used. Overall, this chapter will provide a brief introduction to the medications used in the management of T2D.

CHOICE OF MEDICATION

The efficacy associated with single-drug therapy and with various permutations of multiple drug combinations continues to be evaluated as newer agents are released. The selection of the best medication or combination of medications for the management of hyperglycemia in patients with T2D, while based in science, remains to a large degree in the realm of "art." Although in some situations the choice of medication is relatively simple, in the majority of situations the decision-making process is complex and does not necessarily lead to a clear-cut choice. Algorithms can sometimes provide an overall framework through which decisions can be made, but they often ignore pertinent patient-specific characteristics and are not powerful enough to provide specific recommendations for the best medications in the multitude of complex situations often encountered in clinical practice. However, the new approach originally proffered by the American Diabetes Association and the European Association for the Study of Diabetes (EASD) and updated in the American Diabetes Association 2023 *Standards of Care in Diabetes* provides us with a circumspect perspective and a solid roadmap to the management of hyperglycemia in patients with T2D. This new approach includes consideration of the major factors that are pertinent to choice of medication.[1,2]

Several factors should be considered when choosing a medication, including degree of glycemic lowering needed to get the patient into target goal ranges, renal effects, cardiovascular effects, ease of compliance, effect of the medication on weight and lipids, contraindications, side effects, cost and patient insurance coverage, and the need for dose adjustment with renal and/or hepatic impairment. This chapter will provide a cursory and abbreviated review of the use of the above-mentioned categories of medications. More detailed information regarding specific medications is provided in subsequent chapters and linked monographs.

Using the American Diabetes Association *Standards of Care* schema, patients presenting with T2D should first be treated with metformin and comprehensive lifestyle interventions (Figure 5.1). If metformin monotherapy has been instituted and the patient's glycemic indices are not appropriately controlled, the patient should next be categorized as: *1*) having *a*) established atherosclerotic cardiovascular disease (ASCVD) or indicators of high risk or *b*) congestive heart failure or chronic kidney disease (CKD), or *2*) not having established ASCVD or CKD. In patients with predominately ASCVD, either a GLP-1 RA or an SGLT2i that has been shown to provide cardiovascular disease (CVD) benefit should be used inde-penent of baseline A1C or A1C target. In patients with predominately CKD or HF, an SGLT2i with evidence of the ability to reduce CKD or HF should be used (unless contraindicated). In patients without established ASCVD or CKD, either a DPP-4 inhibitor, GLP-1 RA, SGLT2 inhibitor, TZD, or sulfonylurea should be used. The decision regarding specific agent should be made with consideration to level of hyperglycemia, need for weight loss and risk of hypoglycemia. Additional antihyperglycemic medications may be added as needed to achieve the appropriate level of glycemic control. If the patient's initial A1C is >10%, or the blood glucose concentration is ≥300 mg/dL, there is evidence of ongoing catabolism, or the diagnosis of T1D is possible, the guidelines recommend considering insulin therapy. Also, in patients who are not at their A1C target despite dual or triple therapy, insulin and/or GLP-1 RA should be considered. In most cases a GLP-1 RA or a GIP/GLP-1 RA should be utilized prior to the initiation of insulin. The considerations involved in this decision are articulated in Figure 5.2.[1]

The number of medications available for the management of hyperglycemia has grown consistently since the first use of exogenous insulin in the 1920s. However, the rate of growth of the introduction of new medications and new categories of medications has burgeoned over the past 30 years (Fig. 5.3).

ORAL THERAPY

BIGUANIDES

The biguanide metformin (Glucophage) was first introduced in 1959 as an antihyperglycemic agent for use in patients with T2D but was not approved for use in the U.S. until the 1990s.

Metformin is the usual first choice in the management of hyperglycemia in patients with T2D if it is not contraindicated, is tolerated, and if the patient does not have a presenting initial A1C of >10%.[1,2]

Metformin should be continued if insulin therapy is initiated unless there are contraindications or lack of tolerance. The physiologic effects of this compound on carbohydrate metabolism and disposition occur primarily in the liver via inhi-

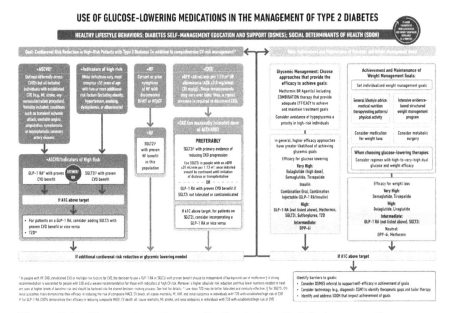

Figure 5.1—Glucose-lowering medication in type 2 diabetes: overall approach. Reprinted with permission from the American Diabetes Association.[1] A larger version of this graphic is found on p. 60.

bition of hepatic glucose production.[3] Additionally, it may also cause a reduction in the intestinal absorption of glucose.[4] At a molecular level, metformin probably elicits its glycemic effects by activation of AMP kinase although other mechanisms may be in play as well.[2]

While it is difficult to assign an expected drop in A1C with any medications because of the myriad confounding factors, generally metformin therapy can be expected to cause about a 1–1.5 percentage point reduction in A1C.[5,6]

Metformin does not typically cause hypoglycemia when used as monotherapy and may be associated with weigh loss.[3] In a medication review carried out by the Agency for Healthcare Research and Quality (AHRQ), metformin was superior to TZDs and sulfonylureas in terms of effect on weight (mean 2.6 kg).[7] It is potentially beneficial in ASCVD and is neutral in its impact on congestive heart failure (CHF).[2] Additionally, metformin was associated with a reduction in LDL compared to pioglitazone, sulfonylureas, and DPP-4 inhibitors.[7]

Conversely, metformin is also associated with gastrointestinal side effects. Patients treated with metformin may experience a 30% higher incidence of abdominal bloating, nausea, cramping, feeling of fullness, and diarrhea.[6] These side effects can be a particular problem during the initiation phases of therapy. However, these side effects are usually self-limiting and transient and can be mitigated by starting with a low dose, titrating up slowly, and taking the medication with food.

Less common side effects include a reduction in cyanocobalamin levels (vitamin B_{12}) and a metallic taste in the mouth. Periodic testing of B_{12} should be con-

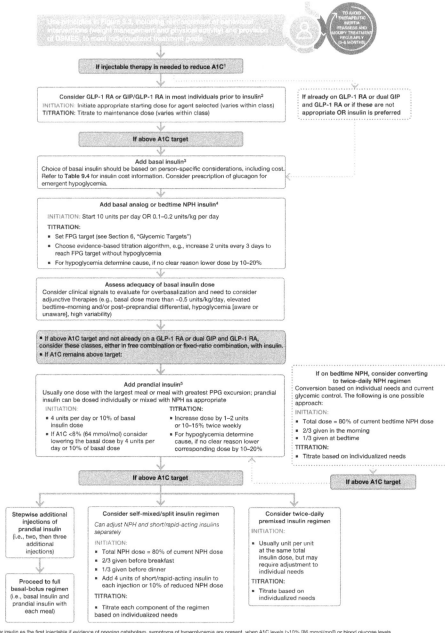

1. Consider insulin as the first injectable if evidence of ongoing catabolism, symptoms of hyperglycemia are present, when A1C levels (>10% [86 mmol/mol]) or blood glucose levels (300 mg/dL [16.7 mmol/L]) are very high, or a diagnosis of type 1 diabetes is a possibility.
2. When selecting GLP-1 RA, consider individual preference, A1C lowering, weight-lowering effect, or fequency of injection. If CVD is present, consider GLP-1 RA with proven CVD benefit. Oral or injectable GLP-1 RA are appropriate.
3. For people on GLP-1 RA and basal insulin combination, consider use of a fixed-ratio combination product (IDegLira or IGlarLixi).
4. Consider switching from evening NPH to a basal analog if the individual develops hypoglycemia and/or frequently forgets to administer NPH in the evening and would be better managed with an A.M. dose of a long-acting basal insulin.
5. If adding prandial insulin to NPH, consider initiation of a self-mixed or premixed insulin regimen to decrease the number of injections required.

Figure 5.2—Reprinted with permission from the American Diabetes Association.[1]

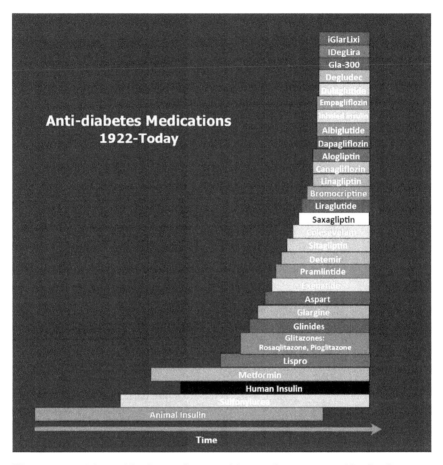

Figure 5.3—Adapted by Dawn Scartozzi from a figure created by Dr. Sam Dagogo-Jack. Reprinted with permission.

sidered in patients treated with metformin, particularly those with peripheral neuropathy or anemia.[2] Lactic acidosis can occur with the administration of metformin, but it is extremely rare (0.03 cases per 1,000 patient-years) and has occurred primarily in patients with significant renal dysfunction.[6]

Metformin is contraindicated in patients with an estimated glomerular filtration rate (eGFR) of ≤30 mL/min/1.73 m^2. Metformin should not be initiated in patients with an eGFR of 30–45 mL/min/1.73 m^2 and its use should be evaluated in any patient with these renal parameters who is already being treated with the drug. Other warnings and contraindications are detailed in chapter 6.

Metformin is available generically and is relatively inexpensive.

SULFONYLUREAS

Sulfonylureas have been widely used in the management of T2D since their introduction in the late 1950s. In the past, it was estimated that 40% of all T2D patients were treated with sulfonylureas. However, since the introduction of newer antihyperglycemic medications, the fraction of patients with T2D treated with sulfonylureas has probably dropped.

Sulfonylureas exhibit both pancreatic and extrapancreatic effects and are clinically useful only in patients with viable β-cells. The primary effect of sulfonylureas is due to direct stimulation of insulin release.[8] In-vivo studies of sulfonylureas show that they sensitize β-cells to glucose, increasing insulin secretion indirectly. Therefore, under the influence of sulfonylureas, more insulin is secreted at all glucose levels than would be expected in the absence of sulfonylureas. Sulfonylureas may also affect glucose metabolism via several extrapancreatic mechanisms, such as increasing insulin's effect by a postreceptor action, decreasing hepatic insulin extraction, and increasing insulin receptor number and receptor binding affinity; however, the relative clinical relevance of each of these mechanisms of action is still subject to research and debate.

In terms of glycemic lowering, sulfonylureas can be expected to reduce A1C values between 1 and 2%.[6]

The sulfonylureas have also been associated with weight gain. Lastly, sulfonylureas are true hypoglycemic agents and can cause significant hypoglycemia. There remains a question regarding cardiovascular risk/outcomes with the use of sulfonylureas. This is well outlined in chapter 8. Generally speaking, validated randomized controlled trials do not demonstrate added cardiovascular risk, but meta-analyses suggest added risk. However, their long track record of relative safety, efficacy in reducing hypoglycemia, and very low cost probably make them a reasonable choice early on in the treatment of some patients with T2D. While there is not a clear drug of choice in this category, the two that are generally preferred are glipizide and glimepiride.

GLINIDES

Repaglinide and nateglinide are nonsulfonylurea insulinotropic agents whose biochemical mechanism of action—closure of ATP-sensitive potassium channels in β-cells—is similar to that of sulfonylureas. Closure of ATP-sensitive potassium channels causes an influx of calcium by way of voltage-dependent calcium channels. Insulin release is stimulated after intercellular calcium concentrations reach a threshold.[8] Therefore, similar to sulfonylureas, the glinides reduce blood glucose levels by stimulating insulin release from the pancreas.

The glycemic lowering afforded by the glinides is generally less than that of the sulfonylureas. Typically, A1C lowering of about 1–1.5% can be expected in a secretagogue-naïve patient.[6] These agents do not work in patients who do not respond to sulfonylureas. The glinides are associated with a lower incidence of hypoglycemia than are sulfonylureas. The major disadvantages of the glinides are the need for multiple daily doses and less A1C-lowering capacity than the sulfonylureas. More information about these agents can be found in chapter 9.

α-GLUCOSIDASE INHIBITORS (AGIs)

Two drugs in the α-glucosidase inhibitor category have been approved for use in the U.S.: acarbose and miglitol. These drugs exhibit mild antihyperglycemic activity. They may be used as monotherapy in newly onset T2D if the hyperglycemia is low grade and metformin was contraindicated—although other agents would likely be preferable. They may also be useful in combination with other antihyperglycemic medications.

The primary mechanism of action of α-glucosidase inhibitors is competitive inhibition of the α-glucosidase enzymes in the brush border of the small intestine.[10] Inhibition of these enzyme systems effectively reduces the rate of absorption of carbohydrates without altering the absolute absorption. The result is reduced PPG levels. There is also a modest effect on fasting glucose.

The most common side effects of the α-glucosidase inhibitors are dose-related gastrointestinal complaints, abdominal pain, flatulence, and diarrhea.[11] In many cases these side effects may be mitigated with continued administration of the drug and with slow stepwise titration.

Elevated hepatic enzymes have been reported at higher doses of acarbose (200 and 300 mg t.i.d.); however, the occurrence of hepatic dysfunction with doses of ≤100 mg t.i.d. is rare.[11] In fact, elevated serum transaminase levels are no more frequent than those observed with placebo when doses of ≤100mg t.i.d. were used.

Contraindications for the use of α-glucosidase inhibitors primarily revolve around gastrointestinal side effects. Acarbose should be avoided in patients with inflammatory bowel disease, colonic ulceration, or obstructive bowel disorders.[7] Relative contraindications include medical conditions that might deteriorate with increased intestinal gas formation and chronic intestinal disorders of digestion or absorption.

Both AGIs should be avoided in patients with significant renal dysfunction: Acarbose, avoid if eGFR <30 mL/min/1.73 m²; miglitol, avoid if eGFR <25 mL/min/1.73 m².[2]

Typically an A1C reduction of about 0.5–1% can be expected with AGIs.[12] However, they must be dosed three times daily and are sometimes avoided due to their gastrointestinal side effects.

More information about these agents can be found in chapter 11.

THIAZOLIDINEDIONES

Currently two TZDs are available for use in the U.S.: pioglitazone and rosiglitazone. These medications appear to work by affecting insulin action without affecting insulin secretion. They are sometimes referred to as insulin sensitizers. Although several mechanisms of action may contribute to their antihyperglycemic properties, it is known that these compounds stimulate receptors on the nuclear surface, PPAR-γ (peroxisome-proliferator-activated receptor γ). Therefore, the TZDs are also referred to as PPAR activators. Stimulation of PPAR-γ leads to increased glucose uptake by upregulation of the genes responsible for the production of GLUT1 and GLUT2.

Several studies have suggested a link between the use of TZDs and reduced bone density and fractures. Because of this, TZDs should be avoided in patients who are at risk for fracture. TZDs have also been associated with mild to moderate weight gain (1–5 kg) in some patients. Initially, this weight gain was thought to be due primarily to edema but has since been shown to be nonedema weight gain.

Rosiglitazone and pioglitazone have different effects on lipid profiles. This difference may be related to relative effect of these agents on the nuclear receptor. Pioglitazone has a higher affinity for PPAR-α and is associated with mild improvements in lipid profiles (reduction of TG and increases in HDL). Both agents may cause an increase in LDL. Indirect comparisons of pioglitazone and rosiglitazone suggest that rosiglitazone probably causes more LDL elevation than pioglitazone.[6]

Both agents can cause edema. This may in turn increase the incidence of exacerbations of CHF in patients who have underlying disease. This effect seems to be more pronounced in patients who are also treated with insulin. Edema, if it occurs, can sometimes be mitigated through the use of diuretics. However, TZDs are contraindicated in patients with New York Heart Association (NYHA) class III or IV failure.

The published conclusions regarding the impact of TZDs on overall cardiovascular mortality are conflicting. A handful of contradictory manuscripts and a plethora of opposing opinions and editorials on this subject have been published. While it is clear that untreated hyperglycemia is a major risk factor for cardiovascular mortality, it is not clear that treating hyperglycemia in patients with TZDs results in significantly more cardiovascular mortality than is encountered in patients treated with other modalities.

A1C lowering can be expected somewhere between 0.5 and 1.5% in most patients. Significant differences between the two available agents, in terms of glycemic lowering, are not obvious. However the TZDs are less effective than insulin and slightly less effective than metformin or sulfonylureas. In most cases, the latter agents should probably be used initially.

More information about these agents can be found in chapter 7.

DPP-4 INHIBITORS

GLP-1 and glucose-dependent insulinotropic polypeptide (GIP) hormone, under normal physiologic conditions, have very short half-lives and short durations of action. These small half-lives are due to degradation of GLP by a dipeptidyl peptidase-4 (DPP-4).[13] Pharmacologic inhibition of this system results in prolonged activity of the incretin hormones, which in turn are associated with enhanced insulin secretion and a reduction in glucagon secretion. Currently, four DPP-4 inhibitors are available in the U.S.: sitagliptin, saxagliptin, alogliptin, and linagliptin.

The four DPP-4 inhibitors differ in terms or pharmacokinetics and drug interactions. For example, linagliptin does not require dosage adjustment with renal dysfunction while the others three agents in this class do.[14] There are other nuances among the four agents with regard to drug interactions. These differences are reviewed in chapter 12.

Therapeutic use of DPP-4 inhibitors generally results in a modest A1C reduction. A reduction in A1C of about 0.4–0.9% can be expected in most cases.[14] These medications, however, do tend to be weight neutral, are taken once daily, and are generally well tolerated. Cardiovascular outcome trials (CVOT) have to date demonstrated no particular cardiovascular benefit, and there has been some concern that DPP-4 inhibitors may be linked to a slight increase in HF.[15-17] Considering their high cost and mild glucose-lowering effect, DPP-4 inhibitors are probably considered by most to be a third- or fourth-line agent.

More information about these agents can be found in chapter 12.

SGLT2 INHIBITORS

Currently, there are five SGLT2 inhibitors on the market in the U.S. (canagliflozin, dapagliflozin, empagliflozin, bexagliflozin, and ertugliflozin) and others are in development. These compounds are analogs to the natural compound phlorizin, which is found in the bark of apple trees.[18] The first SGLT2 inhibitor (canagliflozin) was approved for use in the U.S. in 2013.[19]

The mechanism of action of the SGLT2 inhibitors is through inhibition of the transporter SGLT2, which in turn results in an increase in urine glucose excretion (UGE). These medications essentially lower the renal threshold for glucose excretion. The SGLT2 inhibitors prevent the reabsorption of between 30 and 50% of filtered glucose. The result of this inhibition is renal loss of glucose and a concomitant reduction in blood glucose. It should be noted that a mixed SGLT1 and SGLT2 inhibitor, sotagliflozin, is currently under development. This medication will modulate glucose transport in both the gastrointestinal tract and kidneys.[20]

The SGLT2 inhibitors are generally associated with an A1C reduction (difference from placebo) of approximately 0.8% when used as monotherapy and 0.6% when used as add-on therapy.[21] Individual response will vary, of course, depending on the agent used and patient characteristics.

The SGLT2 inhibitors have grown in popularity for several reasons. They are associated with weight loss, and may have positive cardiovascular and renal effects. Additionally, they are in and of themselves associated with low rates of hypoglycemia. The SGLT2 inhibitors have been consistently associated with weight loss. The level of weight loss varies but may in some cases be as high as 4.7 kg.[22] Although the magnitude of weight loss varies depending on conditions of the study and population evaluated, a positive effect on weight (i.e., loss) has been consistently observed. One of the more exciting and salient findings with the SGLT2 inhibitors has been the correlation between their use and positive renal and cardiovascular outcomes. For these reasons SGLT2 inhibitors should be considered preferentially as a possible therapeutic modality in patients with ASCVD, CHF, and CKD (particularly agents with proven benefit).[1] The cardiovascular and renal findings are detailed in chapter 10.

The SGLT2 inhibitors are associated with the potential for acute kidney injury (probably secondary to volume depletion) and an increase in urogenital infections; they are relatively expensive.

The use of or the need for dose adjustment with these agents in cases of renal or hepatic impairment varies from agent to agent.

Generally speaking, these agents have been widely accepted and used. They offer a unique mechanism of action, are effective in lowering glycemic indices, have low rates of hypoglycemia, and may have positive cardiovascular and renal effects.

More information about these agents can be found in chapter 10.

GLP-1 AGONISTS AND GIP/GLP 1 AGONIST

GLP-1 7–37, is a naturally occurring peptide that stimulates insulin secretion. It, along with GIP, is secreted under the influence of glucose in the L-cells of the small intestine.[23] These compounds both have very short half-lives, rendering them ineffective, or at least not practical, as pharmacologic agents. A compound isolated from the Gila monster, exendin-4, was found to have homology with the human GLP-1 sequence but with a longer circulating half-life. This finding circumvented the issue of short half-life encountered with native GLP-1 and led to the development of the first pharmacologically viable GLP-1 receptor agonist (GLP-1 RA), exenatide (Byetta), a synthetic version of exendin-4. It was approved for use in the U.S. in 2005. Since that time, multiple other GLP-1 RAs have been approved: liraglutide (Victoza, approved 2010), exenatide XR (Bydureon, approved 2012; BCise pen, approved 2017), albiglutide (Tanzeum, approved 2014), dulaglutide (Trulicity, approved 2014), lixisenatide (Adlyxin, approved 2016), semaglutide (Ozempic, approved 2017), and oral semaglutide (Rebelsus, approved 2019). Albiglutide was discontinued in 2017.

The mechanism of action of the GLP-1 RAs is complex and multifaceted. First, they stimulate insulin secretion from functional β-cells. Second, they suppress glucagon secretion and slow gastric motility. They also have a central effect on satiety and are associated with reduced food intake and weight loss.[23]

GLP-1 RAs are associated with significant reductions in A1C. Placebo-subtracted changes from baseline generally range from 0.5–2%, depending on the particular medication and the population being evaluated.[14] Additionally, GLP-1 RAs are associated with weight loss that has been reported to be as high as 6.5 kg (mean).[24] However, across other studies, weight loss ranged from 0.3–4.7 kg (mean).[14] In fact, these agents are now being used for weight loss in individuals without diabetes. GLP-1 RAs are associated with very low rates of hypoglycemia. This is due primarily to their glucose-lowering actions being linked to ambient glucose concentrations.[25] Three of these agents (liraglutide, dulaglutide, and semaglutide) have demonstrated cardiovascular benefits. GLP-1 RAs likely have a positive impact on CKD, as the published trials thus far have included a limited number of patients and relied heavily on those with co-existing ASCVD. More will be known after the publication of the Research Study to See How Semaglutide Works Compared to Placebo in People With Type 2 Diabetes and Chronic Kidney Disease (FLOW) trial, whose primary objective is to evaluate the impact of semaglutide on CKD.[1,2]

GLP-1 RAs are associated with a relatively high frequency of gastrointestinal side effects. These gastrointestinal events are generally mild to moderate in intensity, transient, self-limiting, and do not usually result in the need for discontinuation of the medication.[25] Early in the evolution of GLP-1 RAs, there was concern about a potential correlation with these medications and acute pancreatitis. However, retrospective observational evaluations have concluded that there is essentially no increase in the incidence of pancreatitis with these agents.[25] No prospective trials have conclusively addressed the potential correlation between this category of medication and pancreatitis; it is recommended that they be used cautiously in patients with a history of pancreatitis, and be discontinued in those who develop it. These agents also carry a black box warning for risk of thyroid C-cell tumors. This concern arose from rodent studies, and no cases of tumors caused by GLP-1 RAs have been reported, but these agents are contraindicated in patients with a family or personal history of medullary thyroid cancer or multiple endocrine neoplasia type 2 (MEN2).[26] Other possible adverse event issues include acute kidney injury, hypersensitivity, and injection site reactions.[2,26]

The currently available GLP-1 RAs differ by duration of action, other elements of their pharmacokinetic profiles, A1C-lowering potency, level of weight loss, and potential cardiovascular benefits. All of these characteristics should be considered when choosing a particular agent.

Recently the GIP/GLP-1 RA bi-agonist tirzepatide was introduced to the market.[1] Its pharmacologic effects are similar to the GLP-1 RAs but it has been associated with very good weight loss potential (similar to semaglutide and dulaglutide [high dose]).

More information about these agents can be found in chapter 13.

INSULIN

Insulin has been used widely for monotherapy since its introduction in 1922 and has been used in combination with oral agents since the late 1950s.[6] It is difficult to estimate the fraction of patients with T2D who are treated with insulin, but one study estimated that about 24% of Medicare beneficiaries with T2D were treated with insulin.[27] Although one could argue about the absolute fraction or number of those with T2D treated with insulin, insulin is probably underutilized in this population. It is the one type of therapy that, with appropriate titration, can consistently bring a patient's blood glucose levels into the target range.

Insulin binds to the α-subunit of the insulin receptor, activating tyrosine kinase activity of the α-subunit. Activation of tyrosine kinase initiates a cascade of reactions, resulting in several physiological events, including inhibition of hepatic glucose production, stimulation of hepatic glucose uptake, stimulation of glucose uptake by muscle, and mild stimulation of glucose uptake by adipose tissue. Insulin therapy has been associated with as much as a 44% reduction in hepatic glucose production and between a 17 and 80% increase in peripheral glucose uptake.[6]

The most significant side effects of insulin in patients with T2D include hypoglycemia and weight gain. Severe hypoglycemia, while a major concern in patients with T2D, probably occurs much less frequently than in patients with T1D. In clinical trials where patients were treated toward an A1C of <7%, rates of severe hypoglycemia occurred at about 1/50th (1–3 episodes per 100 patient-years) of the rate encountered in T1D during the Diabetes Control and Complications Trial (DCCT). Insulin has also been associated with significant weight gain. Studies in patients treated with insulin for between 6 and 12 months have reported weight gain of up to 6 kg but are more commonly on the order of 2–4 kg.

The hyperglycemic-lowering capacity of insulin therapy in patients with T2D is limited only by dose and eventual development of hypoglycemia if too much insulin is used. It is very effective in combination with other pharmacologic

Table 5.1—Summary of Antidiabetic Medication Attributes in a Typical Patient

Interventions	Expected decrease in A1C (%)	Advantages	Disadvantages
Metformin	1.5	Weight neutral, inexpensive	GI side effects, rare to questionable lactic acidosis
Insulin	Dose dependent	No dose limit, inexpensive⊠expensive	Injections, monitoring, hypoglycemia, weight gain
Sulfonylureas	1–2	Inexpensive	Weight gain, hypoglycemia
TZDs	0.5–1.5	Low rates of hypoglycemia	Fluid retention, weight gain, may worsen or facilitate CHF, expensive, fractures
GLP-1 RAs, GIP/GLP 1 RA	0.5–2.0	Weight loss, low rates of hypoglycemia, cardiovascular benefits (liraglutide)	Injections, frequent GI side effects, expensive
DPP-4 inhibitors	0.4–0.9	Once-daily oral dosing	Moderate glycemic lowering, expensive
SGLT2 inhibitors	0.8	Weight loss, cardiovascular benefits (empagliflozin)	Genitourinary infections, expensive

GI, gastrointestinal.

modalities. Its titration can be simplified, in many instances, to a point that allows the patient to continue to titrate dose between visits to the provider.

The use of insulin is reviewed in detail in chapter 3.

CONCLUSION

At present, the development of a meaningful, clinically effective, and relevant medication treatment regimen for T2D is complex, and providers do not find it easy to decide which medication to prescribe. The prescriber must consider the patient's weight, diabetes duration, cardiovascular risk, dexterity, and liver and kidney function, as well as the medications that have been tried previously. Fasting plasma glucose, A1C levels, PPG levels, allergies, insurance coverage, cost of therapy, dosing complexity, and the time it takes to titrate to effective doses, degree of insulin resistance, and whether or not the β-cell is still capable of producing and releasing insulin are all additional considerations. For these reasons, an exact step-by-step treatment algorithm is difficult to develop and various clinics follow different guidelines.

As mentioned above, the hyperglycemia encountered in patients with T2D is often accompanied by other metabolic abnormalities, such as hyperlipidemia, hyperinsulinemia, hypertension, and weight gain. In the past several years, many new medications have been introduced that address not only glycemic abnormalities but also other metabolic abnormalities in patients with T2D. Although the cost of medication should be considered, the most effective method of achieving cost savings in the management of T2D is via strict glycemic control with medications that do not adversely affect the patient's metabolic profile and do not carry contraindications to the patient's specific situation. Clinicians presently have an expanded medication tool chest from which to select that will allow achievement of metabolic objectives and still allow patients a flexible and near-normal lifestyle.

REFERENCES

1. American Diabetes, Association, 9. Pharmacologic Approaches to Glycemic Treatment: *Standards of Care in Diabetes—2023. Diabetes Care* 2023. 46(Suppl 1):S140–S157

2. Davies MJK, D'Alessio DA, Fradkin J, et al. Management of hyperglycemia in type 2 diabetes, 2018: a consensus report by the American Diabetes Association (ADA) and the European Association for the Study of Diabetes (EASD). *Diabetes Care* 2018 Sep; dci180033. https://doi.org/10.2337/dci18-0033

3. Bailey CJ, Turner RC. Metformin. *N Engl J Med* 1996;334:574–579 DOI:10.1056/NEJM199602293340906

4. Chung JW, Hartzler ML, Smith A, Hatton J, Kelley K. Pharmacological agents utilized in patients with type-2 diabetes: beyond lowering A1C. *P T* 2018;43;4:214–227

5. Metformin [package insert]. https://dailymed.nlm.nih.gov/dailymed/drugInfo.cfm?setid=2d98aea3-35ba-447a-b88f-a5a20b612b2f&audience=consumer

6. White JR. Biguanides. In *ADA/PDR Medications for the Treatment of Diabetes.* White JR, Campbell RK, Eds. Alexandria, American Diabetes Association, 2008

7. Bennett WL, Wilson LM, Bolen S, et al. Oral diabetes medications for adults with type 2 diabetes: an update. *AHRQ Comparative Effectiveness Reviews* 2011;27:Report No.:11-EHC038-EF

8. Inzucchi SE. Oral antihyperglycemic therapy for type 2 diabetes: scientific review. *JAMA* 2002;287:360–372

9. Guardado-Mendoza R, Prioletta A, Jiménez-Ceja LM, Sosale A, Folli F. The role of nateglinide and repaglinide, derivatives of meglitinide, in the treatment of type 2 diabetes mellitus. *Arch Med Sci* 2013;9;5:936–943

10. Trevor AJ, Katzung BG, Knuidering-Hall M. Pancreatic hormones, antidiabetic agents and glucagon. In *Katzung and Trevor's Pharmacology: Examination and Board Review*, 11th ed. New York, McGraw Hill Education, 2015

11. Krentz AJ, Bailey CJ. Oral antidiabetic agents: current role in type 2 diabetes mellitus. *Drugs* 2005;65:385–411

12. Chiasson JL, Josse RG, Hunt JA, et al. The efficacy of acarbose in the treatment of patients with non-insulin-dependent diabetes mellitus: a multicenter controlled clinical trial. *Ann Intern Med* 1994;121:928–935

13. Neumiller JJ. Incretin pharmacology: a review of the incretin effect and current incretin-based therapies. *Cardiovasc Hematol Agents Med Chem* 2012;10(4):276–288

14. Neumiller JJ. Incretin-based therapies. *Med Clin North Am* 2015;99:107–130

15. White WB, Cannon CP, Heller SR, et al.; EXAMINE Investigators. Alogliptin after acute coronary syndrome in patients with type 2 diabetes. *N Engl J Med* 2013;369:1327–1335

16. Scirica BM, Bhatt DL, Braunwald E. et al.; SAVOR-TIMI 53 Steering Committee and Investigators. Saxagliptin and cardiovascular outcomes in patients with type 2 diabetes mellitus. *N Engl J Med* 2013;369:1317–1326

17. Green JB, Bethel MA, Armstrong PW, et al.; TECOS Study Group. Effect of sitagliptin on cardiovascular outcomes in type 2 diabetes. *N Engl J Med* 2015;373:232–242

18. White J. Apple trees to sodium glucose co-transporter inhibitors: a review of SGLT2 inhibition. *Clin Diabetes* 2010;28(1):5–10

19. Vasilakou D, Karagiannis T, Athanasiadou E, et al. Sodium-glucose cotransporter 2 inhibitors for type 2 diabetes: a systematic review and meta-analysis. *Ann Intern Med.* 2013;159:262–274

20. Garg SK, Henry RR, Banks P, et al. Effects of sotagliflozin added to insulin in patients with type 1 diabetes. *N Engl J Med* 2017;377:2337–2348

21. White JR. Sodium glucose cotransporter 2 inhibitors. *Med Clin North Am* 2015;99:131–144

22. Chao EC. SGLT-2 inhibitors: a new mechanism for glycemic control. *Clin Diabetes* 2014;32(1):4–11

23. Mudaliar S, Henry RR. The incretin hormones: from scientific discovery to practical therapeutics. *Diabetologia* 2012;55:1865–1868

24. Pratley RE, Aroda VR, Lingvay I, Lüdemann J, Andreassen C, Navarria A, Viljoen A; SUSTAIN 7 Investigators. Semaglutide versus dulaglutide once weekly in patients with type 2 diabetes (SUSTAIN 7): a randomised, open-label, phase 3b trial. *Lancet* 2018;6(4):275–286

25. Leiter LA, Nauck MA. Efficacy and safety of GLP-1 receptor agonists across the spectrum of type 2 diabetes mellitus. *Exp Clin Endocrinol Diabetes* 2017;125:419–435

26. Prasad-Reddy L, Isaacs D. A clinical review of GLP-1 receptor agonists: efficacy and safety in diabetes and beyond. *Drugs Context* 2015;4:212283. DOI:10.7573/dic.212283

27. Sargen MR, Hoffstad OJ, Wiebe DJ, Margolis DJ. Geographic variation in pharmacotherapy decisions for U.S. Medicare enrollees with diabetes. *J Diabetes Complications* 2012;26(4):301–307

Chapter 6
Biguanides

Peggy Soule Odegard, BSPharm, PharmD, CDCES
Kam L. Capoccia, PharmD, BCPS, CDCES

INTRODUCTION

Biguanides[1] in some form have been used since medieval times. French lilac, or goat's rue (*galega officinalis*), was used as a folk treatment for diabetes in southern and eastern Europe. Later, *galega officinalis* was found to be rich in the compound guanidine. In 1918, the hypoglycemic activity of guanidine was confirmed. Unfortunately, guanidine was too toxic for human clinical use, but its chemical congeners, such as the alkyldiguanide synthalin A, were introduced in the early 1920s. Further analysis continued with the biguanide group in the 1920s; however, clinical use of these compounds was not pursued. The compounds fell into disfavor because of the discovery and availability of insulin products.

With the advent of sulfonylureas in the 1950s, biguanides were reinvestigated for possible use in the treatment of diabetes. Metformin and phenformin were introduced in 1957, followed by buformin in 1958. No other active compounds in the biguanide category have been discovered, even though significant work on the structure-activity relationship has taken place. Clinical use of buformin was limited, but phenformin was used widely in the 1960s and 1970s. An association between phenformin and lactic acidosis resulted in the withdrawal of this compound from use in many countries. Metformin was introduced in 1995 and has been the only drug in the biguanide category in the U.S. ever since. Metformin is now the most widely used oral antihyperglycemic agent.

Metformin hydrochloride is indicated for management of T2D as an adjunct to nutrition, physical activity, and education. It is used as monotherapy and in combination with other oral agents, such as GLP-1 RAs or SGLT2 inhibitors, and insulin, as part of a treatment plan taking into account person-centered factors including comorbidities, cardiorenal risks, social determinants of health, and goals.[2] Metformin is also used in prevention of diabetes.[3]

PHARMACOLOGY

MECHANISM OF ACTION

Metformin causes a plethora of metabolic effects, including changes in carbohydrate, lipid, and lipoprotein metabolism. The effects of metformin on carbohydrate metabolism occur primarily in the liver and, to a lesser extent, in peripheral muscle tissue. Metformin's main effect is associated with a reduction in basal hepatic glucose production in patients with T2D. Metformin has been shown to enhance insulin-stimulated glucose transport in skeletal muscle, thereby increasing glucose uptake and insulin sensitivity, although this effect is not as significant as that of hepatic glucose production. More recently, study results have suggested that metformin may prolong β-cell function,[4] reduce glucose absorption from the intestines,[5] and stimulate glucagon-like peptide-1 release, which may contribute to its effect on glucose.[6] Emerging research is also revealing an action of metformin on the gut microbiome, producing positive effects on glucose homeostasis.[7,8] Favorable effects on lipids have also been reported for metformin, in that it decreases plasma triglycerides and low-density lipoprotein cholesterol (LDL-C) and increases high-density lipoprotein cholesterol (HDL-C).

PHARMACOKINETICS

The bioavailability of the immediate-release formulation of metformin ranges from 50–60% when fasting, which is slightly decreased when taken with food. Food increases the absorption of the extended-release formulation. The clinical significance of the increased and decreased absorption caused by food intake is questionable, however. The compound is absorbed mainly through the small intestine. For conventional tablets, peak plasma concentration of 0.4–3 μg/mL is reached ~2–4 h after an oral dose of between 500 and 1,000 mg. For extended-release tablets, peak plasma concentration of 0.6–1.8 μg/mL is reached in 4–8 h. The drug undergoes negligible binding to plasma proteins. The average half-life of metformin in individuals with normal renal function is 6 h. No measurable metabolism of metformin occurs.

In terms of elimination, ~90% of the compound is excreted via the urine within 17–24 h of administration. Elimination occurs via glomerular filtration and tubular secretion. Tubular secretion is thought to be a major route of metformin elimination because the renal clearance of this compound is ~3.5 times greater than creatinine clearance. The drug is widely distributed into most tissues in concentrations similar to those found in peripheral plasma. However, the highest concentrations are found in the salivary glands and in the intestinal wall. Relatively high concentrations are found in the liver and the kidney.

TREATMENT ADVANTAGES/DISADVANTAGES

Metformin gained position as the primary oral pharmacologic treatment for T2D because of its ability to reduce A1C and fasting glucose, beneficial effect on weight, and relatively low cost compared to other glucose-lowering therapies. Although it remains standard of care, person-centered treatment factors should be weighed to assure that the benefits of metformin as initial therapy for T2D outweigh the benefits offered by other agents such as their cardiorenal protection.[2] In addition to these improved effects on glucose control, data continue to emerge highlighting other potential health benefits of metformin. Specifically, its impact on polycystic ovary syndrome (PCOS), prevention or slowing progression to T2D in those at high risk, reduction of certain cancer risks and improvement in survival rates, reduction in CV disease, and favorable impact on aging-related conditions, including the potential reduction in the occurrence of dementia. There is limited data evaluating the impact of metformin initiation in subjects without diabetes on risk reduction or treatment benefits for these conditions; however, initial studies are underway to explore the use of metformin as an adjunct therapy in certain cancers. An important emerging area with metformin is its potential impact on inflammation and immune response.

Recently, the efficacy and durability of combination therapy with metformin as an initial treatment of newly diagnosed diabetes has been investigated. Metformin combined with vildagliptin was shown to be successful in producing better glycemic control with a more durable benefit as compared to metformin alone[8] or metformin-glimepiride combination therapy.[10] Another study showed reduced glycemic variability with low-dose metformin plus linagliptin over high-dose metformin alone.[11] These results suggest that a DPP-4 inhibitor may be combined with metformin as primary initial therapy.

SARS-COV-2 COVID INFECTION

A beneficial effect of metformin on reducing mortality in those with diabetes who contract COVID-19 has been noted, with the postulated mechanism, although yet unconfirmed, of chemical mediation of cytokine storm and inflammation.[12] In a meta-analysis, of 17 studies including 20,719 COVID-19 patients with diabetes, metformin was associated with significantly decreased mortality and severity (OR = 0.64, 95% CI = 0.51-0.79 mortality, and OR = 0.81, 95% CI = 0.66-0.99 severity).[13] Ganesh and Randall conducted a meta-analysis of 32 cohort studies including 2,916,231 patients that demonstrated decreased mortality in COVID-19 patients with diabetes taking metformin in both unadjusted (OR = 0.61, 95% CI = 0.53-0.71) and adjusted (OR = 0.78, 95% CI = 0.69-0.88) models.[14]

POLYCYSTIC OVARY SYNDROME

Metformin has demonstrated efficacy in the treatment of PCOS, with effects on fertility.[15] The primary actions of metformin in PCOS include resumption of menses, improvement in menses cyclic frequency, and hormonal and metabolic parameters. In one study of 119 women with PCOS, 24 months of metformin treatment was correlated with improved hormonal profiles for testosterone and luteinizing hormone, increased menstrual frequency, and decreased body mass in both overweight and normal weight women.[16]

Metformin, when used to treat PCOS and induce ovulation, should be discontinued by the end of the first trimester in pregnancy.[17]

PREVENTION OF T2D

The Diabetes Prevention Program, a 3-year multicenter trial (n = 3,234) aimed to prevent T2D, compared intensive lifestyle support intervention to metformin and placebo in people at high risk for diabetes. The results substantially favored the lifestyle intervention (5–7% weight loss and 150 min moderate level physical activity weekly) with a 58% reduction in the incidence of diabetes at

3 years; however, metformin (850 mg twice daily) demonstrated significant benefits on risk reduction as well, with 31% reduced incidence of diabetes as compared to placebo.[18] These findings were reinforced by the 10-year follow-up to the Diabetes Prevention Program study of 924 subjects initially in the metformin group, with an 18% reduction in diabetes incidence for those taking metformin.[19] Another analysis of the data on DPP-4 inhibitors supports the use of metformin for the prevention of progression to T2D, but shows that metformin may be the most beneficial in men[20] or in patients with the highest risk of progression.[21] The American Diabetes Association, in its *Standards of Care in Diabetes*, currently recommends metformin as a pharmacotherapeutic approach for those with prediabetes, especially if BMI is greater than or equal to 35 kg/m^2, in women with a history of gestational diabetes, and for those who are less than 60 years old.[3]

Combination therapy of metformin and lifestyle management does not seem to do better than metformin alone in preventing T2D.[22,23] In Latina patients, lifestyle intervention may be more effective than metformin for prevention of T2D.[21] Other pharmacologic treatments have been evaluated for their efficacy in diabetes prevention; however, metformin continues to be the best option if pharmacotherapy is used and lifestyle continues to show the strongest benefit. In a recent trial, the effect of linagliptin was explored in comparison to metformin for control of glycemic variability in patients with glucose intolerance;[25] however, no distinction between the two was identified. Metformin has been found to be less beneficial for preventing T2D in adolescent youth than in adults.[26]

USE IN PREGNANCY

Metformin is not approved by the FDA for the treatment of diabetes during pregnancy, and it does cross the placenta. Metformin should not be used in pregnant people with hypertension or preeclampsia, or those at risk of intrauterine growth restriction due to the risk of acidosis or potential for growth restriction in the setting of placental insufficiency.[17] Studies have demonstrated the safety of metformin use in patients who are pregnant, and continued research is underway to assess longer-term outcomes for babies. Metformin is associated with a lower risk of neonatal hypoglycemia and less maternal weight gain. Currently, metformin is used in gestational diabetes and pregnant women with T2D as an alternative to insulin, which is usually considered first-line choice of therapy.[27–37]

In a controlled trial of 502 women with T2D taking insulin during pregnancy, the addition of metformin in early pregnancy resulted in improved maternal glucose, less weight gain, fewer Caesarean births, and lower insulin doses as compared to placebo. Although infants of mothers in the metformin group weighed less and had reduced adiposity, a greater proportion (13% vs. 7%) were small for gestational age as compared to those in the placebo group.[36] The authors conclude the need for further investigation to be able to counsel appropriately about this treatment's effect on infants. A meta-analysis of 24 studies, inclusive of 17 studies with quantitative data (n = 2,828 subjects), demonstrated metformin was significantly associated with reduced risks for pregnancy-induced hypertension (RR 0.64 [95%CI 0.44–0.95]; P = 0.03), large-for-gestational-age babies (RR 0.82 [95% CI 0.68–0.99]; P = 0.04), neonatal hypoglycemia (RR 0.72 [95%CI 0.59–0.88]; P = 0.001), and neonatal intensive care unit admission (RR 0.74 [95%CI 0.58–

0.94]; $P = 0.01$). Importantly, this same analysis did not find increased risk of premature delivery or for small-for-gestational-age babies.[37]

CARDIOVASCULAR RISK REDUCTIONS

A positive effect of metformin on cardiovascular health has been reported by multiple studies, although the explicit CV benefit—often attributed to its effects on weight, blood pressure, endothelial function, and lipids—has yet to be specifically confirmed. In the United Kingdom Prospective Diabetes Study (UKPDS) and subsequent follow-up study, metformin treatment was associated with reduced all-cause mortality, including reduction in myocardial infarction.[38,39] In a meta-analysis of 40 trials, metformin reduced risk of CV mortality compared to the other oral diabetes agents studied and placebo.[40,41] In the Diabetes Prevention Program and the Diabetes Prevention Program Outcomes Study, neither metformin nor lifestyle interventions reduced major cardiovascular events or mortality after a median follow-up of 21 years.[42,43] In patients with T1D, metformin has been shown to have beneficial effects on cardiovascular risk, although it does not affect glucose control in these patients.[34] More recently, the contraindication regarding the use of metformin in patients with advanced HF has been removed from the product labeling in light of several studies demonstrating the safety and benefit of metformin use in people with diabetes and HF, including reduction in HF readmissions and mortality.[45] It is still, however, prudent to consider holding metformin therapy in acute HF exacerbations involving substantial reduction in renal function, until stabilized, to mitigate risk.

MITIGATION OF GLUCOCORTICOID-INDUCED DIABETES

Limited research has identified a potential benefit of preventative metformin use to mitigate the metabolic effects on glucose homeostasis in people without diabetes using systemic glucocorticoids. In a randomized, double-blind, placebo-controlled 4-week trial of 34 patients receiving regular glucocorticoids (prednisone, prednisolone, or methylprednisolone), median glucose remained stable for those treated with metformin 850 mg twice daily (after 1 week titration) as compared to those on placebo, with the change significantly different between both groups at 4 weeks ($P = 0.005$).[46] Additionally, in a randomized trial of usual care versus two dose options of metformin, with 18 subjects on high-dose corticosteroids as part of cancer treatment, a significant difference in 2-hour PPG was noted in those receiving metformin, with greater benefit in those taking 1,700 mg versus 850 mg daily.[47] Although initial research was limited to a small group of individuals, this suggests a potential therapeutic advantage to metformin in a population at high risk for diabetes in the future.

IMPACT ON BONE METABOLISM

People with diabetes have been shown to have increased risk of bone fractures.[48,49] However, investigation of metformin's effect on bone metabolism has produced mixed results. Results of one study in 371 patients with T2D over 12 months suggested that metformin may have some beneficial effects on bone metabolism.[50] Another study in 407 patients with T2D over 18 months showed no difference from placebo in bone density.[51] Data from the Diabetes Prevention Program Outcomes Study (DPPOS) revealed that year 10 of metformin use did not reduce the prevalence of frailty.[52] However, metformin use at year 12 in the DPPOS did not result in long-term negative effects on bone mineral density.[53]

IMPACT ON CANCER RISKS AND OUTCOMES

An impact of metformin on cancer risk and survival has been reported in several studies, although current findings are based primarily on studies using a retrospective design. A review of the most recent evidence is reflected in the subsequent sections. Additional prospective, controlled investigations are needed to confirm any potential benefit of metformin in prevention of specific cancers and to more specifically characterize metformin's effects on cancer treatment outcomes. Initial data exploring these effects of metformin is summarized below for certain cancers. Readers are encouraged to conduct updated medical literature searches to confirm the most recent findings to guide therapeutic decision-making.

Breast, Ovarian, and Endometrial Cancer Risk and Outcomes

Current evidence does not support a benefit of metformin in reducing invasive disease-free survival in people with breast cancer. In retrospective studies of ovarian cancer, there appears to be an independent benefit of metformin on lowering overall mortality (HR 0.72 [95% CI 0.55–0.93, $P < 0.01$); however, prospective clinical trials are imperative to define a specific benefit and guide treatment.[54] In a subset of five pooled studies of a meta-analysis of 11 studies involving more than 766,000 subjects conducted by Tang et al., metformin use in individuals with T2D who had endometrial cancer was associated with a reduction of endometrial cancer risk among patients with diabetes (RR 0.87 [95% CI 0.80–0.95]; $P = 0.006$). Additionally, pooled analysis of six retrospective studies identified significantly improved survival in patients with endometrial cancer using metformin compared to nonusers (HR 0.63 [95% CI 0.45–0.87]; $P = 0.006$).[55]

Pancreatic Cancer Risk and Outcomes

Four recent studies have identified a positive impact on survival in people with T2D and pancreatic cancer who were taking metformin. In a systematic review and meta-analysis of nine studies comprising 9,265 subjects taking metformin, Zhou et al. identified a relative survival benefit (overall survival HR 0.84 [95% CI 0.73–0.96]) associated with metformin use compared to no metformin use.[56] In a similar systematic review of 14 studies (12 cohort studies and 2 randomized controlled trials) of over 94,000 patients with pancreatic cancer, metformin use was associated with improved overall survival (adjusted HR 0.77 [95% CI 0.68–0.87]).[57] In the cohort studies, however, no improvement in progression-free survival or overall survival was identified. Separate meta-analyses conducted by Li et al. and Jian-Yu et al. have confirmed these findings with some subanalyses pointing to potential differential effects of this benefit, based on tumor stage.[58,59]

Hepatocellular Carcinoma

Li et al. identified significantly reduced risk (OR/RR = 0.59 [95% CI 0.51–0.68] I2 = 96.5%; $P < 0.001$ from 9 case-control and 15 cohort studies) and decreased all-cause mortality (from 9 cohort studies) of hepatocellular carcinoma in people with diabetes taking metformin using a random effects model (HR = 0.74 [95% CI 0.66–0.83] I2 = 49.6%; $P = 0.037$). Although this finding is positive, prospective studies to further assess this potentially protective benefit of metformin are indicated.[60]

Colorectal Cancer Risk and Outcomes

The risk of colorectal cancer (CRC) in patients with T2D taking metformin has been evaluated in a number of studies with evidence pointing to a reduced incidence of CRC and a survival benefit in those using metformin. In a meta-analysis conducted of 20 studies published prior to 2016, including 12 cohort, 7 case-control, and 1 randomized controlled trial, metformin use was associated with reduced incidence of colorectal adenomas (OR 0.80 [95% CI 0.71–0.90]; $P = 0.0002$).[61] In a similar analysis, Du et al. identified improved overall survival in metformin users with diabetes and CRC as compared to non-metformin users (HR 0.69 [95% CI 0.61–0.77]), with benefit noted in particular for patients with stage II and III CRC disease.[62] Furthering this observation of the positive impact of metformin on CRC, Tian and colleagues conducted a meta-analysis of 81 studies, representing 6,908 cases of CRC patients using metformin and 4,954 CRC patients with T2D not using metformin. This analysis found a significantly improved overall survival (HR 0.82 [95% CI 0.77–0.87]; $P = 0.000$) in patients using metformin, although this benefit was not significant for CRC-specific survival (HR 0.84 [95% CI 0.69–1.02]; $P = 0.079$).[63] Wang and Shi conducted a systematic review and meta-analysis of 28 studies that demonstrated metformin reduced the risk of CRC by 29% compared with nonuse (OR/RR 0.71 [95% CI 0.64-0.80]; $P < 0.001$) and lowered all-cause mortality (HR 0.72 [95% CI 0.62–0.83] $P = 0.014$).[64]

Prostate Cancer Risk and Outcomes

The impact of metformin use on risk reduction for prostate cancer has been reported; however, studies have largely been focused in Asian populations, limiting the ability to generalize findings. With this in mind, Chen and colleagues used a meta-analysis design to investigate this impact further with attention to ethnicity. Of 482 studies identified, 26 were chosen for inclusion (23 Western-based, 3 Asian-based, representing almost 2 million patients). No significant association between metformin use and prostate cancer was identified for Western- or Asian-based studies collectively (RR 1.01 [95% CI 0.86–1.18]). The removal of one large study in an Asian population resulted in similar findings for the Asian-based studies. The authors concluded there is likely no association between metformin and risk of prostate cancer based on the current evidence.[65]

Gastric Cancer Risk and Outcomes

The potential effect of metformin use on the risk of gastric cancer in patients with T2D has been evaluated in limited studies. In a meta-analysis of 7 cohort studies (*n* = 591,077 patients), metformin therapy was associated with a lower incidence of gastric cancer in Asian patients with T2D than that of other therapies for diabetes (HR 0.763 [95% CI 0.642–0.905]). Given these findings were limited to observations in a specific ethnic population, clarity regarding the potential benefit of metformin on reducing the risk of gastric cancer more generally is needed.[66]

More recently, a meta-analysis of 22 RCTs of 5,943 participants with cancer identified no statistically significant benefit in progression-free survival (PFS) (HR 0.97 [95% CI 0.82–1.15] I2 = 50%) or overall survival (OS; HR 0.98 [95% CI 0.86–1.13] I2 = 33%) for patients with any cancer between the metformin and control groups. Subgroup analyses demonstrated that metformin treatment was associated with significantly worse PFS in digestive system cancers (HR 1.45 [95% CI 1.03–2.04]) lending question to any potential benefit of metformin use in diabetes for those with gastric cancers.[67]

Lung Cancer Risk and Outcomes

Several investigations have explored the effect of metformin on OS and PFS in lung cancer; however, no definitive treatment recommendations can be made at this time. The potential benefit of metformin in lung cancer stems from the experimental observation that cancer proliferation rate and tumor progression occur more quickly in patients with diabetes, theoretically due to the influence of hyperinsulinemia, inflammatory cytokines, and hyperglycemia.[68] Cao and colleagues conducted a recent meta-analysis of studies published prior to April 2017. In this analysis of people with T2D and lung cancer, both OS (HR 0.77 [95% CI 0.66–0.9]; *P* = 0.001) and PFS (HR 0.53 [95% CI 0.41–0.68]; *P* < 0.001) improved (23% and 47% reductions, respectively) with metformin use compared to no metformin use. Histological analysis revealed this beneficial effect for both non-small cell lung cancer and small cell lung cancer with statistically significant improvements in OS and PFS.[69]

IMPACT ON AGING-RELATED CONDITIONS

Recently, reports in the popular press hinted at the aging benefits of metformin, suggesting far-reaching benefits of age extension. There is not current evidence to support this suggested benefit; however, some research is underway to characterize this potential, but unproven, benefit.[70,71] The impact of metformin on reducing risk of the occurrence of cognitive decline has recently been identified. In a meta-analysis of 10 studies of over 250,000 subjects, metformin was associated with reduced occurrence of cognitive dysfunction (HR 0.90; 95% CI [0.88, 0.92]) in those with T2D.[72] A similar meta-analysis identified a reduced risk of dementia in those taking metformin as compared to no treatment for hyperglycemia (HR for metformin, 0.75; 95% CI, 0.63-0.86).[73]

In 2022, Malazy and colleagues published a meta-analysis evaluating 19 studies, which included 3,827 records from cross-sectional, cohort, and randomized control trials, that demonstrated no significant effect on improvement of cognitive dysfunction or protection against dementia or cognitive dysfunction.[74]

SIGNIFICANT WARNINGS/PRECAUTIONS

Metformin is contraindicated in patients with

- Acute or chronic metabolic acidosis, including diabetic ketoacidosis.
- Known hypersensitivity to metformin hydrochloride.
- Severe renal impairment (GFR below 30 mL/min).

Metformin should be discontinued temporarily in patients requiring radiological studies using iodinated contrast media, because these agents are known to cause renal dysfunction in some individuals.

Monitoring Renal Function

Metformin is excreted via the kidneys; thus, the risk of accumulation of the medication is greater in patients with reduced renal function. The risk of lactic acidosis is increased in these patients as well. Calculation of GFR is recommended for renal monitoring in patients taking metformin. Metformin use in patients with renal impairment should be monitored closely.[75] When the GFR for a patient taking metformin falls below 45 mL/min, assessing risk versus benefit of continued use is recommended. Normally, the annual assessment of renal function is appropriate, assuming stable health status for the patient. In patients with a GFR of less than 60 mL/min, renal function should be assessed every 3–6 months; in those with a GFR of 30–45 mL/min, the dose should be reduced and they should have more frequent renal monitoring. In patients 65 years of age or older who have the additional risk for age-related decline in renal function, more frequent assessment of renal function when taking metformin is warranted.

Radiological Studies

Until recently, recommendations were that radiological studies involving the use of iodinated contrast media should be undertaken only after metformin has been discontinued. The drug should be withheld on the day of the procedure, and for at least 2–3 days after, until normal renal function has been documented. Recent evaluation of this practice indicates it is possible that a less conservative approach, withholding the drug for renal function at levels of GFR less than 60 ml/min may be sufficient; however, further research to confirm safety of this practice is warranted.

Hypoxic States

Lactic acidosis is associated with cardiovascular collapse, acute congestive heart failure, acute myocardial infarction, and other conditions such as septicemia and dehydration that cause hypoxemia. Therefore, metformin should be discontinued in patients with these acute medical conditions and may be reinstituted once the acute illness has resolved and renal function is normal.

Surgical Procedures

Metformin therapy should be discontinued temporarily for any major surgical procedure and should be restarted only after the patient's oral intake has been resumed and renal function has normalized.

Alcohol Intake

Metformin should be used cautiously in patients who are known to consume excessive alcohol, since this may be a precipitating factor increasing risk for lactic acidosis.

Impaired Hepatic Function

Impaired hepatic function has been associated with some cases of lactic acidosis; therefore, it is recommended that metformin not be used in patients with impaired hepatic function. Recently, metformin, along with other medications used for T2D, has been evaluated for effects on reducing nonalcoholic fatty liver disease (NAFLD), with modest effects on steatosis demonstrated when combined with weight loss; however, no appreciable effect on fibrosis was demonstrated.[76]

Vitamin B$_{12}$ Levels

Among patients treated with metformin, 7–9% experience a reduction in vitamin B$_{12}$ to subnormal levels with long-term use.[77] However, this is rarely associated with anemia and appears to be rapidly reversible with discontinuation of the medication or with vitamin B$_{12}$ supplementation. Patients treated with metformin should therefore undergo measurement of hematological parameters annually. Hematological evaluation is also advised in any patient with apparent abnormalities. Routine serum vitamin B$_{12}$ measurements approximately every 2–3 years may be useful in individuals with inadequate B$_{12}$ or calcium intake and/or absorption.

Hypoglycemia

Hypoglycemia does not occur with metformin monotherapy under normal conditions. However, it may occur in patients in whom caloric intake is deficient, in patients who undertake strenuous exercise, in patients who are treated with other glucose-lowering agents, such as sulfonylureas, or in patients who consume ethanol. Patients taking combination products containing metformin along with other agents, especially sulfonylureas and meglitinides, can experience hypoglycemia.

SPECIAL POPULATIONS

Hepatic Impairment

Patients with hepatic impairment have developed lactic acidosis while taking metformin, perhaps not due to metformin itself but because of reduced hepatic lactate clearance. Nevertheless, metformin should be avoided in patients with hepatic impairment.

Table 6.1 – Antihyperglycemic Medications Containing Metformin

Metformin formulations	Available strengths	Extended or immediate release	Can be cut?	Dosing interval	Maximum therapeutic effect (time)	Maximum daily dose (MDD)	Renal dose adjustments (mL/min/1.73 m²)	Hepatic dose adjustments	Contraindications	Pregnancy category
Extended Release (XR)										
Fortamet; Glucophage XR; Glumetza; Generic	Fortamet: 500 mg, 1,000 mg; Glucophage XR: 500 mg, 750 mg; Glumetza: 500 mg, 1000 mg; Generic: 500 mg, 750 mg, 1,000 mg	Extended release	Do not chew, cut, or crush	Once daily–b.i.d.	May take 4–6 weeks to see full effect	2,000 mg/d	eGFR 30–45: Do not initiate; if eGFR falls to <45, consider benefits/risks of continuing therapy eGFR <30: Do not use	Avoid use of metformin in patients with clinical or laboratory evidence of hepatic disease due to risk of lactic acidosis	Hypersensitivity to metformin; eGFR <30; acute or chronic metabolic acidosis, including diabetic ketoacidosis; use cautiously in patients at risk for lactic acidosis	B
Immediate Release (IR)										
Glucophage; Generic	500 mg, 850 mg, 1,000 mg (scored)	Immediate release	Yes	b.i.d.	May take 4–6 weeks to see full effect	2,000 mg/d	See metformin above	See metformin above	See metformin above	B
Liquid										
Riomet; Generic	500 mg/5 mL	Immediate release	N/A	Once daily–t.i.d.	May take 4–6 weeks to see full effect	2,000 mg/d	See metformin above	See metformin above	See metformin above	B

(continued)

Table 6.1 (continued)

Metformin formulations	Available strengths	Extended or immediate release	Can be cut?	Dosing interval	Maximum therapeutic effect (time)	Maximum daily dose (MDD)	Renal dose adjustments (mL/min/1.73 m²)	Hepatic dose adjustments	Contraindications	Pregnancy category
Metformin & DPP-4 Inhibitors										
Metformin & Alogliptan (Generic)	500 mg/12.5 mg, 1,000 mg/12.5 mg	Immediate release	Do not chew, cut, or crush	b.i.d.	Metformin: 4–6 weeks, Alogliptin: 2–4 weeks	Metformin 2,000 mg/d, Alogliptin 12.5 mg/d	See metformin above	See metformin above	See metformin above, Hypersensitivity to alogliptan	B
Metformin & Linagliptin Brand (Jentadueto)	500 mg/2.5 mg, 850 mg/2.5 mg, 1,000 mg/2.5 mg	Immediate release	Yes	b.i.d.	Metformin: 4–6 weeks, Linagliptin: 2–4 weeks	Metformin 2,000 mg/d, Linagliptin 5 mg/d	See metformin above	See metformin above	See metformin above, Hypersensitivity to linagliptin	B
Metformin Extended Release & Linagliptin Brand (Jentadueto XR)	1,000 mg XR/2.5 mg, 1000 mg XR/5 mg	Extended release	Do not crush, cut, or chew	Once daily	Metformin: 4–6 weeks, Linagliptin: 2–4 weeks	Metformin 2,000 mg/d, Linagliptin 5 mg/d	See metformin above	See metformin above	See metformin above, Hypersensitivity to linagliptin	B
Metformin Extended Release & Saxagliptin Brand (Kombiglyze XR)	500 mg XR/5 mg, 1,000 mg XR/2.5 mg, 1,000 mg XR/5 mg	Extended release	Do not crush, cut, or chew	Once daily	Metformin: 4–6 weeks, Saxagliptin: 2–4 weeks	Metformin 2,000 mg/d, Saxagliptin 5 mg/d	See metformin above, Limit saxagliptin dose to 2.5 mg/d	See metformin above	See metformin above Hypersensitivity to saxagliptin	B
Metformin & Sitagliptin Brand (Janumet)	500 mg/50 mg, 1,000 mg/50 mg	Immediate release	Do not chew, cut, or crush	b.i.d.	Metformin: 4–6 weeks, Saxagliptin: 2–4 weeks	Metformin 2,000 mg/d, Sitagliptin 100 mg/d	See metformin above, Limit sitagliptin dose to 50 mg/day	See metformin above	See metformin above, Hypersensitivity to sitagliptin	B

(continued)

Table 6.1 (continued)

Metformin formulations	Available strengths	Extended or immediate release	Can be cut?	Dosing interval	Maximum therapeutic effect (time)	Maximum daily dose (MDD)	Renal dose adjustments (mL/min/1.73 m²)	Hepatic dose adjustments	Contraindications	Pregnancy category
Metformin Extended Release & Sitagliptin Brand (Janumet XR)	500 mg XR/50 mg, 1,000 mg XR/50 mg, 1,000 mg XR/100 mg	Extended release	Do not chew, cut, or crush	Once daily	Metformin: 4–6 weeks; Sitagliptin: 2–4 weeks	Metformin 2,000 mg/d; Sitagliptin 100 mg/d	See metformin above	See metformin above	See metformin above; Hypersensitivity to sitagliptin	B
Metformin & Meglitinide										
Metformin & Repaglinide (Generic)	500 mg/1 mg, 500 mg/2 mg	Immediate release	Yes	b.i.d.–t.i.d.	Metformin: 4–6 weeks; Repaglinide: 2 weeks	Metformin 2,000 mg/d; Repaglinide 10 mg; Do not exceed 1,000 mg metformin/4 mg repaglinide per meal	See metformin above	See metformin above	See metformin above; Hypersensitivity to repaglinide; Concomitant administration of gemfibrozil	C
Metformin & SGLT2 Inhibitors										
Metformin & Canagliflozin Brand (Invokamet)	500 mg/50 mg, 500 mg/150 mg, 1,000 mg/50 mg, 1,000 mg/150 mg	Immediate release	Yes	b.i.d.	Metformin: 4–6 weeks; Canagliflozin: 2 weeks	Metformin 2,000 mg/d; Canagliflozin 300 mg/d	See metformin above; eGFR 45 to <60: Limit the dose of canagliflozin to 100 mg/day; eGFR <45: Do not use	See metformin above	See metformin above; Hypersensitivity to canagliflozin; eGFR <45, end-stage renal disease or patients on dialysis	C

(continued)

Table 6.1 (continued)

Metformin formulations	Available strengths	Extended or immediate release	Can be cut?	Dosing interval	Maximum therapeutic effect (time)	Maximum daily dose (MDD)	Renal dose adjustments (mL/min/1.73 m²)	Hepatic dose adjustments	Contraindications	Pregnancy category
Metformin Extended Release & Canagliflozin Brand (Invokamet XR)	500 mg XR/50 mg 500 mg XR/150 mg 1,000 mg XR/50 mg 1,000 mg XR/150 mg	Extended release	Do not crush, cut, or chew	Once daily	Metformin: 4–6 weeks Canagliflozin: 2 weeks	Metformin 2,000 mg/d Canagliflozin 300mg/d	See metformin above eGFR 45 to <60: Limit the dose of canagliflozin to 100 mg/day eGFR <45: Do not use	See metformin above	See metformin above Hypersensitivity to canagliflozin eGFR <45, end-stage renal disease or patients on dialysis	C
Metformin Extended Release & Dapagliflozin Brand (Xigduo XR)	500 mg XR/5 mg 500 mg XR/10 mg 1,000 mg XR/5 mg 1,000 mg XR/10 mg	Extended release	Do not crush, cut, or chew	Once daily	Metformin: 4–6 weeks Dapagliflozin: 2 weeks	Metformin 2,000 mg/d Dapagliflozin 10 mg/d	See metformin above Dapagliflozin: eGFR <60: Do not initiate; eGFR that declines persistently in the range of 30 to <60 use is not recommended; eGFR <30 Do not use	See metformin above	See metformin above Hypersensitivity to dapagliflozin Moderate to severe renal impairment (eGFR <60), end-stage renal disease or patients on dialysis	C

(continued)

Table 6.1 (continued)

Metformin formulations	Available strengths	Extended or immediate release	Can be cut?	Dosing interval	Maximum therapeutic effect (time)	Maximum daily dose (MDD)	Renal dose adjustments (mL/min/1.73 m²)	Hepatic dose adjustments	Contraindications	Pregnancy category
Metformin & Empaglifozin Brand (Synjardy)	500 mg/5 mg 1000 mg/5 mg 500 mg/12.5 mg 1,000 mg/12.5 mg	Immediate release	Yes	b.i.d.	Metformin: 4–6 weeks Empagliflozin: 2 weeks	Metformin 2,000 mg/d Empagliflozin 25mg/d	See metformin above Empagliflozin: eGFR ≥45: No dosage adjustment necessary. Monitor renal function at least annually eGFR <45: Do not use	See metformin above	See metformin above Hypersensitivity to empagliflozin eGFR <45, end-stage renal disease or patients on dialysis	C
Metformin Extended Release & Empaglifozin Brand (Synjardy XR)	1,000 mg XR/5 mg 1,000 mg XR/10 mg 1,000 mg XR/12.5 mg 1,000 mg XR/25 mg	Extended release	Do not crush, cut, or chew	Once daily	Metformin: 4–6 weeks Empagliflozin: 2 weeks	Metformin 2,000 mg/d Empagliflozin 25 mg/d	See metformin above Empagliflozin: eGFR ≥45: No dosage adjustment necessary. Monitor renal function at least annually eGFR <45: Do not use	See metformin above	See metformin above Hypersensitivity to empagliflozin eGFR <45, end-stage renal disease or patients on dialysis	C

(continued)

Table 6.1 (continued)

Metformin formulations	Available strengths	Extended or immediate release	Can be cut?	Dosing interval	Maximum therapeutic effect (time)	Maximum daily dose (MDD)	Renal dose adjustments (mL/min/1.73 m²)	Hepatic dose adjustments	Contraindications	Pregnancy category
Metformin & Sulfonylurea										
Metformin & Glipizide Brand (Metaglip) and Generic	250 mg/2.5 mg 500 mg/2.5 mg 500 mg/5 mg	Immediate release	Yes	b.i.d.	Metformin: 4–6 weeks Glipizide: 2 weeks	Metformin 2,000 mg/d Glipizide 10 mg/d	See metformin above Glipizide: ERSD start with 2.5mg and titrate accordingly	See metformin above	See metformin above Hypersensitivity to glipizide eGFR <30	C
Metformin & Glyburide Brand (Glucovance) and Generic	500 mg/2.5 mg 500 mg/5 mg	Immediate release	Yes	b.i.d.	Metformin: 4–6 weeks Glyburide: 2 weeks	Metformin 2,000 mg/d Glyburide 10 mg/d	See metformin above Do not use glyburide in chronic kidney disease	See metformin above	See metformin above Hypersensitivity to glyburide eGFR <30 Concomitant administration of bosentan	C
Metformin & Thiazolidinediones										
Metformin & Pioglitazone Brand (Actoplus Met) and Generic	500 mg/15 mg 850 mg/15 mg	Immediate release	Yes	Once daily or b.i.d.	Metformin: 4–6 weeks Pioglitazone: 3–6 months	Metformin 2,000 mg/d Pioglitazone 45 mg/d	See metformin above	See metformin above Do not initiate if ALT > 2.5 times the ULN at baseline; If ALT levels persist above three times the ULN during therapy, discontinue use	See metformin above Hypersensitivity to pioglitazone NYHA Class III or IV heart failure	C Pioglitazone may cause ovulation in anovulatory premenopausal women, increasing the risk of unintended pregnancy

ALT, alanine aminotransferase; ULN, upper limit of normal; NYHA, New York Heart Association.

Pediatrics

The safety and efficacy of metformin in pediatric patients between the ages of 10 and 16 years has been established. Extended-release metformin has been evaluated in this population. Even though combination products are sometimes used for greater medication adherence, the safety and efficacy of combination products containing metformin have not been established in this population except for one (metformin with glyburide).[78]

Geriatrics

Limited published data on the use of metformin in geriatric patients indicates a potential for changes in its pharmacokinetic profile, primarily due to renal function decline. Yet no overall difference in the safety or efficacy of metformin has been found in geriatric patients compared to younger patients. Since metformin is excreted renally and renal function declines with age, elderly patients have a theoretically increased likelihood of metformin-associated lactic acidosis. Because of this concern about increased risk, monitoring renal function more frequently is recommended for this patient population to assure safety.

Sex

No pharmacokinetic differences have been reported based on sex. Clinically, in controlled trials in patients with T2D, no differences have been observed between males and female patients.

Ethnicity

Although no controlled clinical trials have been conducted evaluating differences in the pharmacokinetics or pharmacodynamics of metformin use among ethnic groups, the effects of metformin have been shown to be comparable in non-Hispanic white, black, and Hispanic subjects.

ADVERSE EFFECTS AND MONITORING

Lactic Acidosis

Lactic acidosis is a very rare but extremely serious condition that can occur secondary to the accumulation of metformin. Lactic acidosis is fatal in ~50% of cases. Currently, the reported incidence of lactic acidosis in patients receiving metformin is extremely low. The majority of these cases have occurred in patients with significant renal insufficiency. The risk of lactic acidosis can be reduced by observing the aforementioned contraindications and precautions. Recent studies have demonstrated that if contraindications are followed, the rates of lactic acidosis in patients treated with metformin are no greater than background rates observed in similar patients not treated with metformin.[79–81]

Gastrointestinal Reactions

Gastrointestinal symptoms, such as abdominal bloating, flatulence, anorexia, diarrhea, nausea, and vomiting, are the most common side effects observed in patients treated with metformin. Importantly, these symptoms may be mitigated by taking with food (e.g., start the dose with the major meal), gradual dose escalation as tolerated against gastrointestinal symptoms, and by using the extended-release (i.e., XR) formulation of the drug. Gastrointestinal complaints are ~30% more frequent in patients on metformin monotherapy than in patients treated with placebo, particularly during the initial phases of therapy. These complaints are generally transient and may resolve with continued treatment and attention to the dosing strategies mentioned above. In some cases, however, temporary dose reduction may be prudent. If significant diarrhea and/or vomiting occur, metformin should be temporarily discontinued or a trial of the extended-release formulation be considered, if not yet attempted.

Recent research on the gut microbiome indicates a shift in bacterial flora related to metformin use.[7] While favoring the formation of bacteria associated with enhanced metabolic effects in the gut, this effect may also result in the formation of some undesirable strains, including those that may mediate increased risk of gastrointestinal side effects of therapy. Overall, gastrointestinal complaints are generally transient and may resolve with continued treatment and attention to the dosing strategies mentioned above. Based on current price comparability of the extended-release and immediate-release metformin products and in light of new evidence suggesting the extended-release formulation may have slightly improved efficacy, it seems prudent that therapy should now be initiated with extended release metformin whenever possible.

Dysgeusia

Approximately 1–5% of patients treated with metformin will complain of an unpleasant or metallic taste in their mouths. This usually resolves spontaneously; if not, some clinicians find it helpful for the patient to try taking metformin with saltine crackers or a lemon hard candy (sugar free) to help reduce the unpleasant taste.

Dermatological Reactions

In controlled trials, the incidence of rash or dermatitis in patients treated with metformin monotherapy was comparable to that of placebo.

Hematological Reactions

As mentioned above, metformin therapy may result in a small reduction in vitamin B_{12} levels; however, reports of megaloblastic anemia secondary to metformin are exceedingly rare. Annual monitoring of hematologic parameters is suggested. In patients at risk for low vitamin B_{12} levels (such as those with inadequate B_{12} or calcium intake), such levels should be checked every 2–3 years. Some recommend vitamin B_{12} supplementation in those with excessive use of alcohol, which may result in depletion of vitamin B_{12} stores.

DRUG INTERACTIONS

Antihyperglycemic Agents

Although metformin alone does not cause hypoglycemia, concomitant therapy with other antihyperglycemic agents can result in hypoglycemia, especially when changes in diet and physical activity occur. In a single-dose study of subjects with T2D, administration of metformin with glyburide did not result in changes in metformin pharmacokinetics or pharmacodynamics but did result in reductions in glyburide area under the curve (AUC) and C_{max}.[1] The clinical significance of this interaction is uncertain. In a single-dose study, administration of metformin with an α-glucosidase inhibitor resulted in a decrease in the bioavailability of metformin.[82] The clinical significance of this interaction is uncertain.

Other Drugs

Corticosteroids, such as prednisone, can cause hyperglycemia and lead to loss of glucose control in patients with diabetes. Concurrent use of these agents or agents with a similar impact on glucose may in effect lower the efficacy of metformin; the discontinuation of such agents could lead to hypoglycemia if metformin use is continued. Other drugs with the potential for causing hyperglycemia include: thiazide diuretics, estrogens, thyroid products, oral contraceptives, phenytoin, phenothiazines, niacin, sympathomimetics, β-blockers, calcium channel blockers, and isoniazid.

Metformin/furosemide interaction was studied in healthy subjects in a single-dose trial where both medications were affected. Furosemide caused an increase in metformin's C_{max} and AUC (22 and 15%, respectively) without altering metformin's renal clearance. Furosemide's C_{max} and AUC were reduced by 31 and 12%, respectively. The terminal half-life of furosemide was reduced by 32%, without any significant alteration in renal clearance.

Telmisartan reduced the AUC and C_{max} of metformin in healthy subjects but did not have an effect on glycemic control.

Agents that Enhance Effects of Metformin

The following drugs have the potential to enhance the glucose-lowering effects of metformin. Patients taking these agents with metformin should perform close monitoring of blood glucose to avoid hypoglycemia.

- Alpha-lipoic acid
- Androgens
- Guanethidine
- Mono-amine oxidase inhibitors
- Nifedipine
- Prothionamide
- Pegvisomant
- Salicylates
- Selective serotonin reuptake inhibitors (SSRIs)

Quinolones

Quinolone antibiotics taken with metformin can have a transient impact on metformin effectiveness, with both increases and decreases in effectiveness reported. Patients taking quinolones while taking metformin should monitor their blood glucose more closely to avoid hyper- or hypoglycemia, and to assure ongoing glucose control during antibiotic therapy.

Trospium

A study in healthy volunteers showed that taking metformin with trospium can decrease absorption of trospium. Patients taking both of these agents should be monitored closely for evidence of reduced trospium efficacy.

Cationic Drugs

An interaction between metformin and cimetidine has been observed in normal healthy subjects, with a 60% increase in peak metformin concentrations and a 40% increase in metformin AUC. However, in one single-dose study, the elimination half-life of metformin was unchanged. Metformin apparently has no effect on cimetidine kinetics.

Other compounds that are eliminated via renal tubular secretion have the potential for causing an interaction with metformin by competing for renal tubular transport systems; therefore, these drugs should be used cautiously. Examples include abemaciclib, amiloride, bictegravir, bupropion, cephalexin, dalfampridine, digoxin, dofetilide, dolutegravir, isavuconazonium, lamotrigine, morphine, ondansetron, procainamide, quinidine, quinine, ranitidine, ranolazine, topiramate, triamterene, trimethoprim, and vancomycin.

Agents with Increased Risk of Lactic Acidosis

The following drugs have potential to increase risk of lactic acidosis alone. When taken with metformin, caution should be taken to monitor for signs and symptoms of lactic acidosis as patients may be at increased risk for it.

- Carbonic anhydrase inhibitors
- Glycopyrrolate
- Topiramate
- Ombitasvir, paritaprevir, and ritonavir

Agents that Decrease Effects of Metformin

The following drugs have been found in small studies to significantly decrease the glucose-lowering effect of metformin. Increased self-monitoring of blood glucose should be performed when starting, stopping, or adjusting any of these agents.

- Patiromer
- Ritodrine
- Vandetanib
- Verapamil

β-Blockers

In a single-dose study of metformin taken with propranolol in healthy patients, neither drug was affected in its pharmacokinetic profile. However, β-adrenergic blocking agents as a class have potential for effects on blood glucose. β-Blockers can impair glucose tolerance, increase frequency and severity of hypoglycemia, alter the hemodynamic response to hypoglycemia, and delay the recovery of blood glucose following hypoglycemia. And, because nonselective β-blockers inhibit some of the typical response to hypoglycemia like tachycardia, the only sign of hypoglycemia patients may recognize is sweating.

Angiotensin-Converting Enzyme Inhibitors

Angiotensin-converting enzyme (ACE) inhibitors have been associated with unexplained hypoglycemia and increased insulin sensitivity. The risk of this effect is low, but patients taking metformin who are newly started on ACE inhibitors or who are adjusting doses or discontinuing them should monitor blood glucose for this potential effect.

Clomiphene

Metformin and other antihyperglycemic agents have been known to cause resumption of ovulation in premenopausal women with PCOS. Patients with this syndrome taking metformin, especially if taking clomiphene, should be aware that fertility and chance of pregnancy may improve.

DOSAGE AND ADMINISTRATION

Based on the reduced risk of gastrointestinal intolerance, current pricing for some extended-release formulations, and data supporting the comparable efficacy of metformin extended-release and immediate-release formulations, it seems prudent to initiate therapy using the extended-release formulation.

The usual starting dose of the extended-release form is 500 mg once a day, given with the largest meal of the day. Doses may be titrated in increments of 1 tablet every week up to a maximum of 2,000 mg daily, given with the evening meal. This formulation may be useful to improve tolerance in individuals experiencing ongoing gastrointestinal side effects on the immediate-release formulation. In patients previously treated with immediate-release metformin, dosage may be safely switched to the extended-release form at the same total daily dose (up to 2,000 mg) given as one daily dose of the extended-release form.

When using immediate-release metformin, the usual starting dose is 500-mg metformin tablets once a day, given with the largest meal of the day. In those with anticipated poor gastrointestinal tolerance, a dose of 250 mg may be useful as a starting point. The importance of initiating metformin dosing with a full meal, especially when the first meal of the day is scant, should be reinforced to minimize gastrointestinal distress. Doses may be titrated in increments of one tablet every week up to a maximum effective dose of 2,000 mg per day, although the total maximum dose is 2,500 mg per day. Metformin is often administered at a dose of 1,000 mg twice a day with the morning and evening meals. If a dose of 2,500 mg is required, the patient may have improved tolerance if it is given three times a day with meals. The usual starting dose of 850-mg metformin tablets is once daily, given with the largest meal of the day. Dosage increases are usually made in increments of one tablet every other week given in divided doses up to a maximum of 2,550 mg per day. The most common maintenance dose is 850 mg given twice a day with the morning and evening meals. However, if necessary, patients may be given 850 mg three times a day with meals.

COMBINATION PRODUCTS

The use of combination products containing metformin and other antihypergly-cemic medications may be especially helpful for individuals with adherence challenges due to the complexity of taking multiple drug regimens and who may benefit from the dual action of two agents. When using a combination product, it is prudent to approach the decision with consideration to the benefit of each individual product on the health of the patient. An initial titration using metformin as a single agent is ideal to assess its efficacy (e.g., A1c reduction of 1–2%) and to reduce the risk of gastrointestinal toxicity that might occur with a fixed-dose combination without the flexibility to titrate the metformin to gastrointestinal tolerance. If efficacy is demonstrated and additional efficacy with a second agent is desired, a combination product can be useful to keep the dosing regimen simplified to one physical product while gaining the treatment advantages of two medications. In choosing a metformin combination product, the mechanism of action of the second product in the combination should be matched to the perceived therapeutic need for the patient. For example, if the patient appears to need enhanced insulin as well as the effects of metformin on hepatic glucose production and insulin sensitivity, the addition of a sulfonylurea to augment physiologic insulin release through a dual-drug product like glipizide/metformin combination may be useful. Table 6.1 provides a list of the currently available combination antihyperglycemic medications containing metformin, their current brand name information, and selected dose or formulation information.

MONOGRAPHS

BIGUANIDES

Metformin (Glucophage) and Metformin XR (Glucophage XR): https://dailymed.nlm.nih.gov/dailymed/drugInfo.cfm?setid=4a0166c7-7097-4e4a-9036-6c9a60d08fc6

REFERENCES

1. Glucophage—4079189 [package insert]. Princeton, NJ, Bristol-Myers Squibb Company, 2018, https://packageinserts.bms.com/pi/pi_glucophage.pdf

2. ElSayed NA, Aleppo G, Aroda VR, et al., American Diabetes Association. 9. Pharmacologic Approaches to Glycemic Treatment: Standards of Care in Diabetes—2023. *Diabetes Care* 2023;46(Suppl. 1):S140–S157

3. ElSayed NA, Aleppo G, Aroda VR, et al., American Diabetes Association. Prevention or Delay of Type 2 Diabetes and Associated Comorbidities:

Standards of Care in Diabetes—2023. *Diabetes Care* 2023;46(Suppl. 1):S41–S48

4. Top W, Stehouwer C, Lehert P, Kooy A. Metformin and β-cell function in insulin-treated patients with type 2 diabetes: A randomized placebo-controlled 4.3-year trial. *Diabetes Obes Metab* 2018 Mar;20(3):730–733. DOI:10.1111/dom.13123. Epub 27 Oct 2017

5. Wu T, Xie C, Wu H, Jones KL, Horowitz M, Rayner CK. Metformin reduces the rate of small intestinal glucose absorption in type 2 diabetes. *Diabetes Obes Metab* 2017;19(2):290–293. DOI:10.1111/dom.12812. Epub 21 Nov 2016

6. Bahne E, Sun EWL, Young RL, Hansen M, Sonne DP, Hansen JS, Rohde U, Liou AP, Jackson ML, de Fontgalland D, Rabbitt P, Hollington P, Sposato L, Due S, Wattchow DA, Rehfeld JF, Holst JJ, Keating DJ, Vilsbøll T, Knop FK. Metformin-induced glucagon-like peptide-1 secretion contributes to the actions of metformin in type 2 diabetes. *JCI Insight* 2018;3(23). pii: 93936. DOI:10.1172/jci.insight.93936

7. Pascale A, Marchesi N, Govoni S, Coppola A, Gazzaruso C. The role of gut microbiota in obesity, diabetes mellitus, and effect of metformin: new insights into old diseases. *Curr Opin Pharmcol* 2019;49:1–5

8. Rodriguiez, J, Hiel S, Delzenne NM. Metformin: old friend, new ways of action—implication of the gut microbiome? *Curr Opin Clin Nutr Metab Care* 2018;21:294–301

9. Matthews DR, Paldánius PM, Proot P, Chiang Y, Stumvoll M, Del Prato S; VERIFY study group. Glycaemic durability of an early combination therapy with vildagliptin and metformin versus sequential metformin monotherapy in newly diagnosed type 2 diabetes (VERIFY): a 5-year, multicentre, randomised, double-blind trial. *Lancet* 2019;394(10208):1519–1529. DOI:10.1016/S0140-6736(19)32131–2. Epub 18 Sep 2019

10. Mokta JK, Ramesh, Sahai AK, Kaundal PK, Mokta K. Comparison of safety and efficacy of glimepiride-metformin and vildagliptin- metformin treatment in newly diagnosed type 2 diabetic patients. *J Assoc Physicians India* 2018 Aug;66(8):30–35

11. Takahashi H, Nishimura R, Tsujino D, Utsunomiya K. Which is better, high-dose metformin monotherapy or low-dose metformin/linagliptin combination therapy, in improving glycemic variability in type 2 diabetes patients with insufficient glycemic control despite lowdose metformin monotherapy? A randomized, cross-over, continuous glucose monitoring-based pilot study. *J Diabetes Investig* 2019;10(3):714–722. DOI:0.1111/jdi.12922. Epub 9 Oct 2018

12. Lukito AA, Pranata R, Henrina J, Lim MA, Lawrensia S, Suastika K. The effect of metformin consumption on mortality in hospitalized COVID-19 patients: a systematic review and meta-analysis. *Diabetes Metab Syndr* 2020 Nov-Dec;14(6):2177-2183. DOI:10.1016/j.dsx.2020.11.006. Epub 2020 Nov 11. PMID: 33395778

13. Yang W, Sun X, Zhang J, et al. The effect of metformin on mortality and severity in COVID-19 patients with diabetes mellitus. *Diab Res Clin Pract* 2021;178:108977. DOI:10.1016/j.diabres.2021.108977

14. Ganesh A and Randall MD. Does metformin affect outcomes in COVID-19 patients with new or pre-existing diabetes mellitus? A systematic review and meta-analysis. *BJCP* 2022;88:2642–2656

15. Morley LC, Tang T, Yasmin E, et al. Insulin sensitising drugs (metformin, rosiglitazone, pioglitazone, D-chiro-inositol) for women with polycystic ovary syndrome, oligo amenorrhoea and subfertility. *Cochrane Database Syst Rev* 2017;11:CDO03053. DOI:10.1002/14651858.CD003053.pub6

16. Yang PK, Hsu CY, Chen MJ, et al. The efficacy of 24-month metformin for improving menses, hormones, and metabolic profiles in polycystic ovary syndrome. *J Clin Endocrinol Metab* 2018;103:890–899

17. ElSayed NA, Aleppo G, Aroda VR, et al., American Diabetes Association. 15. Management of Diabetes in Pregnancy: Standards of Care in Diabetes—2023. *Diabetes Care* 2023;46(Suppl. 1):S254–S266

18. Knowler WC, Barrett-Connor E, Fowler SE, et al. Reduction in the incidence of type 2 diabetes with lifestyle intervention or metformin. *N Engl J Med* 2002;346(6):393–403

19. Diabetes Prevention Program Research Group, Knowler WC. 10-year follow-up of diabetes incidence and weight loss in the Diabetes Prevention Program Outcomes Study. *Lancet* 2009;374(9702):1677–1686

20. Goldberg RB, Aroda VR, Bluemke DA, et al.; Diabetes Prevention Program Research Group. Effect of long-term metformin and lifestyle in the diabetes prevention program and its outcome study on coronary artery calcium. *Circulation* 2017;136(1):52–64. DOI:10.1161/CIRCULATIONAHA.116. 025483. Epub 5May 2017

21. Herman WH, Pan Q, Edelstein SL, et al.; Diabetes Prevention Program Research Group. Impact of lifestyle and metformin interventions on the risk of progression to diabetes and regression to normal glucose regulation in overweight or obese people with impaired glucose regulation. *Diabetes Care* 2017;40(12):1668–1677. DOI:10.2337/dc17-1116. Epub 11 Oct 2017. Erratum in: *Diabetes Care* 2018 Feb 23; *Diabetes Care* 2019;42(4):701

22. Kulkarni S, Xavier D, George B, et al. Effect of intensive lifestyle modification and metformin on cardiovascular risk in prediabetes: A pilot randomized control trial. *Indian J Med Res* 2018;148(6):705–712. DOI:10.4103/ ijmr.IJMR_1201_17

23. Terada T, Boulé NG. Does metformin therapy influence the effects of intensive lifestyle intervention? Exploring the interaction between first line therapies in the Look AHEAD trial. *Metabolism* 2019;94:39–46. DOI:10.1016/j.metabol.2019.01.004. Epub 14 Jan 2019

24. O'Brien MJ, Perez A, Scanlan AB, et al. PREVENT-DM comparative effectiveness trial of lifestyle intervention and metformin. *Am J Prev Med*

2017;52(6):788–797. DOI:10.1016/j.amepre.2017.01.008. Epub 22 Feb 2017

25. González-Heredia T, Hernández-Corona DM, González-Ortiz M, Martínez-Abundis E. Effect of linagliptin versus metformin on glycemic variability in patients with impaired glucose tolerance. *Diabetes Technol Ther* 2017;19(8):471–475. DOI:10.1089/dia.2017.0020. Epub 5 Jun 2017

26. RISE Consortium. Impact of insulin and metformin versus metformin alone on β-cell function in youth with impaired glucose tolerance or recently diagnosed type 2 diabetes. *Diabetes Care* 2018;41(8):1717–1725. DOI:10.2337/dc18-0787. Epub 25 Jun 2018

27. Rowan JA, Hague WM, Gao W, et al. Metformin versus insulin for the treatment of gestational diabetes. *N Engl J Med* 2008;358:2003–2015

28. Nicholson W, Bolen S, Witkop CT, et al. Benefits and risks of oral diabetes agents compared with insulin in women with gestational diabetes: a systematic review. *Obstet Gynecol* 2009;113:193–205

29. Dhulkotia JS, Ola B, Fraser R, Farrell T. Oral hypoglycemic agents vs insulin in management of gestational diabetes: a systematic review and meta-analysis. *Am J Obstet Gynecol* 2010;203(5):457.e1–9

30. Balsells M, García-Patterson A, Solà I, et al. Glibenclamide, metformin, and insulin for the treatment of gestational diabetes: a systematic review and meta-analysis. *BMJ* 2015;350:h102

31. Jiang YF, Chen XY, Ding T, et al. Comparative efficacy and safety of OADs in management of GDM: network meta-analysis of randomized controlled trials. *J Clin Endocrinol Metab* 2015;100:2017–2080

32. Finneran MM, Landon MB. Oral agents for the treatment of gestational diabetes. *Curr Diab Rep* 2018;18(11):119

33. Patti AM, Giglio RV, Pafili K, Rizzo M, Papanas N. Pharmacotherapy for gestational diabetes. *Expert Opin Pharmacother* 2018;19(13):1407–1414.

34. Martis R, Crowther CA, Shepherd E, Alsweiler J, Downie MR, Brown J. Treatments for women with gestational diabetes mellitus: an overview of Cochrane systematic reviews. *Cochrane Database Syst Rev* 2018;8:CD012327

35. Priya G, Kaira S. Metformin in the managements of diabetes during pregnancy and lactation. *Drugs Context* 2018;7:212523

36. Feig DS, Donovan LE, Zinman B, et al. Metformin in women with type 2 diabetes in pregnancy (MITy): a multicenter, international, randomized, placebo-controlled trial. *Lancet Diab Endocrinol* 2020;10:834-844

37. Bao LX, Shi WT, Han YX. Metformin versus insulin for gestational diabetes: a systematic review and meta-anlysis. *J Matern Fetal Neonatal Med* 2021;34(16):2741–2753

38. UK Prospective Diabetes Study (UKPDS) Group. Effect of intensive blood-glucose control with metformin on complications in overweight patients with type 2 diabetes (UKPDS 34). *Lancet* 1998;352(9131):854–865

39. Holman RR, Paul SK, Bethel A, Matthews DR, Neil HA. 10-year follow-up of intensive glucose control in type 2 diabetes. *N Engl J Med* 2008;359(15):1577–1589

40. Rojas LB, Gomez MB. Metformin: an old but still the best treatment for type 2 diabetes. *Diabetol Metab Syndr* 2013;5:6

41. Selvin E, Bolen S, Yeh HC, et al. Cardiovascular outcomes in trials of oral diabetes medications: a systematic review. *Arch Int Med* 2008;168:2070–2080

42. Goldberg RB, Orchard TJ, Crandall JP, et al.; Diabetes Prevention Program Research Group. Effects of long-term metformin and lifestyle interventions on cardiovascular events in the diabetes prevention program and its outcome study. *Circulation* 2022;145:1632–1641

43. Lee CG, Heckman-Stoddard B, Dabelea D, et al.; Diabetes Prevention Program Research Group. Effects of metformin and lifestyle interventions on mortality in the diabetes prevention program and diabetes prevention program outcomes study. *Diabetes Care* 2021;44:2775–2782

44. Petrie JR, Chaturvedi N, Ford I, et al.; REMOVAL Study Group. Cardiovascular and metabolic effects of metformin in patients with type 1 diabetes (REMOVAL): a double-blind, randomised, placebo-controlled trial. *Lancet Diabetes Endocrinol* 2017;5(8):597–609. DOI:10.1016/S2213-8587(17)30194-8. Epub 11 Jun 2017. Erratum in: *Lancet Diabetes Endocrinol* 2017;5(8):e5. *Lancet Diabetes Endocrinol* 2017 Nov;5(11):e7

45. MacDonald MR, Eurich DT, Majumdar S, et al. Treatment of type 2 diabetes and outcomes in patients with heart failure: a nested case–control study from the UK General Practice Research Database. *Diabetes Care* 2010;33:1213–1218

46. Ochola LA, Nyamu DG, Guantai EM, Weru IW. Metformin's effectiveness in preventing prednisone-induced hyperglycemia in hematological cancers. *J Oncol Pharm Pract* 2020;26(4):823-834

47. Seelig E, Meyer S, Timper K, et al. Metformin prevents metabolic side effects during systemic glucocorticoid treatment. *Eur J Endocrinol* 2017;176(3):349–358. DOI:10.1530/EJE-16-0653. Epub 10 Jan 2017

48. Vestergaard, P. Discrepancies in bone mineral density and fracture risk in patients with type 1 and type 2 diabetes—a meta-analysis. *Osteoporosis Int* 2007;18(4):427–444

49. Janghorbani M, Van Dam RM, Willett WC, Hu FB. Systematic review of type 1 and type 2 diabetes mellitus and risk of fracture. *Am J Epidemiol* 2007;166(5):495–505

50. Stage TB, Christensen MH, Jørgensen NR, et al. Effects of metformin, rosiglitazone and insulin on bone metabolism in patients with type 2 diabetes. *Bone* 2018;112:35–41. DOI:10.1016/j.bone.2018.04.004. Epub 12 Apr 2018

51. Nordklint AK, Almdal TP, Vestergaard P, et al. The effect of metformin versus placebo in combination with insulin analogues on bone mineral den-

sity and trabecular bone score in patients with type 2 diabetes mellitus: a randomized placebo-controlled trial. *Osteoporos Int* 2018;29(11):2517–2526. DOI:10.1007/s00198-018- 4637-z. Epub 19 Jul 2018

52. Hazuda HP, Pan Q, Florez H, Luchsinger JA, Crandall JP, Venditti EM, Golden SH, Kriska AM, Bray GA. Association of Intensive Lifestyle and Metformin Interventions With Frailty in the Diabetes Prevention Program Outcomes Study. *J Gerontol A Biol Sci Med Sci* 2021;76(5):929–936

53. Schwartz AV, PanQ, Aroda VR, Crandall JP, Kriska A, Piromalli C, Wallia A, Temprosa M, Florez H. Long-term effects on lifestyle and metformin interventiosn in DPP on bone density. Osteoporos Int. 2021;32(11):2279–2287

54. Guo M, Shang X, Guo D. Metformin Use and Mortality in Women with Ovarian Cancer: An Updated Meta-Analysis. *Int J Clin Pract* 2022:9592969.

55. Tang YL, Zhu LH, Li Y, et al. Metformin use is associated with reduced incidence and improved survival of endometrial cancer: a meta-analysis. *BioMed Res Int* 2017;2017:5905384

56. Zhou PT, Li B, Liu FR, et al. Metformin is associated with survival benefit in pancreatic cancer patients with diabetes: a systematic review and meta-analysis. *Oncotarget* 2017;8(15):25422–25250

57. Zhou DC, Gong H, Chong-Qing T, et al. Prognostic significance of anti-diabetic medications in pancreatic cancer: a meta-analysis. *Oncotarget* 2017;8(37):62349–62357

58. Li X, Li T, Liu Z, et al. The effect of metformin on survival of patients with pancreatic cancer: a meta-analysis. *Sci Rep* 2017;7(1):5825

59. Jian-Yu E, Graber JM, Lu SE, et al. Effect of metformin and statin use on survival in pancreatic cancer patients: a systematic literature review and meta-analysis. *Curr Med Chem* 2018;25(22):2595–2607

60. Li Q, Xu H, Sui C, Zhang H. Impact of metformin use on risk and mortality of hepatocellular carcinoma in diabetes mellitus. *Clin Res Hepatol Gastroenterol* 2022;46(2):101781

61. Liu F, Yan L, Wang Z, et al. Metformin therapy and risk of colorectal adenomas and colorectal cancer in type 2 diabetes mellitus patients: a systematic review and meta-analysis. *Oncotarget* 2017;8(9):16017–16026

62. Du L, Wang M, Kang Y, et al. Prognostic role of metformin intake in diabetic patients with colorectal cancer: an updated qualitative evidence of cohort studies. *Oncotarget* 2017;8(16):26448–26459

63. Tian S, Lei HB, Liu YL, et al. The association between metformin use and colorectal cancer survival among patients with diabetes mellitus: an updated meta-analysis. *Chronic Dis Trans Med* 2017;3(3):169–175

64. Wang Q and Shi M. Effect of metformin use on the risk and prognosis of colorectal cancer in diabetes mellitus: a meta-analysis. *Anticancer Drugs* 2022;33(2):191–199

65. Chen CB, Eskin M, Eurich DT, et al. Metformin, Asian ethnicity and risk of prostate cancer in type 2 diabetes: a systematic review and meta-analysis. *BMC Cancer* 2018;18(1):65

66. Zhou XL, Xue WH, Ding XF, et al. Association between metformin and the risk of gastric cancer in patients with type 2 diabetes mellitus: a meta-analysis of cohort studies. *Oncotarget* 2017;8(33):55622–55631

67. Wen j, Yi Z, Chen Y, et al. Efficacy of metformin therapy in patients with cancer: a meta-analysis of 22 randomised controlled trials. *BMC Med* 2022 Oct 24;20(1):402

68. Giovannucci E, Harlan DM, Archer MC, et al. Diabetes and cancer: a consensus report. *CA Cancer J Clin* 2010;60:207–221

69. Cao X, Wen ZS, Wang XD, et al. The clinical effect of metformin on the survival of lung cancer patients with diabetes: a comprehensive systematic review and meta-analysis of retrospective studies. *J Cancer* 2017;8(13):2532–2541

70. Metformin in Longevity Study (MILES) [Internet], 2018. Available from https://clinicaltrials.gov/ct2/show/study/NCT02432287

71. Targeting Aging with Metformin (TAME) [Internet]. Available from American Federation for Aging Research, https://www.afar.org/research/TAME/

72. Zhang QQ, Li WS, Liu Z, Zhang HL, Ba YG, Zhang RX. Metformin therapy and cognitive dysfunction in patients with type 2 diabetes: a meta-analysis and systematic review. *Medicine* (Baltimore) 2020;99(10):e19378

73. Zhou JB, Tang X, Han M, Yang J, Simo R. Impact of antidiabetic agents on dementia risk: a Bayesian network meta-analysis. *Metabolism*. 2020; 109:154265

74. Malazy OT, Bandarian F, Qorbani M, et al. The effect of metformin on cognitive function: A systematic review and meta-analysis. *J Psychopharm* 2022:36(6);666–679

75. FDA Drug Safety Communication: FDA revises warnings regarding use of the diabetes medicine metformin in certain patients with reduced kidney function. U.S. Food and Drug Administration, April 2017. Available from https://www.fda.gov/Drugs/DrugSafety/ucm493244.htm

76. Mills EP, Brown KPD, Smith JD, et al. Treating nonalcoholic fatty liver disease in patients with type 2 diabetes mellitus: a review of efficacy and safety. *Ther Adv Endocrinol Metab* 2018;9(1):15–28. Published online 2017 Dec 7. DOI:10.1177/2042018817741852

77. de Jager J, Kooy A, Lehert P, et al. Long term treatment with metformin in patients with type 2 diabetes and risk of vitamin B-12 deficiency: randomised placebo controlled trial. *BMJ* 2010;340:c2181

78. Glucovance [package insert]. Princeton, NJ, Bristol-Myers Squibb Company, 2017. Available from https://packageinserts.bms.com/pi/pi_glucovance.pdf

79. Salpeter SR, Greyber E, Pasternak GA, Salpeter EE. Risk of fatal and non-fatal lactic acidosis with metformin use in type 2 diabetes mellitus. *Arch Intern Med* 2003;163:2594–2602

80. Salpeter SR, Greyber E, Pasternak GA, Salpeter EE. Risk of fatal and non-fatal lactic acidosis with metformin use in type 2 diabetes mellitus. *Cochrane Database Syst Rev* 2010(4):CD002967. DOI:10.1002/14651858.CD002967. pub4

81. Bodmer M, Meier C, Krähenbühl S, et al. Metformin, sulfonylureas, or other antidiabetes drugs and the risk of lactic acidosis or hypoglyemia. *Diabetes Care* 2008;31:2086–2091

82. Scheen AJ, Ferreira Alves de Magalhaes AC, Salvatore T, et al. Reduction of the acute bioavailability of metformin by the alpha-glucosidase inhibitor acarbose in normal man. *Eur J Clin Invest* 1993;23(1):A43

Chapter 7
Thiazolidinediones

Kam L. Capoccia, PharmD, BCPS, CDCES
Peggy Soule Odegard, BSPharm, PharmD, CDCES

INTRODUCTION

The first thiazolidinedione (TZD), ciglitazone, was synthesized in 1982. It was soon thereafter discovered that ciglitazone reduced insulin resistance in obese and diabetic animals. Because of their effects on insulin resistance, TZDs have been developed as pharmacological agents for the management of T2D, although they were initially synthesized as potential lipid-reducing agents. Since their discovery, three TZDs have been introduced to the market in the U.S.: troglitazone (Rezulin), rosiglitazone (Avandia), and pioglitazone (Actos). In 2013, the FDA removed the Risk Evaluation and Mitigation Strategy (REMS) program and lifted restrictions on prescribing and dispensing rosiglitazone after concluding that data did not show a higher risk of heart attack with rosiglitazone compared with the standard T2D drugs of metformin and sulfonylurea. Currently, pioglitazone and rosiglitazone are available.

These compounds are taken orally and are unrelated to the other oral antihyperglycemic agents either chemically or by mechanism of action. A thiazolidine-2-4-dione structure is common to these drugs, with differences in potency, receptor binding, metabolic effects, pharmacokinetics, and side effects, governed by modifications in the side chain.[1,2]

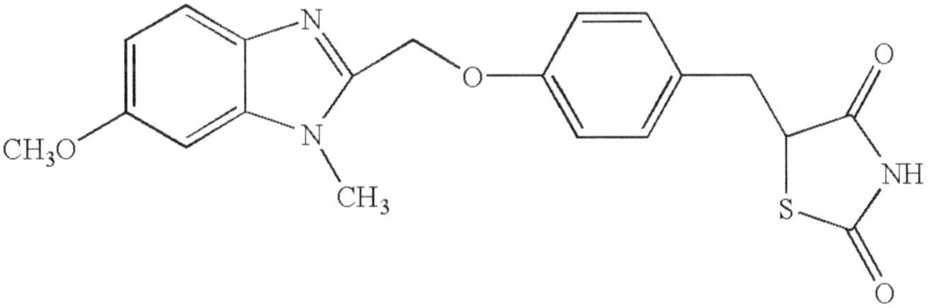

Figure 7.1—Thiazolidine-2-4-dione structure.

TZDs have been used in the management of T2D as monotherapeutic agents and in combination with insulin, GLP-1 RAs, and other oral antihyperglycemic agents (metformin, DPP-4 inhibitors, SGLT2 inhibitors, meglitinides, and sulfonylureas). Additionally, they have been studied and found to be effective in treating insulin-resistace, nonalcoholic steatohepatitis (NASH), as well as having beneficial effects in some cardiovascular conditions. TZDs are sometimes referred to as "insulin sensitizers."

PHARMACOLOGY

MECHANISM OF ACTION

The relative importance of the mechanisms of action of TZDs are related to their effects on gene regulation. The primary mechanism of action appears to be the direct stimulation of a family of receptors on the nuclear surface of cells that are responsible for the modulation of lipid homeostasis, adipocyte differentiation, and insulin action. TZDs are potent and highly selective agonists for one of the isoforms in this family of receptors, known as peroxisome proliferator-activated receptor γ (PPARγ), which is predominantly expressed in white adipose tissue but also found in brown adipose tissue, muscle, kidney, liver, pancreatic β-cells, vascular endothelium, and macrophages. The TZDs also display some cross-reactivity with other isoforms in the PPAR family; PPARα (alpha), which is found in the liver, cardiac, and skeletal muscle, and PPARβ/δ (beta/delta), which is found in the liver, skeletal muscle, kidney, intestines, and esophagus. The effects of TZDs on PPARα and PPAR β/δ on human tissues remain unclear. Different relative affinities of pioglitazone and rosiglitazone for these three receptor types may explain the different effects that these two agents have on lipid profiles and other organ systems in the body.

These drugs improve glycemic control by increasing insulin sensitivity. PPARγ is the most important of these three receptors in terms of the antihyperglycemic action of TZDs. A relationship between the ability to stimulate PPARγ and antihyperglycemic activity is well understood. TZDs stimulate the expression of genes responsible for the production of glucose transporters (GLUT1 and GLUT4). PPARγ stimulation reduces TNF-α (tumor necrosis factor alpha), resulting in an anti-inflammatory effect and reducing hepatic glucokinase expression, which improves glucose homeostasis.

TZDs cause a reduction in the number of large adipocytes and an increase in the number of small adipocytes, leading to lower free fatty acid and triglyceride levels. PPARγ in the muscle and liver accounts for improved insulin sensitivity and glucose metabolism. The pleiotropic effects and implications of the TZDs have been described in the literature. Pioglitazone has been shown to improve endothelial dysfunction and improve dyslipidemia. Notably, there is a difference on cardiovascular outcomes favoring pioglitazone over rosiglitazone.[3] The cardiovascular data describing these differences is discussed further in this chapter.

PHARMACOKINETICS

Pioglitazone

Following the administration of pioglitazone, C_{max} occurs within approximately 2 h. Food may delay the absorption rate and time to C_{max} but not the extent of absorption. Pioglitazone may be taken without regard to meals. It is extensively bound, primarily to albumin (>99%), and its metabolites M-III and M-IV are >98% bound. The apparent mean volume of distribution (Vd) is 0.63 ±0.41 L/kg. Pioglitazone is extensively metabolized via oxidation and hydroxylation, with metabolites being partially converted to glucuronide or sulfate conjugates. Metabolites M-III (keto derivatives) and M-IV (hydroxy derivatives), along with parent pioglitazone, are the predominant species found in human serum at steady state. Approximately 15–30% of pioglitazone can be recovered in the urine and feces following oral administration. The mean serum half-lives of pioglitazone and pioglitazone metabolites are 3–7 h and 16–24 h, respectively. Pioglitazone clearance is 5–7 L/h.[1]

Rosiglitazone

Following the administration of rosiglitazone, C_{max} occurs within 1 h. Food may delay the absorption rate and time to C_{max}, but the extent of absorption is not clinically significantly changed. Rosiglitazone may be taken without regard to meals. It is extensively bound to serum protein (>99.8%), primarily albumin. The apparent mean volume of distribution (Vd) was 17.6 L/kg. Rosiglitazone is extensively metabolized via *N*-demethylation and hydroxylation, followed by conjugation with glucuronic acid or sulfate. No unchanged drug is found in the urine. The metabolites of rosiglitazone are less potent than the parent compound and are not thought to contribute to the insulin-sensitizing effects of the drug. After administration of labeled rosiglitazone, ~64% is eliminated via the urine and 23% is eliminated via the feces. The serum half-life for rosiglitazone is 3–4 h, which is prolonged by approximately 2 h in patients with moderate-to-severe hepatic impairment. Rosiglitazone clearance is ~3 L/h.[2]

While the serum half-lives of pioglitazone and rosiglitazone are several hours, the onset of action and duration of effect is delayed due to their mechanism of action. The initial effect on glucose may be seen within a few weeks but it could take upward of a few months to see the maximum effect of these drugs, due to the time intensive mechanism of altering gene expression. Similarly, when these drugs are discontinued, there is a delayed effect on the subsequent rise in glucose.

TREATMENT ADVANTAGES/DISADVANTAGES

As a class, the TZDs are effective in reducing hyperglycemia in patients with T2D. Reductions in hyperglycemia vary significantly between patients. Some researchers have even suggested the terms "responders" and "non-responders" in the population of patients treated with TZDs. A1C lowering can be expected to fall somewhere between 0.5 and 1.5% in most patients. There is no difference between pioglitazone and rosiglitazone in their glucose-lowering effects.

The advantage of the TZDs is predominantly the durability of their insulin-sensitizing effects. Regardless of the amount of insulin secretion in the body, the TZDs still work to decrease peripheral insulin resistance, while other oral antihyperglycemic agents (sulfonylureas, meglitinides) are dependent on insulin secretion and therefore ineffective when the pancreas is no longer secreting insulin. TZDs enhance insulin sensitivity through a variety of mechanisms in multiple tissues (adipose, liver, muscle). As a result, they are valuable agents in the management of metabolic syndrome, due to the underlying cause of insulin resistance.

TZDs have positive effects on the pancreatic β-cell through increased insulin capacity and protection from oxidative stress. They have been shown to improve or preserve β-cell function. The Diabetes Reduction Assessment With Ramipril and Rosiglitazone Medication (DREAM) study showed a 62% reduction in the development of T2D followed for a median of 3 years, while the Actos Now for the Prevention of Diabetes (ACT NOW) study showed a 72% reduction in the development of diabetes with a median follow-up of 2.4 years.[4,5] The Insulin Resistance Intervention after Stroke (IRIS) trial showed a 52% reduction in the development of diabetes with pioglitazone during a median follow-up of 4.8 years.[6] In a subgroup analysis of people with prediabetes and good adherence in the IRIS trial, pioglitazone reduced new onset diabetes by 80%.[7] These studies demonstrated the preservation of β-cell function as well as the insulin-sensitizing effects of TZDs. This class of drugs is useful if metformin is contraindicated or cannot be used and an insulin-sensitizing agent is needed. TZDs are also beneficial if trying to reduce the risk of hypoglycemia or in those occupations that preclude the use of insulin.

The expression of PPARγ in the kidneys may account for the renal benefits seen with TZDs. Pioglitazone and rosiglitazone have shown reductions in albuminuria in people with T2D.[8,9] In hemodialysis patients, those treated with TZDs and/or insulin experienced a reduction in all-cause mortality compared to those treated with other oral agents.[10]

The expression of PPAR in the liver likely accounts for the benefits seen with TZDs in people with T2D and nonalcoholic fatty liver disease (NAFLD). Improvements in fibrosis and resolution of NASH have been shown with both rosiglitazone and pioglitazone. Continued use of these agents is necessary to sustain these results.[11]

Rosiglitazone and pioglitazone have different effects on lipid profiles. This difference may be related to the relative effect of these agents on the PPARγ nuclear receptor. Pioglitazone has a higher affinity for PPARγ and is associated with improvements in the lipid profile (reduction of triglycerides, increase in HDL-C, and neutral effect on LDL-C). On the other hand, rosiglitazone raises LDL-C levels and the reduction in triglycerides and increase in HDL-C is less than that seen with pioglitazone.

There have been numerous publications with conflicting results suggesting that rosiglitazone is associated with an increased risk of myocardial infarction (MI) and other cardiovascular events. However, several studies have shown that rosiglitazone does not increase cardiovascular mortality or all-cause mortality. In the Rosiglitazone Evaluated for Cardiovascular Outcomes in Oral Agents Combination Therapy for Type 2 Diabetes (RECORD) trial, the primary study endpoint was hospitalization for acute MI, CHF, stroke, unstable angina, transient ischemic attack, unplanned revascularization, amputation of extremities, or any other definitive cardiovascular reason, or cardiovascular mortality. In 4,447 patients with T2D, rosiglitazone was added to metformin or sulfonylurea and compared to a control group of metformin plus sulfonylurea with dose titration to a target A1C of ≤7%. The incidence of HF was greater with rosiglitazone (2.7% compared to control 1.3%, HR 2.10 [CI 1.35–3.27]), but there were no statistically significant differences between rosiglitazone and control groups for MI, stroke, or death.[12] According to a meta-analysis by Mannucci and colleagues, there was no increase in all-cause or cardiovascular mortality observed with rosiglitazone. However, when rosiglitazone was combined with insulin, there was an increased risk of CHF (OR 2.20 [CI 1.28–3.78]).[13] Postmarketing studies indicate the risk of CHF is higher in patients taking TZDs, even with no previously known heart disease. Although change in mortality has not been found to be significant, patients with history of cardiovascular disease, especially those aged 65 years and over, were found to have higher incidence of serious HF requiring hospitalization when taking TZDs.[14-16]

Pioglitazone has been shown to reduce cardiovascular event rates in the PROspective pioglitAzone Clinical Trial In macroVascular Events (PROactive) trial, a large, prospective, randomized, placebo-controlled outcome trial. The study enrolled 5,238 patients with T2D who had a history of a previous cardiovascular event or multiple risk factors for cardiovascular disease. The primary outcome was a composite of seven different cardiovascular endpoints; a 10% reduction was observed but it did not reach statistical significance ($P = 0.09$). However, there was a statistically significant 16% decrease in the secondary endpoint of all-cause mortality, myocardial infarction, and stroke. Pioglitazone was titrated from 15 mg to 45 mg in more than 90% of the patients, compared with at least 95% of those on placebo who reached the maximum dose. Since its original publication in 2005, there have been 19 additional publications from the PROactive investigators describing various subanalyses. Of note, PROactive 04 described a 47% reduction in the incidence of recurrent stroke (HR 0.53 [95% CI 0.34–0.85]; $P = 0.008$).[17,18]

In the IRIS trial, pioglitazone demonstrated a decreased risk of recurring stroke or transient ischemic attack and myocardial infarction in people with insulin resistance who did not have diabetes.[19] A meta-analysis by Lee and colleagues describes three randomized trials of pioglitazone use in stroke patients with insulin resistance, prediabetes, and diabetes.[20] Although there was no evidence of an effect on all-cause mortality, pioglitazone was associated with lower risk of recurrent stroke (HR 0.68 [CI 0.50–0.92]; $P = 0.01$) and a lower risk of future vascular events (HR 0.75 [CI 0.64–0.87]; $P = 0.0001$).[19,20] In the RECORD trial, there was a nonsignificant reduction in stroke events when rosiglitazone was added to either metformin or sulfonylurea compared to the metformin-sulfonylurea combination group.[21]

The disadvantages of TZDs are related to the side-effect profile of this class of drugs and likely outweigh the benefits for the majority of patients. This class of drugs is contraindicated in patients with NYHA class III or IV HF. Fluid retention leading to weight gain and peripheral edema may cause or exacerbate CHF. TZDs should not be used in anyone with a history of or active bladder cancer. They also increase the risk of fractures in postmenopausal women and elderly men and therefore should be avoided in these populations. These side effects are further described below in the "Significant Warnings/Precautions" section.

Generally speaking, the use of pioglitazone is favored over rosiglitazone due to its beneficial effects on the lipid profile, in NASH, at lower doses, as well as its cardiovascular benefit of decreasing the risk of recurring stroke or TIA in people with insulin resistance. Due to its pleiotropic effects that improve endothelial dysfunction, improve pancreatic β-cell function, reduce blood pressure, improve dyslipidemia, reduce proteinuria, and reduce circulating levels of inflammatory cytokines, pioglitazone is the preferred TZD.[22] Lower doses (7.5–15 mg) have demonstrated fewer side effects with significant improvements in A1C reduction, fasting plasma glucose, PPG, lipid profiles, pancreatic β-cell function, and insulin resistance.[23-26] The addition of low-dose pioglitazone could be incredibly helpful to an obese person who has diabetes and a significant degree of insulin resistance. Low dose pioglitazone (7.5 mg) was also shown to be beneficial and safe in people with T2D and chronic kidney disease.[27] The low dose may reduce risk or minimize the unwanted side effects of weight gain and fluid retention, while potentially decreasing negative cardiovascular outcomes and the amount of or need for insulin or other medicines for T2D, while improving glucose homeostasis and reducing A1C. Pioglitazone is a viable option when the primary patient-specific factors are insulin resistance, secondary stroke prevention, cost and/or hypoglycemia.

THERAPEUTIC CONSIDERATIONS

SIGNIFICANT WARNINGS/PRECAUTIONS

T1D

These agents should not be used to treat people with T1D or to manage patients in diabetic ketoacidosis.

Hypoglycemia

The risk of hypoglycemia is increased when a TZD is combined with another agent known to cause hypoglycemia such as insulin or sulfonylureas. A decrease in dose of insulin and/or sulfonylurea will likely be necessary to reduce the risk of hypoglycemia.

Ovulation

TZDs may cause resumption of ovulation in premenopausal women with anovulation secondary to insulin resistance. These patients may be at risk for unintended pregnancy. Contraception is recommended in these premenopausal women. TZDs have been studied as a treatment for anovulation in women with PCOS and have been shown to be effective. However, they are no longer recommended as first-line agents due to weight gain and increased risk of fractures.

Hematology

Dose-related reductions in hemoglobin and hematocrit have been observed in patients treated with pioglitazone and rosiglitazone. Reductions in hemoglobin and hematocrit with the TZDs are ≤4% and ≤1 g/dL, respectively. These changes are possibly due to volume expansion and have not been associated with significant hematological effects. The changes occur within the first 4–8 weeks of therapy and remain unchanged thereafter.

Weight Gain and Edema

Dose-related weight gain is the most common side effect of the TZDs. Pioglitazone and rosiglitazone typically cause weight gain of 1–5 kg when used as monotherapy, in combination with oral antihyperglycemic agents, or in combination with insulin. The mechanism of weight gain is not entirely clear but is likely related to the activation of the PPARγ receptors in adipose tissue, resulting in an increase of deposition, and in the kidney, resulting in the retention of salt and water. Edema, fluid retention, and weight gain are problematic in coexisting CHF and require increased patient monitoring. Of note, there is a favorable shift of fat accumulation from visceral to subcutaneous.

Cardiac

The prescribing information for rosiglitazone and pioglitazone includes a black box warning regarding CHF. TZDs are contraindicated in patients with NYHA class III or IV failure. Use of TZDs is not recommended in patients with symptomatic HF. Fluid retention may lead to or exacerbate CHF. Patients should be observed for signs and symptoms of CHF. If CHF develops, it should be managed according to current standards of care and discontinuation or dose reduction of TZDs must be considered.

Hepatic

No evidence of hepatotoxicity has been observed with either rosiglitazone or pioglitazone. In the phase 3 trials of rosiglitazone, 0.2% of patients treated with rosiglitazone had reversible elevations in alanine transaminase (ALT) greater than three times the upper limit of normal (ULN), compared with 0.2% of patients treated with placebo. In the phase 3 trials of pioglitazone, 0.26% of patients treated with pioglitazone had reversible elevations in ALT greater than three times the ULN, compared with 0.25% of patients treated with placebo. Because of the association between the first-marketed TZD (troglitazone) and fulminate hepatic failure, patients treated with TZDs should have their liver function tested prior to initiation of therapy and periodically thereafter. Troglitazone was removed from the market, leaving behind the concern that the hepatotoxic reaction might be a class effect. Although this concern has not been supported by data from the legions of patients treated with pioglitazone and rosiglitazone, testing is still recommended. Current recommendations state to test liver enzymes prior to initiation and periodically thereafter. Evaluate patients with ALT ≥2.5 times ULN at baseline or during therapy for cause of enzyme elevation. If ALT levels remain greater than three times ULN, therapy should be discontinued.

Bladder Cancer

Pioglitazone should not be used in patients with active or a history of bladder cancer. Associations between cumulative dose or cumulative duration of exposure to pioglitazone and bladder cancer have been unfounded. In the 10-year observational follow-up of patients completing PROactive, bladder cancer was reported in 0.8% of patients ($n = 14$) in the pioglitazone versus 1.2% ($n = 21$) in the placebo group [RR 0.65 [95% CI 0.33–1.28]).[28] Inconsistent findings and limitations inherent in these and other studies preclude conclusive interpretations of the observational data.[1]

Fractures

TZDs have demonstrated an increased incidence of bone fractures, especially peripheral factures in women. In the ADOPT and RECORD trials, rosiglitazone demonstrated an increased risk of limb fractures in the first year of treatment that persisted for the length of the trials.[2] In the PROactive trial, pioglitazone demonstrated an increased incidence of bone fracture in women of 5.1% (44/870) vs. 2.5% (23/905) for the placebo group. Fracture risk in men did not differ between the two groups.[17] Although the majority of data has demonstrated an increased risk of fracture in older women, men and younger patients may be susceptible as well. The mechanism is not entirely clear but studies have shown a change in bone mineral density and changes in biochemical markers of bone turnover.[29] Overall, TZDs should not be used in people who are at an increased risk of fracture.

Pregnancy and Nursing

Pioglitazone and rosiglitazone cross the placenta. However, there is limited information regarding the use of TZDs in pregnancy. Agents other than TZDs are recommended to treat T2D in pregnancy. It is unknown if TZDs are excreted in breast milk. Therefore, breast-feeding women should not take TZDs as the current evidence is inconclusive.

SPECIAL POPULATIONS

TZDs are not recommended as first-line agents in the treatment of T2D. However, they are used as dual- or triple-combination therapy for the management of T2D when cost and/or hypoglycemia are patient-specific considerations. TZDs continue to be studied for new applications and potential effectiveness in the treatment of other conditions and diseases.[30] The various cellular effects of TZDs have led to the evaluation in acromegaly, Alzheimer's, Cushing syndrome, mental health disorders, erectile dysfunction (ED), Huntington's, NASH, Parkinson's, PCOS, polycystic kidney disease, and psoriasis. The following information includes human, clinical trials involving pioglitazone or rosiglitazone and is not intended to be all-inclusive. Pioglitazone and rosiglitazone are not FDA approved for any of the following conditions discussed below.[31]

NAFLD/NASH

NAFLD is a frequent comorbidity in patients with T2D and obesity. These patients are at an even higher risk of the aggressive liver disease NASH, end-stage liver disease, cirrhosis, hepatocellular carcinoma, and death. The treatment of

NAFLD/NASH focuses on the underlying pathology of insulin resistance and dysfunctional adipose tissue that leads to hepatocyte toxicity. The insulin-sensitizing properties of the TZDs are responsible for the beneficial effects seen with this class of drugs. A recent review by Mills and colleagues evaluated the literature on the safety and efficacy of treatment for NAFLD in T2D. They evaluated 23 studies involving metformin, TZDs, statins, and GLP-1 RAs for the treatment of NAFLD. All of the treatment options were safe. TZDs had positive results on fibrosis and resolution of NASH, while the GLP-1 RAs and metformin did not improve fibrosis.[9] Authors Davidson and Pan are calling for the resurrection of the use of pioglitazone due to the small number needed to treat for benefit[2-5,8-12] of histological improvement and radiological resolution of NASH based on their findings in the meta-analysis of epidemiological studies.[32] In a subgroup analysis of the TOSCA.IT trial, low-dose pioglitazone resulted in improvements of systemic and adipose insulin resistance as well as indirect indices of hepatic steatosis and inflammation in T2D after 1-year follow-up, independent of blood glucose management.[33] The American Diabetes Association's *Standards of Care in Diabetes* state pioglitazone has been shown to effectively treat steatohepatitis and may slow the progression of fibrosis in people with T2D and NAFLD and is cost effective in the treatment of NASH.[34] In the clinical practice guidelines for the management of NAFLD by the American Association of Clinical Endocrinology and co-sponsored by the American Association for the Study of Liver Disease (AASLD), pioglitazone or GLP-1 RAs are recommended for people with diabetes who have an elevated probability of NASH, biopsy-proven NASH, or in NAFLD.[35] In the guidelines by the European Associations for the Study of the Liver, Diabetes, and Obesity (EASL, EASD, EASO), pioglitazone is considered a treatment option for select individuals with NASH.[36]

PCOS

Rosiglitazone and pioglitazone have been studied in PCOS because of their insulin-sensitizing properties. Despite positive results, these agents are not commonly used or recommended due to adverse effects, concerns of weight gain, and increased risk of fractures in women.[37]

Secondary Stroke Prevention

The IRIS trial reported that treatment of insulin resistance with pioglitazone (median daily dose each year ranged 29–40 mg) significantly reduced recurrent stroke or MI by 24% compared to placebo (pioglitazone 9.0% vs. placebo 11.8%; HR 0.76 [95% CI 0.62–0.93]; $P = 0.007$) in 3,876 patients who had a recent (<6 months) history of ischemic stroke or transient ischemic attack and insulin resistance without diabetes, HF, or bladder cancer. There was no difference in all-cause mortality between the pioglitazone and placebo groups. Pioglitazone was associated with greater frequency of weight gain (52.2% vs. 33.7%, $P < 0.001$), edema (35.6% vs. 24.9%, $P < 0.001$), and bone fracture requiring surgery or hospitalization (5.1% vs. 3.2%, $P = 0.003$) compared to placebo, respectively. The pioglitazone group was also associated with a lower risk of diabetes (3.8% vs. 7.7%; HR 0.48 [95% CI 0.33–0.69]; $P < 0.001$).[19] This study demonstrates the vascular benefits of pioglitazone in a specific subset of patients without diabetes who have insulin resistance. It also demonstrated a lower risk of T2D. The potential impact of pioglitazone in this trial on reducing the burden of stroke and reducing the burden of diabetes could have a global impact.

A secondary analysis evaluated the IRIS participants without HF upon entry to determine if the addition of pioglitazone increased their risk of HF. Young and colleagues concluded the 5-year risk of HF did not differ by treatment (4.1% pioglitazone, 4.2% placebo). The risk for hospitalized HF was not significantly different between treatment groups (2.9% pioglitazone, 2.3% placebo, $P = 0.36$). The risk of HF with pioglitazone was not altered by the baseline HF risk in these participants.[38]

Kernan and colleagues performed another secondary analysis to determine if the IRIS participants who were at a higher risk (increasing age, history of prior stroke, coronary heart disease, hypertension, currently smoking, or aphasia) of stroke or future MI would derive a greater benefit with the addition of pioglitazone than patients with a lower risk. Among patients at lower baseline risk, the 5-year risk for stroke or MI was 6.0% in the pioglitazone group and 7.9% in the placebo group (absolute risk reduction, 1.9% [95% CI -0.6–4.4]). In those at higher baseline risk, the 5-year risk of stroke or MI was 14.7% in the pioglitazone group and 19.6% in the placebo group (absolute risk reduction, 4.9% [95% CI 1.2–8.6]). However, these higher risk patients had greater rates of bone fracture with pioglitazone (19.6% vs. 10.1% with placebo; absolute risk increase, 6.8% [95% CI 3.3–10.2]) than did those at lower risk (10.6% vs. 7.4% with placebo; absolute risk increase, 3.2% [95% CI 0.4–6.0]).[39] Despite the limitations in a post hoc exploratory analysis of data from the IRIS trial, Spence and colleagues found that daily doses of 15 mg or 30 mg of pioglitazone demonstrated similar efficacy for the prevention of secondary stroke and MI when compared to the 45 mg daily dose with fewer side effects, except for fractures. Larger, randomized trials are needed to determine the lowest effective dose of pioglitazone in the prevention of secondary stroke.[40]

Bone Health

TZDs have demonstrated an increased incidence of bone fractures, especially peripheral factures in women. Rosiglitazone demonstrated an increased risk of limb fractures in the first year of treatment in the ADOPT and RECORD trials that persisted for the length of the trials.[2] In the PROactive trial, pioglitazone demonstrated an increased incidence of bone fracture in women of 5.1% (44/870) vs. 2.5% (23/905) for the placebo group.[17] Fracture risk in men did not differ between the two groups. Although the majority of data has demonstrated an increased risk of fracture in older women, men and younger patients may be susceptible as well. The mechanism is not entirely clear, but studies have shown a change in bone mineral density, inhibition of bone formation by PPAR-mediated diversion of mesenchymal progenitor cells into the adipocytes rather than osteoblasts, and changes in biochemical markers of bone turnover.[29] A 36-month trial investigated the effects of pioglitazone on bone mineral density and bone metabolism in people with prediabetes or T2D and NASH. Ninety-two patients were randomly assigned to pioglitazone (45 mg/day) or placebo for 18 months, followed by an 18 month open label pioglitazone treatment phase. After 18 months of pioglitazone treatment, there were no differences in bone mineral density versus placebo at either the femoral neck ($P = 0.87$), total hip ($P = 0.78$), or one-third radius ($P = 0.44$); however, bone density decreased at the level of the spine with pioglitazone (–3.5%; $P = 0.002$). During the extension phase (18–36 months), patients had no further decreases in bone mineral density or plasma biomarkers of bone turnover during pioglitazone treatment. There were no bone fractures.[41] Given the existing data regarding the effects of TZDs on bone, use of TZDs should be with caution, assuring the benefit of use outweighs the risk in those at increased risk of fracture or who have had a fracture.

Renal Impairment

Dose adjustments for rosiglitazone or pioglitazone are not required in patients with renal dysfunction or renal failure.

Hepatic Impairment

Patients with impaired hepatic function (Child-Pugh grade B/C) have a 45% reduction in pioglitazone and total pioglitazone mean peak concentrations, but no change in mean AUC when compared with normal subjects. In patients with impaired hepatic function (Child-Pugh grade B/C), C_{max} and AUC values for rosiglitazone were increased two- and threefold, respectively, and elimination half-life was increased by 2 h. Rosiglitazone and pioglitazone should not be used in patients with clinical evidence of active liver disease or with serum ALT concentrations greater than three times the ULN.

Pediatrics

Current use of TZDs in pediatrics is not recommended. No pharmacokinetic, safety, or efficacy data for TZDs is available in children.

Geriatrics

Age does not result in clinically significant changes in the effects or pharmacokinetics of rosiglitazone or pioglitazone. No dosage adjustment is needed in this population.

Sex

Rosiglitazone clearance was reported to be 6% lower in males than females of comparable body weight. In monotherapeutic trials with rosiglitazone, a slightly greater therapeutic response (quantitative differences were not reported) was observed in female patients, while no such difference was reported in metformin/rosiglitazone combination trials. Interestingly, sex-related differences were less marked in more obese patients. Women tend to have a greater fat mass than men for a given BMI. The sex-related differences in effect may be due to this difference in fat mass where the molecular target PPARγ is highly expressed in lipid tissue. Although there are slight differences in the effects of both rosiglitazone and pioglitazone in women, no dose adjustment is recommended. Treatment should be individualized for men and women.

Ethnicity

No differences in the effects of these agents have been observed in any ethnic group.

ADVERSE EFFECTS AND MONITORING

Weight Gain and Edema

Dose-related weight gain is the most common side effect of the TZDs. Pioglitazone and rosiglitazone typically cause weight gain of 1–5 kg when used as monotherapy, in combination with oral antihyperglycemic agents, and in combination with insulin. In a 6-month, randomized placebo-controlled dose-response study, pioglitazone 15 mg/day was associated with approximately 1% weight gain, while 45 mg/day demonstrated up to 3–5% weight gain.[42] The mechanism of weight gain is not entirely clear but is likely related to the activation of the PPARγ receptors, resulting in an increase of adipose tissue deposition.

Dose-related edema can be seen with monotherapy, in combination with oral antihyperglycemic agents, and in combination with insulin. Although the mechanism of edema is not clearly understood, it may be due to the activation of the PPARγ receptors in the kidney, which results in the retention of salt and water. Edema, fluid retention, and weight gain are problematic in coexisting CHF and require increased patient monitoring. Rosiglitazone and pioglitazone are contraindicated in NHYA class III or IV HF and should be not be used in patients with symptomatic HF.

Anemia

Dose-related reductions in hemoglobin and hematocrit ($\leq 4\%$ and ≤ 1 g, respectively) have been observed in patients treated with pioglitazone or rosiglitazone. These changes are possibly due to volume expansion and have not been associated with significant hematological effects. The changes occur within the first 4–8 weeks of therapy and remain unchanged thereafter. These effects are usually mild and no routine monitoring for anemia is recommended.

Liver Function Abnormalities

Currently, it is recommended that patients treated with rosiglitazone or pioglitazone undergo serum transaminase monitoring at the initiation of therapy and periodically thereafter, based on the judgment of the clinician. Patients treated with rosiglitazone or pioglitazone who present with ALT levels greater than or equal to 2.5 times the ULN should have their ALT levels assessed with some frequency. Patients treated with rosiglitazone or pioglitazone who present with ALT levels greater than or equal to three times the ULN should have the level repeated and should discontinue the drug if the elevation persists.

Fractures

The risk of fracture should be considered in the care of patients treated with pioglitazone and rosiglitazone, and attention given to assessing and maintaining bone health according to current standards of care. The majority of the observed fractures in the trials were nonvertebral fractures including upper distal limb and lower limb.

Bladder Cancer Risk

Pioglitazone should not be used in patients with active or a history of bladder cancer. Associations between cumulative dose or cumulative duration of exposure to pioglitazone and bladder cancer were not detected in some studies, including the 10-year observational study in the U.S.[27] During the 13 years of both PROactive and observational follow-up, the occurrence of bladder cancer did not differ between patients randomized to pioglitazone or placebo (HR 1.00 [95% CI 0.59–1.72]). Inconsistent findings and limitations inherent in these and other studies preclude conclusive interpretations of the observational data.[1]

Ocular Effects

Rare cases of macular edema have been reported with the use of TZDs, frequently during concurrent peripheral edema. Patients should report any vision changes such as blurred vision or decreased visual acuity. Routine ophthalmological exams should be recommended to all patients with diabetes according to current guidelines.

DRUG INTERACTIONS

Cytochrome P450 enzymes play a role in the metabolism of the TZDs. Rosiglitazone is metabolized predominantly by CYP2C8 and to a lesser degree by CYP2C9. Pioglitazone is metabolized predominantly by CYP2C8 and to a lesser extent by CYP3A4. Inhibitors of CYP2C8 will decrease metabolism of rosiglitazone and pioglitazone and increase serum concentrations. Monitoring for increased hypoglycemia and dose reductions are often needed. CYP2C8 inhibitors include: abiraterone, clopidogrel, deferasirox, gemfibrozil, mifepristone, leflunomide, and teriflunomide. Inducers of CYP2C8 will increase metabolism of rosiglitazone and pioglitazone and thus decrease their effectiveness. Some of the CYP2C8 inducers include: lumacaftor, dabrafenib, ritodrine, and salicylates. In the case of salicylates, this interaction is more likely to occur at doses of 3 g per day or more. Clinical response to TZDs should be monitored when taken in combination with these other agents.

When taken with other antihyperglycemic agents, TZDs can enhance hypoglycemic effects. Risk of hypoglycemia is increased when taken in combination with other antihyperglycemic agents. Doses of the offending drugs may need to be reduced to avoid hypoglycemia.

When taken in combination with other drugs that have been associated with hyperglycemic effects (such as aripiprazole, atazanavir, bumetanide, cortisone, chlorthalidone, clozapine, dexamethasone, epinephrine, estradiol, estrogens, fosamprenavir, furosemide, methylprednisolone, olanzapine, prednisolone, prednisone, quetiapine, risperidone, ritonavir, saquinavir, tacrolimus, thiazide diuretics, torsemide, triamcinolone, ziprasidone), the effectiveness of TZDs can be reduced. The dose of rosiglitazone or pioglitazone may need to be increased to achieve desired effectiveness when taken in combination with these other agents.

When taken in combination with other drugs that have been associated with hypoglycemic effects (such as linezolid, selegiline, monoamine oxidase inhibitors like mebanazine or phenelzine, and serotonin reuptake inhibitors like citalopram, escitalopram, fluoxetine, paroxetine, or sertraline), the effectiveness of TZDs can be enhanced. Increased blood glucose testing should be performed, and the dose of rosiglitazone or pioglitazone may need to be decreased to avoid hypoglycemic effects.

ACE Inhibitors

ACE inhibitors may or may not enhance the hypoglycemic effects of TZDs. Case reports describe episodes of hypoglycemia after taking ACE inhibitors along with antihyperglycemic agents. However, published results are inconsistent and most often reported with sulfonylureas. No action is recommended to manage this potential interaction at this time.

Alpha-Lipoic Acid

Alpha-lipoic acid may enhance the effects of antihyperglycemic agents, including pioglitazone and rosiglitazone. Patients should be monitored closely for signs of hypoglycemia if taking α-lipoic acid with these agents. Intravenous formulations have a greater impact than oral formulations. The dose of rosiglitazone or pioglitazone may need to be reduced to avoid hypoglycemia.

Androgens

Androgen hormones such as fluoxymesterone, mesterolone, methyltestosterone, nandrolone, oxandrolone, oxymetholone, and testosterone may increase the hypoglycemia effect of antihyperglycemic agents like rosiglitazone and pioglitazone. Monitor patients closely for signs of hypoglycemia and reduce the dose of rosiglitazone or pioglitazone if such effects are seen.

Antifungals

Although the AUC of pioglitazone was increased by 34% in a single-dose study administered with ketoconazole, the kinetics of pioglitazone were unaffected when taken with itraconazole in another study.

Clopidogrel

In a study of healthy subjects, clopidogrel was found to significantly increase the AUC and half-life of pioglitazone. Monitor patients closely for increased pioglitazone effects such as hypoglycemia, edema, or hepatotoxicity.

Dabrafenib

Dabrafenib is a strong inducer of CYP2C8, which can decrease serum concentrations of pioglitazone and rosiglitazone. Product labeling recommends finding an alternative to these agents for glucose control in patients taking dabrafenib.

Digoxin

Rosiglitazone and pioglitazone do not alter the pharmacokinetics of digoxin.

Gemfibrozil

Three studies have shown that gemfibrozil increases serum concentrations of pioglitazone when taken together. The dose of pioglitazone should be limited to 15 mg per day when taken with gemfibrozil. Although specific dose limits are not listed, prescribing information for rosiglitazone recommends considering dose reductions when taken with gemfibrozil as well.

Guanethidine

Guanethidine may increase the hypoglycemia effect of antihyperglycemic agents like rosiglitazone and pioglitazone. Monitor patients closely for signs of hypoglycemia and reduce the dose of rosiglitazone or pioglitazone if such effects are seen.

Ethanol

No significant effect has been found between moderate amounts of ethanol and pioglitazone or rosiglitazone.

Leukotriene Receptor Antagonists

In vitro results suggest that leukotriene receptor antagonists may inhibit CYP2C8; however, no change in the kinetics of pioglitazone were seen in a study of 12 healthy subjects.

Oral Contraceptives

When pioglitazone was coadministered with a combination oral contraceptive (ethinyl estradiol/norethindrone) for 21 days, an 11% reduction in ethinyl estradiol AUC and an 11–14% reduction in ethinyl estradiol C_{max} values were reported. The clinical significance of this is unknown. Rosiglitazone has been shown to have no clinically significant effect on the pharmacokinetics of ethinyl estradiol or norethindrone.

Pregabalin

Pregabalin may enhance the fluid-retaining effect of TZDs. Patients taking pregabalin with either rosiglitazone or pioglitazone should be monitored closely for weight gain and edema. Take extra caution in using these agents together in patients at risk for HF.

Quinolones

Quinolone antibiotics may enhance or diminish the effects of blood glucose–lowering agents, such as TZDs. Monitor patients for hypo- or hyperglycemia when initiating a quinolone antibiotic in patients taking rosiglitazone or pioglitazone. Hypoglycemic effects are more likely to occur in the first few days of therapy, while hyperglycemia is at most risk after several days of therapy.

Rifampin

Rifampin has been shown in studies to decrease serum concentrations of both rosiglitazone and pioglitazone. Rifampin likely induces metabolism of these agents, and patients taking them should be monitored for reduced efficacy if therapy with rifampin is initiated.

Topiramate

Concomitant administration with topiramate was found in one study to decrease the serum concentration of pioglitazone. Hypokalemia also occurred

Table 7.1 —Thiazolidinediones

Thiazolidinediones	Available strengths	Can be cut?	Dosing interval	Maximum daily dose (MDD)	Maximum therapeutic effect (time)	Renal dose adjustments (mL/min/1.73 m^2)	Hepatic dose adjustments	Contraindications	Pregnancy category
					Rosiglitazone				
Avandia	2 mg, 4 mg, 8 mg	Yes	1 or 2 divided doses	8 mg/day	May take 3–6 months to see full effect	No dosage adjustment necessary	Do not initiate if ALT > 2.5 times the ULN at baseline; If ALT levels persist above three times the ULN during therapy, discontinue use	Hypersensitivity to rosiglitazone NYHA Class III or IV heart failure	C TZDs may cause ovulation in anovulatory premenopausal women, increasng the risk of unintended pregnancy
					Pioglitazone				
Actos	15 mg, 30 mg, 45 mg	Yes	Once daily	45 mg/day	May take 3–6 months to see full effect	No dosage adjustment necessary	Do not initiate if ALT > 2.5 times the ULN at baseline; If ALT levels persist above three times the ULN during therapy, discontinue use	Hypersensitivity to pioglitazone NYHA Class III or IV heart failure	C TZDs may cause ovulation in anovulatory premenopausal women, increasing the risk of unintended pregnancy
					Pioglitazone Combinations				
Pioglitazone & Alogliptan (Oseni)	15 mg/25 mg 30 mg/12.5 mg 30 mg/25 mg 45 mg/12.5 mg 45 mg/25 mg	Do not split tablets	Once daily	Pio-glitazone 45 mg/day Alogliptan 25 mg/day	Pioglitazone: 3–6 months alogliptin: 2–4 weeks	eGFR >30 to <50: alogliptan 12.5 mg/day eGFR <30 do not use	Do not initiate if ALT > 2.5 times the ULN at baseline; If ALT levels persist above three times the ULN during therapy, discontinue use	Hypersensitivity to alogliptin or pioglitazone; NYHA Class III or IV heart failure	C TZDs may cause ovulation in anovulatory premenopausal women, increasing the risk of unintended pregnancy

(continued)

Table 7.1 (continued)

Thiazolidinediones	Available strengths	Can be cut?	Dosing interval	Maximum daily dose (MDD)	Maximum therapeutic effect (time)	Renal dose adjustments (mL/min/1.73 m²)	Hepatic dose adjustments	Contraindications	Pregnancy category
Pioglitazone & Glimerpiride (Duetact)	30 mg/2 mg 30 mg/4 mg	Yes	Once daily	Pioglitazone 45 mg/day Glimepiride 8 mg/day	Pioglitazone: 3–6 months glimerpiride: 2 weeks	Starting dose of glimepiride in renal insufficiency is 1 mg p.o. daily. Do not use combination product unless dose has been titrated	Do not initiate if ALT > 2.5 times the ULN at baseline; If ALT levels persist above three times the ULN during therapy, discontinue use	Hypersensitivity to pioglitazone or glimepiride; history of allergic reaction to sulfonamide derivatives NYHA Class III or IV heart failure	C TZDs may cause ovulation in anovulatory premenopausal women, increasing the risk of unintended pregnancy
Pioglitazone & Metformin (Actoplus Met)	15 mg/500 mg 15 mg/850 mg	Yes	Once daily or b.i.d.	Pioglitazone 45 mg/day Metformin 2,000 mg/day	Pioglitazone: 3–6 months metformin: 4–6 weeks	eGFR 30–45: Do not initiatiate; if eGFR falls to <45, consider benefits/risks of continuing therapy eGFR <30: Do not use	Do not initiate if ALT > 2.5 times the ULN at baseline; If ALT levels persist above three times the ULN during therapy, discontinue use	Hypersensitivity to pioglitazone or metformin; NYHA Class III or IV heart failure; Lactic acidosis	C TZDs may cause ovulation in anovulatory premenopausal women, increasing the risk of unintended pregnancy

ALT, alanine aminotransferase; ULN, upper limit of normal; NYHA, New York Heart Association.

when topiramate was added to pioglitazone therapy. Clinical significance of this interaction is uncertain, but glycemic control should be monitored in patients taking pioglitazone when topiramate is initiated.

Trimethoprim

The AUC of rosiglitazone was increased in a study of normal subjects after taking a single dose of rosiglitazone during day 3–4 of a course of trimethoprim therapy. This interaction is thought to be caused by inhibition of CYP2C8, and thus is possible to occur with pioglitazone as well. Monitor for increased effects of TZDs when initiating or discontinuing trimethoprim.

Warfarin

No significant effect has been found between warfarin and pioglitazone or rosiglitazone.

DOSAGE AND ADMINISTRATION

Maximum therapeutic results may not be fully observed for several weeks to months following initiation or change in dose of pioglitazone or rosiglitazone due to the time-intensive mechanism of altering gene expression.

Pioglitazone is available in 15-, 30-, and 45-mg tablets. Pioglitazone is given once daily in doses of 15, 30, or 45 mg. Usual initial doses are either 15 or 30 mg; maximum dose is 45 mg daily. Dose escalation is based on re-evaluation of A1C after 3 months of therapy at a given dose, unless rapid deterioration of glycemic control dictates otherwise. Pioglitazone may be given without regard to meals.

Rosiglitazone is given either once or twice daily, and is available in 2-, 4-, or 8-mg tablets. The typical starting dose is 4 mg daily as a single or divided dose. Dose escalations should be made at 8–12-week intervals. In phase 3 trials, the greatest response was observed in patients treated with 4 mg twice daily. The maximum daily dose is 8 mg.

MONOGRAPHS

THIAZOLIDINEDIONES

Pioglitazone (Actos): https://dailymed.nlm.nih.gov/dailymed/drugInfo.
cfm?setid=d2ddc491-88a9-4063-9150-443b4fa4330c

Rosiglitazone (Avandia): https://dailymed.nlm.nih.gov/dailymed/drugInfo.
cfm?setid=ec682aec-e98f-41a1-9d21-eb7580ea3a8a

REFERENCES

1. Actos (pioglitazone) [package insert]. Deerfield, IL, Takeda Pharmaceuticals America, Inc., 2011. Available from https://www.accessdata.fda.gov/drugsatfda_docs/label/2011/021073s043s044lbl.pdf. Accessed 29 March 2020

2. Avandia (rosiglitazone) [package insert]. Research Triangle Park, NC, GlaxoSmithKline, 2016. Available from https://www.gsksource.com/pharma/content/dam/GlaxoSmithKline/US/en/Prescribing_Information/Avandia/pdf/AVANDIA-PI-MG.PDF. Accessed 29 March 2020

3. DeFronzo RA, Mehta RJ, Schnure JJ. Pleiotropic effects of thiazolidinediones: implications for the treatment of patients with type 2 diabetes mellitus. *Hosp Pract* 1995;41(2):132–147

4. The DREAM (Diabetes REduction Assessment with ramipril and rosiglitazone Medication) Trial Investigators. Effect of rosiglitazone on the frequency of diabetes in patients with impaired glucose tolerance or impaired fasting glucose: a randomized controlled trial. *Lancet* 2006;368:1096–1105

5. DeFronzo RA, Tripathy D, Schwenke DC, Banerji M, Bray GA, Buchanan TA, Clement SC, Henry RR, Hodis HN, Kitabchi AE, Mack WJ, Mudaliar S, Ratner RE, Williams K, Stentz FB, Musi N, Reaven PD; ACT NOW Study. Pioglitazone for diabetes prevention in impaired glucose tolerance. *N Engl J Med* 2011;364(12):1104–1115

6. Inzucchi SE, Viscoli CM, Young LM, et al.; IRIS Investigators. Pioglitazone prevents diabetes in patients with insuin resistance and cerebrovascular disease. *Diabetes Care* 2016;39:1684–1692

7. Spence JD, Viscoli CM, Inzucchi SE, et al.; IRIS Investigators. Pioglitazone therapy in patients with stroke and prediabetes. *JAMA Neurol* 2019; 76(5):526–535

8. Sarafidis PA, Stafylas PC, Georgianos PI, Saratzis AN, Lasaridis AN. Effect of thiazolidinediones on albuminuria and proteinuria in diabetes: a meta-analysis. *Am J Kidney Dis* 2010;55(5):835–847

9. Miyazaki Y, Cersosimo E, Triplitt C, DeFronzo RA. Rosiglitazone decreases albuminuria in type 2 diabetic patients. *Kidney Int* 2007;72(11):1367–1373

10. Brunelli SM, Thadhani R, Ikizler TA, Feldman HI. Thiazolidinedione use is associated with better survival in hemodialysis patients with non-insulin dependent diabetes. *Kidney Int* 2009;75(9):961–968

11. Mills EP, Brown KPD, Smith JD, Vang PW, Trotta K. Treating nonalcoholic fatty liver disease in patients with type 2 diabetes mellitus: a review of efficacy and safety. *Ther Adv Endocrinol Metab* 2018;9(1):15–28

12. Home PD, Pocock SJ, Beck-Nielsen H, Curtis PS, Gomis R, Hanefeld M, Jones NP, Komajda M, McMurray JJ; RECORD Study Team. Rosiglitazone evaluated for cardiovascular outcomes in oral agent combination therapy

for type 2 diabetes (RECORD): a multicentre, randomised, open-label trial. *Lancet* 2009;373(9681):2125–2135

13. Mannucci E, Monami M, Di Bari M, Lamanna C, Gori F, Gensini GF, Marchionni N. Cardiac safety profile of rosiglitazone: a comprehensive meta-analysis of randomized clinical trials. *Int J Cardiology* 2010;143:135–140

14. Erdmann E, Charbonnel B, Wilcox RG, et al.; PROactive Investigators. Pioglitazone use and heart failure in patients with type 2 diabetes and pre-existing cardiovascular disease: data from the PROactive study (PROactive 08). *Diabetes Care* 2007;30:2773–2778

15. Nesto RW, Bell D, Bonow RO, et al. Thiazolidinedione use, fluid retention, and congestive heart failure: a consensus statement from the American Heart Association and the American Diabetes Association. *Circulation* 2003;108:2941–2948

16. Lago RM, Singh PP, Nesto RW. Congestive heart failure and cardiovascular death in patients with prediabetes and type 2 diabetes given thiazolidinediones: a meta-analysis of randomised clinical trials. *Lancet* 2007;370:1129–1136

17. Dormandy JA, Charbonnel B, Eckland DJ, Erdmann E, Massi-Benedetti M, Moules IK, Skene AM, Tan MH, Lefèbvre PJ, Murray GD, Standl E, Wilcox RG, Wilhelmsen L, Betteridge J, Birkeland K, Golay A, Heine RJ, Korányi L, Laakso M, Mokán M, Norkus A, Pirags V, Podar T, Scheen A, Scherbaum W, Schernthaner G, Schmitz O, Skrha J, Smith U, Taton J; PROactive Investigators. Secondary prevention of macrovascular events in patients with type 2 diabetes in the PROactive Study (PROspective pioglitAzone Clinical Trial In macroVascular Events): a randomised controlled trial. *Lancet* 2005;366(9493):1279–1289

18. Wilcox R, Bousser MG, Betteridge DJ, Schernthaner G, Pirags V, Kupfer S, Dormandy J; PROactive Investigators. Effects of pioglitazone in patients with type 2 diabetes with or without previous stroke: results from PROactive (PROspective pioglitAzone Clinical Trial In macroVascular Events 04). *Stroke* 2007;38:865–873

19. Kernan WN, Viscoli CM, Furie KL, Young LH, Inzucchi SE, Gorman M, Guarino PD, Lovejoy AM, Peduzzi PN, Conwit R, Brass LM, Schwartz GG, Adams HP Jr., Berger L, Carolei A, Clark W, Coull B, Ford GA, Kleindorfer D, O'Leary JR, Parsons MW, Ringleb P, Sen S, Spence JD, Tanne D, Wang D, Winder TR; IRIS Trial Investigators. Pioglitazone after ischemic stroke or transient ischemic attack. *N Engl J Med* 2016;374(14):1321–1331

20. Lee M, Saver JL, Liao HW, Lin CH, Ovbiagele B. Pioglitazone for secondary stroke prevention: a systematic review and meta-analysis. *Stroke* 2017;48:388–393

21. Bonnet F, Scheen AJ. Impact of glucose-lowering therapies on risk of stroke in type 2 diabetes. *Diabetes Metab* 2017;43:299–313

22. DeFronzo RA. Insulin resistance, lipotoxicity, type 2 diabetes and atherosclerosis: the missing links. *Diabetologia* 2010;53(7):1270–1287

23. Rajagopalan S, Dutta P, Hota D, Bhansali A, Srinivasan A, Chakrabar A. Effect of low dose pioglitazone on glycemic control and insulin resistance in type 2 diabetes: a randomized, double blind, clinical trial. *Diabetes Res Clin Pract* 2015;109(3):e32–e35

24. Kurisu S, Iwasaki T, Ishibashi K, Mitsuba N, Dohi Y, Nishioka K, Kihara Y. Effects of low-dose pioglitazone on glucose control, lipid profiles, renin-angiotensin-aldosterone system and natriuretic peptides in diabetic patients with coronary artery disease. *J Renin Angiotensin Aldosterone Syst* 2013;14(1):51–55

25. Tripathy D, Daniele G, Fiorentino TV, Perez-Cadena Z, Chavez-Velasquez A, Kamath S, Fanti P, Jenkinson C, Andreozzi F, Federici M, Gastaldelli A, DeFronzo RA, Folli F. Pioglitazone improves glucose metabolism and modulates skeletal muscle TIMP-3-TACE dyad in type 2 diabetes mellitus: a randomised, double-blind, placebo-controlled, mechanistic study. *Diabetologia* 2013;56(10):2153–2163

26. Yanai H, Adachi H. The low-dose (7.5 mg/day) pioglitazone therapy. *J Clin Med Res* 2017;9(10):821–825

27. Satirapoj B, Watanakijthavonkul K, Supasyndh O. Safety and efficacy of low dose pioglitazone compared with standard dose pioglitazone in type 2 diabetes with chronic kidney disease: a randomized controlled trial. *PLoSONE* 13(10):e0206722. Available from https://doi.org/10.1371/journal.pone.0206722

28. Erdmann E, Harding S, Lam H, Perez A. Ten-year observational follow-up of PROactive: a randomized cardiovascular outcomes trial evaluating pioglitazone in type 2 diabetes. *Diabetes Obes Metab* 2016;18(3):266–273

29. Billington EO, Grey A, Bolland MJ. The effect of thiazolidinediones on bone mineral density and bone turnover: systematic review and meta-analysis. *Diabetologia* 2015;58:2238–2246

30. American Diabetes Association. 3. Prevention or delay of type 2 diabetes: Standards of Medical Care in Diabetes—2020. *Diabetes Care* 2020;43(Suppl. 1):S32–S36

31. Davidson MA, Mattison DR, Azoulay L, Krewski D. Thiazolidinedione drugs in the treatment of type 2 diabetes mellitus: past, present and future. *Crit Rev Toxicol* 2018;48(1):52–108

32. Davidson MB, Pan D. An updated meta-analysis of pioglitazone exposure and bladder cancer and comparison to the drug's effect on cardiovascular disease and non-alcoholic steatohepatitis. *Diabetes Res Clin Pract* 2018;135:102–110.

33. Della Pepa P, Russo M, Vitale M, Carli F, Vetrani C, Masulli M, Riccardi G, Vaccaro O, Gastaldelli A, Rivellese AA, BozettoL. Pioglitazone even at low

dosage improves NAFLD in type 2 diabetes: clinic and pathophysiological insights from a subgroup of the TOSCA.IT randomised trial. *Diabetes Res and Clin Prac* 2021 Aug;178:108984. DOI:10.1016/j.diabres.2021.108984. Epub 2021 Jul 24

34. ElSayed NA, Aleppo G, Aroda VR, et al., American Diabetes Association. 4. Comprehensive Medical Evaluation and Assessment of Comorbidities: Standards of Care in Diabetes—2023. *Diabetes Care* 2023;46(Suppl. 1):S47–S67

35. American Association of Clinical Endocrinology Clinical Practice Guideline for the Diagnosis and Management of Nonalcoholic Fatty Liver Disease in Primary Care and Endocrinology Clinical Settings, Co-sponsored by the American Association for the Study of Liver Diseases (AASLD). *Endocrine Practice* 2022;28:528–562

36. Chalasani N, Younossi Z, Lavine JE, Charlton M, Cusi K, Rinella M, Harrison SA, Brunt EM, Sanyal AJ. The diagnosis and management of nonalcoholic fatty liver disease: practice guideline from the American Association for the Study of Liver Diseases. *Hepatology* 2018;76(1):328–357

37. Legro RS, Arslanian SA, Ehrmann DA, Hoeger KM, Murad H, Pasquali R, Welt CK; Endocrine Society. Diagnosis and treatment of polycystic ovary syndrome: an Endocrine Society clinical practice guideline. *J Clin Endocrinol Metab* 2013;89(12):4565–4592

38. Young LH, Viscoli CM, Schwartz GG, Inzucchi SE, Curtis JP, Gorman MJ, Furie KL, Conwit R, Spatz E, Lovejoy A, Abbott JD, Jacoby DL, Kolansky DM, Ling FS, Pfau SE, Kernan WN; IRIS Investigators. Heart failure after ischemic stroke or TIA in insulin-resistant patients without diabetes treated with pioglitazone. *Circulation* 2018;138(12):1210–1220

39. Kernan WN, Viscoli CM, Dearborn JL, Kent DM, Conwit R, Fayad P, Furie KL, Gorman M, Guarino PD, Inzucchi SE, Stuart A, Young LH; IRIS Investigators. Targeting pioglitazone hydrochlorothiazide therapy after stroke or transient ischemic attack according to pretreatment risk for stroke or myocardial infarction. *JAMA Neurol* 2017;74(11):1210–1220

40. Spence JD, Viscoli C, Kernan WD, et al. Efficacy of lower doses of pioglitazone after stroke or transient ischaemic attack in patients with insulin resistance. *Diabetes Obes Metab* 2022;24:1150–1158

41. Portillo-Sanchez P, Brill F, Lomonaco R, Barb D, Orsak B, Bruder JM, Cusi K. Effect of pioglitazone on bone mineral density in patients with nonalcoholic steatohepatitis: a 36-month clinical trial. *J Diab* 2019;11(3):223–231

42. Aronoff S, Rosenblatt S, Braithwaite S, Egan J, Mathisen AL, Schneider RL: Pioglitazone 001 Study Group. Pioglitazone hydrochloride monotherapy improves glycemic control in the treatment of patients with type 2 diabetes: A 6-month randomized placebo-controlled dose-response study. *Diabetes Care* 2000;23:1605–1611

Chapter 8
Sulfonylureas

Lisa Kroon, PharmD
Crystal Zhou, PharmD

INTRODUCTION

Sulfonylureas have been a mainstay in the pharmacologic treatment of T2D for over 60 years. Three first-generation sulfonylureas (chlorpropamide, tolbutamide, and tolazamide) are rarely used in the United States. The three second-generation sulfonylureas (glyburide, glipizide, and glimepiride) are the most frequently used, so this chapter will focus on these agents. With the availability of many noninsulin classes of medications for T2D, sulfonylurea usage is on the decline, yet their use persists.[1] They remain some of the most commonly used and effective agents in A1C lowering, are cost effective, and, when dosed appropriately, are well tolerated and easily taken.[1,2,3]

The American Diabetes Association's pharmacologic treatment approach for glycemic control place insulin secretagogues (sulfonylureas and meglitinides) as an option for a second agent after a patient is on metformin and cost is a concern.[4] In clinical practice, sulfonylureas are often initiated as a second or third noninsulin agent. T2D is a progressive disease in which most patients at some point require multiple medications to achieve good glycemic control.[5] As a patient progresses to needing additional pharmacologic therapy, a sulfonylurea is generally discontinued when a patient is advanced to requiring mealtime insulin. At this point, the pancreatic function has declined to a point where the insulin secretagogues likely have no appreciable effect on insulin secretion. In patients with maturity-onset diabetes of the young (MODY), type HNF1A or HNF4A, low-dose sulfonylureas are considered first-line therapy.[6]

PHARMACOLOGY

MECHANISM OF ACTION

Sulfonylureas exert their antihyperglycemic effect by stimulating insulin secretion in the pancreas. Sulfonylureas bind to a high-affinity sulfonylurea receptor on the pancreatic β-cell and increase both basal and meal-stimulated insulin secretion.[7] The second-generation sulfonylureas have greater intrinsic potency than the first-generation agents. Insulin secretion is regulated by ATP-dependent potassium ion channels in the plasma membrane of the β-cell.[7] The ATP-dependent potassium channel consists of two subunits, one containing a sulfonylurea receptor and the other containing the channel. Upon the sulfonylurea binding to its receptor, the ATP-dependent potassium channel closes, blocking the efflux of potassium. As potassium accumulates within the β-cell membrane, the membrane potential lowers, causing depolarization, which opens the voltage-dependent calcium channels; this calcium influx results in increased intracellular calcium, which, in turn, causes insulin granules to migrate to the cell surface, where the granules rupture and release the insulin.[7] Patients with T2D characteristically have defects in both insulin secretion and insulin action. Therefore, sulfonylureas' primary action in improving glycemic control is by affecting the β-cell defect.

With long-term use, sulfonylureas are thought to also exert extrapancreatic effects, including normalizing hepatic glucose production, reducing glucagon levels, enhancing peripheral glucose uptake, enhancing β-cell sensitivity to glucose, and closure of potassium channels in other tissues (e.g., cardiac tissue).[7] These effects are likely due to the improved glycemic control, which then reduces glucose toxicity.[8] The reduction of glucagon levels may be due to the enhanced insulin release, which inhibits α-cell secretion of glucagon. The significance of extrapancreatic potassium channel effects are likely minimal. However, in the heart, the closure of potassium channels on cardiac myocytes can affect ischemic preconditioning, in which vasodilation occurs during an ischemic episode.[9,10]

PHARMACOKINETICS

The sulfonylureas possess differences in their pharmacokinetic profiles. All sulfonylureas are nearly completely absorbed; however, the onset and duration of action are determined by the unique pharmacokinetic features of each agent and its specific formulation.[11] Most sulfonylureas have a relatively short plasma half-life, usually in the range of 4–10 h; only chlorpropamide has a half-life longer than 24 h. All sulfonylureas are highly protein-bound (90–100%), mainly to albumin; however, binding characteristics vary by individual sulfonylurea.[11] Most sulfonylureas effectively maintain glucose control with once- or twice-daily dosing. The longer duration of action seen than would be expected based on plasma half-life is thought to be due to a longer tissue half-life on the β-cell receptor and also the action of any active metabolites.[12] All sulfonylureas are metabolized in the liver, some to weakly active or inactive metabolites.[11] The first-generation sulfonylureas are excreted exclusively by the kidney, whereas the second-generation agents and their metabolites are excreted in differing proportions in the urine and feces. The pharmacokinetic properties of the sulfonylureas are summarized in Table 8.1.

Glyburide (also called glibenclamide) is longer acting compared to glipizide and can be taken once a day. It is metabolized completely by the liver to active metabolites, half of which are excreted in the urine and the rest in the biliary tract. A micronized formulation is available that is not bioequivalent to the conventional tablets. When patients are switched from formulations, they should be carefully monitored for possible dose adjustments.

Glipizide is an intermediate-acting agent, with a duration of action between 12 and 24 h. When taking doses of 20 mg/day or less, patients often can take glipizide once daily. Glipizide is metabolized completely by the liver to inactive metabolites, which are primarily excreted by the kidney. An extended-release formulation is available; the clinical significance on its duration of effect is minimal. Although the FDA-approved maximum dose is 40 mg/day, there is likely little additional glucose-lowering benefit to titrating over 20 mg/day.[13,14] While some clinicians recommend taking sulfonylureas, glipizide in particular, 30 min before the meal, the clinical significance of this on overall glycemic control has not been established and taking at the start of the meal is just as effective.[15]

Glimepiride is a long-acting agent with a duration of action of 24 h, allowing for daily dosing. It is metabolized by the liver to a principle metabolite that has 30% of the activity of glimepiride; metabolites are excreted in the urine and feces. Glimepiride is unique in its selectivity to β-cells. It may be advantageous for use in patients with coronary heart disease, due to the theoretical benefit of not affecting cardiac tissue.

From a pharmacodynamic perspective, sulfonylureas have a rapid onset of effect compared to other noninsulin agents. The full glycemic-lowering effect at a particular dose is seen within 1–2 weeks. Therefore, while most sulfonylureas could be dose adjusted before 1 week, dose titrations are usually done every 1–2 weeks.

TREATMENT ADVANTAGES/DISADVANTAGES

ADVANTAGES

As initial treatment in patients with T2D, sulfonylureas can induce a mean decrease in A1C of 1–2% and can reduce fasting plasma glucose by 60–70 mg/dL (3.3–3.8 mmol/L). Sulfonyureas can be used at diagnosis in patients with severe hyperglycemia and then changed to metformin or other diabetes therapy once glucose levels are in a lower range. However, in most cases, sulfonylureas will be started as an add-on agent to metformin or as a third agent, especially when the cost of therapy is an issue. The ideal candidates for treatment with sulfonylureas are patients with T2D who have significant insulin deficiency (e.g., insulinopenic) but sufficient residual β-cell function to respond to stimulation. Patients are likely to demonstrate a good glycemic response to sulfonylureas if they have a shorter duration of T2D and are not in a state of glucose toxicity (in which insulin therapy may be preferable for short-term use). In the less common condition where a patient with T2D has a thinner phenotype, indicating more insulin secretion defect rather than insulin resistance, a sulfonylurea should be considered.

DISADVANTAGES

The main disadvantages of the sulfonylureas are the side effects of weight gain and hypoglycemia. These are discussed in the "Adverse Effects and Monitoring" section. In addition, with the natural progressive decline in β-cell function associated with T2D over time, the response to sulfonylurea treatment likewise will diminish, and changes to the treatment regimen may be necessary. The ADOPT study assessed the time to monotherapy failure for glyburide, metformin, and rosiglitazone. At 5 years, 34% of patients on a sulfonylurea failed monotherapy, compared to 15 and 21% with rosiglitazone and metformin, respectively.[16] One hypothesis for the lower durability of the sulfonylureas is that the continuous stimulation of β-cells can cause them to fail sooner. This has been studied mainly in animal models and more clinical data is needed to prove this theory.[17] The Glycemia Reduction Approaches in Diabetes: A Comparative Effectiveness Study (GRADE) is assessing the long-term efficacy of a sulfonylurea (glimepiride), insulin glargine, a GLP-1 RA (liraglutide), and a DPP-4 inhibitor (sitagliptin) in patients already on metformin.[18] The primary metabolic outcome in this open label clinical trial is time to primary failure (i.e., A1C ≥7%). This head-to-head comparison study, funded by the National Institute of Diabetes and Digestive and Kidney Diseases (NIDDK), hopes to provide important information about optimal combinations of glucose-lowering medications, effect on cardiovascular outcomes, and how to individualize treatment.

The progressive decrease in β-cell function is not the only possible cause of the reduced effectiveness of an antihyperglycemic medication regimen. Patient-specific factors, including poor adherence to the medication(s) or factors that can increase the insulin-resistance component of hyperglycemia such as weight gain, physical inactivity, stress, or intercurrent illness can also reduce the effectiveness of the medication regimen. Medication-related factors are another possible reason for lack of (or diminished) response, such as not uptitrating the dose or initiation of a diabetogenic drug (e.g., glucocorticoids or certain antipsychotics).

THERAPEUTIC CONSIDERATIONS

SIGNIFICANT WARNINGS/PRECAUTIONS

The sulfonylureas are contraindicated in patients with a known hypersensitivity to the drug and in those with DKA, with or without coma. DKA should be treated with insulin. Sulfonylureas should not be used in patients with T1D.

The product information for sulfonylureas contains a special warning that the administration of oral antidiabetic agents has been reported to be associated with increased risk of cardiovascular mortality compared with treatment with nutrition therapy alone or nutrition therapy plus insulin. This warning is based on the results of the long-term, prospective clinical trial, the University Group Diabetes Program that was published in 1970.[19] Although only tolbutamide was included in this study, this warning has been applied to all sulfonylureas. The validity of this finding has been questioned due to design flaws and more recent long-term, randomized, controlled trials, such as the UKPDS and ADVANCE studies, which found no increased cardiovascular mortality in patients on sulfonylureas and provide reassuring evidence.[20,21] However, meta-analyses continue to be published that show an association of sulfonylureas and cardiovascular risk (see "Special Populations").

Hypoglycemia

The most serious acute complication of sulfonylurea therapy is hypoglycemia, and all sulfonylureas are capable of producing severe hypoglycemia. Appropriate patient selection, dosage, and patient education are important to avoid hypoglycemic episodes. Debilitated or malnourished patients and those with adrenal, pituitary, or hepatic insufficiency are particularly susceptible to the hypoglycemic action of insulin secretagogues. Hypoglycemia may be difficult to recognize in the elderly and in people taking β-blockers or other sympatholytic drugs. For patients taking a β-blocker, particularly a nonselective one such as propranolol, hypoglycemic symptoms of tachycardia and shakiness can be blunted, resulting in sweating being the most pronounced symptom. Hypoglycemia is more likely to occur when caloric intake is reduced or deficient, after severe or prolonged exercise, when alcohol is ingested, or when more than one glucose-lowering medication is used.

SPECIAL POPULATIONS

Hypoglycemia

Hypoglycemia is the most significant risk when using sulfonylureas and other antihyperglycemic agents in elderly patients and those with multiple comorbidities. Both renal and hepatic insufficiency are substantial risk factors for the development of severe hypoglycemia during sulfonylurea treatment in the elderly. Sulfonylureas should be initiated at lower doses and titrated slowly in elderly patients. See "Adverse Effects and Monitoring" for in-depth discussion.

Pregnancy and Lactation

The sulfonylureas are categorized as pregnancy category C. Glipizide and glimepiride have been found to be fetotoxic in rats at doses that produced maternal hypoglycemia. In some studies in rats, nonteratogenic skeletal deformities were observed after exposure during gestation and lactation. Because a higher incidence of congenital abnormalities is associated with abnormal maternal blood glucose levels during pregnancy, insulin therapy is most often the recommended choice of therapy during pregnancy to maintain blood glucose levels as close to normal as possible.

Pediatrics

The safety and effectiveness of sulfonylureas in pediatric patients has not been established.

Hepatic or Renal Impairment

Because sulfonylureas are major CYP2C9 substrates, caution should be exercised when using this class of medications in patients with hepatic impairment. Due to chlorpropamide and glyburide's longer elimination half-life, they should be avoided in patients with impaired renal function due to the increased risk for hypoglycemia. Glipizide and glimepiride can be initiated at lower doses to avoid hypoglycemia in renal impairment and are the preferred second-generation agents.

Food Insecurity and Homelessness

Patients who are homeless or do not have a reliable source of food may experience more frequent hypoglycemia if taking a longer-acting sulfonylurea. Therefore, in patients with food insecurities who may benefit from sulfonylureas, it is recommended to use glipizide due to its relatively short half-life. In order to prevent hypoglycemia, patients can take glipizide only prior to a meal, as they may not have to plan for future meals. Providers should also help these patients seek local resources to assist them in obtaining regularly distributed food.[22]

Cardiovascular Disease and Increased Cardiovascular Risk

Meta-analyses comparing sulfonylureas to other antidiabetic medications show conflicting results with regard to cardiovascular risk. Two meta-analyses found an increased cardiovascular-related mortality associated with sulfonylureas, with a Mantel-Haenszel odds ratio of 1.22 for patients on glyburide (glibenclamide) specifically in one study and a hazard ratio of 1.46 in another study.[23,24]

A network meta-analysis found that sulfonylureas were associated with greater cardiovascular risk, which was partly attributable to a concomitant increased risk of severe hypoglycemia.[25] In another meta-analysis that assessed 47 trials in which patients were on sulfonylureas or other classes of antihyperglycemic medications for at least 52 weeks, no increase in cardiovascular mortality was found.[26]

Since 2008, the FDA has required cardiovascular disease outcomes trials to be conducted for new antihyperglycemic medications. A cardiovascular trial was conducted with linagliptin comparing it to glimepiride. The Cardiovascular Outcome Study of Linagliptin vs. Glimepiride in Type 2 Diabetes (CAROLINA) trial compared the effect of linagliptin, a DPP-4 inhibitor, to glimepiride on cardiovascular safety. The CAROLINA study was a randomized, multicenter, noninferiority trial where patients with relatively early T2D (i.e., mean diabetes duration 6.3 years and mean age 64 years) at high risk for cardiovascular disease were randomized to linagliptin or glimepiride. Patients could be on background therapy of any antihyperglycemic except a DPP4- inhibitor, GLP-1 RA, or insulin. At baseline, approximately 42% of patients had established cardiovascular disease; therefore, for 58% of enrolled patients, this was a primary prevention trial. After a median duration of 6.3 years of follow-up, the incidence of cardiovascular death, nonfatal myocardial infarction, or nonfatal stroke (3-point MACE) was no different in the linagliptin or glimepiride groups (11.8% and 12.0%, respectively). Linagliptin was noninferior to glimepiride in the prevention of MACE. Therefore, using a sulfonylurea, such as glimepiride, did not increase the risk of a future cardiovascular event compared to a DPP-4 inhibitor.[27]

Two retrospective cohort studies studying the outcomes of medications in relation to sulfonylureas were recently published. In one, using data from the Veterans Affairs system, sulfonylureas (mostly glipizide) were compared with SGLT2 inhibitors (mostly empagliflozin) for efficacy in patients with T2D.[28] Over 23,000 individuals who were started on SGLT2 inhibitors and over 104,000 individuals who were started on sulfonylureas after metformin were included in the study. The authors found that participants who were starting on an SGLT2 inhibitor experienced a reduced risk of all-cause mortality compared to those on sulfo-nylureas (HR 0.81 [95% CI 0.75-0.87]). In another longitudinal retrospective cohort study using the Catalan database SIDIAP (Information System for the Development of Research in Primary Care), the authors found that compared to metformin, sulfonylurea use increased risk of MACE (HR 1.55 [95% CI 1.42-1.68]).[29] Given that these were both retrospective cohort studies, it is difficult to draw clear conclusions; however, they both had large sample sizes and showed a similar trend with sulfonylureas resulting in worse outcomes.

Although the data are inconclusive, and until additional RCT evidence is available, it is reasonable to weigh the benefits (e.g., improved glycemic control) and possible risks when using a sulfonylurea in a patient with known cardiovascu-lar disease.

ADVERSE EFFECTS AND MONITORING

Sulfonylureas are usually well tolerated and the frequency of side effects, other than hypoglycemia, is low. The most common adverse events associated with sul-fonylurea treatment, other than hypoglycemia, are dizziness, headache, and nau-sea. In comparative clinical trials, common adverse events occurred at similar rates with glimepiride and glipizide but were less likely to occur with glimepiride than glyburide.[30] Hematological complications, including thrombocytopenia, agranu-locytosis, and hemolytic anemia, have been described with tolbutamide and chlor-propamide but appear to be very rare with the second-generation sulfonylureas. Other rare adverse effects include allergic skin reactions (e.g., rash, urticarial, pru-ritus), photosensitivity, abnormal liver function tests, and icterus.[12] In the rare event that a patient develops a severe rash or reports a sulfa allergy (although the risk of cross-reactivity is likely extremely low), a meglitinide can be safely used as an alternative.

Certain side effects are unique to the specific agents because of their individ-ual chemical structures. For example, chlorpropamide can increase the secretion of antidiuretic hormone leading to water retention and hyponatremia.[12] A rare, disulfiram-like reaction can occur when patients take chlorpropamide and drink ethanol.[31]

The two adverse effects that are the primary disadvantages of sulfonylureas are weight gain and hypoglycemia.[2,32] Weight gain associated with sulfonylurea use is approximately 2 kg.[12] The weight gain can be attributed to two factors: improved glycemic control and hypoglycemia. Inherent in improving glycemic control is weight gain, as fewer calories are spilling into the urine. Also, a patient consumes additional calories when treating hypoglycemia. Therefore, it is impor-tant not only to reduce the risk of hypoglycemia from a safety perspective, but also to limit weight gain associated with sulfonylureas. Data from several studies have suggested that the second-generation sulfonylurea glimepiride may be associated with a lower incidence of hypoglycemia and less weight gain, and may improve insulin sensitivity compared to other sulfonylureas.

In the UKPDS 6-year follow-up, the proportion of patients on sulfonylurea monotherapy reporting at least one episode per year of hypoglycemia (defined as temporarily incapacitated but a patient is able to control symptoms without help, incapacitated and required assistance to control symptoms, or required medical attention) was 1.2% compared to 0.3% with metformin.[33] In a retrospective analysis of a large, national cohort of T2D, use of a sulfonylurea or meglitinide increased the risk of severe hypoglycemia about twofold.[34] This analysis also found that patients with high complexity (i.e., age 75 years and older or multiple comorbidities) on intensive treatment also had nearly double the risk of severe hypoglycemia. A comparable analysis determined that the rate of severe hypoglycemia (defined as requiring an emergency department visit or hospitalization) was between 1.8 and 2.1 events per 100 person-years; again, rates were highest in older patients and those with multiple comorbidities.[35] In addition, an observational study in elderly patients ≥70 years old also confirmed that a majority of the elderly subjects with T2D on a sulfonylurea and/or insulin experienced severe hypoglycemia (defined as an admission to the hospital) with a hazard ratio of 2.52 (95% CI 2.23, 2.84).[36] Chlorpropamide and glyburide are identified in the Beers Criteria as potentially inappropriate medications in people 65 and older.[37] Sulfonylureas should be used with caution in the elderly and those with multiple comorbidities.

Patients on sulfonylureas should be educated on how to self-monitor their blood glucose (and to monitor regularly), on hypoglycemic symptoms and values, and on how to self-treat for a hypoglycemic episode. A quick-acting source of glucose should be used. Glucagon, while effective for hypoglycemia cause by exogenous insulin, can cause a paradoxical lowering of blood glucose when used with a sulfonylurea, as it stimulates insulin secretion.[38,39] Patients should also be educated to not skip meals, as this, along with irregular eating patterns, will increase the risk of hypoglycemia. Patients who are purposefully trying to eat less, increase physical activity, or lose weight may need their sulfonylurea dose reduced.

Although the sulfonylureas have important side effects to consider, the newer noninsulin agents also have significant side effects (i.e., newer doesn't necessarily mean better or safer). When developing a T2D medication regimen, it is important to tailor the medication selection(s) to the patient, taking into account the unique side effects of the various classes of medications and patient factors (e.g., concurrent medication conditions, ability to adhere, and ability to pay for the medication).

DRUG INTERACTIONS

The hypoglycemic action of sulfonylureas may be enhanced by certain drugs, including nonsteroidal anti-inflammatory drugs (NSAIDs) and other drugs that are highly bound to protein, such as salicylates, sulfonamides, chloramphenicol, warfarin, probenecid, monoamine oxidase inhibitors, and β-blockers (see "Hypoglycemia"). Although the risk is greater with the first-generation sulfonylureas, patients given these drugs concomitantly with any sulfonylurea should be monitored closely for hypoglycemia. Similarly, when these drugs are discontinued, patients on sulfonylurea therapy should be observed closely for worsening of glycemic control.

Pharmacodynamic interactions with all antihyperglycemics include drugs that can cause hyperglycemia, and when taken may lead to worsening of glycemic control. Examples of these drugs include thiazide diuretics, statins, glucocorticoids, phenothiazines, certain antipsychotics (e.g., chlorpromazine, olanzapine, clozapine), HIV protease inhibitors, estrogens and hormonal contraceptives, phenytoin, immunosuppressive therapies, sympathomimetics, and isoniazid.

DOSAGE AND ADMINISTRATION

A sulfonylurea is typically started at a low dose and then titrated until the glycemic response is achieved. The dose should generally be increased at no shorter than weekly intervals. Most patients will achieve the maximum therapeutic benefit with one-half of the FDA-approved maximum dose. Typical dosing and administration regimens are shown in Table 8.2.

A number of factors influence the choice of a sulfonylurea, including the duration of action and frequency of administration, patterns of metabolism and excretion, and the side effect profiles. The duration of action of a sulfonylurea is an important consideration. Of the first-generation agents, tolbutamide has a very short duration of action and needs to be taken two or three times a day. Most of the second-generation agents, which have a duration of 16–24 h, can be administered once daily at the usual therapeutic doses, but maximal doses may need to be divided into two daily doses. Glipizide is typically dosed twice daily with breakfast and dinner. Glyburide and glimepiride are usually dosed daily with breakfast, or the first meal of the day. It is important to educate patients to not take a sulfonylurea at bedtime as this can increase the risk of hypoglycemia.

The patterns of metabolism and excretion are also important to the risk of hypoglycemia. Because sulfonylureas are metabolized by and inactivated in the liver, the risk of hypoglycemia is significantly increased in patients with hepatic impairment. Sulfonylureas that are metabolized to active metabolites, such as glyburide, should be avoided in renal dysfunction, as the active metabolites can accumulate, increasing the hypoglycemia risk. Glipizide is preferred for use in renal dysfunction due to its shorter duration of action compared to glyburide and glimepiride, and is metabolized to inactive metabolites.

If a patient is experiencing hypoglycemia on a particular sulfonylurea, their eating pattern should be assessed. Hypoglycemia could occur due to one skipped meal, and thus is explainable. If the hypoglycemia is consistent, the dose should be reduced. If hypoglycemia persists, a meglitinide, a shorter-acting insulin secretagogue, can be used instead of a sulfonylurea.

Sulfonylurea therapy is used most in patients already on metformin, as second- or third-line treatment. Sulfonylureas can be combined with other antidiabetic medications that have different or complementary mechanisms of action. They should not be used in combination with the meglitinides, as these are also insulin secretagogues. When used with a GLP-1 RA or DPP-4 inhibitor, it is recommended to reduce the dose of the sulfonylurea (e.g., by half) when adding either of these agents to reduce the risk of hypoglycemia. When using combination therapy with noninsulin agents and a patient experiences hypoglycemia, the sulfonylurea should be the first consideration in dosage reduction versus other agents, as it is the sulfonylurea's insulin secretory effect that causes hypoglycemia.

Table 8.1 Sulfonylurea Pharmacokinetic Properties

Sulfonylurea	Peak effect (h)	Approximate duration of action (h)	Protein binding	Metabolism	Half-life (h)	Excretion
Chlorpropamide	3 to 6	36	90%	Hepatic via CYP2C9 (~80%) to metabolites (inactive and active)	~36	Urine (unchanged drug and metabolites)
Glimepiride	2 to 3	24	>99.5%	Hepatic oxidation via CYP2C9 to M1 metabolite (one-third activity compared to parent); further oxidative metabolism to M2 metabolite (inactive)	5 to 9	Urine (60%; 80%–90% as M1 and M2 metabolites); feces (40%; 70% as M1 and M2 metabolites)
Glipizide	IR: 1 to 3 ER: 6 to 12	12 to 24	98% to 99%, primarily to albumin	Hepatic via CYP2C9 to inactive metabolites	IR: 2 to 4 ER: 4–13	Urine (<10% unchanged drug; 80% as metabolites); feces (10%)
Glyburide	2 to 4	≤24	Extensive, primarily to albumin	Hepatic via CYP2C to metabolites (weakly active)	~10; Glynase PresTab: ~4	Urine (50%, as metabolites); feces (50%, as metabolites)
Tolazamide	3 to 4	10 to 24	94%	Extensively hepatic to 5 major metabolites (some active)	7	Urine (85%); feces (7%)
Tolbutamide	3 to 4	6 to 24	~95% (concentration dependent)	Hepatic via CYP2C9 to 2 inactive metabolites	4.5 to 6.5	Urine (75% to 85%, primarily as metabolites); feces

Source: Individual drug monographs on DAILYMED

Table 8.2 Sulfonylurea Dosage Information

Sulfonylurea	Available strengths	Usual starting dose	Dose titration	Dosage range
Chlorpropamide	100 mg, 250 mg	100–250 mg daily	50–125 mg every 1–2 weeks	100–500 mg daily
Tolazamide	250 mg, 500 mg	100–250 mg daily*	100–250 mg every 1–2 weeks	250–1,000 mg daily (if >500 mg, take twice daily)
Tolbutamide	500 mg	250–500 mg twice daily	250 mg every 1–2 weeks	0.25–3 g daily (taken with meals two to three times daily; usual maintenance dose is up to 2 g)
Glimepiride	1 mg, 2 mg, 4 mg	1–2 mg daily*	2 mg every 1–2 weeks	1–8 mg daily (usual maintenance dose is up to 4 mg)
Glipizide	IR: 5 mg, 10 mg	IR: 5 mg daily*	IR: 2.5–5 mg at intervals of at least several days	IR: 10–40 mg once daily (if >15 mg, take twice daily)
	ER: 2.5 mg, 5 mg, 10 mg	ER: 2.5–10 daily*	ER: 2.5 mg at intervals of at least a week	ER: 2.5–20 mg daily
Glyburide (Glibenclamide)	1.25 mg, 2.5 mg, 5 mg	2.5–5 mg daily*	2.5 mg every 1–2 weeks	1.25–20 mg daily (or twice daily)
	Micronized: 1.5 mg, 3 mg, 6 mg	Micronized: 1.5–3 mg daily	Micronized: 1.5 mg every 1–2 weeks	Micronized: 1.5–12 mg daily (if >6 mg, take twice daily)

* Daily is usually at breakfast or with first main meal. *Source*: Individual drug monographs at DAILYMED.

Sulfonylureas and insulin have been used extensively in combination therapy. Based on the American Diabetes Association's treatment algorithm for initiating insulin, basal insulin is usually started first and used in combination with other noninsulin medications.[4] At this point in treatment, a sulfonylurea is usually continued, as it still may have some therapeutic benefit. In fact, an older term for this therapy was BIDS: bedtime insulin (with a basal insulin), daytime sulfonylurea. As a patient progresses to needing mealtime insulin, then the sulfonylurea is typically discontinued.

COMBINATION PILLS CONTAINING A SULFONYLUREA

Available combination tablets with sulfonylureas are listed below. They can be considered for patients on stable doses of each medication, which can assist with adherence and possibly lower drug costs. However, if the dose of either agent is being dose adjusted, it is best to for a patient to take each medication as a separate pill. This will avoid any confusion on how much of each medication to take and even medication errors.

Glyburide/metformin (generics)

- 1.25 mg/250 mg: Glyburide 1.25 mg and metformin hydrochloride 250 mg
- 2.5 mg/500 mg: Glyburide 2.5 mg and metformin hydrochloride 500 mg
- 5 mg/500 mg: Glyburide 5 mg and metformin hydrochloride 500 mg
- Glipizide/metformin (generics)
- Glipizide 2.5 mg and metformin hydrochloride 250 mg
- Glipizide 2.5 mg and metformin hydrochloride 500 mg
- Glipizide 5 mg and metformin hydrochloride 500 mg
- Pioglitazone/glimepiride (Duetact; generics)
- Pioglitazone 30 mg and glimepiride 2 mg
- Pioglitazone 30 mg and glimepiride 4 mg

MONOGRAPHS

Glimepiride (Amaryl): https://dailymed.nlm.nih.gov/dailymed/drugInfo. cfm?setid=222b630b-7e09-43b4-9894-3d87f10add91

Glipizide (Glucotrol): https://dailymed.nlm.nih.gov/dailymed/drugInfo. cfm?setid=3e21bcc7-6f0d-4d63-befd-aa3ac8c63e37

Glipizide extended-release (Glucotrol XL): https://dailymed.nlm.nih.gov/dailymed/drugInfo.cfm?setid=8438b406-9259-46d1-b26a-90fdcb5cbc50

Glyburide: https://dailymed.nlm.nih.gov/dailymed/drugInfo.cfm?setid=5c391b11-68e9-4040-8408-56b43ee853f5

Glyburide-micronized (Glynase PresTab): https://dailymed.nlm.nih.gov/dailymed/drugInfo.cfm?setid=a7fce80a-2f13-43cc-8e1c-561f7d3ec3d5

Tolazamide: https://dailymed.nlm.nih.gov/dailymed/drugInfo.cfm?setid=f82dcff5-4afa-45d8-bc8c-f0f7c0c96272

REFERENCES

1. Le P, Chaitoff A, Misra-Herbert AD, et al. Use of antihyperglycemic medications in U.S. adults: An analysis of the national health and nutrition examination survey. *Diabetes Care* 2020;43:1227–1233

2. Bennett WL, Maruthur NM, Singh S, et al. Comparative effectiveness and safety of medications for type 2 diabetes: an update including new drugs and 2-drug combinations. *Ann Intern Med* 2011;154:602–613

3. UK Prospective Diabetes Study (UKPDS) Group. Intensive blood glucose control with sulfonylureas or insulin compared with conventional treatment

and risk of complications in patients with type 2 diabetes (UKPDS 33). *Lancet* 1998;352:837–853

4. American Diabetes Association. 9. Pharmacologic approaches to glycemic treatment: Standards of Medical Care in Diabetes—2022. *Diabetes Care* 2022;45(Suppl. 1):S125–S143

5. Turner RC, Cull CA, Frighi V, Holman RR;UKPDS Group. Glycemic control with diet, sulfonylurea, metformin, or insulin in patients with type 2 diabetes mellitus: progressive requirement for multiple therapies (UKPDS 49). *JAMA* 1999;281:2005–2012

6. American Diabetes Association. 2. Classification and diagnosis of diabetes: Standards of Medical Care in Diabetes—2022. *Diabetes Care* 2022; 45(Suppl. 1):S17–S38

7. Masharani U, Kroon L. Pancreatic hormones and glucose-lowering drugs. In *Basic & Clinical Pharmacology*, 15th ed. Katzung BG, VanderahTW, Eds. New York, McGraw-Hill, 2021. Available from https://accesspharmacy. mhmedical.com/content.aspx?bookid=2988&sectionid=250601239. Accessed 22 March 2021

8. Inzucchi SE. Oral antihyperglycemic therapy for type 2 diabetes: scientific review. *JAMA* 2002;287:360–372

9. Klepzig H, Kober G, Matter C, et al. Sulfonylureas and ischaemic preconditioning: a double-blind, placebo-controlled evaluation of glimepiride and glibenclamide. *Eur Heart J* 1999;20:439–436

10. Quast U, Stephan D, Bieger S, Russ U. The impact of ATP-sensitive K+ channel subtype selectivity of insulin secretagogues for the coronary vasculature and the myocardium. *Diabetes* 2004;53(Suppl. 3): S156–164

11. Groop LC. Sulfonylureas in NIDDM. *Diabetes Care* 1992;15:737

12. Sola D, Rossi L, Schianca GPC, et al. Sulfonylureas and their use in clinical practice. *Arch Med Sci* 2015;11:840–848

13. Groop LC, Barzilai N, Ratheiser K, et al. Dose-dependent effects of glyburide in insulin secretion and glucose uptake in humans. *Diabetes Care* 1991;14:724–727

14. Stenman S, Melander A, Groop PH, Groop LC. What is the benefit of increasing the sulfonylurea dose? *Ann Intern Med* 1993;118:169–172

15. Faber OK, Beck-Nielsen H, Binder C, et al. Acute actions of sulfonylurea drugs during long-term treatment of NIDDM. *Diabetes Care* 1990;13(Suppl. 3):26–31

16. Kahn SE, Haffner SM, Heise MA, et al.; ADOPT Study Group. Glycemic durability of rosiglitazone, metformin, or glyburide monotherapy. *N Engl J Med* 2006;355:2427–2443

17. van Raalte DH, Verchere CB. Improving glycemic control in type 2 diabetes: stimulate insulin secretion or provide beta-cell rest? *Diabetes Obes Metab* 2017;19:1205–1213

18. Nathan DM, Buse JB, Kahn SE, et al.; GRADE Study Research Group. Rationale and design of the glycemia reduction approaches in diabetes: a comparative effectiveness study (GRADE). *Diabetes Care* 2013;36:2254–2261

19. The University Group Diabetes Program. A study of the effects of hypoglycemic agents on vascular complications in patients with adult-onset diabetes I. Design, methods, and baseline results. *Diabetes* 1970;19(Suppl. 2):747–830

20. ADVANCE Collaborative Group. Intensive blood glucose control and vascular outcomes in patients with type 2 diabetes. *N Engl J Med* 2008;358:2560–2572

21. Holman RR, Paul SK, Bethel MA, et al. 10-year follow-up of intensive glucose control in type 2 diabetes. *N Engl J Med* 2008;359:1577–1589

22. Seligman HK, Schillinger D. Hunger and socioeconomic disparities in chronic disease. *N Engl J Med* 2010;363:6–9

23. Monami M, Genovese S, Mannucci E. Cardiovascular safety of sulfonylureas: a meta-analysis of randomized clinical trials. *Diabetes Obes Metab* 2013;15:938–953

24. Bain S, Druyts E, Balijepalli C, et al. Cardiovascular events and all-cause mortality associated with sulphonylureas compared with other antihyperglycaemic drugs: a Bayesian meta-analysis of survival data. *Diabetes Obes Metab* 2017;19:329–335

25. Zhuang XD, He X, Yang DY, et al. Comparative cardiovascular outcomes in the era of novel anti-diabetic agents: a comprehensive network meta-analysis of 166,371 participants from 170 randomized controlled trials. *Cardiovasc Diabetol* 2018;17:79. DOI:10.1186/s12933-018-0722-z

26. Rados DV, Pinto LC, Remonti LR, et al. The association between sulfonylurea use and all-cause and cardiovascular mortality: A meta-analysis with trial sequential analysis of randomized clinical trials. *PLoS Med* 2016;13(4): e1001992. DOI:10.1371/journal.pmed.1001992

27. Rosenstock J, Kahn SE, Johansen OE, et al. Effect of linagliptin vs glimepiride on major adverse cardiovascular outcomes in patients with type 2 diabetes: the CAROLINA Randomized Clinical Trial. *JAMA* 2019;322:1155–66

28. Xie Y, Bowe B, Gibson AK, McGill JB, Maddukuri G, Al-Aly Z. Comparative effectiveness of sodium-glucose cotransporter 2 inhibitors vs sulfonylureas in patients with type 2 diabetes. *JAMA Intern Med* 2021;181(8):1043–1053

29. Herrera Comoglio R, Vidal Guitart X. Cardiovascular events and mortality among type 2 diabetes mellitus patients newly prescribed first-line blood

glucose-lowering drugs monotherapies: A population-based cohort study in the Catalan electronic medical record database, SIDIAP, 2010-2015. *Prim Care Diabetes* 2021;15(2):323–331

30. Korytkowski MT. Sulfonylurea treatment of type 2 diabetes: focus on glimepiride. *Pharmacotherapy* 2004;24:606–620

31. Towell J, Garthwaite T, Wang R. Erythrocyte aldehyde dehydrogenase and disulfiram-like side effects of hypoglycemics and antianginals. *Alcohol Clin Exp Res* 1985;9:438–442

32. Maruthur NM, Tseng E, Hutfless S, et al. Diabetes medications as monotherapy or metformin-based combination therapy for type 2 diabetes: a systematic review and meta-analysis. *Ann Intern Med* 2016;164:740–751

33. Wright AD, Cull CA, Macleod KM, Holman RR; UKPDS Group. Hypoglycemia in type 2 diabetic patients randomized to and maintained on monotherapy with diet, sulfonylurea, metformin, or insulin for 6 years from diagnosis: UKPDS73. *J Diabetes Complications* 2006;20:395–401

34. McCoy RD, Lipska KJ, Yao X, et al. Intensive treatment and severe hypoglycemia among adults with type 2 diabetes. *JAMA Intern Med* 2016;176(7):969–978

35. Lipska KJ, Yao X, Herrin J, et al. Trends in drug utilization, glycemic control, and rates of severe hypoglycemia, 2006–2013. *Diabetes Care* 2017;40:468–475

36. Ling S, Zaccardi F, Lawson C, Seidu SI, Davies MJ, Khunti K. Glucose control, sulfonylureas, and insulin treatment in elderly people with type 2 diabetes and risk of severe hypoglycemia and death: An observational study. *Diabetes Care* 2021:dc200876.

37. American Geriatrics Society 2015 Beers Criteria Update Expert Panel. American Geriatrics Society 2015 updated Beers Criteria for potentially inappropriate medication use in older adults. *J Am Geriatr Soc* 2015;63:2227–2246

38. Graudins A, Linden CH, Ferm RP. Diagnosis and treatment of sulfonylurea-induced hyperinsulinemic hypoglycemia. *Am J Emerg Med* 1997;15:95–96

39. Cryer PE, Davis SN, Shamoon H. Hypoglycemia in diabetes. *Diabetes Care* 2003;26:1902–1912

Chapter 9
Glinides

Lisa Kroon, PharmD
Crystal Zhou, PharmD

The meglitinides are insulin secretagogues that are structurally different from the sulfonylureas and have different pharmacokinetics. The meglitinides (or "glinides," as they will be referred to in this chapter) have a similar mechanism of action as the sulfonylureas, causing an increase in insulin release from the β-cells in the pancreas. They are taken at the time of a meal, and thus require multiple daily dosing for patients, but also allow for more flexibility in dose administration with the timing of their meals. Because of their short half-life, they have a reduced risk of hypoglycemia. Although glinides are some of the less frequently used antihyperglycemic medications, they do offer a niche in T2D therapy that will be reviewed.[1,2] Two compounds are available in this class of antihyperglycemics: nateglinide and repaglinide, which are analogs of meglitinide. The glinides are FDA approved to improve glycemic control in adults with T2D as an adjunct to diet and exercise.

The American Diabetes Association's pharmacologic treatment approach for glycemic control places insulin secretagogues (sulfonylureas and glinides) as an option for a second agent after a patient is on metformin and cost is a concern.[3] In clinical practice, the glinides are often used after a patient is not able to tolerate a sulfonylurea (usually due to hypoglycemia), where the sulfonylurea is discontinued and switched to a glinide. Thus, their place in therapy is generally as a second or third noninsulin agent. T2D is a progressive disease in which most patients at some point require multiple medications to achieve good glycemic control.[4] As a patient progresses to needing additional pharmacologic therapy, a glinide is generally discontinued when a patient is advanced to requiring mealtime insulin. At this point, the pancreatic function has declined to a point where the insulin secretagogues likely have no appreciable effect on insulin secretion. In patients with MODY, type HNF1A or HNF4A, while low-dose sulfonylureas are considered first-line therapy, meglitinides could be considered as well.[5,6]

MECHANISM OF ACTION

The glinides are structurally different from the sulfonylureas; however, similar to that class, they lower blood glucose levels by stimulating insulin release from the pancreas.[7,8] As with the sulfonylureas, release of insulin is dependent on functioning β-cells in the pancreatic islets. Repaglinide is a derivative of benzoic acid and is a meglitinide analog. Nateglinide is a derivative of the amino acid D-phenylalanine.

The glinides' effect on the β-cell is glucose-dependent and diminishes at lower glucose concentrations.[8] Glinides bind to the sulfonylurea receptor on the β-cell but in a different configuration than the sulfonylureas and at a separate distinct binding site on the β-cell.[7–9] As with the sulfonylureas, the glinides close ATP-dependent potassium channels in the β-cell membrane, blocking the efflux of potassium.[7] As potassium accumulates within the β-cell membrane, the membrane potential lowers causing depolarization, which opens the voltage-dependent calcium channels; the calcium influx results in increased intracellular calcium. The increased concentration of calcium causes insulin granules to migrate to the cell surface, where the granules rupture and release the insulin.[7]

Patients with T2D characteristically have defects in both insulin secretion and insulin action. Glinides' primary action in improving glycemic control is by affecting the β-cell defect, enhancing (and restoring) early-phase insulin release.[8] Glinides thus reduce postprandial glucose excursions.[10] Since they have a more rapid onset and a shorter duration of action than the sulfonylureas, glinides' niche in therapy is to improve glycemic control postprandially while reducing the risk of late hypoglycemia.

PHARMACOKINETICS

Both repaglinide and nateglinide have a rapid onset and short duration of action. They are extensively metabolized to primarily inactive metabolites. The pharmacokinetic properties of glinides are summarized in Table 9.1.

Peak plasma concentrations of repaglinide are reached within 1 h following oral administration.[11] Repaglinide has an absolute bioavailability of 56–63%.[11] Administration with food does not affect the time to peak level, but it reduces the mean peak concentration by 20% and the area under the plasma time concentration curve by 12.4%. Repaglinide should be taken within 30 min before a meal. The volume of distribution of repaglinide is 31 L, and it is highly protein-bound (>98%).[11]

Repaglinide is rapidly and completely metabolized via oxidative biotransformation and direct conjugation with glucuronic acid. CYP2C8 and CYP3A4 isoenzymes are involved in its metabolism to the M1 and M2 metabolites, which are both inactive. Repaglinide's elimination half-life is about 1 h, and its duration of action is 4–7 h.[7,9] The majority of the drug is excreted in the feces (90%) with 8% excreted in urine. Less than 2% of repaglinide is excreted unchanged in the feces.[11]

Nateglinide is rapidly and almost completely absorbed (about 90%) with a peak plasma concentration within 1 h.[12] Peak levels of nateglinide are lower when it is taken after a meal than when taken shortly before a meal. Nateglinide's absolute bioavailability is about 73%, and its volume of distribution is approximately 10.5 L.[12] It should be taken within 30 min before a meal. Similar to repaglinide and the sulfonylureas, nateglinide is highly bound (98%), mainly to albumin.[12]

Table 9.1—Glinide Pharmacokinetic Properties

Glinide	Peak effect (h)	Approximate duration of action (h)	Protein binding	Metabolism	Half-life (h)	Excretion
Nateglinide	~1	4	98%	Hepatic via CYP2C9 (70%) and CYP3A4 (30%) to metabolites (inactive and 1 active with similar activity to parent)	~1.5	Urine (83%, 16% unchanged drug); feces (10%)
Repaglinide	~1	4–7	>98%	Hepatic via CYP3A4 and CYP2C8 to metabolite (inactive)	~1	Urine (~8%; 0.1% unchanged drug); feces (90%; <2% unchanged drug)

Source: Individual drug monographs on DAILYMED.

Nateglinide is extensively metabolized by hydroxylation and then glucuronide conjugation. The CYP enzymes, CYP3A4 (30%) and CYP2C9 (70%), convert nateglinide to several inactive metabolites, with only one metabolite (M1) having similar pharmacologic activity to nateglinide. However, the overall exposure to the M1 metabolite is less than 5% compared to nateglinide.[12] The metabolites are primarily excreted in the urine (84–87%) with 8–10% excreted in the feces. Approximately 16% of nateglinide is excreted unchanged in the urine. Nateglinide's elimination half-life is about 1.5 h, and its duration of action is 4 h.[7,12]

TREATMENT ADVANTAGES/DISADVANTAGES

ADVANTAGES

As monotherapy in patients with T2D, glinides can induce a mean decrease in A1C of 0.5–1.5% from baseline, with nateglinide typically having a lesser effect on A1C. The expected A1C lowering of the glinides is generally less than that of the sulfonylureas. A Cochrane review found that repaglinide and nateglinide (specifically the 120-mg dose in three studies) reduced A1C by 0.5–2.1% and 0.5%, respectively, compared to placebo.[13] In a head-to-head, open-label, 16-week study, the mean reduction in A1C was significantly greater with repaglinide monotherapy compared to nateglinide (–1.57 vs. –1.04%).[14] The mean change in fasting blood glucose was also significantly greater with repaglinide (–57 vs. –18 mg/dL). Their effects on postprandial glucose AUC were similar.

Given their rapid onset of action and effect on first-phase insulin release, glinides are effective in lowering postprandial glucose excursions. Repaglinide has been shown to reduce postprandial glucose levels by approximately 100 mg/dL and nateglinide by 85 mg/dL.[15–17] In a study comparing nateglinide and glyburide, nateglinide had a greater effect on mealtime glucose excursions, whereas glyburide was more effective in reducing fasting plasma glucose.[18]

Postprandial hyperglycemia has been shown to contribute to cardiovascular risk in patients with T2D. The Diabetes Epidemiology: Collaborative analysis of Diagnostic criteria in Europe (DECODE) and Diabetes Epidemiology: Collaborative analysis of Diagnostic criteria in Asia (DECODA) studies showed that high 2-h postprandial glucose following an oral-glucose tolerance test was an independent risk factor for all-cause mortality and cardiovascular death in patients with T2D.[19,20] Therefore, postprandial blood glucose control and postprandial glucose monitoring can be an important component of T2D management.[21,22] Glinides can play a unique role in this strategy, given their primary effect in lowering postprandial glucose excursions.

Glinides have a relatively low incidence of hypoglycemia and may be preferable over a sulfonylurea in patients who are predisposed to hypoglycemia, such as the elderly. In patients for whom sulfonylureas are effective, but they are experiencing hypoglycemia, glinides can be used in place of sulfonylureas, which are longer-acting insulin secretagogues. It is important to note that glinides will have little, if any, effect when substituted for a sulfonylurea in a patient who is not responding adequately to a sulfonylurea, due to their same mechanism of action. Glinides and sulfonylureas should not be used in combination for the same reason.

Since glinides do not contain a sulfa moiety, they can be used instead of a sulfonylurea in patients with a history of a serious sulfa allergy or patients who experience an allergic reaction to a sulfonylurea.

From a pharmacodynamics perspective, glinides have a rapid onset of effect compared to other noninsulin agents. While general dose titrations are usually made every 1–2 weeks, in practice, the dose is sometimes adjusted daily or at a particular meal.

DISADVANTAGES

The main disadvantages of glinides are the need for multiple daily doses, which can affect adherence, and less A1C efficacy compared to other antihyperglycemic medications. In addition, with the natural progressive decline in β-cell function associated with T2D over time, the response to glinide treatment likewise will diminish, and changes to the treatment regimen may be necessary. Please see the "Sulfonylureas" chapter for further discussion.

SIGNIFICANT WARNINGS/PRECAUTIONS

Glinides are contraindicated in patients with DKA, T1D, or known hypersensitivity to either nateglinide or repaglinide. Unlike the sulfonylureas, glinides do not carry a special warning about an associated increased risk of cardiovascular mortality. Repaglinide has a specific warning about an increased risk of MI with the concurrent use with NPH insulin, based on older literature. Clinical studies have since been published demonstrating safety and efficacy when repaglinide is used with this particular insulin.[9]

Hypoglycemia

Due to their mechanism of action of stimulating insulin release, glinides can cause hypoglycemia. The frequency of hypoglycemia is less with the glinides than with the sulfonylureas primarily due to their pharmacokinetics (e.g., shorter duration of action and conversion to inactive metabolites).[2,10] See further discussion below in "Patients at Risk for Hypoglycemia."

SPECIAL POPULATIONS

Hypoglycemia

The most serious complication of glinide therapy is hypoglycemia. Appropriate patient selection, dosage, and patient education are important to avoid hypoglycemic episodes. Debilitated or malnourished patients and those with adrenal, pituitary, or hepatic insufficiency are particularly susceptible to the hypoglycemic action of insulin secretagogues. Hypoglycemia may be difficult to recognize in the elderly and in people taking β-blockers, particularly nonselective ones. Hypoglycemia is more likely to occur when caloric intake is reduced, meals are skipped (and the glinide still taken), after severe or prolonged exercise, when alcohol is ingested, or when more than one glucose-lowering drug is used. Elderly patients and those with multiple comorbidities are at greater risk of hypoglycemia (see "Adverse Effects and Monitoring" for in-depth discussion on hypoglycemia).

Irregular Eating Patterns

Due to the rapid onset and shorter duration of action, glinides are ideal for patients who eat meals at differing times day to day. For these patients, glinides should be taken just before the meal (0–30 min prior) regardless of the time of the meal. The ability to change the dose timing of these insulin secretagogues to when a patient eats is a niche for glinides in antihyperglycemic medication options.

Pregnancy and Lactation

Repaglinide is categorized as pregnancy category C. Repaglinide has not been found to be teratogenic in animal studies; however, nonteratogenic skeletal deformities were observed following exposure during gestation and lactation. Nateglinide is also categorized as pregnancy category C. Adverse effects have been observed in some animal reproduction studies. As the studies on the effects of glinides on pregnancy outcomes is limited, it is not recommended to use them during pregnancy.

Although it is not known whether or not the glinides are excreted in human milk, some animal studies do suggest secretion into the milk of lactating animals. It is recommended that neither glinide be used in nursing women, due to the possible risk of hypoglycemia in nursing infants.

Hepatic or Renal Impairment

Because glinides are metabolized by CYP isoenzymes, caution should be exercised when using this class of medications in patients with hepatic impairment. Patients with moderate to severe impairment of liver function will have higher serum concentrations and more unbound repaglinide and metabolites than will patients with normal hepatic function. However, the altered serum concentrations and unbound fraction have not been shown to alter the response to repaglinide. Since some patients with hepatic dysfunction could respond differently, it is reasonable to start with lower doses of repaglinide. Peak concentration and overall drug exposure to nateglinide were increased by about 30% in nondiabetic subjects with mild hepatic dysfunction when compared to healthy volunteers. No dosage adjustment is recommended in patients with mild to moderate hepatic dysfunction; nateglinide should be used with caution in patients with severe hepatic failure.

In patients for whom insulin secretagogue therapy is effective, glinides can be useful for those with renal dysfunction, due to their short duration of action and their reduced risk of hypoglycemia. No adjustment in the initial dose of repaglinide is required in patients with mild to moderate renal dysfunction. In those with severe renal dysfunction, it is recommended to start with the 0.5-mg dose. Although no dosage adjustment is needed for nateglinide in patients with renal dysfunction, patients with severe renal impairment could be more susceptible to hypoglycemia, due to accumulation of the M1 active metabolite. Therefore, it would be reasonable to start with the 60-mg dose in this population.

Pediatrics

The safety and effectiveness of repaglinide and nateglinide has not been established in children.

Geriatrics

The pharmacokinetics of either glinide are not significantly affected by age, and no dose adjustment is recommended in elderly patients.

Patients with Food Insecurities and Homelessness

Patients who are homeless or who do not have a reliable source of food may experience more frequent hypoglycemia if taking a sulfonylurea, particularly a longer-acting one. Therefore, in patients with food insecurities who may benefit from an insulin secretagogue, the glinides may be advantageous, as they are only taken if a meal is available. Use of glinides can therefore help to prevent hypoglycemia in patients who may not have a plan for future meals, whereas use of a sulfonylurea could put these patients at risk for hypoglycemia. Providers should also help these patients seek local resources to assist them in obtaining regularly distributed food.[23]

Patients with Cardiovascular Disease and Increased Cardiovascular Risk

In the Nateglinide And Valsartan in Impaired Glucose Tolerance Outcomes Research (NAVIGATOR) study, nateglinide was evaluated in patients with impaired glucose tolerance to see if its use could reduce the risk of cardiovascular outcomes; nateglinide was not found to reduce the risk of cardiovascular events.[24]

In a longitudinal, retrospective cohort study using the Catalan database SIDIAP (Information System for the Development of Research in Primary Care), repaglinide use, compared to metformin, was associated with an increased risk of MACE, with a hazard ratio of 2.01 (95% CI 1.29-3.12).[25] Although there were well over 100,000 patients included in the study, the retrospective nature does not allow for definitive conclusions; therefore, randomized controlled trials are needed to confirm these results. Given this data, glinides should be used with caution in patients with existing cardiovascular disease.

ADVERSE EFFECTS AND MONITORING

Glinides are usually well tolerated, and the frequency of side effects, including hypoglycemia, is low. The most common adverse effects associated with glinide treatment other than hypoglycemia are upper respiratory infections, sinusitis, nausea, diarrhea, constipation, arthralgia, weight gain, and headache.[11] Rare side effects include hypersensitivity reactions and hepatic enzyme elevations.[11,26]

The two adverse effects that are the primary disadvantages of glinides are weight gain and hypoglycemia.[2] In a retrospective analysis of a large, national cohort of T2D, use of a sulfonylurea or glinide increased the risk of severe hypoglycemia about twofold.[27] This analysis also found that patients with high complexity (i.e., age 75 years and older or multiple comorbidities) on intensive treatment also had nearly double the risk of severe hypoglycemia. Monitoring blood glucose levels and only taking a glinide when eating a meal can help to reduce the risk of hypoglycemia. Unlike some of the sulfonylureas, glinides do not appear in the Beers Criteria as potentially inappropriate medications in people 65 years and older.[28]

Glinides can cause a weight gain of 1–3 kg compared to baseline. In a pooled analysis of studies, sulfonylureas and glinides increased weight similarly.[2] The weight gain can be attributed to two factors: improved glycemic control and hypoglycemia. Inherent in improving glycemic control is weight gain, as fewer calories are spilling into the urine. Also, a patient consumes additional calories when treating hypoglycemia. Therefore, it is important not only to reduce the risk of hypoglycemia from a safety perspective, but also to limit weight gain associated with glinides.

Patients on glinides should be educated on how to self-monitor their blood glucose (and to monitor regularly), hypoglycemic symptoms and values, and how to self-treat for a hypoglycemic episode. A quick-acting source of glucose should be used. Patients should also be educated to only take a glinide with the meal; if the meal is skipped, the glinide dose is also skipped. Patients who are purposefully trying to eat less, increase physical activity, or lose weight may need their glinide dose reduced.

DRUG INTERACTIONS

Repaglinide's metabolism can be inhibited by CYP3A4 inhibitors, such as keto-conazole, itraconazole, cyclosporine, and erythromycin.[29,30] When used with cyclo-sporine, the maximum daily dose of repaglinide is 6 mg. Agents that induce CYP3A4 metabolism, such as rifampin, barbiturates, and carbamazepine, may reduce repaglinide levels. The combination of repaglinide and atazanavir should be avoided, as atazanavir is a CYP2C8 substrate.

Coadministration of repaglinide with the CYP450 inhibitor clarithromycin resulted in significantly higher concentrations of repaglinide.[31,32] This increase may necessitate a dosage reduction of repaglinide in cases when these drugs are used together. Gemfibrozil causes a significant increase in repaglinide serum levels, and their concomitant use is considered a contraindication.[33,34] Itraconazole has been shown to augment the interaction with gemfibrozil and repaglinide.[32]

Clopidogrel can inhibit CYP2C8 and thus increase repaglinide levels.[35] It is recommended to avoid their concomitant use; if it is necessary to use together, the starting dose of repaglinide is 0.5 mg with each meal, and the total daily dose should be limited to 4 mg or less.

The hypoglycemic action of repaglinide may be enhanced by certain drugs, including NSAIDs and other agents that are highly bound to protein, such as salicylates, sulfonamides, chloramphenicol, warfarin, probenecid, monoamine oxidase inhibitors, and β-blockers. Therefore, if using repaglinide with any of the aforementioned drugs, blood glucose should be monitored and the dose adjusted accordingly.

Even though nateglinide is metabolized by CYP2C9 (major) and CYP3A4 (minor), few clinically significant drug-drug interactions exist with nateglinide. Nateglinide's metabolism can be inhibited by CYP2C9 inhibitors, such as amiodarone, fluconazole, and voriconazole; therefore, the dose of nateglinide may need to be reduced. Although nateglinide is highly protein-bound, in vitro displacement studies have found that nateglinide does not have a significant effect on other highly bound drugs.[12]

Pharmacodynamic interactions with all antihyperglycemics include drugs that can cause hyperglycemia, and when taken may lead to worsening of glycemic control. Examples of these drugs include thiazide diuretics, statins, glucocorticoids, phenothiazines, certain antipsychotics (e.g., chlorpromazine, olanzapine, clozapine), HIV protease inhibitors, estrogens and hormonal contraceptives, phenytoin, immunosuppressive therapies, sympathomimetics, and isoniazid.

DOSAGE AND ADMINISTRATION

For patients whose A1C is <8%, the starting dose of repaglinide is 0.5 mg before each meal. For patients whose A1C is ≥8%, the initial dose is 1 or 2 mg before each meal. Dosage adjustments are determined by blood glucose response. The preprandial dose should be increased (typically doubled) until glycemic control is achieved or until a maximum dose of 4 mg per meal or 16 mg daily is reached. The usual starting dose of nateglinide is 120 mg before each meal. For patients who are close to their target A1C goal, nateglinide can be initiated at the lower 60-mg dose and then titrated up to 120 mg or until the glycemic response is achieved.

Doses should be taken 0–30 min before a meal. Patients who skip a meal or add an extra meal should be instructed to skip or add a dose for that meal, respectively. Most glinide dosage adjustments are typically done at weekly intervals or longer. Monitoring the preprandial and postprandial (e.g., 2 h after the start of the meal) glucose is particularly effective in assessing the dose response to a glinide. Typical dosing and administration regimens are shown in Table 9.2. In practice, depending on a patient's blood glucose profile, a different dose of a glinide may be taken at particular mealtimes, taking into account different types of meals (e.g., the amount of carbohydrates in the meal) and/or the premeal blood glucose.

When switching from a sulfonylurea to a glinide, the first glinide dose may be administered on the day after the final dose of the sulfonylurea. After changing to a glinide, patients should closely monitor their blood glucose, watching for any hypoglycemia, in case there is a residual effect of the sulfonylurea or an enhanced response to the glinide.

Table 9.2—Glinide Dosage Information

Glinide	Available strengths	Usual starting dose	Dose titration	Dosage range
Nateglinide	60 mg, 120 mg	120 mg three times daily before meals 60 mg three times daily before meals if close to A1C goal	Weekly, if started on 60 mg dose	180–360 mg daily
Repaglinide	0.5 mg, 1 mg, 2 mg	A1C <8%: 0.5 mg three times daily before meals A1C ≥8%: 1 or 2 mg three times daily before meals	0.5–2 mg each meal on a weekly basis (mealtime dose is typically doubled)	0.5–4 mg before meals or up to 16 mg daily

Source: Individual drug monographs at DAILYMED.

COMBINATION PILLS CONTAINING A GLINIDE

Repaglinide/metformin (generics)

- 1 mg/250 mg: Repaglinide 1 mg and metformin hydrochloride 250 mg
- 2 mg/500 mg: Repapglinide 2 mg and metformin hydrochloride 500 mg

MONOGRAPHS

Nateglinide: https://dailymed.nlm.nih.gov/dailymed/drugInfo.cfm?setid =a7e9f62e-32f8-4a89-8588-74d029c8f6a2

Repaglinide: https://dailymed.nlm.nih.gov/dailymed/drugInfo.cfm?setid =68064989-47ea-4ed5-a20e-43c4ef6ec271

REFERENCES

1. Le P, Chaitoff A, Misra-Herbert AD, et al. Use of antihyperglycemic medications in U.S. adults: An analysis of the national health and nutrition examination survey. *Diabetes Care* 2020;43:1227–1233

2. Bennett WL, Maruthur NM, Singh S, et al. Comparative effectiveness and safety of medications for type 2 diabetes: an update including new drugs and 2-drug combinations. *Ann Intern Med* 2011;154:602–613

3. American Diabetes Association. 9. Pharmacologic approaches to glycemic treatment: Standards of Medical Care in Diabetes—2022. *Diabetes Care* 2022;45(Suppl. 1):S125–S143

4. Turner RC, Cull CA, Frighi V, Holman RR; UKPDS Group. Glycemic control with diet, sulfonylurea, metformin, or insulin in patients with type 2 diabetes mellitus: progressive requirement for multiple therapies (UKPDS 49). *JAMA* 1999;281:2005–2012

5. American Diabetes Association. 2. Classification and diagnosis of diabetes: Standards of Medical Care in Diabetes—2022. *Diabetes Care* 2022; 45(Suppl. 1):S17–S38

6. Tuomi T, Honkanen EH, Isomaa B, Sarelin L, Groop LC. Improved prandial glucose control with lower risk of hypoglycemia with nateglinide than with glibenclamide in patients with maturity-onset diabetes of the young type 3. *Diabetes Care* 2006;29:189–194

7. Masharani U, Kroon L. Pancreatic hormones and glucose-lowering drugs. In *Basic & Clinical Pharmacology*, 15th ed. Katzung BG, Vanderah TW, Eds. New York, McGraw-Hill, 2021. Available from https://accesspharmacy. mhmedical.com/content.aspx?bookid=2988&sectionid=250601239. Accessed 22 March 2021

8. Dornhorst A. Insulinotropic meglitinide analogues. *Lancet* 2001;358: 1709–1716

9. Guardado-Mendoza R, Prioletta A, Jiménez-Ceja LM, Sosale A, Folli F. The role of nateglinide and repaglinide, derivatives of meglitinide, in the treatment of type 2 diabetes mellitus. *Arch Med Sci* 2013;9:936–943

10. Inzucchi SE. Oral antihyperglycemic therapy for type 2 diabetes: scientific review. *JAMA* 2002;287:360–372

11. Scott LJ. Repaglinide: a review of its use in type 2 diabetes mellitus. *Drugs* 2012;72:249–272

12. McLeod JF. Clinical pharmacokinetics of nateglinide: a rapidly-absorbed, short-acting insulinotropic agent. *Clin Pharmacokinet* 2004;43:97–120

13. Black C, Donnelly P, McIntyre L, Royle PL, Shepherd JP, Thomas S. Meglitinide analogues for type 2 diabetes mellitus. *Cochrane Database Syst Rev* 2007;(2):CD004654

14. Rosenstock J, Hassman DR, Madder RD, et al.; Repaglinide Versus Nateglinide Comparison Study Group. Repaglinide versus nateglinide monotherapy: a randomized, multicenter study. *Diabetes Care* 2004;27:1265–1270

15. Van Gaal LF, Van Acker KL, De Leeuw IH. Repaglinide improves blood glucose control in sulphonylurea-naive type 2 diabetes. *Diabetes Res Clin Pract* 2001;53:141–148

16. Hezarkhani S, Bonakdaran S, Rajabian R, Shahini N, Marjani A. Comparison of glycemic excursion in patients with new onset type 2 diabetes mellitus before and after treatment with repaglinide. *Open Biochem J* 2013;7:19–23

17. Islas-Andrade S, Revilla-Monsalve MC, Martínez de Hurtado E, et al.; Latin American Study Group. Evaluation of the effects of nateglinide on postprandial glycemia in patients with type 2 diabetes mellitus: a multicenter, multinational, non-randomized, non-controlled Latin American study. *Pharmacology* 2003;68:89–95

18. Hollander PA, Schwartz SL, Gatlin MR, Haas SJ, et al. Importance of early insulin secretion: comparison of nateglinide and glyburide in previously diet-treated patients with type 2 diabetes. *Diabetes Care* 2001;26:983–988

19. The DECODE Study Group on behalf of the European Diabetes Epidemiology Group. Glucose tolerance and mortality: comparison of WHO and American Diabetes Association diagnostic criteria. *Lancet* 1999;354:617–621

20. Nakagami T; DECODA Study Group. Hyperglycaemia and mortality from all causes and from cardiovascular disease in five populations of Asian origin. *Diabetologia* 2004;47:385–394

21. Fonseca V. Clinical significance of targeting postprandial and fasting hyperglycemia in managing type 2 diabetes mellitus. *Curr Med Res Opin* 2003;19:635–641

22. Aronoff SL. Rationale for treatment options for mealtime glucose control in patients with type 2 diabetes. *Postgrad Med* 2017;129:231–241

23. Seligman HK, Schillinger D. Hunger and socioeconomic disparities in chronic disease. *N Engl J Med* 2010;363:6–9

24. Herrera Comoglio R, Vidal Guitart X. Cardiovascular events and mortality among type 2 diabetes mellitus patients newly prescribed first-line blood glucose-lowering drugs monotherapies: A population-based cohort study in the Catalan electronic medical record database, SIDIAP, 2010-2015. *Prim Care Diabetes* 2021;15(2):323–331

25. Derosa G. Nateglinide does not reduce the incidence of diabetes or cardiovascular outcomes in people with impaired glucose tolerance and cardiovascular disease or risk factors. *BMJ Evid Based Med* 2011;16:7–8

26. Nan DN, Hernández JL, Fernández-Ayala M, Carrascosa M. Acute hepatotoxicity caused by repaglinide. *Ann Intern Med* 2004;141:823

27. McCoy RD, Lipska KJ, Yao X, et al. Intensive treatment and severe hypoglycemia among adults with type 2 diabetes. *JAMA Intern Med* 2016; 176:969–978

28. American Geriatrics Society 2015 Beers Criteria Update Expert Panel. American Geriatrics Society 2015 updated Beers Criteria for potentially inappropriate medication use in older adults. *J Am Geriatr Soc* 2015;63: 2227–2246

29. Scheen AJ. Drug-drug and food-drug pharmacokinetic interactions with new insulinotropic agents repaglinide and nateglinide. *Clin Pharmacokinet* 2007;46:93–108

30. Kudo T, Hisaka A, Sugiyama Y, Ito K. Analysis of the repaglinide concentration increase produced by gemfibrozil and itraconazole based on the inhibition of the hepatic uptake transporter and metabolic enzymes. *Drug Metab Dispos* 2013;41:362–371

31. Khamaisi M, Leitersdorf E. Severe hypoglycemia from clarithromycin-repaglinide drug interaction. *Pharmacotherapy* 2008;28:682–684

32. Niemi M, Neuvonen PJ, Kivistö KT. The cytochrome P4503A4 inhibitor clarithromycin increases the plasma concentrations and effects of repaglinide. *Clin Pharmacol Ther* 2001;70:58–65

33. Gan J, Chen W, Shen H, et al. Repaglinide-gemfibrozil drug interaction: inhibition of repaglinide glucuronidation as a potential additional contributing mechanism. *Br J Clin Pharmacol* 2010;70:870–880

34. Honkalammi J, Niemi M, Neuvonen PJ, Backman JT. Dose-dependent interaction between gemfibrozil and repaglinide in humans: strong inhibition of CYP2C8 with subtherapeutic gemfibrozil doses. *Drug Metab Dispos* 2011;39:1977–1986

35. Tornio A, Filppula AM, Kailari O, et al. Glucuronidation converts clopidogrel to a strong time-dependent inhibitor of CYP2C8: a phase II metabolite as a perpetrator of drug-drug interactions. *Clin Pharmacol Ther* 2014;96: 498–507

Chapter 10
SGLT2 Inhibitors

John R. White, Jr., PA-C, PharmD

INTRODUCTION

The kidney has been considered primarily an organ of elimination for several hundred years, as well as a modulator of salt and ion balance. Our construct of the kidney has evolved significantly over the past 2 decades. At one time, it was considered to be the structural cause of diabetes. Later, its role in glucose homeostasis, while recognized, was all but ignored. Today, however, it is recognized for its salient role in the regulation of glucose homeostasis. As the elucidation of the physiology of glucose transport via specific carriers such as the SGLTs developed, the idea that the natural compound phlorizin (which was isolated in the early 1800s) or its analogs could possibly be used pharmacologically began to be investigated.[1] This work led to the development of several SGLT2 inhibitors. Currently, there are five FDA-approved SGLT2 inhibitors on the market in the U.S.: canagliflozin, dapagliflozin, empagliflozin, bexagliflozin, and ertugliflozin.

PHARMACOLOGY

MECHANISM OF ACTION

The mechanism of action of these agents is novel and unique. The kidney is involved in glucose homeostasis via several mechanisms, including gluconeogenesis, glucose utilization, glomerular filtration, and reabsorption of glucose in the proximal convoluted tubules.[2] However, the primary effect of the kidney on glucose homeostasis is by glomerular filtration, reabsorption, and urine glucose excretion (UGE). UGE can simply be calculated by subtracting the amount of glucose that is reabsorbed from the amount filtered. Under typical conditions, normal healthy adults filter approximately 180 g of glucose daily. In nondiabetic individuals under euglycemic conditions, the majority of glucose (99%) is reabsorbed with only a small fraction being excreted in the urine.

The reabsorption of glucose from the urine begins with the transport of glucose from the tubule (lumen) into the tubular epithelial cells by way of SGLTs. These SGLTs include a number of membrane proteins that transport many compounds across the lumen membrane of renal tubules as well as from the lumen of the intestine across the intestinal epithelium. The two most well-characterized members of this family are SGLT1 and SGLT2. The first of these, SGLT1, is a low-capacity, high-affinity Na^+/glucose transporter, located primarily in the gastrointestinal tract and also found in the S3 segment of the proximal tubule. Although the role of SGLT1s in the kidney is relatively small—accounting for only about 10% of glucose reabsorption there—it is the most important transport mechanism for glucose absorption in the gastrointestinal tract. Conversely, SGLT2 is a high-capacity, low-affinity transporter found primarily in the kidney. It accounts for approximately 90% of glucose reabsorption in the kidney. This transporter is found at a relatively high density on the lumen (brush-border) membrane of the S1 segment of the proximal convoluted tubule. This transporter binds with glucose and Na^+ in the tubular filtrate and actively transports glucose across the membrane through Na^+ coupling. This process is fueled by the Na^+ gradient established between the tubular filtrate and the cell (secondary active transport).[2]

After glucose is transported via SGLT2 into the luminal epithelium, it is transported by GLUTs (glucose transporter proteins) through the basolateral membrane along with Na^+ back into the peritubular capillary. This basolateral membrane–peritubular capillary transfer uses both GLUT1 transporters in the late proximal tubule and GLUT2 transporters in the early proximal tubule (see Figure 10.1).[2]

The mechanism of action of the SGLT2 inhibitors is through inhibition of SGLT2, which in turn results in an increase in UGE. These medications essen-

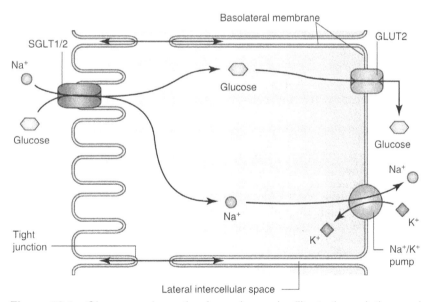

Figure 10.1—Glucose reabsorption from glomerular filtrate through the proximal tubule epithelial cell into the blood. Abbreviations: GLUT, glucose transporter protein. *Source*: Bakris.[3]

tially lower the renal threshold for glucose excretion. The SGLT2 inhibitors prevent the reabsorption of between 30 and 50% of filtered glucose.[4] The result of this inhibition is renal loss of glucose and a concomitant reduction in blood glucose. Also, it should be noted that a mixed SGLT1 and SGLT2 inhibitor, sotagliflozin, is currently under development.[5] This medication will modulate glucose transport in both the gastrointestinal tract and the kidney.

PHARMACOKINETICS

Canagliflozin

Canagliflozin has a mean oral bioavailability of 65%. Although it can probably be taken with or without food, it is recommended that it be taken before the first meal of the day. The mean volume of distribution is approximately 83.5 L, and the drug is 99% bound to plasma proteins. The metabolism of canagliflozin is primarily via uridine diphosphate glucuronosyltransferase (UGT) (1A2 and 2B4) to inactive metabolites, but about 7% is metabolized by CYP3A4. The metabolites are excreted primarily by the fecal route, with about one-third being excreted through the urine. Mean systemic clearance of canagliflozin is 192 mL/min in healthy subjects. The mean terminal half-life ranges from approximately 10–13 h.[6]

Dapagliflozin

The mean bioavailability of dapagliflozin following a 10-mg dose is 78%.[7] Some alterations in C_{max} and T_{max} are observed when the medication is administered with a high-fat meal, but the AUC is unchanged. The observed changes are not considered to be clinically relevant, and this medication can be administered with or without food. Dapagliflozin is extensively metabolized via UGT to an inactive metabolite (~61%). The parent compound and related metabolites are excreted via the kidneys (75%) and the feces (21%). Approximately 2% of the dose is excreted unchanged in the urine, and approximately 15% is excreted in the feces. The mean terminal half-life following a single oral dose of 10 mg is 12.9 h.

Empagliflozin

Administration of empagliflozin with a meal resulted in a slightly reduced AUC (16%) and C_{max} (37%) compared to administration in the fasting state. This difference was deemed not clinically significant, and this medication may be administered with or without food. The apparent mean volume of distribution is estimated to be 73.8 L. Empagliflozin is metabolized via UGT and is also partially excreted unchanged in the urine (11–19%) and feces.[8,9] The mean terminal half-life is estimated to be 12.4 h, and the oral clearance is estimated to be 10.6 L/h (based on population kinetics).

Ertugliflozin

The mean bioavailability of ertugliflozin following a 15-mg dose was 100%.[10] Some alterations in C_{max} and T_{max} are observed when the medication is administered with a high-fat meal, but the AUC is unchanged. The observed changes are not considered to be clinically relevant, and this medication can be administered with or without food. The mean steady-state volume of distribution of ertugliflozin after the administration of an intravenous dose is 85.5 L. Ertugliflozin is primarily metabolized via UGT to two inactive glucuronide metabolites. Approximately 12% of ertugliflozin is metabolized by CYP enzymes. Approximately 1.5% of the parent compound is excreted through the urine, and approximately 33.8% is excreted unchanged in the feces. It is thought that this "unchanged" fecal fraction may actually be secondary to the biliary excretion of the glucuronide metabolite, which is then hydrolyzed back to the parent compound. The mean clearance following an intravenous dose of 100 µg was 11.2 L/h. The mean terminal half-life in patients with T2D was 16.6 h (based on population kinetics).

Bexagliflozin

Maximum concentrations of bexagliflozin are seen 2–4 h post dose and can be delayed if the medication is taken with food.[10,11] When taken after consumption of a high-fat, high-caloric meal C_{max} and AUC are increased by 31% and 10% respectively. This drug is approximately 93% bound to plasma protein and has an apparent volume of distribution of 262 L. Bexagliflozin is metabolized via UGT1A9 and CYP3A without metabolites that have clinically relevant effects. Bexagliflozin has a clearance of 19.1 L/h and a terminal half-life of 12 h.

TREATMENT ADVANTAGES/DISADVANTAGES

ADVANTAGES

There are several characteristics of the SGLT2 inhibitors that could be considered advantageous. These include cardiovascular effects, potential renal protective effects, low rates of hypoglycemia, and weight loss.

Cardiovascular and Renal Outcomes

One of the more exciting and salient findings with the SGLT2 inhibitors has been the correlation between their use (canagliflozin, empagliflozin, and dapagliflozin) and positive cardiovascular outcomes.[12,13,14] Three landmark trials have suggested cardiovascular benefit with the use of the SGLT2 inhibitors studied. The first trial, Empagliflozin, Cardiovascular Outcomes, and Mortality in Type 2 Diabetes (EMPA-REG), was a large, multicenter, randomized, double-blind, placebo-controlled trial that evaluated over 7,000 patients with T2D who were at high risk for cardiovascular events. These patients were randomized to either 10 or 25 mg of empagliflozin or placebo against a background of standard diabetes care. The primary composite outcome of the study was cardiovascular death, nonfatal MI, and stroke. The pooled empagliflozin group realized a significant reduction in the composite outcome (14% risk reduction), in the risk of death from cardiovascular causes (38% relative risk reduction), hospitalization for HF (35% relative risk reduction), and death from any cause (32% relative risk reduction). There was no significant difference in the rates of MI or stroke when analyzed singularly.[12] The findings of this study led the American Diabetes Association to recommend that empagliflozin (and also liraglutide) be considered after lifestyle management and metformin in order to reduce cardiovascular events and mortality.[15] The second trial, Canagliflozin Cardiovascular Assessment Study (CANVAS), evaluated more than 10,000 patients with T2D who were at high risk for cardiovascular events. Patients were randomized to receive canagliflozin or placebo. Patients were treated with either 100 or 300 mg of canagliflozin. The primary outcome of this trial was the same as with EMPA-REG (composite of death from cardiovascular causes, nonfatal MI, stroke). The patients receiving canagliflozin compared to those receiving placebo had a hazard ratio of 0.86 for the composite outcome. The study also demonstrated a possible renal benefit related to canagliflozin, with a hazard ratio of 0.73 for progression of albuminuria and a hazard ratio of 0.6 for the composite renal outcome of 40% reduction in glomerular filtration rate, the need for renal replacement therapy, and death due to renal causes. Unfortunately, the study also reported an almost twofold increase in the risk of lower limb amputation in the patients receiving canagliflozin. The third trial evaluated the impact of dapagliflozin on cardiovascular outcomes in patients with known atherosclerotic cardiovascular disease (ASCVD) and those at risk for ASCVD.[14] The study concluded that treatment with dapagliflozin did not result in a higher or lower rate of major adverse cardiovascular events but it was correlated with a reduced rate of cardiovascular death or hospitalizations secondary to heart failure. Based on these studies the ADA currently recommends that an SGLT2 inhibitor with evidence of benefit be considered for use (independent of baseline A1C or target A1C) in patients with T2D who have indicators or high risk for or established ASCVD (empagliflozin and canagliflozin), CKD (empagliflozin, canagliflozin, and dapagliflozin), or HF (empagliflozin, canagliflozin, and dapagliflozin).[15]

Renal Protection

SGLT2 inhibition has shown promise in several studies evaluating the impact of these agents on renal disease. One recent review stated that the two studies cited above demonstrated overall cardiovascular benefit and "suggest the possibility of dramatic kidney protection in DM2."[16] Several major trials evaluating this question are currently underway, including Cardiovascular Outcomes Following Ertugliflozin Treatment in Type 2 Diabetes Mellitus Participants With Vascular Disease [VERTIS] and A Study to Evaluate the Effect of Dapagliflozin on Renal Outcomes and Cardiovascular Mortality in Patients With Chronic Kidney Disease [DAPA-CKD]. The Canagliflozin and Renal Outcomes in Type 2 Diabetes and Nephropathy (CREDENCE) study evaluated the renal and cardiovascular disease effects of canagliflozin in 4,401 patients with both T2D and albuminuric CKD.[17] The trial was stopped early after an interim analysis demonstrated striking positive effects of canagliflozin. The primary outcome analyzed in this study was a composite of end-stage kidney disease (dialysis, transplantation, or a sustained estimated GFR of <15 mL/min per 1.73 m^2). The relative risk of this primary outcome was 30% lower in those subjects who were treated with canagliflozin.

Low Rates of Hypoglycemia

SGLT2 inhibitors are not associated with high rates of hypoglycemia, in part because they do not completely block renal glucose reabsorption. They inhibit reabsorption of 30–50% of filtered glucose.[4] The reason for this has not been elucidated but may be due to a saturation in the transport mechanism that delivers the medication to the active site. Generally speaking, low rates of hypoglycemia have been consistently reported in clinical trials with SGLT2 inhibitors, except in patients receiving background insulin or sulfonylureas. A meta-analysis of 58 clinical trials reported an odds ratio of 0.44 for hypoglycemia in patients treated with SGLT2 inhibitors when compared to other antihyperglycemic medications.[18]

Weight Loss

The SGLT2 inhibitors have been consistently associated with weight loss. The level of weight loss varies but may in some cases be as high as 4.7 kg.[4] Although the magnitude of weight loss varies depending on conditions of the study and population evaluated, a positive effect on weight (i.e., loss) has been consistently observed in multiple studies. The SGLT2 inhibitors may in some cases be effective in mitigating the increase in weight caused by other medications. In one trial that included the TZD pioglitazone (which is linked to weight gain), dapagliflozin attenuated the TZD-associated weight gain.[19] Another study evaluating weight loss secondary to SGLT2 inhibitors reported that 66% of the weight loss linked to the SGLT2 inhibitor dapagliflozin was due to loss of both visceral and subcutaneous fat.[20]

DISADVANTAGES

There are also several characteristics that could be considered to be disadvantages, including cost, a potential greater risk of lower limb amputation, and other well-recognized adverse events.

Cost

Although the cost of the SGLT2 inhibitors is less than that of GLP-1 RAs, they are higher than most of the other commonly utilized oral antihyperglycemic agents.[21] The average wholesale price for a 1-month supply of canagliflozin, dapagliflozin, ertugliflozin, or empagliflozin ranges from $338 to $593. The national average acquisition cost ranges from $271 to $475.

Black Box Warning (Lower Limb Amputation)—Canagliflozin

One of the findings of the CANVAS and Canagliflozin Cardiovascular Assessment Study-Renal (CANVAS-R) trials was a twofold increased risk of lower limb amputations in patients with T2D who had established cardiovascular disease. The most frequent types of amputations involved the toe or the midfoot. However, some patients had multiple amputations, in some cases involving both limbs. Prior to initiation of therapy, it is suggested that multiple factors be considered, including history of prior amputation, peripheral vascular disease (PVD), neuropathy, and diabetes-related foot ulcers. Additionally, patients taking this agent should be provided with appropriate caution regarding the early reportage of any signs or symptoms that might be associated with lower limb problems.[6,13]

SIGNIFICANT WARNINGS/PRECAUTIONS

Lower Limb Amputations

This warning is described in the section above. The numbers of cases per 1,000 patients per year treated with canagliflozin and placebo in the CANVAS study were 5.9 and 2.8, respectively. The numbers of cases per 1,000 patients per year treated with canagliflozin and placebo in the CANVAS-R study were 7.5 and 4.2, respectively. Appropriate cautions as mentioned above should be instituted.[6,13]

Hypotension/Acute Kidney Injury and Impairment in Renal Function

These agents cause intravascular volume contraction by virtue of their mechanism of action and the diuresis that occurs when they are used. This volume depletion may lead to hypotension and a temporary or transient reduction in glomerular filtration. The package inserts from the currently marketed SGLT2 inhibitors all contain warnings about this potential adverse event and suggest care with patients at high risk for side effects related to intravascular volume contraction.[6–8,10] The greatest increase in incidence of volume contraction–related events has occurred in the elderly, patients with reduced GFRs, patients treated with loop diuretics or renin-angiotensin-aldosterone system modulators, and patients with low systolic blood pressure. Volume status should be addressed and corrected prior to initiation of therapy.

Ketoacidosis

DKA has been observed in both T1D and T2D patients treated with SGLT2 inhibition. The increased risk seems to be greater in patients treated with exogenous insulin. Also, the increased risk is more clearly defined in patients with T1D. As many as 9.4% of patients with T1D enrolled in trials evaluating SGLT2 inhibition developed ketosis while 6% developed DKA.[22] The relationship between ketoacidosis and SGLT2 inhibitors in patients with T2D is less clear. Still, appropriate vigilance should be exercised in patients with T2D being treated with SGLT2 inhibition. SGLT2 inhibition in patients with T1D is being evaluated in well-controlled studies and should probably not be used in the general practice setting until more is known about the risk/benefit ratio of these medications in patients with T1D.

Urogenital Infections

Glucosuria has historically been recognized as a risk factor for urinary tract and other genital infections. Thus, these potential adverse events were anticipated with the SGLT2 inhibitors and have been well documented. Multiple studies have demonstrated that urogenital infections typically occur at a higher rate in patients treated with SGLT2 inhibitors than in those treated with placebo or other medications.[2] However, the incidence of infections in patients treated with SGLT2s varied greatly across those published studies and was even similar to placebo in some.

A meta-analysis of SGLT2 studies reported an odds ratio of 1.34 for the development of urinary tract infections (UTIs) in patients treated with SGLT2 inhibitors when compared to placebo. The study reported an odds ratio of 1.42 in patients treated with SGLT2 inhibitors versus other antihyperglycemic agents.[18] Another study evaluated the rates of UTIs from 12 randomized placebo-controlled trials involving the SGLT2 inhibitor dapagliflozin. The overall rates of UTIs in 3,152 patients treated with dapagliflozin 2.5, 5, 10 mg, or placebo in these trials were 3.6%, 5.7%, 4.3%, and 3.7%, respectively.[23] The overall rates of UTIs in patients treated with empagliflozin 10, 25 mg, or placebo in the phase 3 trials (2,971 patients) were 9.3%, 7.6%, and 7.6%, respectively.[8] The overall rates of UTIs in 2,313 patients treated with canagliflozin 100, 300 mg, or placebo were 5.9%, 4.3%, and 4.0%, respectively.[6] The overall rates of UTIs in 1,544 patients treated with ertugliflozin 5, 15 mg, or placebo in the phase 3 trials were 4.0%, 4.1%, and 3.9% respectively.[10] Females are linked to a higher incidence of UTIs than are males with all of the SGLT2 inhibitors currently on the market.

Genital infections (vulvovaginitis, balanitis, and others) also occur at a higher rate in patients treated with SGLT2 inhibitors than in those treated with placebo.[2] A meta-analysis of pertinent studies reported an odds ratio of 3.5 for the development of genital infections in patients treated with SGLT2 inhibitors versus placebo and an odds ratio of 5.06 for the development of genital infections in patients treated with SGLT2 inhibitors versus active comparators.[18]

Generally speaking, both UTIs and genital infections that are associated with SGLT2 inhibition are mild and rarely result in discontinuation of the medication. However, there have been occasional reports of urosepsis and pyelonephritis in patients treated with SGLT2 inhibitors.

SPECIAL POPULATIONS

Canagliflozin[6]

Pregnancy
Not recommended during second or third trimesters. There are insufficient data to determine drug-associated risk of major birth defects or miscarriage.

Lactation
No information is available regarding the presence of canagliflozin in human milk, the breast-fed infant, or the effects on milk production.

Pediatrics
Safety and effectiveness in patients under 18 years old has not been established.

Geriatrics
This drug has been studied in the geriatric population in multiple clinical trials. These patients experienced a higher incidence of intravascular volume–related

adverse events (particularly at a higher dose of 300 mg/day) and experienced smaller reductions in A1C than were observed in their younger counterparts.

Renal Impairment

Patients with moderate renal dysfunction (eGFR 45–60 mL/min/1.73 m^2) experienced reduced glycemic efficacy, a higher incidence of intravascular volume–related adverse events, and a higher rate of hyperkalemia. The dose should be limited to 100 mg/day in these patients. Canagliflozin has not been studied and is not recommended in patients with an eGFR of <45 mL/min/1.73 m^2.

Hepatic Impairment

No dosage adjustment is required in patients with mild to moderate hepatic impairment. This drug has not been studied and is not recommended in patients with severe hepatic impairment.

Dapagliflozin[7]

Pregnancy

Not recommended during second or third trimesters. There are insufficient data to determine drug-associated risk of major birth defects or miscarriage.

Lactation

No information is available regarding the presence of dapagliflozin in human milk, the breast-fed infant, or the effects on milk production.

Pediatrics

Safety and effectiveness in patients under 18 years old has not been established.

Geriatrics

This drug has been studied in the geriatric population in multiple clinical trials. These patients experienced a higher incidence of intravascular volume and renal-related adverse events. After controlling for changes in eGFR, elderly patients treated with dapagliflozin experienced similar reductions in A1C as were observed in their younger counterparts.

Renal Impairment

Patients with moderate renal dysfunction (eGFR 30–60 mL/min/1.73 m^2) treated with dapagliflozin did not experience an improvement in glycemic control when compared to placebo. They did, however, experience a higher incidence of renal-related adverse events and more bone fractures. Initiation of this drug is not recommended in patients with an eGFR of <60 mL/min/1.73 m^2.

Hepatic Impairment

No dosage adjustment is required in patients with mild, moderate, or severe hepatic impairment. However, this drug has not been studied in patients with severe hepatic impairment and therefore the benefit/risk ratio of its use in this population should be individually assessed.

Empagliflozin[8]

Pregnancy

Not recommended during second or third trimesters. There are insufficient data to determine drug-associated risk of major birth defects or miscarriage.

Lactation
No information is available regarding the presence of empagliflozin in human milk, the breast-fed infant, or the effects on milk production.
Pediatrics
Safety and effectiveness in patients under 18 years old has not been established.
Geriatrics
This drug has been studied in the geriatric population in multiple clinical trials. It is expected that these patients will realize less glycemic impact with renal impairment. No adjustment of dose is recommended for empagliflozin in this population. A subgroup of these patients (>75 years old) experienced a dose-related (2.3%—10 mg daily; 4.4%—25 mg daily) higher incidence of intravascular volume–adverse events.
Renal Impairment
Empagliflozin was studied in patients with mild to moderate renal dysfunction (eGFR 30–90 mL/min/1.73 m^2). The glycemic-lowering effect of this drug was diminished with worsening renal function. These patients experienced a higher incidence of renal- and volume-related adverse events and UTIs as renal function declined. The efficacy and safety of empagliflozin has not been established in patients with severe renal impairment, end-stage renal disease (ESRD), or in those receiving dialysis.
Hepatic Impairment
Empagliflozin may be used in patients with hepatic impairment.

Ertugliflozin[10]

Pregnancy
Not recommended during second or third trimesters. There are insufficient data to determine drug-associated risk of major birth defects or miscarriage.
Lactation
No information is available regarding the presence of ertugliflozin in human milk, the breast-fed infant, or the effects on milk production.
Pediatrics
Safety and effectiveness in patients under 18 years old has not been established.
Geriatrics
This drug has been studied in the geriatric population in clinical trials. It is expected that these patients will realize less glycemic impact from ertugliflozin with renal impairment. No adjustment of dose is recommended for ertugliflozin in this population. These patients (>65 years old) experienced a higher incidence of volume depletion–related adverse events than was reported for younger patients.
Renal Impairment
In patients with T2D and moderate renal impairment, those treated with ertugliflozin did not have an improvement in their glycemic control and had a greater risk of renal impairment, renal-related adverse events, and intravascular volume–related adverse events. Therefore, ertugliflozin is not recommended in patients with mod-

erate renal impairment. Ertugliflozin is contraindicated in patients with severe renal impairment, ESRD, or in those receiving dialysis. No dose adjustment or increased monitoring is needed in patients with mild renal impairment.

Hepatic Impairment

Dose adjustment of ertugliflozin is not needed in patients with mild to moderate hepatic dysfunction. It has not been studied and should not be used in those with severe hepatic impairment.

Bexagliflozin[10, 11]

Pregnancy

Not recommended during second or third trimesters. There are insufficient data to determine drug-associated risk of major birth defects or miscarriage.

Lactation

No information is available regarding the presence of bexagliflozin in human milk, the breast-fed infant, or the effects on milk production.

Pediatrics

Safety and effectiveness in pediatric patients has not been established.

Geriatrics

This drug has been studied in the geriatric population in multiple clinical trials (1,047 patients 65 years or older). In one study these patients experienced a slightly higher incidence of intravascular volume depletion (9.8% on bexagliflozin versus 7.6% on placebo).

Renal Impairment

Patients with an eGFR <30 mL/min/1.73 m^2 or those treated with dialysis should not be treated with bexagliflozin due to a decline in therapeutic effect and a reduction in urine output in these patients. Patients with eGFRs of 30–60 mL/min/1.73 m^2 experienced more adverse reactions but do not require dosage adjustments.

Hepatic Impairment

No dosage adjustment is required in patients with mild to moderate hepatic impairment. However, this drug has not been studied in patients with severe hepatic impairment and its use is not recommended in this group.

PHARMACOGENOMICS

There are several potential areas of interest with regard to the intersection of pharmacogenomics and the clinical use of SGLT2 inhibitors. First, genetic variations in UGTs and/or in their expression could potentially be related to clinically significant differences in SGLT2 inhibition response. Second, the SGLT2 gene (SLC5) and many mutations have been identified and mapped. One or more of these SLC5 variants could be related to level of observed response to SGLT2 inhibition. However, at this point there are no studies that have demonstrated a clinically significant relationship between SGLT2 inhibition response and genetic variants.[23]

ADVERSE EFFECTS AND MONITORING[6–8,10]

HYPOTENSION

This adverse effect is possible with all four of the currently approved SGLT2 inhibitors. Greater risk of hypotension is seen in elderly, in patients with renal impairment, and in patients treated with diuretics. Monitor for signs and symptoms of hypotension during initiation and dose escalation.

KETOACIDOSIS

Please see "Significant Warnings/Precautions" above.

LOWER LIMB AMPUTATION

Canagliflozin and ertugliflozin only—please see "Significant Warnings/Precautions" above.

ACUTE KIDNEY INJURY AND IMPAIRMENT

Please see "Significant Warnings/Precautions" above.

HYPERKALEMIA

Canagliflozin only—Use of this medication can lead to hyperkalemia. Those who are at increased risk for this adverse effect are patients with moderate renal impairment who are also taking medications that interfere with potassium excretion (K^+-sparing diuretics) or medications that modulate the renin-angiotensin-aldosterone system. Serum monitoring of potassium is indicated in patients with the risk of developing hyperkalemia. Also, please consider that hyperkalemia in the settings described above could be theoretically possible with any of the SGLT2 inhibitors.

UROSEPSIS AND PYELONEPHRITIS

Please see "Significant Warnings/Precautions: Urogenital Infections" above.

HYPOGLYCEMIA WITH CONCOMITANT USE OF INSULIN AND INSULIN SECRETAGOGUES

Use of any of the SGLT2 inhibitors in the setting of concomitant insulin and/or secretagogue therapy results in an increased risk of hypoglycemia. A lower dose of insulin or secretagogue may be appropriate when used with an SGLT2 inhibitor.

GENITAL MYCOTIC INFECTIONS

Please see "Significant Warnings/Precautions: Urogenital Infections" above.

HYPERSENSITIVITY REACTIONS

Severe hypersensitivity reactions have been reported with canagliflozin and empagliflozin. When this occurs, the medication should be discontinued, and the patient should be treated promptly per standards of care. Also, please note that hypersensitivity reactions are possible with any medication.

BONE FRACTURE

Canagliflozin only—An increased risk of fracture has been observed with the administration of canagliflozin. This effect can occur as early as 12 weeks after initiation of therapy.

BLADDER CANCER

Dapagliflozin only—A slight increase in the incidence of bladder cancer was seen across 22 studies that evaluated dapagliflozin versus placebo (0.17% vs. 0.03%, respectively). The association between bladder cancer and this medication is unclear because there were so few cases. Currently it is recommended that patients with active bladder cancer not be treated with dapagliflozin. The benefit/risk ratio should be considered for those with a prior history of bladder cancer.

INCREASES IN LDL-C

Slight increases in LDL-C have been observed with the four currently marketed SGLT2 inhibitors.

DRUG INTERACTIONS

PHARMACODYNAMICS

One should consider the potential for two types of pharmacodynamic interactions with all four of the currently available SGLT2 inhibitors on the market. First, these medications can potentially interact in a pharmacodynamic manner with diuretics, ACE inhibitors, angiotensin II receptor blockers (ARBs), or aldosterone antagonists to facilitate or cause the worsening of volume depletion–related adverse events. Second, although these medications are associated with a very low risk of hypoglycemia when used as monotherapy, the potential for a pharmacodynamic interaction resulting in an increase in the incidence and level of hypoglycemia exists with insulin and secretagogues.

PHARMACOKINETICS

The primary metabolic pathway for all four SGLT2 inhibitors is via UGT.[6–8,10,24] These drugs are therefore not likely to be involved in the typical

CYP450-mediated interactions that are commonly encountered. Still, SGLT2 inhibitors are likely to be frequently used with multiple other medications; thus, the potential for drug-drug interactions, as with all medications, is present to some degree. The four SGLT2 inhibitors have been evaluated with varying rigor for potential interactions with multiple medications in myriad studies. A review of the interactions related to canagliflozin, dapagliflozin, and empagliflozin has been published elsewhere and provides a more detailed evaluation than is found here.[24] The pharmacokinetic studies were, in most cases, carried out on healthy volunteers and evaluated the potential impact of interactions after the administration of a single dose of an SGLT2 inhibitor. The exposure to SGLT2 inhibitors (as measured by C_{max} and AUC) was not clinically significantly altered by the concomitant administration of cardiovascular agents or antihyperglycemic medications commonly encountered in patients with T2D (metformin, glimepiride, pioglitazone, sitagliptin, linagliptin, voglibose, simvastatin, valsartan, ramipril, hydrochlorothiazide, torasemide, verapamil, warfarin—note that not all of these medications have been evaluated with all four SGLT2 inhibitors). Also, the SGLT2 inhibitors studied did not significantly affect the pharmacokinetic parameters of the second drug studied (those listed above). One exception to this is digoxin and canagliflozin. Canagliflozin has been shown to increase the AUC (20%) and the C_{max} (36%) of digoxin when the two are coadministered.[6]

Additionally, the SGLT2 inhibitors have been evaluated in the context of UGT modulators. Dapagliflozin is primarily metabolized through the UGT1A9 pathway. Dapagliflozin kinetics have been shown to be altered by two UGT1A9 pathway modulators (rifampicin [an inducer] and mefenamic acid [an inhibitor]). Rifampin coadministration with dapagliflozin resulted in a significant reduction in dapagliflozin exposure (AUC reduction of 22%).[7] When mefenamic acid was coadministered with dapagliflozin, a significant increase in dapagliflozin exposure (AUC increase of 51%) was observed. Canagliflozin has been evaluated in combination with rifampicin (600 mg/day × 8 days). In this setting, canagliflozin exposure was significantly reduced (AUC reduction—51%, C_{max} reduction—28%). Empagliflozin is metabolized via multiple UGTs (1A3, 1A8, 1A9, and 2B7). A slight increase in empagliflozin AUC and C_{max} was observed when it was administered with rifampin.[8] The change was deemed to be non-clinically relevant. Ertugliflozin is primarily metabolized via UGT1A9 and 2B7. When evaluated in combination with rifampin, a reduction in AUC (39%) and C_{max} (15%) was observed.[10] These changes were deemed to be non-clinically relevant.

Generally, the SGLT2 inhibitors appear to be relatively free of clinically significant interactions with commonly used medications. This is likely due to the nonexistent to relatively small impact of CYP metabolism on the disposition of these drugs. Still, care should always be taken, particularly when coadministering these agents with modulators of UGT.

Table 10.1—Dosage and Administration[6–8,10]

Medication	Available doses	Initial dose and range	Renal impairment	Hepatic impairment
Canagliflozin	Tablets: 100 mg, 300 mg	Initial Dose: 100 mg daily Range: 100–300 mg daily	eGFR ≥60 mL/min/1.73 m²: No dosage adjustment needed eGFR 45–59 mL/min/1.73 m²: Do not exceed 100 mg/day by mouth eGFR <45 mL/min/1.73 m²: Do not initiate; discontinue in patients currently receiving drug	No adjustment needed for mild or moderate impairment, not recommended with severe impairment
Dapagliflozin	Tablets: 2.5 mg, 5 mg, 10 mg	Initial Dose: 5 mg daily Range: 5–10 mg daily	eGFR <60 mL/min/1.73 m² Initiation is not recommended eGFR 30–60 mL/min/1.73 m²: Not recommended Contraindicated in those with severe renal impairment, ESRD, or dialysis	No dose adjustment recommended for mild, moderate, or severe impairment. Efficacy and safety has not been studied in severe impairment
Empagliflozin	Tablets: 10 mg, 25 mg	Initial Dose: 10 mg daily Range: 10–25 mg daily	eGFR ≥45 mL/min/1.73 m²: No dosage adjustment needed eGFR <45 mL/min/1.73 m²: Do not initiate; discontinue in patients currently receiving drug	May be used in patients with hepatic impairment
Ertugliflozin	Tablets: 5 mg, 15 mg	Initial Dose: 5 mg daily Range: 5–15 mg daily	eGFR 30–60 mL/min/1.73 m²: Initiation and use is not recommended Contraindicated in those with severe renal impairment, ESRD, or dialysis	No dose adjustment recommended for mild or moderate impairment. Efficacy and safety has not been studied in severe impairment and is not recommended in this population

(continued)

Table 10.1 (continued)

Medication	Available doses	Initial dose and range	Renal impairment	Hepatic impairment
Bexagliflozin	Tablets: 20 mg	Initial and maintenance dose: 20 mg daily	eGFR <30 mL/min/1.73 m² or dialysis: Not recommended	No dose adjustment recommended for mild or moderate impairment. Efficacy and safety has not been studied in severe impairment and is not recommended in this population

Source: Invokana [prescribing information],[6] Farxiga [prescribing information],[7] Jardiance [prescribing information],[8] Steglatro [prescribing information],[10] and Bexa [prescribing information].[11]

COMBINATION PRODUCTS

- Canagliflozin
    - Canagliflozin plus metformin hydrochloride
- Dapagliflozin
    - Dapagliflozin plus metformin hydrochloride
    - Dapagliflozin plus saxagliptin
- Empagliflozin
    - Empagliflozin plus metformin hydrochloride
    - Empagliflozin plus linagliptin
- Ertugliflozin
    - Ertugliflozin plus metformin hydrochloride
    - Ertugliflozin plus sitagliptin

MONOGRAPHS

Canagliflozin: https://dailymed.nlm.nih.gov/dailymed/drugInfo.cfm?setid=b9057d3b-b104-4f09-8a61-c61ef9d4a3f3&audience=consumer

Dapagliflozin: https://dailymed.nlm.nih.gov/dailymed/drugInfo.cfm?setid=72ad22ae-efe6-4cd6-a302-98aaee423d69&audience=consumer

Empagliflozin: https://dailymed.nlm.nih.gov/dailymed/drugInfo.cfm?setid=5777b8a8-ada6-4950-8548-43a1de11f075&audience=consumer

Ertugliflozin: https://dailymed.nlm.nih.gov/dailymed/drugInfo.cfm?setid=e6f3e718-bb99-48f1-ab94-b9f0af05fed6&audience=consumer

Bexagliflozin: not available via daily med

REFERENCES

1. White J. Apple trees to sodium glucose co-transporter inhibitors: a review of SGLT2 inhibition. *Clin Diabetes* 2010;28(1):5–10

2. White J. Sodium glucose cotransporter 2 inhibitors. *Med Clin North America* 2015;99:131–143

3. Bakris GL, Fonseca VA, Sharma K, Wright EM. Renal sodium-glucose transport: role in diabetes mellitus and potential clinical implications. *Kidney Int* 2009;75:1272–1277

4. Chao E. SGLT-2 inhibitors: a new mechanism for glycemic control. *Clin Diabetes* 2014;32(1):4–11

5. Garg S, Henry R, Banks P, et al. Effects of sotagliflozin added to insulin in patients with type 1 diabetes. *N Engl J Med* 2017;377:2337–2348

6. Invokana (canagliflozin tablet, film coated) [prescribing information]. Raritan, NJ, Janssen Pharmaceuticals, Inc. Available from https://dailymed.nlm.nih.gov/dailymed/drugInfo.cfm?setid=b9057d3b-b104-4f09-8a61-c61ef9d4a3f3&audience=consumer. Accessed 29 March 2020

7. Farxiga (dapagliflozin propanediol tablet, film coated) [prescribing information]. Princeton, NJ, E. R. Squibb & Sons, LLC. Available from https://dailymed.nlm.nih.gov/dailymed/drugInfo.cfm?setid=72ad22ae-efe6-4cd6-a302-98aaee423d69&audience=consumer. Accessed 29 March 2020

8. Jardiance (empagliflozin tablets, for oral use) [prescribing information]. Ridgefield, CT, Boehringer Ingelheim Pharmaceuticals, Inc. Available from https://dailymed.nlm.nih.gov/dailymed/drugInfo.cfm?setid=faf3dd6a-9cd0-39c2-0d2e-232cb3f67565&audience=consumer. Accessed 29 March 2020

9. Macha S, Mattheus M, Halabi A, et al. Pharmacokinetics, pharmacodynamics and safety of empagliflozin, a sodium glucose cotransporter 2 (SGLT2) inhibitor, in subjects with renal impairment. *Diabetes Obes Metab* 2014;16:215–222

10. Steglatro (ertugliflozin) [prescribing information]. Kenilworth, NJ, Merck Sharp & Dohme Corp. Available from https://dailymed.nlm.nih.gov/dailymed/drugInfo.cfm?setid=e6f3e718-bb99-48f1-ab94-b9f0af05fed6&audience=consumer. Accessed 29 March 2020

11. Brenzavvy (bexagliflozin) tablets [prescribing information]. TheracosBio, LLC, 2023

12. Zinman B, Wanner C, Lachin JM, et al. Empagliflozin, cardiovascular outcomes, and mortality in type 2 diabetes. *New Engl J Med* 2015;373(22):2117–2128

13. Neal B, Perkovic V, Mahaffey KW, et al. Canagliflozin and cardiovascular and renal events in type 2 diabetes. *New Engl J Med* 2017;377(7):644–657

14. Wiviott SD, et al., Dapagliflozin and cardiovascular outcomes in type 2 diabetes. *New Engl J Med* 2019;380(4):347–357

15. American Diabetes Association. 9. Pharmacologic Approaches to Glycemic Treatment: Standards of Medical Care in Diabetes—2022. *Diabetes Care* 2022;45(Suppl. 1):S125–S143

16. Pecoits-Filho R, Perkovic V. Are SGLT2 inhibitors ready for prime time in CKD? *CJASN*. February 2018;13(2):318–320

17. Perkovic V, et al. Canagliflozin and renal outcomes in type 2 diabetes and nephropathy. *New Engl J Med* 2019;380(24):2295–2306

18. Vasilakou D, Karagiannis T, Athanasiadou E, et al. Sodium-glucose cotransporter 2 inhibitors for type 2 diabetes: a systematic review and meta-analysis. *Ann Intern Med* 2013;159(4):262–274

19. Rosenstock J, Vico M, Wei L, et al. Effects of dapagliflozin, an SGLT2 inhibitor, on HbA1c, body weight, and hypoglycemia risk in patients with type 2 diabetes inadequately controlled on pioglitazone monotherapy. *Diabetes Care* 2012;35:1473–1478

20. Bolinder J, Ljunggren Ö, Kullberg J, et al. Effects of dapagliflozin on body weight, total fat mass, and regional adipose tissue distribution in patients with type 2 diabetes mellitus with inadequate glycemic control on metformin. *J Clin Endocrinol Metab* 2012;97:1020–1031

21. American Diabetes Association. 8. Pharmacologic Approaches to Glycemic Treatment: Standards of Medical Care in Diabetes—2018. *Diabetes Care* 2018;41(Suppl. 1):S73–S85

22. Handelsman Y, Henry R, Bloomgarden Z, Dagogo-Jack S, et al. American Association of Clinical Endocrinologists and American College of Endocrinology Position Statement on the association of SGLT-2 inhibitors and diabetic ketoacidosis. *Endocrine Pract* 2016;22(6):753–762

23. Johnsson KM, Ptaszynska A, Schmitz B, et al. Urinary tract infections in patients with diabetes treated with dapagliflozin. *J Diabetes Complications* 2013;27:473–478

24. Scheen AJ. Precision medicine: the future in diabetes care? *Diabetes Res Clin Pract* 2016;117:12–21

25. Scheen AJ. Drug-drug interactions with sodium-glucose cotransporters type 2 (SGLT2) inhibitors, new oral glucose-lowering agents for the management of type 2 diabetes mellitus. *Clin Pharmacokinet* 2014;53:295–304

Chapter 11

α-Glucosidase Inhibitors

KIMBERLY C. MCKEIRNAN, PHARMD, BCACP
NICOLE M. RODIN, PHARMD, MBA

INTRODUCTION

α-Glucosidase inhibitors are a versatile class of medications that have been used in a variety of treatment settings since they were first approved by the FDA in 1995 for patients with T1D. α-Glucosidase inhibitors have a unique mechanism of action that allows the drug to alter the rate at which the body absorbs carbohydrates. This allows for the medication to be applied across several spectrums. Of note, α-glucosidase inhibitors are traditionally used in the management of T2D. They can, however, be used in the management of T1D as well. There are two medications available in the U.S. within this class: acarbose (Precose, Bayer) and miglitol (Glyset, Pfizer Inc.). Voglibose (Volix, Ranbaxy Laboratories Limited) is a third medication in this class available outside the U.S.

Several large clinical trials with acarbose, including the large postmarketing PROTECT (Precose Resolution of Optimal Titration to Enhance Current Therapies) trial, have shown a decrease in A1C values of ~0.5–0.7%, or ~0.6–1.1% from baseline when compared to placebo.[1] In the PROTECT trial, which enrolled over 6,000 patients, postprandial glucose levels decreased 40–50 mg/dL (2.2–2.8 mmol/L), and fasting plasma glucose levels decreased 25–30 mg/dL (1.4–1.7 mmol/L).[1] On average, these medications have been shown to reduce A1C by about 0.5–1%.[2] α-Glucosidase inhibitors have the biggest impact on postprandial blood glucose, creating a niche for this class within the many options used to treat diabetes mellitus.

PHARMACOLOGY

MECHANISM OF ACTION

α-Glucosidase inhibitors are named for their ability to competitively inhibit the α-glucosidase enzyme in the brush borders of the intestines through reversible binding.[3] α-Glucosidase enzymes maltase, isomaltase, sucrase, and glucoamylase break down complex carbohydrates into monosaccharides that can then be absorbed.[4] Inhibition of α-glucosidase enzymes leads to the delayed breakdown of oligosaccharides and disaccharides into monosaccharides suitable for absorption.[3] The delayed absorption of carbohydrates from the small intestine results in reduction of the postprandial hyperglycemia that occurs during digestion of a meal.[3]

190

This slower rise in postprandial blood glucose concentrations is beneficial to patients with T1D or T2D.

PHARMACOKINETICS

Following oral administration, acarbose has very low bioavailability. Minimal absorption by the small intestine leads to <2% of the acarbose being systemically active.[5] Acarbose peak plasma concentration occurs 1 h after administration, while miglitol peak concentrations are reached in 2–3 h.[5,6] Miglitol absorption is also saturable at high doses because miglitol is absorbed via an active transport mechanism, a rate-limiting step, which impacts both the bioavailability and onset of action. A dose of 25 mg, for example, is completely absorbed, but a dose of 100 mg only achieves 50–70% absorption.[6] At higher doses, absorption is also delayed and may take up to 7 h. However, the absorption rate of miglitol does not influence clinical efficacy, since the site of action is the brush border of the intestines.

Acarbose is metabolized exclusively by the intestines. Natural intestinal bacteria and digestive enzymes break acarbose into 13 different metabolites, although only one metabolite inhibits α-glucosidase.[5] Miglitol is not metabolized in humans or any of the animals studied. Miglitol metabolites have not been detected in plasma, urine, or feces, demonstrating the lack of metabolization.[6] Protein binding of miglitol is very low (<4%), and the volume of distribution is 0.18 L/kg, consistent with distribution largely into extracellular fluid.[6] Miglitol also has very low permeability of the blood-brain barrier.

Most of the acarbose dose—approximately 51%—is excreted in the feces, while 34% of the metabolized drug is absorbed systemically and is eliminated in the urine as sulfate, methyl, and glucuronide conjugates.[5] The active metabolite accounts for only 2% of the administered dose and is completely excreted via the kidney. Miglitol is eliminated through renal excretion, and the small amount of miglitol absorbed systemically in the small intestine is excreted in feces. Following a dose of 25 mg, >95% of the dose is recovered in the urine within 24 h.[6] After a 100-mg dose, the amount of drug recovered after 24 h is lower due to the incomplete bioavailability.[6] The elimination half-life for both miglitol and acarbose is approximately 2 h.[5,6]

TREATMENT ADVANTAGES/DISADVANTAGES

Acarbose and miglitol appear to be similar in terms of efficacy. However, there are no head-to-head clinical trials comparing the two drugs, so it is difficult to judge whether there is any advantage for one product over the other. Patients typically do not experience weight gain or hypoglycemia unless α-glucosidase inhibitors are taken in combination with other glucose-lowering medications. α-Glucosidase inhibitors may also have a positive impact on prevention of negative cardiovascular outcomes due to the weight loss seen while on the medication. This impact was seen more in populations in the Eastern Hemisphere. Further research is needed to confirm this theory.[7]

Some studies show patients taking α-glucosidase inhibitors may experience weight loss. A 2014 meta-analysis showed acarbose had a small but statistically significant incidence of weight loss (0.5 kg on average) compared with placebo.[8] The weight loss effect from acarbose was superior to both nateglinide and metformin. Additionally, a significantly greater weight loss (0.92 kg) was seen in Eastern populations compared to Western populations.[8]

α-Glucosidase inhibitors may be used as monotherapy or in combination with other agents. When used in combination, α-glucosidase inhibitors can enhance glycemic control because they have a different mechanism of action than other agents. A study by Wang published in 2013 showed treatment with a combination of acarbose and metformin brought proportionally more patients to goal A1C, had superior effects in lowering blood glucose, and reduced body weight when compared to acarbose alone.[9] Acarbose may be used with insulin, metformin, or sulfonylureas, and miglitol has been approved for use with sulfonylureas.

α-Glucosidase inhibitors are effective at lowering A1C levels by 0.5–1%, which can play a significant role in the treatment of T2D.[10] However, gastrointestinal side effects make these medications challenging to tolerate and unsuitable for patients with chronic intestinal disorders.[11] Slow titration over 10–12 weeks may reduce the likelihood of side effects, but many patients still choose to discontinue use due to these issues. Other classes of medication reduce A1C levels more substantially and have fewer gastrointestinal side effects, relegating α-glucosidase inhibitors to one of the less commonly used classes of medications for diabetes in the U.S.[12]

THERAPEUTIC CONSIDERATIONS

SIGNIFICANT WARNINGS/PRECAUTIONS

Both miglitol and acarbose are contraindicated for patients with inflammatory bowel disease, colonic ulceration, partial intestinal obstruction, predisposition to intestinal obstruction, or chronic intestinal diseases involving digestion or absorption.[5,6] α-Glucosidase inhibitors should not be used for patients with DKA or with any known hypersensitivity to a medication in this class. Acarbose is also contraindicated for patients with liver cirrhosis.

α-Glucosidase inhibitors do not cause hypoglycemia. However, when used in combination with oral sulfonylureas or insulin, hypoglycemia may result. Because α-glucosidase inhibitors block the absorption of dietary carbohydrates, patients experiencing hypoglycemia must use glucose tablets or gels instead of foods containing complex carbohydrates to raise blood glucose levels.[5,6] In the case of severe hypoglycemia, a glucagon injection or intravenous glucose may be necessary. Patients must remember to monitor blood glucose levels, particularly in stressful situations such as illness, trauma, or surgery, all of which can impact blood glucose levels.

SPECIAL POPULATIONS

No significant differences in pharmacokinetics have been observed in either pediatric or geriatric patients or by sex. However, appropriate studies have not been conducted on a pediatric population, so safe and effective use in children has not been established.[13] Following administration of acarbose, the mean steady-state AUC and maximum concentrations were approximately 1.5 times higher in the elderly population, but this difference was not statistically significant.[5]

In controlled clinical studies of acarbose in patients with T2D in the U.S., reductions in A1C were similar between Caucasians (n = 478) and African-Americans (n = 167), with better responses in Latin Americans (n = 132).[5] A 2014 review of 10 large studies of acarbose use in 21 countries around the world (total n = 30,730) showed acarbose was effective across all ethnicities and regions examined.[14] However, the most pronounced effects were seen in Southeast and East Asians and those patients with a higher baseline A1C.[14]

Both medications should be used with caution in patients with renal impairment. Participants with severe renal impairment (CrCl <25 mL/min) who took acarbose exhibited a peak plasma concentration five times higher and an AUC six times higher than participants with normal renal function. Subjects with CrCl <25 mL/min taking 25 mg of miglitol three times daily attained a greater than twofold increase in plasma levels compared to subjects with CrCl >60 mL/min.[5,6]

Both medications are pregnancy category B. Studies in rats given miglitol at doses corresponding to 1.5, 4, and 12 times the maximum recommended human dose, and rabbits given doses corresponding to 0.5, 3, and 10 times the maximum recommended human dose, showed no evidence of fetal malformations attributed to miglitol.[6] However, there are no adequate and well-controlled studies in humans. In 2000, a case report in Mexico showed that six pregnant women successfully took acarbose without issue through the pregnancy, delivering what were considered "normal newborns," while a 1998 case report in England showed that out of five women who took acarbose early in pregnancy, two miscarried.[15,16] Both medications should be used in pregnancy only after weighing the risks and benefits of this and other medication options. Miglitol is excreted in human milk, with 0.02% of a 100-mg maternal dose detected. Use of both miglitol and acarbose is not recommended for nursing mothers, even though the amount of drug found in milk is very small.

ADVERSE EFFECTS AND MONITORING

The most common adverse effects from α-glucosidase inhibitors are gastrointestinal symptoms, including flatulence (acarbose 74%, miglitol 41.5%), diarrhea (acarbose 31%, miglitol 28.7%), and abdominal pain (acarbose 19%, miglitol 11.7%).[5,6] These symptoms occur because of intestinal gas from the formation of short-chain fatty acids resulting from undigested carbohydrates in the colon.[3] Both acarbose and miglitol exert their action locally in the small intestine, blocking the breakdown and absorption of complex carbohydrates. The delayed absorption results in the complex sugars moving to the large intestine. The natural flora of the large intestine ferment the carbohydrates, resulting in the production of gas. These drugs are less popular among patients as a result of these gastrointestinal side effects. However, these side effects can be minimized by slowly titrating doses and encouraging patients to eat meals containing complex, rather than simple, carbohydrates.[11]

α-Glucosidase inhibitors may also impact serum iron. Small reductions in serum iron were found in 9.2% of patients taking miglitol versus 4.2% taking placebo.[6] Changes were not associated with reductions in hemoglobin or other hematologic indices. Similar results were seen with acarbose.[6] Patients with known iron deficiency anemia should be monitored when starting an α-glucosidase inhibitor.

Elevated liver function tests have also been observed in patients taking doses above the manufacturer's recommendations. Increased serum transaminases were detected in 4% of patients taking acarbose at doses of 600–900 mg per day. Patients were asymptomatic, and elevated transaminases were reversible with discontinuation of therapy.[12]

A dermatologic rash was reported in 4.3% of patients taking miglitol compared with 2.4% taking placebo. Rashes were found by physician investigators to be transient and likely unrelated to taking the medication, but are included within the package insert along with a recommendation to monitor liver function tests every 3 months during the first year taking acarbose.[6]

DRUG INTERACTIONS

As described previously in the "Significant Warnings/Precautions" section, an additive hypoglycemic effect may occur when α-glucosidase inhibitors are used in combination with sulfonylureas or insulin. A study of combination therapy with α-glucosidase inhibitors and insulin demonstrated a decreased need for insulin, sometimes requiring a reduction in insulin dosage to avoid a hypoglycemic event.[6,17] Patients taking both an α-glucosidase inhibitor and insulin should be closely monitored to prevent a hypoglycemic event.[13]

Medications that elevate glucose levels may also reduce the efficacy of α-glucosidase inhibitors. These may include thiazide diuretics, corticosteroids, estrogen, and calcium channel blockers, among others.

Miglitol taken in combination with glyburide has been shown to reduce the AUC and peak concentrations of glyburide, but the clinical significance of this interaction is unknown. A similar interaction occurs with metformin, but the reduction was minimal.[13] Acarbose has no effect on the absorption and distribution of glyburide but does cause a significant reduction in the acute bioavailability of metformin. However, after a 24 h urine collection, it was found that overall bioavailability of metformin is not affected by this interaction, so it is not clinically significant.[18]

Results from administering the combination of miglitol and digoxin have been contradictory, showing a reduction of digoxin levels by 19–28% in healthy volunteers but not in patients with diabetes.[19] The reason for this discrepancy is unknown, but providers may wish to consider monitoring digoxin levels periodically in patients taking these two drugs concomitantly. Miglitol also significantly reduces the bioavailability of propranolol by 40% and ranitidine by 60%, but has no drug interactions with nifedipine, antacids, or warfarin.[6,19] Acarbose does not interact with digoxin, nifedipine, or propranolol, so it may be the better choice in patients with a heart condition.

There is no fixed dosage regimen for treatment of diabetes mellitus with either α-glucosidase inhibitor. Treatment must be individualized for each patient based on effectiveness and tolerance to assure maximal clinical efficacy with minimal adverse effects. Both medications should be given with the first bite of each meal, since α-glucosidase inhibitors work in the small intestine when dietary carbohydrates are present. The gastrointestinal side effects can be reduced by starting with a low initial daily dose and titrating slowly to the appropriate maintenance dose.

Initial treatment with acarbose is suggested at a dose of 25 mg orally three times daily with a gradual increase if needed to achieve glycemic control up to the maximum dose of 100 mg three times a day. However, some patients may benefit from a slower titration, starting with 25 mg once per day and titrating up to 25 mg three times a day to reduce gastrointestinal adverse events. The usual maintenance dose is 50 mg three times a day, but some patients may need up to 100 mg three times a day.[3] Patients with body weight below 60 kg should not be considered for doses above 50 mg three times a day because of higher risk for elevated serum transaminases.[5] Once the effective and tolerable dose has been established, it should be maintained.

Miglitol should be started at 25 mg orally three times a day and gradually increased until the minimum dose needed to achieve adequate glycemic control is identified. This titration may also reduce the gastrointestinal adverse effects. During this initiation phase, 1 h postprandial plasma glucose can be used to determine response to the medication. A1C should be measured after 3 months to confirm efficacy and appropriateness. The maximum recommended dose of 100 mg three times a day should not be exceeded.[6] Available products and recommended dosing is described in Table 11.1.

Table 11.1—Product Strengths and Dosing Recommendations for α-Glucosidase Inhibitors

Drug name	How supplied	Initial dose*	Usual maintenance dose	Maximum dose
Acarbose (Precose)	25-mg, 50-mg, 100-mg tablets	25 mg t.i.d.	50 mg t.i.d.	For patients ≤60 kg: 50 mg t.i.d.; for patients >60 kg: 100 mg t.i.d.
Miglitol (Glyset)	25-mg, 50-mg, 100-mg tablets	25 mg t.i.d.	50 mg t.i.d.	100 mg t.i.d.

* Some patients may need to begin with once-daily dosing to decrease potential for adverse effects.
Source: Precose [prescribing information][5] and Glycet [prescribing information].[6]

MONOGRAPHS

Acarbose: https://dailymed.nlm.nih.gov/dailymed/drugInfo.cfm?setid=c445953d-c20a-4b70-8173-009bffc5777b

Miglitol: https://dailymed.nlm.nih.gov/dailymed/drugInfo.cfm?setid=192e6ed7-9e8c-4772-9e3b-5912a1c63a31

REFERENCES

1. Buse J, Hart K, Minasi L. The PROTECT Study: final results of a large multicenter postmarketing study in patients with type 2 diabetes. Precose Resolution of Optimal Titration to Enhance Current Therapies. *Clin Ther* 1998;20(2):257–269

2. Drent ML, Tollefsen AT, van Heusden FH, Hoenderdos EB, et al. Dose-dependent efficacy of miglitol, an alpha-glucosidase inhibitor, in type 2 diabetic patients on diet alone: results of a 24-week double-blind placebo-controlled study. *Diabetes Nutr Metab* 2002;15:152–159

3. Trevor AJ, Katzung BG, Knuidering-Hall M. Pancreatic hormones, antidiabetic agents and glucagon. In *Katzung and Trevor's Pharmacology: Examination and Board Review*, 11th ed. New York, McGraw Hill Education, 2015

4. Triplitt CL, Repas T, Alvarez C. Diabetes mellitus. In *Pharmacotherapy: A Pathophysiologic Approach*, 10th ed. DiPiro JT, Talbert RL, Yee GC, et al., Eds. New York, McGraw-Hill, 2017, p. 1173

5. Precose (acarbose) [prescribing information]. Whippany, NJ, Bayer Health-Care Pharmaceuticals, March 2015

6. Glycet (miglitol) [prescribing information]. Whippany, NJ, Bayer Health-Care Pharmaceuticals, August 2016

7. Standl E, Theodorakis MJ, Erbach M, Schnell O, Tuomilehto J. On the potential of acarbose to reduce cardiovascular disease. *Cardiovasc Diabetol* 2014;13:81

8. Li Y, Tong Y, Zhang Y, Huang L, et al. Acarbose monotherapy and weight loss in Eastern and Western populations with hyperglycaemia: an ethnicity-specific meta-analysis. *Int J Clin Pract* 2014;68(11):1318–1332

9. Wang JS, Huang CN, Hung YJ, Kwok CF, et al.; acarbose/metformin fixed-dose combination study investigators. Acarbose plus metformin fixed-dose combination outperforms acarbose monotherapy for type 2 diabetes. *Diabetes Res Clin Pract* 2013;102(1):16–24

10. Krentz AJ, Bailey CJ. Oral antidiabetic agents: current role in type 2 diabetes mellitus. *Drugs* 2005;65:385–411

11. Linn WD. Diabetes Mellitus Management. In *Pharmacotherapy in Primary Care*. Linn WD, Wofford MR, O'Keefe ME, Posey LM, Eds. New York, McGraw-Hill Education, 2009

12. Chiasson JL, Josse RG, Hunt JA, et al. The efficacy of acarbose in the treatment of patients with non-insulin-dependent diabetes mellitus: a multicenter controlled clinical trial. *Ann Intern Med* 1994;121:928

13. Campbell LK, Baker DE, Campbell RK. Miglitol: assessment of its role in the treatment of patients with diabetes mellitus. *Ann Pharmacother* 2000;34:1291–1301

14. Weng J, Soegondo S, Schnell O, Sheu W, et al. Efficacy of acarbose in different geographical regions of the world: analysis of a real-life database. *Diabetes Metab Res Rev* 2015;31:155–167

15. Zárate A, Ochoa R, Hernández M, Basurto L. Effectiveness of acarbose in the control of glucose tolerance worsening in pregnancy. *Ginecol Obstet Mex* 2000;68:42–45

16. Wilton LV, Pearce GL, Martin RM, Mackay FJ, Mann RD. The outcomes of pregnancy in women exposed to newly marketed drugs in general practices in England. *Br J Obstet Gynaecol* 1998;105:882–889

17. Dimitriadis G, Hatziagellaki E, Alexopoulos E, Kordonouri O, et al. Effects of α-glucosidae inhibition on meal glucose tolerance and timing of insulin administration in patients with type I diabetes mellitus. *Diabetes Care* 1991;14:393–398

18. Scheen AJ, de Magalhaes AC, Salvatore T, Lefebvre PJ. Reduction of the acute bioavailability of metformin by the alpha-glucosidase inhibitor acarbose in normal man. *Eur J Clin Invest* 1994;24(Suppl. 3):50–54

19. Schall R, Müller FO, Hundt HK, Duursema L, et al. Study of the effect of miglitol on the pharmacokinetics and pharmacodynamics of warfarin in healthy males. *Arzneimittelforschung* 1996;46:41–46

Chapter 12

Dipeptidyl Peptidase-4 (DPP-4) Inhibitors

Kimberly C. McKeirnan, PharmD, BCACP
Joshua J. Neumiller, PharmD, CDCES, FADCES, FASCP

INTRODUCTION

D PP-4 inhibitors improve glycemic control by preventing the proteolytic degradation of endogenous incretin hormones. Enhancement of the effects of these hormones leads to increased glucose-dependent insulin secretion by pancreatic β-cells, reduction in glucagon secretion from pancreatic α-cells, and the slowing of gastric emptying.[1] This class of medication is effective at reducing A1C and plays an important role as an antihyperglycemic treatment option in the management of people with T2D.[2] DPP-4 inhibitors are generally used in combination with other antihyperglycemic medications, such as metformin, TZDs, sulfonylureas, SGLT2 inhibitors, and insulin.

DPP-4 inhibitors are approved as adjunct to diet and exercise to improve glycemic control in adults with T2D.[3-6] Sitagliptin was the first DPP-4 inhibitor approved by the FDA in October 2006. Since the approval of sitagliptin, several more agents have followed within the class. There are currently four DPP-4 inhibitors approved for use in the U.S.: sitagliptin (Januvia, Merck & Co.), which was FDA approved in 2006; saxagliptin (Onglyza, AstraZeneca), FDA approved in 2009; linagliptin (Tradjenta, Eli Lilly and Boehringer Ingelheim), FDA approved in 2011; and alogliptin (Nesina, Takeda Pharmaceuticals), FDA approved in 2013.[3-6] Vildagliptin (Glavus) was approved by the European Medicine Agency in 2008 and is available in Europe. Gemigliptin, anagliptin, teneligliptin, trelagliptin, omarigliptin, evogliptin, and gosogliptin are also available in other countries. This section will review the pharmacology of DPP-4 inhibitors, as well as the properties, considerations, and role of these agents in the treatment of T2D.

PHARMACOLOGY

MECHANISM OF ACTION

The incretin effect is mediated via gut hormones that induce insulin secretion from the β-cells of the pancreas in response to oral glucose administration.[1] DPP-4 inhibitors were developed to augment the incretin effect for the treatment of T2D. Dipeptidyl peptidase-4 is an enzyme responsible for breaking down the endogenous incretin hormones GLP-1 and GIP, resulting in decreased endogenous levels of these two peptides.[7] GLP-1 and GIP are important physiological mediators of prandial insulin release and maintenance of glucose homeostasis, responsible for up to 60% of the prandial insulin response.[8] GLP-1 has been shown to lower blood glucose by several mechanisms, including induction of glucose-dependent insulin secretion, decreasing plasma glucagon concentrations, and delaying gastric emptying.[9,10] DPP-4 inhibitors ultimately contribute to improved glycemia via prolonging the half-life of endogenously produced GLP-1 and GIP by slowing enzymatic degradation of these hormones.[7] After a meal, DPP-4 inhibition has been shown to result in a two- to threefold increase in circulating levels of active GLP-1 and GIP, decreased glucagon levels, and increased glucose-dependent insulin secretion.[11]

Currently available GLP-1 RAs, such as exenatide, are susceptible to degradation within the digestive tract. For this reason, most GLP-1 RAs are administered via injection, with the exception of oral semaglutide. Unlike most GLP-1 RAs, DPP-4 inhibitors can be administered orally, which may result in increased ease of use and patient acceptability in some circumstances. That said, DPP-4 inhibitors have less robust glycemic effects when compared to GLP-1 RAs, and are considered weight neutral.

PHARMACOKINETICS

Alogliptin

After administration of a single dose of alogliptin, peak plasma concentrations were achieved within 1–2 h.[12] Peak inhibition of DPP-4 occurred within 2–3 h after dosing, with peak inhibition ranging from 93–98%. Enzyme inhibition ranged from 74–97% 24 h after administration and from 47–83% after 72 h. At the maximum recommended clinical dose of 25 mg, alogliptin was eliminated with a mean terminal half-life of approximately 21 h.[12] Alogliptin has an absolute bioavailability of approximately 100%, even when taken with a high-fat meal, so it can be administered with or without food.[3] The volume of distribution following a 12.5-mg intravenous infusion of alogliptin was 417 L, indicating the agent is well distributed into tissues.[3] The majority of the drug, 60–71%, is excreted unchanged in the urine within 24–72 h. Alogliptin is mainly metabolized by CYP2D6 and 3A4 and is primarily excreted in urine (76%).[12]

Linagliptin

Linagliptin is rapidly absorbed and has a modest oral bioavailability of approximately 30%.[13] Peak plasma concentrations are achieved approximately 1.5 h after oral administration, and are seemingly not impacted by ingestion of a high-fat meal. Linagliptin has a long elimination half-life of 131 h, although the effective half-life is approximately 12 h. While most DPP-4 inhibitors exhibit low binding to plasma proteins, linagliptin is extensively protein-bound in a dose-dependent manner.[14] Linagliptin is primarily eliminated via the hepatic system (80%). A study of linagliptin use in patients with renal compromise concluded that dose adjustment is not required in various degrees of renal impairment.[13]

Saxagliptin

Saxagliptin reaches peak plasma concentration approximately 2 h (4 h for the active metabolite) after a 5-mg oral dose.[5] When administered with a high-fat meal, a 20-min delay to peak concentration was observed. Saxagliptin is metabolized primarily by CYP450 3A4/5, so strong CYP3A4/5 inhibitors and inducers will alter the pharmacokinetics. Both renal and hepatic elimination are involved, and the terminal half-life for saxagliptin and its active metabolite are 2.5 h and 3.1 h, respectively.[5,11] Dose adjustment is not necessary for patients with mild renal impairment, but the dosage should be reduced to 2.5 mg orally once a day for patients with an eGFR of less than 45 mL/min/1.73 m².[5,11] Accordingly, the manufacturer recommends the assessment of renal function prior to the initiation of saxagliptin and periodically thereafter.

Sitagliptin

Sitagliptin given orally has a bioavailability of over 85%, achieving peak concentration within 1–4 h.[15] Following administration of a single oral 100-mg dose of sitagliptin in healthy volunteers, peak serum levels were achieved in approximately 1–4 h. The mean volume of distribution at steady state is 198 L after a single dose of sitagliptin, with approximately 38% of sitagliptin reversibly bound to plasma proteins.[6] Sitagliptin is approximately 79% excreted unchanged in the urine via active tubular secretion. In vitro studies indicate that sitagliptin is modestly metabolized via CYP450 enzyme 3A4 with some contribution from the 2C8 isoenzyme.[15] Because sitagliptin is largely eliminated renally, dosage adjustment to 50 mg orally is recommended in those with moderate renal impairment (eGFR 30–49 mL/min/1.73 m²) and to 25 mg in patients with severe renal impairment (eGFR <30 mL/min/1.73 m²).[6] The terminal half-life of a single dose of 100 mg sitagliptin was found to be 12.4 h, on average, in healthy volunteers. When examined, the presence of moderate hepatic impairment did not show significant alterations in the pharmacokinetic profile of sitagliptin.[15]

TREATMENT ADVANTAGES/DISADVANTAGES

All four DPP-4 inhibitors currently marketed in the U.S. are generally well tolerated, with a low risk of contributing to hypoglycemia due to their glucose-dependent mechanism of action.[16] Considering their low risk of hypoglycemia, excellent tolerability profile, oral administration, and once-daily dosing, DPP-4 inhibitors can be useful antihyperglycemic agents in certain clinical circumstances where hypoglycemic risk and convenience are key considerations. That said, it should be noted that DPP-4 inhibitors result in modest A1C reduction when compared to many other antihyperglycemic medication classes. Although the risk of treatment-emergent hypoglycemia is low with the use of DPP-4 inhibitors, reducing the dose of background insulin secretagogues when beginning initial therapy with a DPP-4 inhibitor may be warranted to prevent hypoglycemia. DPP-4 inhibitors are not approved for treatment of T1D or for the treatment of DKA.[3–6]

The DPP-4 inhibitors currently available for use in the U.S. have unique differentiating factors that should be considered when selecting an agent for use in a given individual. Saxagliptin is a substrate of CYP3A4/5, and a dose reduction is recommended when given in combination with a strong CYP3A4/5 inhibitor, such as ketoconazole.[11] Linagliptin has a longer half-life (131 h) than the other DPP-4 inhibitors due to extensive binding to plasma proteins and is primarily eliminated hepatically (~85%), with an estimated 5% of a given dose undergoing renal elimination.[13] Dose adjustment is therefore not required with linagliptin in the setting of renal impairment, which is unique when compared to other currently available DPP-4 inhibitors.[13]

The effect of DPP-4 inhibitor use on cardiovascular outcomes has also been evaluated. Dedicated CVOTs have been reported for alogliptin, sitagliptin, saxagliptin, and linagliptin (EXAMINE, TECOS, SAVOR-TIMI 53, and CARMELINA, respectively), none of which showed a benefit of preventing major cardiovascular outcomes when compared to placebo, bud did demonstrate cardiovascular safety.[17–20] Findings from these CVOTs have raised questions about the relationship between DPP-4 inhibitor use and HF. The SAVOR-TIMI 53 trial reported that patients treated with saxagliptin were more likely to be hospitalized for HF when compared to participants given placebo (3.5% vs. 2.85%, respectively).[19] The EXAMINE, TECOS, and CARMELINA studies, in contrast, did not show associations between DPP-4 inhibitor use and HF.[17,18,20] While the FDA reported that the hospital admission rates for HF in the EXAMINE trial were 3.9% for patients assigned to alogliptin, versus 3.3% for those on placebo,[21] a post hoc analysis of the trial reported that alogliptin had no effect on the composite endpoint of cardiovascular death and hospitalization for HF.[22] In support of these CVOT findings, one meta-analysis concluded that there is no statistically significant evidence that DPP-4 inhibitors reduce negative cardiovascular outcomes, including acute coronary syndrome, stroke, or overall cardiovascular mortality, and showed an increased risk of HF with DPP-4 inhibitors compared to placebo.[23] Given questions surrounding DPP-4 inhibitor use and HF risk, DPP-4 inhibitors currently carry warnings and/or precautions in their labeling related to HF and associated symptoms.

A 2015 review reported the cost-effectiveness of DPP-4 inhibitors from both a payer and societal standpoint.[24] The study concluded that DPP-4 inhibitors, when compared to sulfonylureas and insulin, are a cost-effective option for patients who are not achieving glycemic targets with monotherapy.[24] This study accounted for the costs related to side effects of insulin and sulfonylureas, such as weight gain and hypoglycemia, which are not as problematic with DPP-4 inhibitors. Of note, this study did not compare the cost-effectiveness of DPP-4 inhibitors to other agents with hypoglycemia and weight benefits, such as GLP-1 RAs or SGLT2 inhibitors. While the DPP-4 inhibitor class has clear benefits in terms of weight neutrality, low hypoglycemia risk, and general tolerability, these benefits must be weighed against cost and a generally modest A1C-lowering potential.

SIGNIFICANT WARNINGS/PRECAUTIONS

All four FDA-approved DPP-4 inhibitors carry warnings for acute pancreatitis within their respective prescribing information.[3-6] Postmarketing reports of fatal and nonfatal hemorrhagic or necrotizing pancreatitis have been reported with sitagliptin.[6] However, a large retrospective study determined the relative risk of pancreatitis in people receiving sitagliptin to be 1.0 (95% CI 0.5–2.0) compared with matched controls receiving metformin or glyburide.[25] CVOT trials with saxagliptin, alogliptin, and sitagliptin reported clear numerical imbalances in cases of acute pancreatitis, yet the numerical increase in cases of acute pancreatitis observed in patients taking a DPP-4 inhibitor did not reach statistical significance in these trials.[17-19] Although causation has not been established, manufacturers of all four products recommend monitoring for signs and symptoms of pancreatitis after initiation, and recommend immediate discontinuation of the medication if pancreatitis is suspected.[3-6] Postmarketing surveillance efforts are underway by the FDA to evaluate the risk of pancreatitis with DPP-4 inhibitor use.

Prescribing information for sitagliptin, saxagliptin, linagliptin, and alogliptin all include warnings/precautions to use with caution in patients with HF and/or to monitor patients for signs and symptoms due to CVOT findings from some agents in the DPP-4 inhibitor class.[3-6] As noted previously, a CVOT with over 16,000 participants with T2D compared the use of saxagliptin and placebo on rates of a cardiovascular-related death, MI, or ischemic stroke. Although saxagliptin did not demonstrate an increased risk of cardiovascular-related death, more participants in the saxagliptin group were hospitalized for HF, raising concerns about DPP-4 inhibitor use and HF occurrence.[19] A 2014 meta-analysis of randomized clinical trials of DPP-4 inhibitors was conducted showing the overall risk of acute HF to be higher in patients treated with DPP-4 inhibitors versus those treated with placebo or an active comparator.[26] Similar to the recommendations for pancreatitis, manufacturers of sitagliptin, alogliptin, linagliptin, and saxagliptin suggest monitoring patients who have recently begun treatment with DPP-4 inhibitors for signs and symptoms of HF.[3-6]

Renal and hepatic considerations also exist for the DPP-4 inhibitor class of medications. Sitagliptin is eliminated largely via the kidneys, and thus dose reduction is warranted in patients with renal disease. Furthermore, renal function should be assessed in patients under consideration for sitagliptin therapy prior to drug initiation.[6] Reports of fatal and nonfatal hepatic failure in patients taking alogliptin have raised concerns.[3] Patients with liver failure or elevated liver enzymes should consider one of the other DPP-4 inhibitors. Liver function tests should be conducted for any patient taking alogliptin who reports symptoms indicative of liver injury.[3]

Postmarketing reports of serious allergic and hypersensitivity reactions have been reported in patients taking all four DPP-4 inhibitors.[3-6] These reactions included cases of anaphylaxis, angioedema, and exfoliative skin conditions including Stevens-Johnson syndrome. Although the occurrences of these drug reactions are rare, patients should be aware of any abnormal skin lesions or changes upon initiation, and should report any unusual reactions to their healthcare provider. DPP-4 inhibitors are contraindicated in patients with a documented hypersensitivity reaction to the medication or any of its components. Additionally, DPP-4 inhibitors are not indicated for T1D and are not intended for use in the treatment of DKA.

SPECIAL POPULATIONS

Alogliptin

The pharmacokinetic properties of alogliptin appear unaffected by age, sex, race, and BMI, although pediatric dosing has not been established.[3] Dose reduction to 12.5 mg once daily is recommended in patients with mild renal impairment (CrCl ≥30 to <60 mL/min) and 6.25 mg once daily for patients with severe renal impairment or ESRD (CrCl <30 mL/min). The prescribing information for alogliptin states that there is insufficient data to determine a drug-associated risk for major birth defects or miscarriage.[3] In animal studies, doses of greater than 180 times the respective human dose were administered to rabbits and rats and did not demonstrate any adverse developmental effects. Alogliptin is present in rat milk during animal studies, but information about presence in human milk and impact on breast-feeding is not available.[3]

Linagliptin

Linagliptin is the only DPP-4 that does not require dose adjustment in patients with renal impairment. Adjustments for patients with hepatic impairment are also not required.[4] Pediatric use has not been established, but there are no adjustment requirements for elderly patients. The prescribing information for linagliptin states that there is insufficient data to determine a drug-associated risk for major birth defects and miscarriage.[4] Studies in rats demonstrate the presence of linagliptin in milk, although the effects have not been tested in humans. Risks and benefits of breast-feeding should be considered.[4]

Saxagliptin

Dosage adjustments are not needed for saxagliptin based on sex, race, BMI, or age, although safe and effective use in pediatric patients has not been established. A dose of 2.5 mg once daily is recommended for patients with moderate or severe renal impairment. The 2.5-mg dose is also recommended when coadministered with strong CYP450 3A4/5 inhibitors (ketoconazole, clarithromycin, ritonavir, etc.) due to saxagliptin's metabolic pathway.[5] Lowering the dose of sulfonylureas may also be required when adding saxagliptin to reduce the risk of hypoglycemia.[5] The prescribing information for saxagliptin indicates there is insufficient data to determine a drug-associated risk for major birth defects or miscarriage.[5] Saxagliptin crosses the placenta into the fetus in animal studies.[27] There is no information available about the presence of saxagliptin in human milk, the effect on the breast-fed infant, or the effect on milk production, although studies with rats do show presence of the drug in milk.[5]

Sitagliptin

Little clinical information is available regarding sitagliptin use in older adults with T2D; however, dose adjustment is recommended for patients with renal compromise. Dosage adjustments are not recommended for patients with mild to moderate hepatic impairment, although sitagliptin has not been formally evaluated in patients with advanced hepatic disease.[6] The prescribing information for sitagliptin states there is insufficient data to determine a drug-associated risk for major birth defects and miscarriage.[6] Caution is advised in women who are nursing, as it is currently unknown if sitagliptin is secreted into human breast milk. Safety and efficacy in patients under 18 years of age has not been studied.[6]

ADVERSE EFFECTS AND MONITORING

Clinical trial adverse event data identified three common side effects occurring with more frequency with DPP-4 inhibitors than events seen in control subjects: nasopharyngitis, upper respiratory tract infection, and headache. In a review of 8,500 patients treated with alogliptin, the most reported side effects were nasopharyngitis (4.4%), headache (4.2%), and upper respiratory tract infection (4.2%).[16] The overall incidence of adverse event was 66%, compared to 62% with placebo and 70% with an active comparator.[16] However, the overall discontinuation was quite low, 4.7%, compared to 4.5% with placebo. Similar side-effect profiles were seen with alogliptin, saxagliptin, and sitagliptin.[3,5,6]

Additionally, the overall incidence of hypoglycemia in subjects receiving DPP-4 inhibitors as monotherapy was similar to that of placebo controls. Alogliptin monotherapy had a hypoglycemia incidence of 1.5%, and alogliptin added to insulin or glyburide did not have a statistically significant increase in incidence of hypoglycemia when compared to placebo.[16] Some of the less common but more serious side effects reported with DPP-4 inhibitors are acute pancreatitis and serious hypersensitivity, including anaphylaxis, angioedema, and severe cutaneous rash.

Therapeutic monitoring recommendations for patients receiving DPP-4 inhibitors include periodic monitoring of A1C and self-monitoring of blood glucose. Patients under consideration for DPP-4 inhibitor therapy should receive the appropriate renal and/or hepatic function testing prior to therapy and periodically during treatment.

DRUG INTERACTIONS

Alogliptin

Alogliptin is not an inducer or inhibitor of CYP450 enzymes and has not been observed to interact with any renally excreted drugs.[3] Interactions were also not observed during coadministration of alogliptin and warfarin.[28]

Linagliptin

Linagliptin efficacy may be reduced when administered with a strong CYP450 3A4 inducer, such as rifampin. Choosing an alternative treatment when the prospective patient is already taking a 3A4 inducer is strongly suggested in the pre-scribing information.[4] Linagliptin did not interact with ethinyl estradiol, levonorgestrel, digoxin, warfarin, glyburide, pioglitazone, simvastatin, or metfor-min in respective studies.[13,29-34]

Saxagliptin

Saxagliptin is significantly impacted by strong CYP3A4/5 inhibitors.[5] Keto-conazole increased saxagliptin exposure when coadministered. The dose of saxa-gliptin should be limited to 2.5 mg when given in combination with a strong CYP3A4/5 inhibitor.[5] Choosing an alternative DPP-4 inhibitor may also be appropriate.

Sitagliptin

Despite the limited metabolism of sitagliptin by CYP450 3A4 and 2C8, it is considered unlikely that any clinically relevant interactions exist with other drugs that utilize the CYP450 system. Sitagliptin did not alter the pharmacokinetics of metformin, glyburide, simvastatin, digoxin, rosiglitazone, warfarin, or oral contra-ceptives.[16] Sitagliptin given in combination with digoxin for 10 days resulted in an 11% increase in the AUC and an 18% increase in peak plasma levels of digoxin.[6] While dosage adjustments of digoxin are not recommended when given in com-bination with sitagliptin, patients receiving these agents in combination should receive periodic monitoring of serum digoxin levels to prevent toxicity.

DOSAGE AND ADMINISTRATION

Alogliptin

Alogliptin is available commercially in 6.25-mg (light pink), 12.5-mg (yellow), and 25-mg (light red) tablets.[3] Alogliptin is FDA approved for the treatment of T2D as an adjunct to diet and exercise to improve glycemic control in adults. The recom-mended dose of alogliptin is 25 mg once daily. A dose of 12.5 mg daily is recom-mended for patients with moderate renal impairment and 6.25 mg daily for patients with severe renal impairment. Alogliptin may be taken with or without food.[3]

Linagliptin

Linagliptin is also indicated as an adjunct to diet and exercise to improve gly-cemic control in adults with T2D. Linagliptin is available as a light 5-mg (red) tablet.[4] The recommended dose is 5 mg once daily with or without food. When linagliptin is coadministered with a sulfonylurea or insulin, adjusting the dose of the secretagogue or insulin may be needed.

Saxagliptin

Saxagliptin is available as a 2.5-mg pale (yellow) or 5-mg (pink) tablet.[5] Saxa-gliptin is indicated as monotherapy or combination therapy for treating T2D in conjunction with diet and exercise. The recommended dosage is 2.5 mg or 5 mg taken once daily regardless of meals. The 2.5-mg strength is recommended for patients taking strong CYP3A4/5 inhibitors or with moderate to severe renal impairment.[5]

Sitagliptin

Sitagliptin is available commercially in 25-mg (pink), 50-mg (light beige), and 100-mg (beige) tablets.[6] For T2D patients with normal renal function, sitagliptin is dosed at 100 mg once daily as monotherapy or in combination with metformin, a TZD, a sulfonylurea, or metformin plus a sulfonylurea. Sitagliptin can be taken with or without food, and because sitagliptin is eliminated via renal excretion, dosage adjustments are required for patients with moderate to severe renal impairment. For patients with an eGFR ≥30 to <45 mL/min/1.73 m², the recommended dose of sitagliptin is 50 mg once daily. For patients with an eGFR <30 mL/min/1.73 m² or with end-stage renal disease requiring dialysis, the recommended dose of sitagliptin is 25 mg once daily.[6]

Table 12.1 — DPP-4 Inhibitor Dosing Recommendations

Generic (brand)	How supplied	Initial dosing	Maintenance dosing	Maximum dosing	Dosing adjustments
Alogliptin (Nesina)	6.25-mg (light pink), 12.5-mg (yellow), and 25-mg (light red) tablets	6.25–25 mg daily	6.25–25 mg daily	25 mg daily	12.5 mg if CrCl ≥30 to <60 mL/min, 6.25 mg if CrCl <30 mL/min or ESRD
Linagliptin (Tradjenta)	5-mg (light red) tablet	5 mg daily	5 mg daily	5 mg daily	None
Saxagliptin (Onglyza)	2.5-mg (pale yellow) or 5-mg (pink) tablet	2.5–5 mg daily	2.5–5 mg daily	5 mg daily	2.5 mg daily if taking strong CYP3A4/5 inhibitors or eGFR <45 mL/min/1.73 m² or ESRD
Sitagliptin (Januvia)	25-mg (pink), 50-mg (light beige), and 100-mg (beige) tablets	25–100 mg daily	25–100 mg daily	100 mg daily	50 mg daily if eGFR ≥30 to <45 mL/min/1.73 m², 25 mg daily if eGFR <30 mL/min/1.73 m² or ESRD

Source: refs. 3–6.

Table 12.2—DPP-4-Containing Combination Products

Brand name	Generic names	How supplied
Kazano	Alogliptin/metformin	12.5 mg alogliptin and 500 mg metformin HCl 12.5 mg alogliptin and 1,000 mg metformin HCl
Oseni	Alogliptin/pioglitazone	12.5 mg alogliptin and 15 mg pioglitazone 12.5 mg alogliptin and 30 mg pioglitazone 12.5 mg alogliptin and 45 mg pioglitazone 25 mg alogliptin and 15 mg pioglitazone 25 mg alogliptin and 30 mg pioglitazone 25 mg alogliptin and 45 mg pioglitazone
Glyxambi	Linagliptin/ empagliflozin	5 mg linagliptin and 10 mg empagliflozin 5 mg linagliptin and 25 mg empagliflozin
Jentadueto	Linagliptin/metformin	2.5 mg linagliptin and 500 mg metformin HCl 2.5 mg linagliptin and 850 mg metformin HCl 2.5 mg linagliptin and 1,000 mg metformin HCl
Jentadueto XR	Linagliptin/metformin	2.5 mg linagliptin and 1,000 mg metformin HCl extended-release 5 mg linagliptin and 1,000 mg metformin HCl extended-release
Trijardy XR	Linagliptin/ empagliflozin/ metformin	2.5 mg linagliptin, 5 mg empagliflozin, and 1,000 mg metformin HCl biphasic release 2.5 mg linagliptin, 12.5 mg empagliflozin, and 1,000 mg metformin HCl biphasic release 5 mg linagliptin, 10 mg empagliflozin, and 1,000 mg metformin HCl biphasic release 5 mg linagliptin, 25 mg empagliflozin, and 1,000 mg metformin HCl biphasic release
Kombiglyze XR	Saxagliptin/metformin	2.5 mg saxagliptin and 1,000 mg metformin HCl extended release 5 mg saxagliptin and 500 mg metformin HCl extended release 5 mg saxagliptin and 1,000 mg metformin HCl extended release
QTERN	Saxagliptin/ dapagliflozin	5 mg saxagliptin and 5 mg dapagliflozin 5 mg saxagliptin and 10 mg dapagliflozin
Janumet	Sitagliptin/metformin	50 mg sitagliptin and 500 mg metformin HCl 50 mg sitagliptin and 1,000 mg metformin HCl
Janumet XR	Sitagliptin/metformin	50 mg sitagliptin and 500 mg metformin HCl extended-release 50 mg sitagliptin and 1,000 mg metformin HCl extended-release 100 mg sitagliptin and 1,000 mg metformin HCl extended-release
Steglujan	Sitagliptin/ertugliflozin	100 mg sitagliptin and 5 mg ertugliflozin 100 mg sitagliptin and 15 mg ertugliflozin

Source: refs. 35–45.

COMBINATION THERAPY

Several combination products containing a DPP-4 inhibitor are available.[35-45] All four DPP-4 inhibitors are available in combination with metformin. A meta-analysis showed DPP-4 inhibitors plus metformin as initial combination therapy was associated with greater reduction in A1C, greater reduction in fasting plasma glucose level, and lower weight loss compared to metformin monotherapy.[41] The combination was also not statistically significant for any increase in gastrointestinal adverse effects or hypoglycemia.[46]

MONOGRAPHS

Alogliptin: https://dailymed.nlm.nih.gov/dailymed/drugInfo.cfm?setid=b25f155a -1259-47c2-aa3b-7c1356e4c7f6

Linagliptin: https://dailymed.nlm.nih.gov/dailymed/drugInfo.cfm?setid= c797ea5c-cab7-494b-9044-27eba0cfe40f

Saxagliptin: https://dailymed.nlm.nih.gov/dailymed/drugInfo.cfm?setid =c5116390-e0fe-4969-94cb-e9de5165fbab

Sitagliptin: https://dailymed.nlm.nih.gov/dailymed/search.cfm?labeltype =all&query=januvia

REFERENCES

1. Neumiller JJ. Incretin pharmacology: a review of the incretin effect and current incretin-based therapies. *Cardiovasc Hematol Agents Med Chem* 2012;10(4):276–288

2. ElSayed NA, Aleppo G, Aroda VR, et al. American Diabetes Association. 9. Pharmacologic approaches to glycemic treatment: Standards of Care in Diabetes – 2023. *Diabetes Care* 2023;46(Suppl. 1):S140–S157

3. Nesina (alogliptin) [prescribing information]. Deerfiled, IL, Takeda Pharmaceuticals America, Inc., 2019. Available from https://general.take-dapharm.com/NESINAPI. Accessed 12 February 2022

4. Tradjenta (linagliptin) [prescribing information]. Ridgefield, CT, Boehringer Ingelheim Pharmaceuticals, Inc., 2020. Available from http://docs. boehringer-ingelheim.com/Prescribing%20Information/PIs/Tradjenta/ Tradjenta.pdf?DMW_FORMAT=pdf. Accessed 12 February 2022

5. Onglyza (saxagliptin) [prescribing information]. Wilmington, DE, Astra-Zeneca Pharmaceuticals LP, 2019. Available from http://www.azpicentral. com/pi.html?product=onglyza&country=us&popup=no. Accessed 12 February 2022

6. Januvia (sitagliptin) [prescribing information]. Whitehouse Station, NJ, Merck & Co., Inc., 2019. Available from https://www.merck.com/product/usa/pi_circulars/j/januvia/januvia_pi.pdf. Accessed 12 February 2022

7. Ahrén B. Clinical results of treating type 2 diabetic patients with sitagliptin, vildagliptin or saxagliptin—diabetes control and potential adverse events. *Best Pract Res Clin Endocrinol Metab* 2009;23(4):487–498

8. Nauck MA, Homberger E, Siegel EG, Allen RC, et al. Incretin effects of increasing glucose loads in man calculated from venous insulin and C-peptide responses. *J Clin Endocrinol Metab* 1986;63(2):492–498

9. Holst JJ, Orskov C, Nielsen OV, Schwartz TW. Truncated glucagon-like peptide 1, an insulin-releasing hormone from the distal gut. *FEBS Lett* 1987;211(2):169–174

10. Kreymann B, Williams G, Ghatei MA, Bloom SR. Glucagon-like peptide-1 7–36: a physiological incretin in man. *Lancet* 1987;2(8571):1300–1304

11. Nowicki M, Rychlik I, Haller H, et al. Long-term treatment with the dipeptidyl peptidase-4 inhibitor saxagliptin in patients with type 2 diabetes mellitus and renal impairment: a randomised controlled 52-week efficacy and safety study. *Int J Clin Pract* 2011;65:1230–1239

12. Covington P, Christopher R, Davenport M, et al. Pharmacokinetic, pharmacodynamic, and tolerability profiles of the dipeptidyl peptidase–4 inhibitor alogliptin: a randomized, double-blind, placebo-controlled, multiple-dose study in adult patients with type 2 diabetes. *Clin Ther* 2008;30:499–512

13. Graefe-Mody U, Huettner S, Stähle H, Ring A, Dugi KA. Effect of linagliptin (BI 1356) on the steady-state pharmacokinetics of simvastatin. *Int J Clin Pharmacol Ther* 2010;48:367–374

14. Fuchs H, Tillement JP, Urien S, Greischel A, Roth W. Concentration-dependent plasma protein binding of the novel dipeptidyl peptidase 4 inhibitor BI 1356 due to saturable binding to its target in plasma of mice, rats and humans. *J Pharm Pharmacol* 2009;61:55–62

15. Subbarayan S, Kipnes M. Sitagliptin: a review. *Expert Opin Pharmacother* 2011;12:1613–1622

16. Chen XW, He ZX, Zhou ZW, Yang T, et al. Clinical pharmacology of dipeptidyl peptidase 4 inhibitors indicated for the treatment of type 2 diabetes mellitus. *Clin Exp Pharmacol Physiol* 2015;42:999–1024

17. White WB, Cannon CP, Heller SR, et al.; EXAMINE Investigators. Alogliptin after acute coronary syndrome in patients with type 2 diabetes. *N Engl J Med* 2013;369:1327–1335

18. Green JB, Bethel MA, Armstrong PW, et al.; TECOS Study Group. Effect of sitagliptin on cardiovascular outcomes in type 2 diabetes. *N Engl J Med* 2015;373:232–242

19. Scirica BM, Bhatt DL, Braunwald E, et al.; SAVOR-TIMI 53 Steering Committee and Investigators. Saxagliptin and cardiovascular outcomes in patients with type 2 diabetes mellitus. *N Engl J Med* 2013;369:1317–1326

20. Rosenstock J, Perkovic V, Johansen OE, et al.; Effect of linagliptin vs placebo on major cardiovascular events in adults with type 2 diabetes and high cardiovascular and renal risk: The CARMELINA randomized clinical trial. *JAMA* 2019;321:69–79

21. U.S. Food and Drug Administration. FDA drug safety communication: FDA adds warning about heart failure risk to labels of type 2 diabetes medications containing saxagliptin and alogliptin [Internet]. Available from https://www.fda.gov/drugs/drug-safety-and-availability/fda-drug-safety-communication-fda-adds-warnings-about-heart-failure-risk-labels-type-2-diabetes. Accessed 30 January 2023

22. Zannad F, Cannon CP, Cushman WC, et al.; EXAMINE Investigators. Heart failure and mortality outcomes in patients with type 2 diabetes taking alogliptin versus placebo in EXAMINE: a multicentre , randomized, double-blind trial. *Lancet* 2015;385:2067–2076

23. Wu S, Hopper I, Skiba M, Krum H. Dipeptidyl peptidase-4 inhibitors and cardiovascular outcomes: meta-analysis of randomized clinical trials with 55,141 participants. *Cardiovascular Ther* 2014;32:147–158

24. Geng J, Yu H, Yiwei M, Zhandg P, Yingyao C. Cost effectiveness of dipeptidyl-peptidase-4 inhibitors for type 2 diabetes. *Pharmacoeconomics* 2015;33:581–597

25. Dore DD, Seeger JD, Arnold Chan K. Use of a claims-based active drug safety surveillance system to assess the risk of acute pancreatitis with exenatide or sitagliptin compared to metformin or glyburide. *Curr Med Res Opin* 2009;25(4):1019–1027

26. Monami M, Dicembrini I, Mannucci E. Dipeptidyl peptidase-4 inhibitors and heart failure: a meta-analysis of randomized clinical trials. *Nutr Metab Cardiovasc Dis* 2014;24(7):689–697

27. Lam S, Saad M. Saxagliptin: a new dipeptidyl peptidase-4 inhibitor for type 2 diabetes. *Cardiol Rev* 2010;18(4):213–217

28. Scheen AJ. Dipeptidylpeptidase–4 inhibitors (gliptins): focus on drug-drug interactions. *Clin Pharmacokinet* 2010;49:573–588

29. Friedrich C, Port A, Ring A, et al. Effect of multiple oral doses of linagliptin on the steady-state pharmacokinetics of a combination oral contraceptive in healthy female adults: an open-label, two-period, fixed-sequence, multiple-dose study. *Clin Drug Investig* 2011;31:643–653

30. Friedrich C, Ring A, Brand T, Sennewald R, et al. Evaluation of the pharmacokinetic interaction after multiple oral doses of linagliptin and digoxin in healthy volunteers. *Eur J Drug Metab Pharmacokinet* 2011;36:17–24

31. Graefe-Mody EU, Brand T, Ring A, et al. Effect of linagliptin on the pharmacokinetics and pharmacodynamics of warfarin in healthy volunteers. *Int J Clin Pharmacol Ther* 2011;49:300–310

32. Graefe-Mody U, Rose P, Ring A, Zander K, et al. Assessment of the pharmacokinetic interaction between the novel DPP-4 inhibitor linagliptin and a sulfonylurea, glyburide, in healthy subjects. *Drug Metab Pharmacokinet* 2011;26:123–129

33. Graefe-Mody EU, Jungnik A, Ring A, Woerle HJ, Dugi KA. Evaluation of the pharmacokinetic interaction between the dipeptidyl peptidase-4 inhibitor linagliptin and pioglitazone in healthy volunteers. *Int J Clin Pharmacol Ther* 2010;48:652–661

34. Scheen AJ. Linagliptin plus metformin: a pharmacokinetic and pharmacodynamic evaluation. *Expert Opin Drug Metab Toxicol* 2013;9:363–377

35. Kazano (alogliptin and metformin HCl) [prescribing information]. Deerfield, IL, Takeda Pharmaceuticals America, Inc., 2019. Available from https://general.takedapharm.com/KAZANOPI. Accessed 12 February 2022

36. Janumet (sitagliptin and metformin HCl) [prescribing information]. Whitehouse Station, NJ, Merck & Co., Inc. 2021. Available from https://www.merck.com/product/usa/pi_circulars/j/janumet/janumet_pi.pdf. Accessed 30 January 2023

37. Kombiglyze XR (saxagliptin and metformin HCl extended-release) [prescribing information]. Princeton, NJ, Bristol-Myers Squibb Company, and Wilmington, DE, AstraZeneca Pharmaceuticals LP, 2019. Available from http://www.azpicentral.com/pi.html?product=kombiglyzexr&country=us&popup=no. Accessed 30 January 2023

38. Jentadueto (linagliptin and metformin hydrochloride) [prescribing information]. Ridgefield, CT, Boehringer Ingelheim Pharmaceuticals, Inc., 2022. Available from https://docs.boehringer-ingelheim.com/Prescribing%20Information/PIs/Jentadueto/Jentadueto.pdf. Accessed 30 January 2023

39. Oseni (alogliptin and pioglitazone) [prescribing information]. Deerfield, IL, Takeda Pharmaceuticals America, Inc., 2019. Available from https://general.takedapharm.com/OSENIPI. Accessed 30 January 2023

40. Glyxambi (empagliflozin and linagliptin) [prescribing information]. Ridgefield, CT, Boehringer Ingelheim Pharmaceuticals, Inc., and Indianapolis, IN, Eli Lilly and Company, 2022. Available from http://docs.boehringer-ingelheim.com/Prescribing%20Information/PIs/Glyxambi/Glyxambi.pdf. Accessed 30 January 2023

41. Jentadueto XR (linagliptin and metformin hydrochloride extended-release) [prescribing information]. Ridgefield, CT, Boehringer Ingelheim Pharmaceuticals, Inc., 2021. Available from https://docs.boehringer-ingelheim.com/Prescribing%20Information/PIs/Jentadueto%20XR/Jentadueto%20XR.pdf?DMW_FORMAT=pdf. Accessed 30 January 2023

42. Trijardy XR (empagliflozin, linagliptin, and metformin hydrochloride extended-release) [prescribing information]. Ridgefield, CT, Boehringer Ingelheim Pharmaceuticals, Inc., 2022. Available from https://docs.boehringer-ingelheim.com/Prescribing%20Information/PIs/Trijardy%20XR/Trijardy%20XR.pdf?DMW_FORMAT=pdf. Accessed 30 January 2023

43. Qtern (dapagliflozin and saxagliptin) [prescribing information]. Wilmington, DE, AstraZeneca Pharmaceuticals LP, 2022. Available from http://www.azpicentral.com/pi.html?product=qtern&country=us&popup=no%E2%80%8B. Accessed 30 January 2023

44. Janumet XR (sitagliptin and metformin hydrochloride extended-release) [prescribing information]. White-house Station, NJ, Merck & Co., Inc. 2022. Available from https://www.merck.com/product/usa/pi_circulars/j/janumet_xr/janumet_xr_pi.pdf. Accessed 30 January 2023

45. Steglujan (ertugliflozin and sitagliptin) [prescribing information]. Whitehouse Station, NJ, Merck & Co., Inc. 2022. Available from https://www.merck.com/product/usa/pi_circulars/s/steglujan/steglujan_pi.pdf. Accessed 30 January 2023

46. Wu D, Li L, Liu C. Efficacy and safety of dipeptidyl peptidase-4 inhibitors and metformin as initial combination therapy and as monotherapy in patients with type 2 diabetes mellitus: a meta-analysis. *Diabetes Obes Metab* 2014;16:30–37

Chapter 13
Glucagon-Like Peptide-1 Receptor Agonists

Jennifer M. Trujillo, PharmD, BCPS, FCCP, CDCES, BC-ADM

INTRODUCTION

Incretin hormones are glucoregulatory neurohormones, and GLP-1 and GIP account for about 90% of the incretin effect.[1] GLP-1 and GIP are secreted in response to food ingestion and act on the pancreas to stimulate glucose-dependent insulin secretion and blunt inappropriate glucagon secretion.[2] GLP-1 is predominantly secreted from the L cells of the distal ileum and colon, but plasma levels of GLP-1 increase within minutes of eating, which suggests that GLP-1 is also released from L cells, present in small number, in the upper gut.[2,3] GLP-1 receptors are expressed on the pancreas as well as in the gastrointestinal tract, brain, and cardiac tissue.[4]

Abnormalities in the incretin system contribute to the pathophysiology of T2D. In T2D, there is a deficiency of GLP-1 and resistance to the action of GIP.[1] The deficiency of GLP-1 occurs early in the natural history of the disease and worsens as the disease progresses.[1]

At pharmacologic doses, exogenous GLP-1, administered intravenously, can restore insulin secretion in response to glucose rises and normalize glucose concentrations in patients with T2D.[3,5] However, GLP-1 is degraded within minutes by the ubiquitous DPP-4, which limits its therapeutic value. This has led to the development of GLP-1 RAs that are resistant to degradation by DPP-4.[4]

Exendin-4, a 39-amino acid GLP-1 RA, was derived from the salivary gland venom of the gila monster and is resistant to the degradation by DPP-4. It shares roughly 50% of its amino acid sequence with mammalian GLP-1. Exenatide is a synthetically derived peptide of exendin-4 and was the first GLP-1 RA approved in the U.S. by the FDA in 2005.[3] Since then, several additional GLP-1 RAs have been developed to provide similar effects of GLP-1 while being resistant to the degradation by DPP-4, thereby extending the duration of action.[5] Currently available injectable GLP-1 RAs, in order of approval by the FDA, include exenatide (Byetta), liraglutide (Victoza, approved 2010), exenatide XR (Bydureon, approved 2012; BCise pen approved 2017), dulaglutide (Trulicity, approved 2014), lixisenatide (Adlyxin, approved 2016), and semaglutide (Ozempic, approved 2017). Of note, due to steady decline in sales, the manufacturing of albiglutide (Tanzeum, approved 2014) was discontinued in 2017. For this reason, albiglutide will not be discussed in detail within this chapter. The first oral formulation of a GLP-1 RA (semaglutide [Rybelsus]) was approved in 2019. Tirzepatide (Mounjaro) was approved for T2D in 2022 and is unique compared to the other GLP-1 RAs because it is a dual agonist of both GLP-1 RA and GIP. In this chapter, tirzepatide will be included when referring to the GLP-1 RA class as a whole and any unique characteristics will be indicated.

GLP-1 RAs are treatment options at multiple points in the T2D disease process and can be used in combination with many other agents including metformin, TZDs, sulfonylureas, SGLT2 inhibitors, and basal insulin. They can be used as monotherapy in patients who cannot tolerate or take other first-line therapy options and some are recommended in some patient populations, such as those with ASCVD or kidney disease, independent of A1C or metformin use, based on other benefits.[6-7] GLP-1 RAs are all administered via subcutaneous injections, except for oral semaglutide, with varying dosing schedules ranging from twice daily to once weekly. They are attractive treatment options as they target multiple pathophysiologic defects and reduce glucose and weight with minimal risk of hypoglycemia. Some agents have also demonstrated CV and renal benefit.[6,8] Disadvantages such as gastrointestinal adverse effects, subcutaneous administration requirements, and cost can impact adherence and persistence, and may limit their use.

PHARMACOLOGY

MECHANISM OF ACTION

The GLP-1 RA class mimics the action of endogenous GLP-1. GLP-1 RAs stimulate insulin secretion from pancreatic β-cells in a glucose-dependent manner. In addition, during hyperglycemia, GLP-1 RAs reduce inappropriately elevated levels of glucagon, which results in decreased hepatic glucose output. These agents also have a direct effect on the stomach through the autonomic nervous system to slow gastric emptying, thereby reducing meal-related glucose excursions. Additionally, agents that penetrate the blood-brain barrier increase satiety via the central nervous system (CNS). These actions result in both a reduction in glucose and weight.[1,3,6,0] GLP-1 RAs also potentially preserve pancreatic β-cell function and protect against cytokine-induced apoptosis.[1-3,10]

Beyond their actions related to glycemic control, GLP-1 RAs also appear to have anti-atherosclerotic effects including improved substrate uptake and ischemia tolerance in the heart to vasodilation, reduced inflammation, and improved plaque stability.[11] A reduction in both systemic and local inflammation may also explain the kidney benefits seen with the GLP-1 RAs.[12]

The GIP/GLP-1 RA, tirzepatide, also stimulates insulin secretion and reduces glucagon levels in a glucose-dependent manner by selectively binding to and activating both GIP and GLP-1 receptors. Tirzepatide also delays gastric emptying and slows post-meal glucose absorption.[13]

PHARMACOKINETICS

Multiple differences exist in the characteristics of the individual agents within the GLP-1 RA class, including molecular structure and size, half-life, duration of action, ability to penetrate different tissue compartments, and homology to native

Table 13.1—Pharmacology/Pharmacokinetics/Pharmacodynamics of GLP-1 RAs

	Name	Base	Homology to native GLP-1	Dose/range	Route	T_{max}	Half-life	Antidrug anti-bodies (%)
Short-acting	Exenatide	Exendin-4	53%	5–10 µg twice daily	SC	2.1 h	2.4 h	44
	Lixisenatide	Exendin-4	50%	10–20 µg once daily	SC	1–3.5 h	3 h	70
Long-acting	Liraglutide	Human GLP-1	97%	0.6–1.8 mg once daily	SC	8–12 h	13 h	8.6
	Exenatide XR	Exendin-4	53%	2 mg once weekly	SC	2.1–5.1 h	NR	42.2
	Dulaglutide	Human GLP-1	90%	0.75–4.5 mg once weekly	SC	24–72 h	5 days	1.6
	Semaglutide	Human GLP-1	94%	0.25–1 mg once weekly	SC	1–3 days	1 week	1.0
	Oral semaglutide	Human GLP-1	94%	3–14 mg once daily	PO	1 h	1 week	0.5
	Tirzepatide	Human GIP and GLP-1	—	2.5–15 mg once weekly	SC	8–72 h	5 days	51

Source: refs. 10,14–21.

GLP-1, which, in turn, lead to important clinical differences such as efficacy, rates of adverse events, dosing schedule, and impact on glucose profile (see Table 13.1).[14–21]

GLP-1 RAs can be categorized as either exendin-4 based or human GLP-1 based. They can also be categorized as short-acting or long-acting. Short-acting GLP-1 RAs predominantly lower PPG levels, likely due to their effect on gastric emptying. Long-acting GLP-1 RAs demonstrate larger effects on FPG levels and appear to lower both FPG and PPG.[4]

SHORT-ACTING GLP-1 RAs

Exenatide

Exenatide is a synthetic form of exendin-4 that shares 53% amino acid homology with mammalian GLP. It is a short-acting, twice-daily GLP-1 RA that has a more pronounced effect on PPG levels than FPG levels.[3,4,14,22] At therapeutic concentrations, exenatide restores both first- and second-phase insulin secretion in response to food in patients with T2D.[4] Exenatide has a terminal half-life of 2.4 h, and, in most individuals, concentrations are measurable for approximately 10 h post dose. Rate of absorption is similar when injected into the upper arm, abdomen, or thigh. Exenatide is predominantly eliminated by glomerular filtration with subsequent proteolytic degradation. Mean exenatide exposure increased by 3.37 times in patients with ESRD on dialysis; therefore, exenatide is not recommended in this patient population.[14,22]

Lixisenatide

Lixisenatide is a once-daily, exendin-4-based GLP-1 RA composed of a 44-amino-acid peptide that differs from exendin-4 by the addition of 6 lysine residues at the C-terminal. It presents an approximately fourfold higher affinity for the GLP-1 receptor than native human GLP-1. Lixisenatide reaches peak concentrations after 1–3.5 h and has an elimination half-life of 3 h. Rate of absorption is similar when injected into the upper arm, abdomen, or thigh.[15,23] Lixisenatide has been shown to cross the blood-brain barrier to bind to GLP-1 receptors. Because of its shorter duration of action, it primarily improves glucose by a pronounced effect on PPG levels following administration. The PPG reductions are most notable after the first meal of the day, and effects attenuate with later meals in the day.[15,23,24] Lixisenatide is presumed to be eliminated through glomerular filtration and proteolytic degradation. Plasma AUC was increased by 34%, 69%, and 124% in patients with mild, moderate, and severe renal impairment, respectively. Close monitoring is recommended in patients with mild to moderate renal insufficiency, and lixisenatide use is not recommended in patients with ESRD.[15,23]

LONG-ACTING GLP-1 RAs

Liraglutide

Liraglutide is a once-daily, acylated human GLP-1 RA with 97% homology to native GLP-1. Liraglutide is made by substituting arginine for lysine at position 34 and attaching a C-16 fatty acid with a glutamic acid spacer to lysine at position 26. Following subcutaneous administration, maximum concentrations are achieved at 8–12 h post dosing. The elimination half-life is approximately 13 h. Absorption was similar between upper arm and abdomen and between upper arm and thigh, but was 22% lower from the thigh than from the abdomen.[16,25] Liraglutide restores both first- and second-phase insulin response. It also crosses the blood-brain barrier and binds to GLP-1 receptors in the hypothalamus.[4] Because of its half-life of 13 h, liraglutide reduces both PPG and FPG and is thus considered a long-acting GLP-1 RA. Liraglutide is endogenously metabolized in a similar manner to large proteins without a specific organ as a major route of elimination.[16,25]

Exenatide Extended Release (XR)

Exenatide XR is a once-weekly, extended-release formulation of the exendin-4-based GLP-1 RA exenatide. The product contains microspheres of exenatide encapsulated in a biodegradable polymer for gradual drug delivery. Following a single subcutaneous dose of exenatide XR, there is an initial period of release of surface-bound exenatide followed by gradual release from the microspheres. This results in a peak concentration at week 6–7 following once-weekly administration and a steady-state concentration reached at week 10. Concentrations of exenatide XR are below minimal quantifiable concentrations approximately 10 weeks after discontinuation. Exenatide is predominantly eliminated by glomerular filtration with subsequent proteolytic degradation. Exenatide XR is not recommended for use in patients with severe renal impairment or ESRD.[17,26]

Dulaglutide

Dulaglutide is a long-acting, once-weekly GLP-1 RA consisting of two GLP-1 analogs that have been linked to a human immunoglobulin class 4 constant fragment. This reduced the renal clearance of the drug because of the increased size of the protein. The amino acid sequence has been modified in both analogs at positions 8, 22, and 26 to protect from DPP-4 degradation. Dulaglutide decreases both FPG and PPG. Maximum concentrations of dulaglutide are seen 24–72 h after dosing. Steady-state concentrations are achieved after 2–4 weeks with once-weekly administration. The site of subcutaneous injection (abdomen, upper arm, or thigh) does not change the exposure to dulaglutide. The elimination half-life is approximately 5 days. Dulaglutide is presumed to be degraded by general protein catabolism pathways, and no dose adjustments are needed for renal or hepatic impairment.[18,27,28]

Semaglutide

Semaglutide is a long-acting, once-weekly GLP-1 RA with 94% structural homology to native human GLP-1. It is structurally similar to liraglutide; however, it has structural modifications, which give it a longer half-life and make it suitable for once-weekly dosing. Amino acid substitutions occur at positions 8 and 34, with the substitution at position 8 rendering semaglutide less susceptible to degradation by DPP-4. Acylation of the lysine at position 26, a spacer, and a C-18 fatty diacid chain improve binding to albumin. Like other long-acting GLP-1 RAs, semaglutide lowers both FPG and PPG. Maximum concentrations are reached 1–3 days post dose. Steady state is achieved following 4–5 weeks of once-weekly administration. The elimination half-life is approximately 1 week, so semaglutide will be present in the circulation for about 5 weeks after the last dose. The primary route of elimination is metabolism following proteolytic cleavage of the peptide and sequential β-oxidation of the fatty acid sidechain. Renal impairment does not have significant effects on the pharmacokinetics of semaglutide.[19,29]

Oral Semaglutide

The first oral GLP-1 RA, semaglutide, was approved in 2019 for adults with T2D as an adjunct to diet and exercise.[20,30] To allow for successful oral administration, semaglutide is co-formulated with an absorption enhancer, SNAC (sodium N-[8-(2-hydroxybenzoyl)amino] caprylate), which noncovalently binds to semaglutide, increasing its lipophilicity and protecting it from pH-dependent degradation. Oral semaglutide is less bioavailable and has more patient-to-patient absorption variability than injectable semaglutide, which is why a higher dose and daily administration are needed for the oral formulation. Maximum concentrations are reached after 1 hour and the elimination half-life is approximately 1 week. The primary route of elimination is the same as injectable semaglutide and renal impairment does not have significant effects on the pharmacokinetics of oral semaglutide.[20,30]

Tirzepatide

Tirzepatide is a long-acting, once-weekly dual agonist that binds to both GIP and GLP-1 receptors but favors GIP receptor agonism over GLP-1. It is a 39-aminio-acid peptide, similar in size to GIP and GLP-1. The C20 fatty diacid moiety enables albumin binding and prolongs the half-life to 5 days, allowing for once-weekly dosing. Maximum concentration is reached in 8–72 h. Steady state is

Table 13.2 — Efficacy and Safety Outcomes in Phase 3 Clinical Studies

Drug	Phase 3 clinical program	Change in A1C (%)	Change in weight (kg)	Gastrointestinal adverse effects (%)^	Injection site reactions (%)
Exenatide	AMIGO	−0.4 to −1.1	−0.3 to −2.8	Nausea 8–44* Vomiting 4–18* Diarrhea 6–18*	5.1
Lixisenatide	GETGOAL	−0.46 to −0.99	+0.3 to −2.96	Nausea 25 Vomiting 10 Diarrhea 8	3.9
Liraglutide	LEAD	−0.84 to −1.5	+0.3 to −3.24	Nausea 18–20 Vomiting 6–9 Diarrhea 10–12	2.0
Exenatide XR	DURATION	−1.48 to −1.9	−2.0 to −4.0	Nausea 8.2 Vomiting 3.4 Diarrhea 4	23.9
Dulaglutide	AWARD	−0.71 to −1.9	+0.2 to −4.7	Nausea 12.4–21.1 Vomiting 6–12.7 Diarrhea 8.9–12.6	0.5
Semaglutide	SUSTAIN	−1.1 to −2.2	−1.4 to −6.5	Nausea 15.8–20.3 Vomiting 5–9.2 Diarrhea 8.8–8.9	0.2
Oral semaglutide	PIONEER	−0.6 to −1.4	−1.2 to −4.4	Nausea 11–20 Vomiting 6–8 Diarrhea 9–10	N/A
Tirzepatide	SURPASS	−1.87 to −2.58	−5.4 to −12.9	Nausea 12–24 Vomiting 2–13 Diarrhea 12–22	3.2

^ Averages from phase 3 trials taken from prescribing information. Ranges based on different doses, except for exenatide. * Ranges based on reported data from separate studies based on background therapy. *Source:* refs. 4,10,14–31,33.

reached after 4–5 days. Tirzepatide is metabolized by proteolytic and the pharmacokinetics are not influenced by renal or hepatic impairment. Dual agonism adds to the effect of glucose-dependent insulin secretion and the ability to decrease inappropriate glucagon secretion, which may result in improved glycemic lowering and weight loss effects compared to other GLP-1 RAs.[13,31]

TREATMENT ADVANTAGES/DISADVANTAGES

The GLP-1 RAs have many favorable attributes compared to other antidiabetic medications. First, the GLP-1 RAs potentially preserve β-cell function and target multiple pathophysiologic defects caused by T2D including insulin secretion, glucagon secretion, gastric motility, and satiety. The GLP-1 RAs have demonstrated robust A1C-lowering efficacy in a wide array of patients with T2D. The class has been studied extensively with varying background therapies and in comparison with a variety of active comparators, and reductions in A1C range generally from 0.4–2.58%. Studies have consistently shown better A1C lowering with GLP-1 RAs than with DPP-4 inhibitors[32] and similar or better A1C lowering with GLP-1 RAs than with sulfonylureas, TZDs, and basal insulin.[13,22–31,33–34] The GLP-1 RAs also have a body-weight advantage and are associated with changes in weight ranging from +0.3 to –6.5 kg in diabetes studies. Weight loss with tirzepatide in Phase 3 trials was more pronounced, ranging from –5.4 to –12.9 kg. The GLP-1 RAs also confer a low risk of hypoglycemia because their effect on insulin secretion is glucose-dependent.[4] Efficacy and safety results of phase 3 clinical trials are summarized in Table 13.2.

Several phase 3 trials have compared GLP-1 RAs in a head-to-head fashion and have demonstrated that differences exist in terms of magnitude of effect on A1C and weight, as well as frequency and severity of adverse effects. In terms of A1C lowering, high dose dulaglutide, semaglutide, and tirzepatide have very high efficacy, while the remaining GLP-1 RAs have high efficacy. In terms of weight loss, tirzepatide and semaglutide have very high efficacy, dulaglutide and liraglutide have high efficacy, and the remaining agents have intermediate efficacy.[6,35,36] Of note, two GLP-1 RAs are also approved at higher doses specifically for weight loss (Saxenda [liraglutide 3 mg SC daily] and Wegovy [semaglutide 2.4 mg SC weekly]).

Through large-scale outcome trials, three of the GLP-1 RAs (liraglutide, semaglutide, and dulaglutide) have also demonstrated CV benefits in addition to their benefits in glycemic control and weight. In the Liraglutide Effect and Action in Diabetes: Evaluation of Cardiovascular Outcome Results (LEADER) trial, liraglutide reduced the risk of a composite endpoint of CV death, nonfatal MI, and nonfatal stroke by 17% compared to placebo (HR 0.87 [95% CI 0.78–0.97]) in patients with T2D at high CV risk. This result was driven by a significant reduction in CV death (HR 0.78 [95% CI 0.66–0.93]). Liraglutide also resulted in a reduction in all-cause mortality.[8,37]

In the Trial to Evaluate Cardiovascular and Other Long-Term Outcomes with Semaglutide in Subjects with Type 2 Diabetes (SUSTAIN-6) trial, semaglutide reduced the risk of a composite endpoint of CV death, nonfatal MI, and nonfatal stroke by 26% compared to placebo (HR 0.74 [95% CI 0.58–0.95]) in patients with T2D at high CV risk. There was also a reduction in the individual endpoint of nonfatal stroke with semaglutide compared to placebo and a reduction in the progression of renal disease. No significant differences were seen between groups in CV death or all-cause mortality.[8,38]

In the Researching Cardiovascular Events With a Weekly Incretin in Diabetes (REWIND) trial, dulaglutide reduced the risk of a composite endpoint of CV death, nonfatal MI, and nonfatal stroke by 12% compared to placebo (HR 0.88 [95% CI 0.79–0.99]) in patients with T2D and a history of cardiovascular disease (CVD) or at risk for CVD. This study was unique in that only 32% of subjects had prior CVD, and the results were consistent across subgroups of those with and without prior CV events.[8,39]

Based on these CV outcome trials, liraglutide, injectable semaglutide, and dulaglutide all have additional FDA indications related to CV-event reduction. Liraglutide and semaglutide are indicated to reduce the risk of major adverse CV events in adults with T2D and established CVD. Dulaglutide is indicated to reduce the risk of major adverse CV events in adults with established CVD or multiple CV risk factors.[16,18,19]

Three additional CV outcome trials have been published and have demonstrated CV safety, but not benefit, with exenatide XR (EXSCEL), lixisenatide (ELIXA), and oral semaglutide (PIONEER-6).[8] The CV outcome trial for tirzepatide is ongoing.

Some GLP-1 RAs have also been shown to delay the decline in renal function and reduce the onset and progression of albuminuria in patients with T2D. Most of the current evidence demonstrating the renal benefits of GLP-1 RAs is from secondary outcome analysis of the major CV outcome trials.[4,8]

The GLP-1 RAs are suggested by the American Diabetes Association *Standards of Care in Diabetes* as a treatment option in several situations.[6] According to the American Diabetes Association, GLP-1 RAs with proven CVD benefit (liraglutide, dulaglutide, or injectable semaglutide) are preferred treatment options (along with SGLT2 inhibitors) in patients with established ASCVD or those with indicators of high risk, independent of metformin use, baseline A1C, or individualized A1C target, due to the evidence supporting a reduction in major adverse CV events. They are also recommended in patients with CKD and albuminuria if an SGLT2 inhibitor is not tolerated or is contraindicated, or if the estimated glomerular filtration rate is less than adequate for SGLT2 inhibitor use. In the absence of these compelling comorbidities, GLP-1 RAs are recommended when a high glucose-lowering efficacy approach is needed to achieve glucose targets or when there is a compelling need to reduce weight or avoid weight gain. Finally, GLP-1 RAs are preferred over basal insulin and recommended as the first injectable agent.[6] Similarly, the American Association of Clinical Endocrinologists (AACE) guidelines recommend initiating a long-acting GLP-1 RA or SGLT2 inhibitor with proven efficacy as preferred treatment if established or high ASCVD risk, stage 3 CKD, or HF with reduced ejection fraction is present, independent of glycemic control.[7,40]

GLP-1 RAs can be used in combination with many other antidiabetic agents to provide glycemic control and target multiple pathophysiologic defects. Current guidelines, however, do not recommend using GLP-1 RAs in combination with DPP-4 inhibitors due to duplication of mechanism of action and lack of clinical outcomes and experience with this combination.[6,7,34] A significant amount of evidence shows the beneficial effect of the combination of a GLP-1 RA and a basal insulin. This combination offers complementary effects on the glucose profile and improved glycemic control with potentially lower risks of hypoglycemia and weight gain, providing a safe and effective alternative to basal-bolus insulin with lower treatment burden.[41] Two fixed-ratio combination products have been approved by the FDA and contain both a basal insulin and a GLP-1 RA in one delivery device. iDegLira combines insulin degludec and liraglutide (Xultophy, approved 2016) and iGlarLixi combines insulin glargine and lixisenatide (Soliqua, approved 2017).[42,43] These agents were initially only approved for use in patients with T2D who have not achieved adequate glycemic control on basal insulin or a GLP-1 RA. In 2019, the FDA expanded the indication, and now both are approved for use as adjuncts to diet and exercise, and thus, can be prescribed as the first injectable agent. They offer better glycemic control than the individual components, less required injections, and lower rates of gastrointestinal adverse effects, likely due to the slow dose titration.[44–47]

Disadvantages of GLP-1 RAs are the gastrointestinal adverse effects, including nausea, vomiting, and diarrhea, which usually occur early in the treatment course, are mild in nature, and are transient. But, in a small number of patients, the adverse effects are significant enough to require discontinuation. The shorter-acting agents, exenatide and lixisenatide, have more effect on gastric emptying and therefore cause more gastrointestinal adverse effects than the once-weekly options. Other disadvantages include safety concerns such as the immunogenicity risk, a potential risk of pancreatitis, cholelithiasis, worsening retinopathy, and the black box warning regarding thyroid C-cell tumors. These risks are discussed in more detail in the following section. Most GLP-1 RAs require subcutaneous administration, which is a disadvantage for patients who are resistant to injections. Each agent uses a unique injection pen device with unique administration requirements. In addition, the short-acting agents require specific dosing schedules before meals. Another potential disadvantage is cost. The GLP-1 RAs are expensive treatment options with average wholesale price for a 1-month supply ranging from $814 to $1,169.[6] Finally, although this medication class is appealing for many reasons, the uptake of prescribing has been slow. For reasons not entirely clear, the GLP-1 RAs are still not commonly used, especially in the primary care setting, and long-term persistence is low.

THERAPEUTIC CONSIDERATIONS

SIGNIFICANT WARNINGS/PRECAUTIONS

Thyroid C-Cell Carcinoma

Most of the GLP-1 RAs, excluding exenatide twice daily and lixisenatide, carry a black box warning for potential risk of thyroid C-cell tumors. GLP-1 RAs cause an increase in the incidence of thyroid C-cell tumors in rodents in a dose-related, duration-dependent fashion. Medullary thyroid carcinoma (MTC) in humans is very rare, and no cases of thyroid C-cell tumors or MTC have been reported in humans to date. Nonetheless, dulaglutide, exenatide XR, liraglutide, semaglutide, and tirzepatide are all contraindicated in patients with a personal or family history of MTC or multiple endocrine neoplasia type 2 (MEN2).[16–21]

Acute Pancreatitis

Cases of acute pancreatitis have been reported in animals and humans taking GLP-1 RAs as well as DPP-4 inhibitors. Retrospective and observational studies have been inconsistent, with some showing positive associations and some showing no association between incretin agents and pancreatitis. Some studies suggested that the risk may be related to T2D itself and not the specific drug treatment. However, early postmarketing reports led the FDA to release warnings that there may be a link between the use of these medication classes and acute pancreatitis. Ultimately, the FDA concluded that a causal relationship could not be established and there was insufficient evidence to modify treatment. The large-scale, prospective CV outcome trials have provided more insight into this potential association. Recent systematic reviews and meta-analyses of randomized controlled trials have concluded that treatment with GLP-1 RAs was not associated with an increased risk of acute pancreatitis or pancreatic cancer.[48,49] Nonetheless, current prescribing information, FDA guidance, and treatment guidelines recommend to use GLP-1 RAs cautiously in patients with a history of pancreatitis. Patients treated with GLP-1 RAs should be monitored for signs and symptoms of pancreatitis and, if pancreatitis develops while taking a GLP-1 RA, therapy should be discontinued and not re-initiated.[6,14–21,50]

Diabetic Retinopathy Complications

A significant increase in retinopathy complications including vitreous hemorrhage, blindness, or need for treatment with photocoagulation or an intravitreal agent was seen in patients receiving semaglutide during the SUSTAIN-6 trial (3% vs. 1.8%; $P = 0.02$).[38] Of the patients with retinopathy complications, 83.5% had a history of retinopathy at baseline. In a recent meta-analysis of four CV outcome trials (dulaglutide, liraglutide, oral semaglutide, subcutaneous semaglutide), GLP-1 RA use was associated with increased risk of rapidly worsening retinopathy (OR 1.23, 95% CI 1.05–1.44).[51] In another meta-analysis, GLP-1 RA use was not independently associated with increased risk of retinopathy, but there was an association with magnitude of A1C reduction.[52] Rapid glucose lowering has previously been associated with worsening of diabetic retinopathy. It is unclear if this is due to the drug itself or an effect of the change or rate of change in blood glucose levels or a combination of both. Caution should be taken when using a GLP-1 RA, particularly semaglutide, in patients with diabetic retinopathy, and the patient should be monitored closely for progression of retinopathy.[19]

Hypoglycemia

Although GLP-1 RAs independently carry a low risk of hypoglycemia, the risk of hypoglycemia is increased when they are used in combination with insulin or insulin secretagogues. Patients may require a lower dose of insulin or the secretagogue to reduce the risk of hypoglycemia in this situation.[14-21]

Acute Kidney Injury

There have been postmarketing reports of acute kidney injury and worsening of chronic renal failure in patients taking GLP-1 RAs. Some reports were in patients who did not have existing kidney disease. A majority of the cases occurred in patients who experienced nausea, vomiting, diarrhea, or dehydration. It remains unclear whether a true causal relationship exists in these case reports, but it is recommended to use caution when starting or increasing the dose of GLP-1 RAs in patients with renal insufficiency.[14-21]

Hypersensitivity

Hypersensitivity reactions have been reported with GLP-1 RAs. If a hypersensitivity reaction occurs, the drug should be stopped immediately, and the patient should be promptly treated until symptoms resolve.

SPECIAL POPULATIONS

T1D

GLP-1 RAs are not indicated for the treatment of T1D or DKA, and cannot replace insulin therapy in this population. The physiologic actions and secretion of GLP-1 in T1D are not well understood, but it is appreciated that T1D is associated with defective counterregulation, including unregulated secretion of glucagon postprandially. Thus, GLP-1 RA therapy has the potential for benefit in T1D by inhibiting inappropriate glucagon secretion after a meal.[24] To date, studies of GLP-1 RAs in combination with insulin in T1D have shown modest improvements in A1C and weight, but currently, no agent has an FDA indication for use in T1D.[53]

Pregnancy and Lactation

Limited data are available to guide the use of GLP-1 RAs in pregnant women. Based on animal studies, there may be risks to the fetus from exposure to GLP-1 RAs during pregnancy. Animal studies demonstrated embryo-fetal mortality as well as structural abnormalities, birth defects, growth alterations, and marked maternal weight loss. Women using GLP-1 RAs should discontinue use prior to a planned pregnancy to allow for washout of the medication. This time frame varies between products, with requirements of 1–2 months for once-weekly agents. No data exists with use of GLP-1 RAs in lactation, and it is not known whether GLP-1 RAs are excreted in human milk.[14-21]

Pediatrics

In 2019, the FDA approved an expanded indication for liraglutide as an adjunct to diet and exercise in children and adolescents aged 10 to 17 years old with T2D. The approval was primarily based on a study comparing liraglutide to placebo in 134 patients aged 10–17 with T2D. After 26 weeks of therapy, liraglutide lowered A1C significantly while placebo increased A1C (–0.64% vs. +0.42%,

Table 13.3— Availability, Dosing, and Administration Requirements

Drug	Availability, storage, preparation	Dosing	Missed dose recommendations	Use in renal impairment
Exenatide	■ Mutidose pen (5 µg/dose, 10 µg/dose, 60 doses per pen) ■ Pen needles not supplied with pen ■ Keep refrigerated ■ After first use, store at room temperature; discard 30 days after first use ■ No reconstitution required	■ Start with 5 µg twice daily ■ Increase to 10 µg twice daily after one month if needed for additional A1C lowering ■ Inject within 60 min prior to morning and evening meals (or before the two main meals of the day; ≥6 h apart)	■ Skip the dose and resume next dose at the prescribed time	■ Not recommended with severe renal impairment (eGFR or CrCl <30 mL/min); use with caution when initiating or escalating dose in patients with CrCl 30–50 mL/min
Lixisenatide	■ Multidose pen (10 µg/dose, 20-µg/dose, 14 doses per pen) ■ Pen needles not supplied with pen ■ Keep refrigerated ■ After first use, store at room temperature; discard 14 days after first use ■ No reconstitution required	■ Start with 10 µg once daily for 14 days ■ Increase to 20 µg once daily ■ Inject within 1 h prior to first meal of the day	■ Skip the dose and resume next dose at the prescribed time	■ No dose adjustment recommended; limited experience in severe renal impairment; avoid if eGFR <15 mL/min/1.73 m²
Liraglutide	■ Multidose pen (6 mg/mL, 3 mL; each pen delivers doses of 0.6 mg, 1.2 mg, or 1.8 mg) ■ Pen needles not supplied with pen ■ Keep refrigerated ■ After first use, store at room temperature; discard 30 days after first use ■ No reconstitution required	■ Start with 0.6 mg once daily for 1 week; then increase to 1.2 mg once daily ■ Increase to 1.8 mg once daily if needed for additional A1C lowering ■ Inject at any time of day, with or without meals	■ Skip the dose and resume next dose at the prescribed time	■ No dose adjustment recommended; limited experience in severe renal impairment

(continued)

Table 13.3 (continued)

Drug	Availability, storage, preparation	Dosing	Missed dose recommendations	Use in renal impairment
Exenatide XR	<ul><li>Single-dose pen (2 mg)</li><li>Pen needle supplied with pen</li><li>Keep refrigerated</li><li>Store flat in original packaging, protected from light</li><li>May store at room temperature for 4 weeks</li><li>Remove from refrigerator 15 min prior to mixing</li><li>Requires reconstitution</li><li>Dose should be administered immediately once reconstituted</li></ul>	<ul><li>2 mg once weekly</li><li>Inject at any time of day, with or without meals</li></ul>	<ul><li>If within 3 days of missed dose, give right away; resume dosing on usual day of administration</li><li>If 3 days have passed, skip dose and resume on usual day of administration</li></ul>	<ul><li>Not recommended with severe renal impairment (eGFR or CrCl <30 mL/min); use with caution in patients with CrCl 30–50 mL/min (Bydureon)</li><li>Not recommended with an eGFR<45 mL/min/1.73m² (Bydureon BCise)</li></ul>
Dulaglutide	<ul><li>Single-dose pen (0.75 mg, 1.5 mg, 3 mg, 4.5 mg)</li><li>Pen needle attached</li><li>Keep refrigerated</li><li>May store at room temperature for 14 days</li><li>No reconstitution required</li></ul>	<ul><li>Start with 0.75 mg once weekly</li><li>Increase to 1.5 mg once weekly if needed for additional A1C lowering; increase to 3 mg and then 4.5 mg once weekly if needed after at least 4 weeks on the previous dose</li><li>Inject at any time of day, with or without meals</li></ul>	<ul><li>If within 3 days of missed dose, give right away. Resume dosing on usual day of administration</li><li>If 3 days have passed, skip dose and resume on usual day of administration</li></ul>	<ul><li>No dose adjustment recommended; limited experience in severe renal impairment</li></ul>
Semaglutide	<ul><li>Multidose pen: 2 mg/1.5 mL, lower-dose pen delivers 0.25 mg or 0.5 mg doses; higher dose pen delivers 1 mg dose or 4 mg/3 mL pen, delivers 1 mg dose</li><li>Pen needles supplied with pen</li><li>Keep refrigerated</li><li>After first use, store at room temperature; discard 56 days after first use</li><li>No reconstitution required</li></ul>	<ul><li>Start with 0.25 mg once weekly</li><li>Increase to 0.5 mg once weekly after 4 weeks</li><li>May increase to 1 mg once weekly after 4 weeks, if needed for additional A1C lowering</li><li>Inject at any time of day, with or without meals</li></ul>	<ul><li>If within 5 days of missed dose, give right away; resume dosing on usual day of administration</li><li>If 5 days have passed, skip dose and resume on usual day of administration</li></ul>	<ul><li>No dose adjustment recommended</li></ul>

(continued)

Table 13.3 (continued)

Drug	Availability, storage, preparation	Dosing	Missed dose recommendations	Use in renal impairment
Oral Semaglutide	■ Oral tablets (3 mg, 7 mg, 14 mg)	■ Start with 3 mg once daily for 30 days ■ Increase to 7 mg once daily ■ May increase to 14 mg once daily after 30 days, if needed for additional A1C lowering ■ Take at least 30 minutes before the first food, beverage, or other oral medication of the day with no more than 4 ounces of plain water only ■ Swallow tablets whole; do not crush or chew	■ Skip the missed dose and resume regular schedule	■ No dose adjustment recommended
Tirzepatide	■ Single-dose pen (2.5 mg, 5 mg, 7.5 mg, 10 mg, 12.5 mg, 15 mg) ■ Pen needle attached ■ Keep refrigerated ■ May store at room temperature for 21 days ■ No reconstitution required	■ Start with 2.5 mg once weekly for 4 weeks ■ Increase to 5 mg once weekly ■ Increase the dose in 2.5 mg increments after at least 4 weeks on the current dose if additional glycemic control is needed ■ Inject at any time of day, with or without meals	■ If within 4 days of missed dose, give right away. Resume dosing on usual day of administration ■ If 4 days have passed, skip dose and resume on usual day of administration	■ No dose adjustment recommended

Source: refs. 10,14–21

$P < 0.001$).[54] In 2021, the FDA approved a similar expanded indication for once-weekly exenatide XR. Because of these recent expanded indications, the American Diabetes Association *Standards of Care in Diabetes* recommends consideration of liraglutide or exenatide XR in this patient population if glycemic targets are not met with metformin (with or without basal insulin) if they have no contraindication.[55]

Older Adults

The phase 3 clinical trials of all GLP-1 RAs did include patients over the age of 65 and a small percentage of patients over the age of 75. No meaningful differences were observed in safety and efficacy between younger and older adults. Small sample sizes could limit these conclusions. Since older patients may have declined renal function, care should be taken with product and dose selection based on renal function status.[14–21]

Renal or Hepatic Impairment

Dose adjustments are not recommended for most of the GLP-1 RAs with the exception of exenatide and exenatide XR, which are not recommended for use in patients with severe renal impairment (CrCl <30 mL/min). There is limited experience with the use of GLP-1 RAs in patients with ESRD. Clinicians should use caution in this patient population and in those at risk for worsening renal function, such as patients experiencing dehydration. Recommendations on the use and dose of specific GLP-1 RAs in renal impairment are in Table 13.3. There is limited experience in patients with hepatic impairment, and dose adjustments are not recommended in this patient population. Exenatide and exenatide XR undergo renal elimination, so hepatic impairment would not be expected to affect blood concentrations.[34]

Gastroparesis

GLP-1 RAs have not been studied in patients with severe gastrointestinal disease, including gastroparesis. Since these agents delay gastric emptying, they are not recommended in patients with gastroparesis.

ADVERSE EFFECTS AND MONITORING

Gastrointestinal Adverse Effects

The most commonly reported adverse effects of the GLP-1 RAs are gastrointestinal in nature, including nausea, vomiting, and diarrhea, which usually occur early in the treatment course, are transient, are mild in nature, and rarely require discontinuation.[4] Rates of nausea, vomiting, and diarrhea range from 8–44% for nausea, from 2–18% for vomiting, and from 4–22% for diarrhea with the GLP-1 RAs (Table 13.2).[14–21] These varying rates are dependent not only on the specific drug, but also on the dose, background therapy, and adverse event reporting process in each clinical trial. In head-to-head clinical studies, exenatide XR was associated with lower rates of nausea and vomiting than liraglutide and exenatide twice daily. Lixisenatide had lower rates compared to exenatide twice daily; dulaglutide and liraglutide had similar rates.[4,5,35,36] The shorter-acting agents, exenatide and lixisenatide, have more effect on gastric emptying and therefore may cause more gastrointestinal adverse effects than the once-weekly options.[35,36] Slow dose titration can minimize the gastrointestinal adverse effects. Patients should also be encouraged to eat slowly and reduce portion sizes to help minimize the gastrointestinal adverse effects.

Hypoglycemia

Because GLP-1 RAs increase insulin secretion from pancreatic β-cells in a glucose-dependent manner in response to food intake, the risk of hypoglycemia is low. Clinical studies done with GLP-1 RAs alone or in combination with other low hypoglycemia risk agents such as metformin have reported low rates of hypoglycemia, typically under 5%.[22-31] Episodes of severe hypoglycemia are rare. Rates of hypoglycemia are consistently lower with GLP-1 RAs than with insulin or sulfonylureas in clinical studies. In head-to-head trials, there have been no significant differences in the rates of hypoglycemia among GLP-1 RAs.[5,35,36]

The risk of hypoglycemia is increased when GLP-1 RAs are used in combination with insulin or insulin secretagogues such as sulfonylureas or meglitinides. However, a meta-analysis evaluating the combination of a GLP-1 RA and basal insulin showed no significant increase in hypoglycemia in patients taking the combination versus other treatments.[56] Studies have also demonstrated that the fixed-ratio combinations of basal insulin and GLP-1 RAs can achieve better A1C lowering with similar or lower rates of hypoglycemia compared to basal insulin alone.[44-46] Nonetheless, care should be taken when initiating a GLP-1 RA in a patient already taking basal insulin. The basal insulin dose may need to be decreased as the GLP-1 RA starts to take effect.[41] Across clinical studies, there were varying approaches to adjusting basal insulin doses, with some empirically decreasing the dose by 10–20% when the GLP-1 RA was initiated. This dose adjustment should depend on baseline glucose and A1C levels, as well as the onset of action, dose titration schedule, and expected impact on glucose profile of the specific GLP-1 RA.[41]

Injection Site Reactions

Injection site reactions range from 0.2–23.9% in patients taking injectable GLP-1 RAs (Table 13.2).[14-19,21] Some evidence suggests that injection site reactions are more common in patients with high drug antibody titers.[4] Rates were also more pronounced with exenatide than other GLP-1 RAs. Exenatide XR can also cause injection site nodules, likely due to its formulation. Exenatide XR is encapsulated in microspheres made of a biodegradable polymer that release the drug over a sustained time interval. The microspheres can lead to injection site nodules described as pea-sized, hard, subcutaneous, lumps, masses, or indurations.[57]

Immunogenicity

Immunogenicity is a potential concern with all therapeutic proteins. The detection of antibody formation in assays is influenced by several factors including assay methodology, sample handling, concomitant medications, and underlying disease; therefore, caution must be taken when comparing rates of antibody formation between studies. Antidrug antibodies occurred in 1–70% of patients taking injectable GLP-1 RAs during phase 3 clinical trials and occurred more frequently with the exendin-4-based agents (exenatide and lixisenatide) than with other agents (Table 13.1).[4,14–21] Patients with antibody formation may have an attenuated A1C response. In the phase 3 clinical program, 70% of patients taking lixisenatide had antibody formation, and an attenuated glycemic response was seen in the subset of patients with the highest antibody titers.[15] Similarly, 20–38% of patients taking exenatide twice daily had low titer antibodies in the phase 3 studies and 2–9% had high titer antibodies, with about half of the patients with high titer antibodies having an attenuated glycemic response.[14]

Increased Heart Rate

Although GLP-1 RAs have been associated with a mild decrease in blood pressure, they also are associated with an increased heart rate of 2–4 beats per minute. The clinical significance of this effect has not been established.[58]

Gallbladder or biliary disease

GLP-1 RAs are also associated with increased risk of gallbladder and biliary disease, including cholelithiasis and cholecystitis. In an evaluation of over 90 clinical trials involving 17,232 patients taking a GLP-1 RA versus 14,872 patients taking a comparator, there was a small but significantly increased risk of cholelithiasis in patients taking a GLP-1 RA versus a comparator (141 vs. 99 cases; HR 1.3 [95% CI 1.01–1.68, $P = 0.041$]).[51] A more recent meta-analysis reported an additional 27 cases per 10,000 patients per year. Although the absolute risk appears small, this may underrepresent the true risk, as many studies did not report biliary-related events.[59] The mechanism of this adverse effect is not understood and warrants further investigation. The risk appears higher with higher medication doses, longer duration of use, and when used for weight loss rather than glycemic control. Caution is warranted with the use of GLP-1 RAs in patients at high risk for biliary complications.

Monitoring

Monitoring for efficacy should include A1C every 3–6 months and weight. Blood glucose monitoring (BGM) can be useful to determine whether FPG or PPG levels are more problematic. Since some of the GLP-1 RAs are affected by renal impairment, routine monitoring of serum creatinine is warranted. Although hypoglycemia is rare with GLP-1 RAs, the risk is increased when used with insulin or secretagogues. Therefore, hypoglycemia occurrence, frequency, and severity should be evaluated. Other monitoring should include close follow-up to assess injection site reactions and gastrointestinal adverse effects such as nausea, vomiting, and diarrhea. Although pancreatitis and cholelithiasis are rare, patients should be educated about the symptoms, including extreme abdominal pain.[34]

DRUG INTERACTIONS

The risk of hypoglycemia is increased when GLP-1 RAs are used concomitantly with insulin or insulin secretagogues (e.g., sulfonylureas or meglitinides). The risk can be decreased by reducing the dose of the concomitant medication.[14–21]

GLP-1 RAs cause delayed gastric emptying and thereby have the potential to impact the absorption of other medications administered concomitantly. In clini-

Table 13.4—Combination GLP-1 RA and Basal Insulin Products

Drug	Availability, storage, preparation	Dosing
iDegLira 100/3.6 (Insulin degludec and liraglutide)	■ Multi-dose pens (insulin degludec 100 units/mL and liraglutide 3.6 mg/mL; 3 mL) ■ Each pen delivers doses based on insulin units; doses range from 10–50 units ■ Pen needles not supplied with pen ■ Keep refrigerated ■ After first use, store at room temperature; discard 21 days after first use	■ If patient is insulin and GLP-1 RA naïve: start with 10 units insulin degludec/0.36 mg liraglutide once daily ■ If patient is currently on insulin or GLP-1 RA: discontinue current basal insulin or GLP-1 RA prior to initiation; start with 16 units insulin degludec/0.58 mg liraglutide once daily ■ Increase dose by 2 units every 3–4 days until FPG goal is reached; maximum dose is 50 units insulin degludec/1.8 mg liraglutide ■ Inject at any time of day, with or without meals
iGlarLixi 100/33 (Insulin glargine and lixisenatide)	■ Multi-dose pens (insulin glargine 100 units/mL and lixisenatide 33 µg/mL; 3 mL) ■ Each pen delivers doses based on insulin units; doses range from 15–60 units ■ Pen needles not supplied with pen ■ Keep refrigerated ■ After first use, store at room temperature; discard 14 days after first use	■ If patient is insulin and GLP-1 RA naïve or on <30 units of basal insulin or on a GLP-1 RA: discontinue current basal insulin or GLP-1 RA prior to initiation; start with 15 units insulin glargine/5 µg lixisenatide once daily ■ If on 30–60 units of basal insulin: discontinue current basal insulin prior to initiation; start with 30 units insulin glargine/10 µg lixisenatide once daily ■ Increase dose by 2–4 units every week until FPG goal is reached; maximum dose is 60 units insulin glargine/20 µg lixisenatide ■ Inject within 1 h before first meal of the day

Source: Xultophy [product information][42] and Soliqua [product information].[43]

cal trials, most of the GLP-1 RAs did not affect the absorption of orally administered drugs to any clinically meaningful degree. However, since GLP-1 RAs delay gastric emptying, caution should be taken when oral medications are given concomitantly with GLP-1 RAs, particularly when a slower rate of absorption could be clinically meaningful.[14–21] Drugs that have a narrow therapeutic index should be adequately monitored when given with a GLP-1 RA. A drug interaction study of exenatide and warfarin did not show any significant interaction; however, there have been postmarketing reports of increased international normalized ratio (INR) with concomitant use of exenatide and warfarin. Therefore, INR should be monitored more frequently after initiating exenatide and can return to normal intervals once stable.[17]

For patients taking a short-acting GLP-1 RA (exenatide and lixisenatide), oral medications that are dependent on threshold concentrations (e.g., antibiotics and contraceptives) should be taken at least 1 h prior to the GLP-1 RA injection (or at least 11 h after the dose for lixisenatide). Drugs that should be taken with food should be taken with a meal or snack when the GLP-1 RA is not administered.[14,15]

Given the strict administration requirements with oral semaglutide, concerns have been raised regarding its use with other oral medications and potential drug-drug interactions. Taking other oral medications at the same time as oral semaglutide could significantly decrease the absorption of oral semaglutide and should be avoided. This could create challenges for patients who take other commonly prescribed medications such as levothyroxine and oral bisphosphonates that also have similar, strict administration requirements. In addition, exposure to levothyroxine was increased by 33% when co-administered with oral semaglutide. In other drug interaction studies, oral semaglutide did not have any clinically relevant effects on the exposure of lisinopril, warfarin, metformin, digoxin, furosemide, or rosuvastatin.[20]

DOSING AND ADMINISTRATION

The availability, storage, dosing, and administration requirements for the GLP-1 RAs are compared in Table 13.3. Availability and dosing of fixed-ratio combination products are summarized in Table 13.4. The injectable GLP-1 RAs are all available in injectable pen devices and administered subcutaneously into the abdomen, thigh, or upper arm. Dosing schedules vary between agents and range from twice daily to once weekly. The short-acting agents, exenatide and lixisenatide, have specific timing requirements in relation to meals since their mechanisms are more targeted toward slowing gastric emptying postprandially. If the dose of exenatide or lixisenatide is missed, it should not be taken after the meal. The long-acting agents have more flexibility with timing of doses and can be taken at any time of day, with or without food. Most of the GLP-1 RAs have recommended lower doses when initiating the drug, followed by titration to higher doses if needed for glycemic control. This is to minimize gastrointestinal adverse effects, since studies have found that the gastrointestinal adverse effects are dose related and transient.

Specific administration requirements must be followed to ensure absorption of oral semaglutide. It must be taken at least 30 minutes before the first food, beverage, or other oral medication of the day with 4 ounces of plain water only. Failure to follow these administration recommendations will likely result in lower systemic absorption and decreased efficacy of oral semaglutide. The tablets should not be crushed or chewed.[20]

Each GLP-1 RA requires medication counseling and self-administration education specific to the product. Preparation steps, administration, and storage requirements are all unique to each product. Some pen devices are single use, while others are multi-use. Exenatide XR requires reconstitution prior to administering the dose, which involves several steps including shaking the pen vigorously for at least 15 seconds. Some require pen needle attachment, while others come with the pen already attached. Therefore, each patient requires education on the agent prescribed and occasional review of administration technique and medication-taking behaviors. Regardless of product, all patients should be instructed that pen devices should never be shared between patients, even if the needle is changed, as it poses a risk for the transmission of blood-borne pathogens.

Adherence and persistence are particularly challenging with the GLP-1 RAs. Several barriers have been identified to consistent use of these agents, including clinical inertia, cost, gastrointestinal adverse effects, and injection concerns. These issues underscore the need for better provider-patient communication to set expectations appropriately, discuss the patient's willingness and ability to take the medication, and address additional barriers that may arise.[59] Several real-world studies have demonstrated variability in patient preference, adherence, and persistence among GLP-1 RA agents. Higher adherence and persistence rates have been demonstrated with dulaglutide than with exenatide XR and liraglutide.[60] Higher adherence has been demonstrated with exenatide XR than with exenatide and liraglutide.[62,63]

The GLP-1 RAs offer an attractive treatment option for T2D with high glycemic-lowering efficacy, weight loss, and low risk of hypoglycemia. Some agents also lower major adverse CV outcomes and slow the progression of kidney disease. Clinicians should use a patient-centered approach when considering the utility, advantages, and disadvantages of a GLP-1 RA compared to other medication classes for the treatment of T2D. When selecting a specific GLP-1 RA within the class, the decision-making process should incorporate evidence on comparative efficacy (A1C, weight, CV and renal outcomes), safety (gastrointestinal adverse effects, injection site reactions), as well as other practical considerations such as self-administration requirements, ease of use, and cost.

MONOGRAPHS

Adlyxin: https://dailymed.nlm.nih.gov/dailymed/drugInfo.cfm?setid=1727cc16-4f86-4f13-b8b5-804d4984fa8c

Bydureon BCise: https://dailymed.nlm.nih.gov/dailymed/drugInfo.cfm?setid=2d18cfc4-e0de-4814-a712-c1b7c504bff5

Byetta: https://dailymed.nlm.nih.gov/dailymed/drugInfo.cfm?setid=53d03c03-ebf7-418d-88a8-533eabd2ee4f

Mounjaro: https://dailymed.nlm.nih.gov/dailymed/drugInfo.cfm?setid=d2d7da5d-ad07-4228-955f-cf7e355c8cc0

Ozempic: https://dailymed.nlm.nih.gov/dailymed/drugInfo.cfm?setid=adec4fd2-6858-4c99-91d4-531f5f2a2d79

Rybelsus: https://dailymed.nlm.nih.gov/dailymed/drugInfo.cfm?setid=27f15fac-7d98-4114-a2ec-92494a91da98

Soliqua: https://dailymed.nlm.nih.gov/dailymed/drugInfo.cfm?setid=4bba538b-cf7c-4310-ae8f-cb711ed21bcc

Trulicity: https://dailymed.nlm.nih.gov/dailymed/drugInfo.cfm?setid=463050bd-2b1c-40f5-b3c3-0a04bb433309

Victoza: https://dailymed.nlm.nih.gov/dailymed/drugInfo.cfm?setid=5a9ef4ea-c76a-4d34-a604-27c5b505f5a4

Xultophy: https://dailymed.nlm.nih.gov/dailymed/drugInfo.cfm?setid=21335fe4-d395-4501-ac2a-2f20d7520da9

REFERENCES

1. DeFronzo RA. From the triumvirate to the ominous octet: a new paradigm for the treatment of type 2 diabetes mellitus. *Diabetes* 2009;58:773–795

2. Mudaliar S, Henry RR. The incretin hormones: from scientific discovery to practical therapeutics. *Diabetologia* 2012;55:1865–1868

3. Drucker DJ, Nauck MA. The incretin system: glucagon-like peptide-1 receptor agonists and dipeptidyl peptidase-4 inhibitors in type 2 diabetes. *Lancet* 2006;368:1696–1705

4. Leiter LA, Nauck MA. Efficacy and safety of GLP-1 receptor agonists across the spectrum of type 2 diabetes mellitus. *Exp Clin Endocrinol Diabetes* 2017;125:419–435

5. Madsbad S. Review of head-to-head comparisons of glucagon-like peptide-1 receptor agonists. *Diabetes Obes Metab* 2016;18:317–332

6. ElSayed NA, Aleppo G, Aroda VR, et al., American Diabetes Association. 9. Pharmacologic Approaches to Glycemic Treatment: Standards of Care in Diabetes—2023. *Diabetes Care* 2023;46(Suppl. 1):S140–S157

7. Garber AJ, Handelsman Y, Grunberger G, et al. Consensus statement by the American Association of Clinical Endocrinologists and American College of Endocrinology on the comprehensive type 2 diabetes management algorithm. *Endocr Pract* 2020;26(1):107–139

8. ElSayed NA, Aleppo G, Aroda VR, et al., American Diabetes Association. 10. Cardiovascular disease and risk management: Standards of Care in Diabetes—2023. *Diabetes Care* 2023;46(Suppl. 1):S158–S190

9. Nauck M. Incretin therapies: highlighting common features and differences in the modes of action of glucagon-like peptide-1 receptor agonists and dipeptidyl peptidase-4 inhibitors. *Diabetes Obes Metab* 2016;18:203–216

10. DeFronzo RA, Eldor R, Abdul-Ghani M. Pathophysiologic approach to therapy in patients with newly diagnosed type 2 diabetes. *Diabetes Care* 2013;36(Suppl. 2):S127–S138

11. Nauck MA and Meier JJ. Are all GLP-1 agonists equal in the treatment of type 2 diabetes? *Eur J Endocrinol* 2019;181(6):R211–R234

12. Alicic RZ, Cox EJ, Neumiller JJ, Tuttle KR. Incretin drugs in diabetic kidney disease: biological mechanisms and clinical evidence. *Nat Rev Nephrol* 2021;17:227–244. DOI:10.1038/s41581-020-00367-2

13. Tall Bull S, Nuffer W, Trujillo JM. Tirzepatide: a novel, first-in-class, dual GIP/GLP-1 receptor agonist. *J Diabetes Complications* 2022;36(12):108332

14. Byetta (exenatide) injection [product information]. Wilmington, DE, AstraZeneca Pharmaceuticals LP, February 2015

15. Adlyxin (lixisenatide) injection [product information]. Bridgewater, NJ, Sanofi-aventis U.S. LLC, July 2017

16. Victoza (liraglutide) injection [product information]. Plainsboro, NJ, Novo Nordisk Inc., November 2020

17. Bydureon BCise (exenatide extended release) injectable suspension [product information]. Wilmington, DE, AstraZeneca Pharmaceuticals LP, December 2020

18. Trulicity (dulaglutide) injection [product information]. Indianapolis, IN, Eli Lilly and Company, September 2020

19. Ozempic (semaglutide) injection [product information]. Plainsboro, NJ, Novo Nordisk Inc., September 2020

20. Rybelsus (semaglutide) tablets [product information]. Plainsboro, NJ, Novo Nordisk Inc., January 2020

21. Mounjaro (tirzepatide) injection [product information]. Indianapolis, IN, Eli Lilly and Company, September 2022

22. Yoo BK, Triller DM, Yoo DJ. Exenatide: a new option for the treatment of type 2 diabetes. *Ann Pharmacother* 2006;40:1777–1784

23. Trujillo JM, Goldman J. Lixisenatide, a once-daily prandial glucagon-like peptide-1 receptor agonist for the treatment of adults with type 2 diabetes. *Pharmacotherapy* 2017;37(8):927–943

24. Trujillo JM, Nuffer W. GLP-1 receptor agonists for type 2 diabetes mellitus: recent developments and emerging agents. *Pharmacotherapy* 2014;34(11):1174–1186

25. Montanya E, Sesti G. A review of efficacy and safety data regarding the use of liraglutide, a once-daily human glucagon-like peptide 1 analogue, in the treatment of type 2 diabetes. *Clin Ther* 2009;31(11):2472–2488

26. Genovese S, Mannucci E, Ceriello A. A review of the long-term efficacy, tolerability, and safety of exenatide once weekly for type 2 diabetes. *Adv Ther* 2017;34:1791–1814

27. Thompson AM, Trujillo JM. Advances in the treatment of type 2 diabetes: impact of dulaglutide. *Diabetes Metab Syndr Obes* 2016;9:125–136

28. Frias JP, Bonora E, Ruiz LN, et al. Efficacy and safety of dulaglutide 3.0 mg and 4.5 mg versus dulaglutide 1.5 mg in metformin-treated patients with type 2 diabetes in a randomized controlled trial (AWARD-11). *Diabetes Care* 2021;44(3):765–773

29. Tuchscherer RM, Thompson AM, Trujillo JM. Semaglutide: the newest once-weekly GLP-1 RA for type 2 diabetes. *Ann Pharmacother* 2018;52(12):1224–1232

30. Anderson SL, Beutel TR, Trujillo JM. Oral semaglutide in type 2 diabetes. *J Diabetes Complications* 2020;34(4):107520. Published online 2020 Jan 8 DOI:10.1016/j.jdiacomp.2019.107520

31. Nauck MA, D-Alessio DA. Tirzepatide, a dual GIP-GLP-1 receptor co-agonist for the treatment of type 2 diabetes with unmatched effectiveness regrading glycemic control and body weight reduction. *Cardiovasc Diabetol* 2022;21:169

32. Tran S, Retnakaran R, Zinman B, Kramer CK. Efficacy of glucagon-like peptide-1 receptor agonists compared to dipeptidyl peptidase-4 inhibitors for the management of type 2 diabetes: a meta-analysis of randomized clinical trials. *Diabetes Obes Metab* 2018;20(Suppl. 1):68–76

33. Tran KL, Park YI, Pandya S, et al. Overview of glucagon-like peptide-1 receptor agonists for the treatment of patients with type 2 diabetes. *Am Health Drug Benefits* 2017;10(4):178–188

34. Prasad-Reddy L, Isaacs D. A clinical review of GLP-1 receptor agonists: efficacy and safety in diabetes and beyond. *Drugs Context* 2015;4:212283. DOI:10.7573/dic.212283

35. Trujillo JM, Nuffer W, Ellis SL. GLP-1 receptor agonists: a review of head-to-head clinical studies. *Ther Adv Endocrinol Metab* 2015;6:19–28

36. Trujillo JM, Nuffer W, Smith BA. GLP-1 receptor agonists: an updated review of head-to-head clinical studies. *Ther Adv Endocrinol Metab* 2021;Mar 9:12:2042018821997320

37. Marso SP, Daniels GH, Brown-Frandsen K, et al. Liraglutide and cardiovascular outcomes in type 2 diabetes. *N Engl J Med* 2016;375:311–322

38. Marso SP, Bain SC, Consoli A, et al. Semaglutide and cardiovascular outcomes in patients with type 2 diabetes. *N Engl J Med* 2016;375:1834–1844

39. Gerstein HC, Colhoun HM, Dagenais GR, et al.; REWIND Investigators. Dulaglutide and cardiovascular outcomes in type 2 diabetes (REWIND): a double-blind, randomized placebo-controlled trial. *Lancet* 2019;394: 121–130

40. Blonde L, Umpierrez GE, Reddy SS, et al. American Association of Clinical Endocrinology Clinical Practice Guideline: Developing a Diabetes Mellitus Comprehensive Care Plan - 2022 update. *Endocr Pract* 2022;28:923–1049

41. Anderson SL, Trujillo JM. Basal insulin use with GLP-1 receptor agonists. *Diabetes Spectr* 2016;29(3):152–160

42. Xultophy 100/3.6 (insulin degludec and liraglutide) injection [product information]. Plainsboro, NJ, Novo Nordisk Inc., November 2016

43. Soliqua 100/33 (insulin glargine and lixisenatide) injection [product information]. Bridgewater, NJ, Sanofi-aventis U.S. LLC, October 2017

44. Goldman J, Trujillo JM. iGlarLixi: a fixed-ratio combination of insulin glargine 100 U/mL and lixisenatide for the treatment of type 2 diabetes. *Ann Pharmacother* 2017;51(11):990–999

45. Gough SCL, Jain R, Woo VC. Insulin degludec/liraglutide (iDegLira) for the treatment of type 2 diabetes. *Expert Rev Endocrinol Metab* 2016; 11(1):7–18

46. Nuffer W, Guesnier A, Trujillo JM. A review of the new GLP-1 receptor agonist/basal insulin fixed-ratio combination products. *Ther Adv Endocrinol Metab* 2018;9(3):69–79

47. Trujillo JM, Roberts M, Dex T, et al. Low incidence of gastrointestinal adverse events over time with a fixed-ratio combination of insulin glargine and lixisenatide versus lixisenatide alone. *Diabetes Obes Metab* 2018;20(11):2690–2694

48. Storgaard H, Cold F, Gluud LL, et al. Glucagon-like peptide-1 receptor agonists and risk of acute pancreatitis in patients with type 2 diabetes. *Diabetes Obes Metab* 2017;19:906–908

49. Monami M, Nreu B, Scatena A, et al. Safety issues with glucagon-like peptide-1 receptor agonists (pancreatitis, pancreatic cancer and cholelithiasis): data from randomized controlled trials. *Diabetes Obes Metab* 2017; 19:1233–1241

50. FDA Drug Safety Communication: FDA investigating reports of possible increased risk of pancreatitis and pre-cancerous findings of the pancreas from incretin mimetic drugs for type 2 diabetes. Available from https://www.fda.gov/Drugs/DrugSafety/ucm343187.htm. Accessed 29 March 2020

51. Yoshida Y, Joshi P, Barri S, et al. Progression of retinopathy with glucagon-like peptide-1 receptor agonists with cardiovascular benefits in type 2 diabetes - A systematic review and meta-analysis. *J Diabetes Complications* 2022;36(8):108255

52. Bethel MA, Diaz R, Castellana N, et al. HbA(1c) change and diabetic retinopathy during GLP-1 receptor agonist cardiovascular outcome trials: Ameta-analysis and meta-regression. *Diabetes Care* 2021;44(1):290-96

53. Wang W, Liu H, Xiao S, et al. Effects of insulin plus glucagon-like peptide-1 receptor agonists (GLP-1RAs) in treating type 1 diabetes mellitus: a systematic review and meta-analysis. *Diabetes Ther* 2017;8(4):727–738

54. Tamborlane WV, Barrientos-Perez M, Fainburg U, et al.; Ellipse Trial Investigators. Liraglutide in children and adolescents with type 2 diabetes. *New Engl J Med* 2019;381(7):637-646

55. ElSayed NA, Aleppo G, Aroda VR, et al., American Diabetes Association. 14. Children and adolescents: Standards of Care in Diabetes—2023. *Diabetes Care* 2023;46(Suppl. 1):S230–S253

56. Eng C, Kramer CK, Zinman B, Retnakaran R. Glucagon-like peptide-1 receptor agonist and basal insulin combination treatment for the management of type 2 diabetes: a systematic review and meta-analysis. *Lancet* 2014;384(9961):2228–2234

57. Jones SC, Ryan DL, Pratt VSW, et al. Injection site nodules associated with the use of exenatide extended-release reports to the U.S. Food and Drug Administration adverse event reporting system. *Diabetes Spectr* 2015;28(4):283–288

58. Sun F, Wu S, Guo S, et al. Impact of GLP-1 receptor agonists on blood pressure, heart rate, and hypertension among patients with type 2 diabetes: a systematic review and network meta-analysis. *Diabetes Res Clin Pract* 2015;110:26–37

59. He L, Wang J, Ping F, et al. Association of glucagon-like peptide-1 receptor agonist use with risk of gallbladder and biliary diseases: A systematic review and meta-analysis of randomized clinical trials. *JAMA Intern Med* 2022;182(5):513–519

60. Spain CV, Wright JJ, Hahn RM, et al. Self-reported barriers to adherence and persistence to treatment with injectable medications for type 2 diabetes. *Clin Ther* 2016;38(7):1653–1664

61. Alatorre C, Fernández Landó L, Yu M, et al. Treatment patterns in patients with type 2 diabetes mellitus treated with glucagon-like peptide-1 receptor agonists: higher adherence and persistence with dulaglutide compared with once-weekly exenatide and liraglutide. *Diabetes Obes Metab* 2017; 19:953–961

62. Nguyen H, Dufour R, Caldwell-Tarr A. Glucagon-like peptide-1 receptor agonist (GLP-1RA) therapy adherence for patients with type 2 diabetes in a Medicare population. *Adv Ther* 2017;34(3):658–673

63. Qiao Q, Ouwens MJ, Grandy S, et al. Adherence to GLP-1 receptor agonist therapy administered by once-daily or once-weekly injection in patients with type 2 diabetes in Germany. *Diabetes Metab Syndr Obes* 2016;9:201–205

Chapter 14
Pramlintide

Jennifer M. Trujillo, PharmD, BCPS, FCCP, CDCES, BC-ADM

INTRODUCTION

Pramlintide is an amylin analog and is the only approved medication in this class. Amylin is a 37-amino acid peptide neurohormone that is co-secreted with insulin from pancreatic β-cells. Amylin plasma levels, similar to insulin, are lower during the fasting state and rise in response to calorie intake. Amylin works in concert with insulin and glucagon to maintain glucose homeostasis by blunting inappropriate glucagon secretion after meals, slowing gastric emptying, and increasing satiety via a centrally mediated mechanism.[1,2]

Amylin secretion is significantly altered in both T1D and T2D. In normal healthy adults, amylin levels rise after calorie intake and return to baseline by 2 h. In patients with T1D, the amylin rise after calorie intake is absent, similar to insulin, due to the destruction of the pancreatic β-cells.[3] Similar to the insulin response in T2D, amylin levels could be increased, normal, or reduced in patients with T2D, depending on the level of β-cell function. In patients with impaired glucose tolerance, amylin increases after calorie intake and remains above baseline 2 h later. Patients with T2D who require insulin therapy have a diminished amylin response to calorie intake.[2]

Amylin can play an additional role in the pathophysiology of T2D when the native type aggregates to form amyloid fibrils in the pancreas. These amylin deposits are thought to be cytotoxic and may contribute to pancreatic β-cell death in T2D.[2]

Amylin is insoluble and viscous and tends to aggregate; thus, it is not viable as an injectable medication. Pramlintide is a synthetic analog of amylin, differing from amylin by three amino acids. It was approved by the FDA in 2005 and is indicated for patients with T1D or T2D who use mealtime insulin and have failed to achieve desired glycemic control despite optimal insulin therapy.[4] Pramlintide was the first noninsulin agent approved for patients with T1D. Pramlintide is effective at lowering PPG levels and A1C and can be an attractive option for some patients, as it can also decrease weight and may allow for lower mealtime insulin doses. It is administered by subcutaneous injection immediately before meals.

MECHANISM OF ACTION

Pramlintide mimics the action of amylin and regulates glucose by three key mechanisms: reducing glucagon secretion, slowing gastric emptying, and increasing satiety.

In normal glucose homeostasis, glucagon is secreted from pancreatic α-cells to signal the liver to stimulate glycogenolysis and gluconeogenesis to ultimately increase glucose output from the liver. This counter-regulatory hormone response is to maintain normal glucose levels during fasting conditions or times of high energy consumption. In patients with diabetes, glucagon secretion occurs inappropriately after meals, ultimately leading to excessive hepatic glucose output postprandially. Pramlintide reduces the release of glucagon from the pancreas, and thus decreases this postprandial hepatic glucose output. Importantly, pramlintide does not appear to blunt the counter-regulatory glucagon response to hypoglycemia.[1,2]

Pramlintide signals the stomach to slow gastric emptying, which allows for more gradual absorption of glucose from the small intestine into the circulation and thereby reduces postprandial spikes in blood glucose levels. Slowing gastric emptying may also lead to a quicker feeling of fullness, which could decrease calorie intake and ultimately promote weight loss.[1,2]

Pramlintide also increases satiety by stimulating the satiety center of the brain. This effect may decrease PPG levels by decreasing the amount of carbohydrates and calories consumed in the meal. This reduction may ultimately promote weight loss, which may further improve glucose control.[1,2]

PHARMACOKINETICS

The bioavailability of pramlintide after a single subcutaneous injection is 30–40%. There is a linear dose-dependent increase in the maximum plasma concentration and overall exposure (AUC) of pramlintide after subcutaneous administration into the abdomen or thigh (Table 14.1).[4] In healthy individuals, the plasma half-life of pramlintide is approximately 48 min and maximum concentration occurs about 20 min after injection. Overall exposure to pramlintide is relatively constant with repeat dosing, indicating no accumulation.[4]

Injection into the arm in obese patients with T1D or T2D showed higher exposure and greater variability compared to injection into the abdomen or thigh. Bioavailability was not significantly different between obese and nonobese patients and was not impacted by skin thickness or injection needle size.[4]

The advantages of pramlintide in the treatment of diabetes include modest reductions in A1C and PPG levels in patients not able to achieve glucose control with insulin alone. In addition, pramlintide may allow for lower doses of insulin and has

Table 14.1—Pharmacokinetics of Pramlintide Following a Single Subcutaneous Dose (Product Information)

Dose (µg)	AUC (pmol*min/L)	C_{max} (pmol/L)	T_{max} (min)	Half-life (min)
30	3,750	39	21	55
60	6,778	79	20	49
90	8,507	102	19	51
120	11,970	147	21	48

more favorable effects on weight compared to continued insulin titration. Pramlintide may also result in less glucose variability.

The efficacy and safety of pramlintide in patients with T1D was evaluated in three large, randomized controlled trials (Table 14.2).[5-7] Reductions in A1C were significantly better in patients taking pramlintide compared to placebo, and mean body weight was decreased in patients taking pramlintide compared to placebo. These improvements were not accompanied by increased rates of severe hypoglycemia. However, in the study conducted by Whitehouse et al., the A1C lowering was more significant earlier in the study and waned over the 52 weeks. Changes in A1C from baseline with pramlintide versus placebo were –0.67% versus –0.16% at week 13, –0.58% versus –0.18% at week 26, and –0.39% versus –0.12% at week 52. The open-label extension of that study showed that patients who continued pramlintide maintained reductions in A1C from week 52 to week 104.[5] Similarly, in the study conducted by Ratner et al., the A1C lowering was most pronounced in the earlier weeks of the study and waned at the end of the study.[6] The study conducted by Edelman et al. specifically investigated whether increasing the pramlintide dose progressively with concomitant reduction in mealtime insulin would increase tolerability and reduce the risk of severe hypoglycemia. Both the pramlintide and placebo groups achieved similar A1C reductions and low rates of severe hypoglycemia, but pramlintide led to reductions in PPG and weight beyond that seen with insulin alone. The authors concluded that pramlintide dose escalation with simultaneous reduced mealtime insulin was effective during therapy initiation in T1D compared to placebo.[7]

Smaller studies have also demonstrated reductions in PPG in patients taking pramlintide.[8,9] Weyer et al. showed reductions in postprandial excursions by more than 100% versus placebo in patients taking regular insulin and by 75% versus placebo in patients taking insulin lispro. The optimal time of administration was immediately with the meal.[8] Hinshaw et al. also demonstrated significant reductions in PPG levels in patients with T1D and determined this effect was due to inhibition of glucagon and gastric emptying.[9]

In a post hoc analysis of the clinical studies in T1D, pramlintide was found to be safe and effective in patients specifically on insulin pump therapy. Pramlintide improved glycemic control while significantly reducing the patient's daily insulin dose and body weight. Thus, pramlintide can be a treatment option in patients on insulin pump therapy who are not achieving optimal glycemic control with insulin alone. Similar to patients on multiple daily injections, pramlintide would be an

Table 14.2—Efficacy and Safety of Pramlintide in Patients with T1D and T2D

Study	Patients and study duration	Treatment arms	A1C, change from baseline (%)	Weight, change from baseline (kg)	Insulin TDD, change from baseline (%)	Severe hypoglycemia (%)	Nausea (%)
T1D (added to premeal insulin)							
Whitehouse F, et al.	n = 480 52 weeks	30–60 µg t.i.d. Placebo	-0.39 -0.12	+0.5 +1.0	+2.3 +10.3	2.12, 0.74, 0.43* 2, 1.37, 1.24*	46.5 21.9
Ratner RE, et al.	n = 479 52 weeks	60 µg t.i.d. 60 µg q.i.d. Placebo	-0.29 -0.34 -0.04	-0.4 -0.4 +0.7	-3.0 -6.0 ±0.0	3.78, 1.13, 0.74* 3.41, 0.98, 0.79* 0.87, 0.80, 0.45*	47 47 12
Edelman S, et al.	n = 296 29 weeks	60 µg t.i.d. Placebo	-0.5 -0.5	-1.3 +1.2	-28.0 +4.0	0.57 0.30	63 36
T2D (added to premeal insulin)							
Ratner RE, et al.	n = 538 52 weeks	30 µg t.i.d. 75 µg t.i.d. 150 µg t.i.d. Placebo	-0.3 -0.5 -0.6 -0.2	-0.3 -0.4 -1.2 +1.0	+10.9 +7.9 NR +15.4	1.5 4.1 2.2 2.8	16.9 14.8 26.5 22.9
Hollander PA, et al.	n = 498 52 weeks	90 µg b.i.d. 120 µg b.i.d. Placebo	-0.35 -0.62 -0.22	-0.5 -1.4 +0.7	2.9 1.4 2.7	0.1 0.3 0.3	31 30 14
T2D (added to basal insulin)							
Riddle M, et al. 2007	n = 212 16 weeks	60–120 µg b.i.d./t.i.d. Placebo	-0.7 -0.36	-1.6 +0.7	+11.7 units +13.1 units	1 event 0	31 10
Riddle M, et al. 2009	n = 113 24 weeks	120 µg t.i.d. RAIA	-1.1 -1.3	+0.0 +4.7	+28 units +67 units	0 0	21 0

RAIA, rapid-acting insulin analog; TDD, total daily dose. * Reported for weeks 0–4, weeks 4–26, weeks 26–52, respectively.

appealing option for patients on insulin pump therapy with continued difficulty controlling PPG levels or body weight.[10]

Another post hoc analysis of clinical studies in T1D demonstrated that pramlintide was effective at lowering A1C regardless of diabetes duration at baseline. Longer disease duration appeared to augment the insulin sparing and weight loss seen with pramlintide. Therefore, pramlintide could be a therapeutic option at any point in the disease.[11]

The efficacy and safety of pramlintide in patients with T2D was evaluated in four large randomized controlled trials (Table 14.2).[12–15] Two of these studies evaluated pramlintide versus placebo in addition to background insulin therapy, which usually included mealtime insulin.[12,13] Both studies found that pramlintide in conjunction with insulin resulted in significant reductions in A1C that were sustained throughout the study. The improvements were achieved without increases in insulin dose or additional hypoglycemia risk. Modest weight loss was also achieved.[12,13] The other two studies evaluated pramlintide versus rapid-acting insulin added to basal insulin.[14,15] In this setting, pramlintide resulted in less hypoglycemia and lower total daily doses of insulin compared to the rapid-acting insulin group.[14,15] Despite these results, pramlintide does not have a specific FDA indication for use with basal insulin alone.

Disadvantages of pramlintide include the potential risk of hypoglycemia when added to insulin therapy and the need for insulin dose adjustments, close glucose monitoring, subsequent dose titrations, and routine follow-up to ensure the safety and efficacy of this combination. Other disadvantages include the subcutaneous injection requirement, increased total number of daily injections, inconvenience, nausea, and cost. Although pramlintide use requires up to three additional daily injections, in one study, pramlintide-treated patients reported greater treatment satisfaction than did patients in the placebo group despite similar reductions in A1C. This suggests that reductions in insulin dose and weight may be more meaningful to many patients than number of injections per day or overall A1C reductions.[16]

Another disadvantage is that the overall efficacy of pramlintide is small with mild reductions in PPG, A1C, and weight, which may not persist. Current treatment guidelines also do not classify pramlintide as a preferred agent for T2D because of its lower effectiveness compared to other agents, the limited clinical evidence, the benefit/risk ratio, and the cost.[17,18]

THERAPEUTIC CONSIDERATIONS

SIGNIFICANT WARNINGS/PRECAUTIONS

The prescribing information for pramlintide includes a black box warning for severe hypoglycemia. Pramlintide itself has a low risk of hypoglycemia. However, pramlintide is only indicated for use in conjunction with insulin, and this combination has been associated with an increased risk of hypoglycemia, particularly in patients with T1D. Hypoglycemia usually occurs within the first 2–3 h following injection. The manufacturer suggests that the hypoglycemia risk can be reduced by appropriate patient selection, patient education, frequent blood glucose monitoring, and an initial insulin dose reduction. The prescribing information recommends an initial insulin dose reduction of 50% when pramlintide is initiated.[4]

Pramlintide slows gastric emptying; therefore, it is contraindicated in patients who have confirmed gastroparesis. Pramlintide is also contraindicated in patients who have had a prior serious hypersensitivity reaction to pramlintide. The prescribing information also warns against mixing pramlintide with insulin due to the potential for altered pharmacokinetics and warns against the potential for drug interactions due to slowed gastric motility. Both of these are discussed in more detail in the "Drug Interactions" section.[4]

Appropriate patient selection is important to ensure the efficacy and safety of pramlintide. Before initiating pramlintide, the patient's A1C, glucose monitoring data, hypoglycemia history, current insulin regimen, and body weight should be reviewed. Pramlintide should be considered only in patients with T1D or T2D who are using mealtime insulin and have failed to achieve glycemic control despite individualized insulin management and are receiving consistent, ongoing diabetes care by a healthcare provider skilled in insulin management and supported by a diabetes educator. Pramlintide should not be used in the following patients:[2,4]

- Poor compliance with insulin regimen.
- Poor compliance with SMBG.
- A1C >9%.
- Recurrent severe hypoglycemia requiring assistance within the past 6 months.
- Hypoglycemia unawareness.
- Confirmed diagnosis of gastroparesis.
- Requiring the use of drugs that stimulate gastric motility.
- Pediatric patients.

SPECIAL POPULATIONS

Pregnancy and Lactation

Pramlintide is a pregnancy category C medication. Studies in pregnancy have not been conducted. Pramlintide has a low potential to cross the maternal/fetal placental barrier. Embryofetal studies in rats and rabbits show increases in congenital abnormalities (neural tube defect, cleft palate, exencephaly) with 10 and 47 times the exposure resulting from the human dose of 360 µg/day. Doses up to nine times the human dose of 360 µg/day given to pregnant rabbits had no effect on embryofetal development.[4]

It is unknown whether pramlintide is excreted in human milk, but there is a high likelihood that it is, based on its structure. Pramlintide should only be used in women who are breast-feeding if it is determined that the benefit outweighs the potential risk to the infant.[4]

Pediatrics

Pramlintide has shown promise in a few small studies in children and adolescents with T1D. PPG levels improved, and pramlintide demonstrated reasonable tolerability in these studies.[19,20] However, the safety and efficacy of pramlintide have not been established in large-scale, long-term studies in this patient population. Thus, pramlintide is not currently recommended in pediatric patients.

Geriatrics

Pramlintide has been studied in patients up to age 85 years. No consistent differences in efficacy and safety were observed in older patients. However, older patients may be more susceptible to hypoglycemia; therefore, caution should still be taken when using pramlintide in this population.[4] It may be appropriate to start with a lower dose and titrate the dose more slowly than for a younger adult. Because pramlintide is administered subcutaneously using an injection pen device, the clinician should ensure that the patient has adequate vision and dexterity to allow for correct self-administration.

Renal Insufficiency

Dose adjustments are not needed in patients with mild (CrCl 60–89 mL/min), moderate (CrCl 30–59 mL/min), or severe (CrCl 15–29 mL/min) renal insufficiency. Pramlintide has not been studied in patients with ESRD.[4]

Hepatic Insufficiency

Studies have not been conducted in patients with hepatic impairment. No changes would be expected, however, since pramlintide is almost exclusively eliminated through the kidneys.[4]

Sex, Race, Ethnicity

No consistent differences in efficacy and safety were observed between men and women in initial pramlintide clinical studies. Similarly, no consistent differences were observed among differing races or ethnicities included in the studies (Caucasian, black, Hispanic, and Asian populations), though smaller sample sizes for non-Caucasian subjects may limit this conclusion.[4]

ADVERSE EFFECTS AND MONITORING

Hypoglycemia

Although hypoglycemia is a concern with pramlintide used in conjunction with insulin, the rates of severe hypoglycemia in clinical studies are low (Table 14.2).

As discussed in the "Significant Warnings/Precautions" section, to minimize the risk of hypoglycemia, patients should be screened carefully to determine if pramlintide is appropriate. Patients must be willing and able to self-monitor their blood glucose, recognize signs and symptoms of hypoglycemia and adhere to patient instructions. The mealtime insulin dose should be reduced by 50% when initiating pramlintide. The dose can be titrated up if needed after a stable dose of pramlintide is reached. Patients should SMBG frequently and should be educated on the prevention, detection, and treatment of hypoglycemia.

Gastrointestinal Effects

The most common adverse effects of pramlintide in clinical trials were gastrointestinal in nature and included nausea, anorexia, vomiting, and abdominal pain. Nausea occurred in 14.8–63% of patients taking pramlintide compared to 10–36% of patients taking placebo (Table 14.2).[5–7,12–15] Nausea can be minimized by initiating pramlintide at a low dose and titrating the dose gradually. If nausea is a significant concern, pramlintide can be initiated with just one meal of the day and increased from there. Administering the first dose before the evening meal may allow patients to evaluate how well they tolerate pramlintide and better manage symptoms of nausea while they are at home.[21]

Injection Site Reactions

Injection site reactions have been reported by patients taking pramlintide. Patients should use proper technique when administering pramlintide and should rotate injection sites.[4]

Cardiovascular Safety

The cardiovascular safety of pramlintide was evaluated in a post hoc analysis of five randomized, controlled phase 3 and 4 trials. The incidence of major adverse cardiovascular outcomes was similar between pramlintide and comparator arms (4.7% vs. 4.5%; RR 1.034 [95% CI 0.694–1.540]). The authors concluded that pramlintide conferred no increased risk of cardiovascular adverse events in patients with diabetes using insulin.[22]

DRUG INTERACTIONS

Because the pH of pramlintide is 4.0 and the pH of most insulin products is 7.8, it is assumed that pramlintide is not compatible with insulin. However, studies evaluating the pharmacokinetic effects of mixing pramlintide with different insulins (regular, NPH, 70/30 premixed, and recombinant human) have produced variable results, with decreases up to 40% in maximum concentrations of pramlintide, increases up to 36% in pramlintide AUC, increases up to 15% in maximum concentrations of insulin, and increases up to 20% in insulin AUC. One randomized, controlled study in 51 patients with T1D did show that mixing pramlintide in the same syringe with regular insulin did not affect the pharmacokinetics or efficacy of either the insulin or pramlintide. Ultimately, mixing pramlintide and insulin in the same syringe is not recommended.[4,23]

Since pramlintide slows gastric emptying, it has the potential to impact the absorption of other medications administered concomitantly. Caution should be taken when oral medications are given concomitantly with pramlintide, particularly when a slower rate of absorption could be clinically meaningful. Other oral medications should be administered at least 1 h before or 2 h after administration of pramlintide, particularly if the onset of effect or threshold concentration is critical. Pramlintide may also impair the efficacy of agents that stimulate gastric motility.[4]

Table 14.3 — Availability, Dosing, and Administration Requirements of Pramlintide

Availability, storage, preparation	Dosing	Missed-dose recommendations	Use in renal impairment
■ Multi-dose pen (1,000 µg/mL, 1.5 mL for 15-µg, 30-µg, 45-µg, and 60-µg doses or 1,000 µg/mL, 2.7 mL for 60-µg and 120-µg doses) ■ Pen needles not supplied ■ Keep refrigerated ■ After first use, store in refrigerator or at room temperature; bring to room temperature before injecting; discard 30 days after first use ■ No reconstitution needed	■ T1D: Start with 15 µg before major meals; increase in 15-µg increments to a maximum of 30–60 µg before major meals ■ T2D: Start with 60 µg before major meals; increase to 120 µg before meals, as tolerated ■ Upon initiation, reduce mealtime insulin by 50%; monitor glucose frequently and adjust insulin do,ses as needed ■ Wait at least 3 days between dose titrations to minimize nausea ■ Do not inject if you have hypoglycemia, do not plan to eat, plan to eat less than 250 calories or 30 g carbohydrates, or are sick and cannot eat usual meal	■ Skip the dose and resume next dose at the prescribed time	■ No dose adjustment recommended; has not been studied in patients with ESRD (CrCl <15 mL/min)

DOSAGE AND ADMINISTRATION

A summary of the dosage and administration recommendations for pramlintide are in Table 14.3. Different doses are recommended for T1D and T2D. However, in both groups, the dose of mealtime insulin should be initially reduced by 50% when pramlintide is initiated to avoid hypoglycemia. The dose of basal insulin does not usually need to be adjusted. The pramlintide dose is then titrated over time based on efficacy and tolerability. Once the maintenance dose of pramlintide is reached, mealtime insulin dose adjustments can be made according to standard clinical practice based on glucose profile data.[2,4]

The recommended starting dose for patients with T1D is 15 µg given with each major meal (at least 250 calories or 30 g carbohydrates). If the patient is tolerating the medication without significant nausea after 3–7 days, the dose can be increased by 15-µg increments to a maximum dose of 30–60 µg before major meals. For patients with T2D, the recommended starting dose is 60 µg before major meals. This can be increased to 120 µg as tolerated after 3–7 days. If a meal has fewer than 250 calories or 30 g carbohydrates, or if the patient does not plan to eat or has hypoglycemia, then the pramlintide dose should be skipped. The dose of pramlintide should be taken immediately prior to major meals.[4]

Pramlintide is available in two different pen devices: one with a maximum dose of 60 µg, primarily indicated for T1D, and one with a maximum dose of 120 µg, primarily indicated for T2D. Pramlintide should be injected into either the abdomen or the thigh. It is not recommended for injection into the arm due to inconsistent absorption from that site. Pramlintide and insulin should not be injected into the same site. Patients should be instructed to inject pramlintide into a site at least 2 inches away from the site of insulin injection. The pen device that is actively being used can be stored at room temperature or in the refrigerator for up to 30 days. If stored in the refrigerator, it should be brought up to room temperature before injecting. Additional pens should be stored in the refrigerator.[4]

MONOGRAPHS

Pramlintide: https://dailymed.nlm.nih.gov/dailymed/drugInfo.cfm?setid= 4aea30ff-eb0d-45c1-b114-3127966328ff

REFERENCES

1. Ryan GJ, Jobe LJ, Martin R. Pramlintide in the treatment of type 1 and type 2 diabetes mellitus. *Clin Ther* 2005;27(10):1500–1512

2. Hieronymus L, Griffin S. Role of amylin in type 1 and type 2 diabetes. *Diabetes Educ* 2015;41(Suppl. 1):47S–56S

3. Koda JE, Fineman M, Rink TJ, et al. Amylin concentrations and glucose control. *Lancet* 1992;339:1179–1180

4. Symlin (pramlintide acetate injection) [product information]. Wilmington, DE, AstraZeneca Pharmaceuticals LP, June 2014

5. Whitehouse F, Kruger DF, Fineman M, et al. A randomized study and open-label extension evaluating the long-term efficacy of pramlintide as an adjunct to insulin therapy in type 1 diabetes. *Diabetes Care* 2002;25:724–730

6. Ratner RE, Dickey R, Fineman M, et al. Amylin replacement with pramlintide as an adjunct to insulin therapy improves long-term glycemic and weight control in type 1 diabetes mellitus: a 1-year, randomized controlled trial. *Diabet Med* 2004;21:1204–1212

7. Edelman S, Garg S, Frias J, et al. A double-blind, placebo-controlled trial assessing pramlintide treatment in the setting of intensive insulin therapy in type 1 diabetes. *Diabetes Care* 2006;29:2189–2195

8. Weyer C, Gottlieb A, Kim DD, et al. Pramlintide reduces postprandial glucose excursions when added to regular insulin or insulin lispro in subjects with type 1 diabetes: a dose-timing study. *Diabetes Care* 2003;26:3074–3079

9. Hinshaw L, Schiavon M, Dadlani V, et al. Effect of pramlintide on postprandial glucose fluxes in type 1 diabetes. *J Clin Endocrinol Metab* 2016;101(5):1954–1962

10. Herrmann K, Frias JP, Edelman SV, et al. Pramlintide improved measures of glycemic control and body weight in patients with type 1 diabetes mellitus undergoing continuous subcutaneous insulin infusion therapy. *Postgrad Med* 2013;125(3):136–144

11. Herrmann K, Brunell SC, Li Y, et al. Impact of disease duration on the effects of pramlintide in type 1 diabetes: a post hoc analysis of three clinical trials. *Adv Ther* 2016;33:848–861

12. Ratner RE, Want LL, Fineman MS, et al. Adjunctive therapy with the amylin analogue pramlintide leads to a combined improvement in glycemic and weight control in insulin-treated subjects with type 2 diabetes. *Diabetes Technol Ther* 2002;4:51–61

13. Hollander PA, Levy P, Fineman MS, et al. Pramlintide as an adjunct to insulin therapy improves long-term glycemic and weight control in patients with type 2 diabetes: a 1-year randomized controlled trial. *Diabetes Care* 2003;26:784–790

14. Riddle M, Frias J, Zhang B, et al. Pramlintide improved glycemic control and reduced weight in patients with type 2 diabetes using basal insulin. *Diabetes Care* 2007;30:2794–2799

15. Riddle M, Pencek R, Charenkavanich S, et al. Randomized comparison of pramlintide or mealtime insulin added to basal insulin treatment for patients with type 2 diabetes. *Diabetes Care* 2009;32:1577–1582

16. Marrero DG, Crean J, Zhang B, et al. Effect of adjunctive pramlintide treatment on treatment satisfaction in patients with type 1 diabetes. *Diabetes Care* 2007;30(2):210–216

17. American Diabetes Association. 9. Pharmacologic approaches to glycemic treatment: Standards of Medical Care in Diabetes—2022. *Diabetes Care* 2022;45(Suppl. 1):S125–S143

18. Garber AJ, Handelsman Y, Grunberger G, et al. Consensus statement by the American Association of Clinical Endocrinologists and American College of Endocrinology on the comprehensive type 2 diabetes management algorithm—2020 executive summary. *Endocr Pract* 2020;26(1):107–139

19. Chase HP, Lutz K, Pencek R, et al. Pramlintide lowered glucose excursions and was well-tolerated in adolescents with type 1 diabetes: results from a randomized, single-blind, placebo-controlled, crossover study. *J Pediatr* 2009;155:369–373

20. Hassan K, Heptulla RA. Reducing postprandial hyperglycemia with adjuvant premeal pramlintide and postmeal insulin in children with type 1 diabetes mellitus. *Pediatr Diabetes* 2009;10:264–268

21. Alrefai HA, Latif KA, Hieronymus LB, et al. Pramlintide: clinical strategies for succzess. *Diabetes Spectr* 2010;23:124–130

22. Herrmann K, Zhou M, Wang A, de Bruin TWA. Cardiovascular safety assessment of pramlintide in type 2 diabetes: results from a pooled analysis of five clinical trials. *Clin Diabetes Endocrinol* 2016;2(12):1–8

23. Weyer C, Fineman M, Strobel S, et al. Properties of pramlintide and insulin upon mixing. *Am J Health Syst Pharm* 2005;62:816–822

Chapter 15
Bile Acid Sequestrants

CHRISTINA R. BUCHMAN, PHARMD, BCACP

INTRODUCTION

B ile acid sequestrants (BAS), also known as bile acid resins, were initially approved in 1973 to treat hyperlipidemia—more specifically, to reduce LDL-C levels.[1] BAS are most frequently used in combination with statins for hyperlipidemia (although their use is declining) and have been associated with modest decreases in A1C in patients with T2D as monotherapy or in combination with other antidiabetic agents.[2-4] There are three FDA-approved BAS in use in the U.S.[1] Of these, the first-generation agents include cholestyramine and colestipol, while the only second-generation agent is colesevelam.[1] There is another second-generation BAS, colestimide, that is available only in Japan and has a similar safety and efficacy profile to colesevelam.[4] Colesevelam is the only BAS that has received FDA approval to treat T2D, but is not indicated for T1D.[1] Although colesevelam is the only FDA-approved agent for patients with T2D, all agents in the class have been shown in studies to decrease FPG and A1C.[5] BAS decreased A1C by 0.5–1% in clinical studies and can be used safely in conjunction with other antidiabetic agents.[4,6] In patients with elevated LDL-C who have not been able to reach target A1C levels, adding a BAS may be a valuable option in helping patients reach their goals and possibly in reducing micro- and macrovascular complications of T2D and hypercholesterolemia.

PHARMACOLOGY

The studies that showed treatment with BAS reduced LDL and cardiovascular risk also showed a reduction in FPG and A1C in patients with T2D.[4,5] This improvement led to further studies in patients with T2D and the eventual FDA approval of colesevelam to treat T2D. Studies have demonstrated an average decrease in A1C of 0.5% with a range of 0.4–1%, depending on the agent taken.[4,5] Among the BAS that are approved in the U.S., colesevelam produces the most marked decrease in FPG and A1C due to its higher affinity for binding bile acids.[5]

MECHANISM OF ACTION

BAS are highly polarized large molecules that tightly bind bile acids to form a nonabsorbable complex that is then excreted in the feces.[7-10] As a response to the increased excretion of bile acids, the body compensates by increasing the synthesis of new bile acids and consumption of LDL-C. The exact mechanism of lowering blood glucose is not completely understood, but it is thought to be multifactorial and surprisingly complex.[7-10]

Historically, it has been hypothesized that BAS administration decreases glucose and carbohydrate absorption, but this proposed mechanism has since been disproven in several studies.[9] Instead of this classical model of blocked absorption, current evidence suggests a much more complex, hormone-related mechanism that involves multiple receptors and organs.[9]

Bile acids are known to be independent signaling molecules that activate farnesoid X receptors (FXR) and a transmembrane G-protein coupled receptor (TGR5).[7-10] FXR is located in the gastrointestinal tract and liver and is involved in the feedback loop of bile acid synthesis. When bile acids interact with FXR, they act as the "brakes" by inhibiting further synthesis of bile acids. Essentially, the body uses FXR to sense existing bile acid levels, and when levels are high, there is no need for further production. When bile acids are bound to BAS, they can no longer interact with FXR, and this leads to the body continuing to synthesize bile acids, leading to changes in the bile acid pool and alterations in bile acid composition. TGR5 is widely expressed in the gastrointestinal tract, liver, pancreas, and gallbladder, and activation of TGR5 leads to increases in cyclic adenosine monophosphate (cAMP), activation of protein kinase A, and many subsequent downstream effects. TGR5 activation is involved in incretin hormone secretion via GLP-1 secretion, leading to decreases in plasma glucose and A1C. Interestingly, unlike with FXR, bile acids continue to interact and activate TGR5 even while bound to BAS, leading to increases in GLP-1 and subsequent decreases in plasma glucose. In conclusion, the lack of FXR activation and the preserved activation of TGR5 (and the related increase of GLP-1 activity) are key to the lowering of plasma glucose and A1C that is observed in studies of patients treated with BAS.[7-10]

PHARMACOKINETICS/PHARMACODYNAMICS

BAS are hydrophilic polymers that are not hydrolyzed by digestive enzymes and are largely not absorbed from the gastrointestinal tract.[11,12] Since BAS are primarily unabsorbed, the distribution is limited to the gastrointestinal tract. BAS are not metabolized systemically and do not interfere with any metabolizing enzymes or CYPs. Excretion is primarily in the feces. Cholestyramine is 100% excreted in the feces. Approximately 0.05% of the doses of colesevelam and colestipol are excreted renally, while the remainder is excreted in the feces. Onset of action in the gastrointestinal tract is immediate for bile acid sequestration, but it takes 4–6 weeks to see initial changes in A1C and 12–18 weeks for maximal effect.[11,12]

TREATMENT ADVANTAGES/DISADVANTAGES

Per the American Diabetes Association *Standards of Care in Diabetes*, BAS are not recommended as a standard part of therapy but may be tried in patients resistant to other treatments or in whom there are other indications for BAS therapy.[2] Per the

AACE/American College of Endocrinology (ACE) guidelines, BAS are an acceptable add-on therapy, but BAS are the sixth class of agents in order of preference, falling just ahead of bromocriptine, α-glucosidase inhibitors, and sulfonylureas.[13]

BAS only have modest efficacy on FPG and A1C. In recent meta-analyses, the average decrease in FPG was found to be between 19.3 and 37.8 mg/dL.[4,2] The average decrease in A1C was found to be between 0.55 and 0.83% with a range of 0.3–1.4%. BAS are associated with an LDL decrease of 15–25% and moderate increases in triglycerides.[14] The combination of effects on LDL and A1C make the use of BAS appealing in patients with comorbid T2D and hyperlipidemia not achieving their goals on standard therapies.

BAS have been used safely with many different oral antidiabetic agents and insulin, as well as monotherapy in diabetes. In the initial study that discovered the A1C-lowering effects of cholestyramine, the patients were stable on either glyburide or insulin therapy with no instances of drug interactions or hypoglycemia noted.[14] In studies, colesevelam was used as an add-on therapy with sulfonylureas, TZDs, metformin, and insulin, with only rare, mild cases of hypoglycemia noted.[15–19] BAS are not recommended in the treatment of prediabetes or as monotherapy for the treatment of T2D due to the modest effects and the presence of better alternative therapies.[2]

BAS should not be used in the treatment of T1D or DKA.[20] They were not studied in this population. If a patient with T1D has comorbid hyperlipidemia that is not responding to statin therapy, the use of BAS is not contraindicated and can be recommended.[20–22] BAS may theoretically affect FPG and A1C in patients with T1D due to the potential effects of GLP-1 action, but further research is needed to determine if this conceptual benefit holds true.

Both T2D and hyperlipidemia are independent risk factors for cardiovascular events, but the use of BAS has not consistently been shown to decrease this risk.[23–25] However, there are several studies and models that propose there are cardiovascular benefits when BAS are used in patients with comorbid diabetes and hyperlipidemia.[23–25] Although it is assumed that BAS may contribute to decreased cardiovascular risk, further studies are needed to verify this assumption.

The major barriers to the consistent use of BAS in standard practice are the undesirably large tablets or taste of the suspensions, dosing frequency, and the side effects and possible drug interactions.[20–22] The tablets of colesevelam are rather large and have been associated with dysphagia; when combined with the number of tablets needed to reach a therapeutic dose, this is a significant barrier to patient adherence.[20] The other BAS are all powder formulations for suspension; for cholestyramine and colestipol, several packets/scoops are needed for a therapeutic dose, leading to patient nonadherence.[21,22] The primary side effects of gastrointestinal disturbances, although generally mild, may inhibit some patients from wanting to take BAS.[20–22] The last barrier is the large list of drug interactions seen with BAS, which may limit the patient population able to take them.[20–22]

In general, BAS are a useful drug class to have in the tool chest of T2D oral antidiabetic agents, and they are especially important for patients with comorbid hyperlipidemia.

SIGNIFICANT WARNINGS/PRECAUTIONS

Decreased Absorption of Fat-Soluble Vitamins

BAS have been shown to cause decreased absorption of fat-soluble vitamins A, D, E, and K.[20-22] To avoid this interaction, patients should take any supplements at least 4 h prior to or after BAS administration and, when reasonable, the longest dosing gap possible is recommended. Caution should be used when treating any patient susceptible to deficiencies or changes in vitamin K absorption (e.g., patient taking warfarin or with malabsorption syndromes). Chronic use of BAS may be associated with an increased risk of bleeding due to hyperprothrombinemia from vitamin K deficiency, which is typically corrected by intravenous administration of vitamin K and further oral supplementation with vitamin K.[20-22]

Serum Triglycerides

BAS are contraindicated in patients with serum triglyceride concentrations greater than 500 mg/dL, and caution should be used for any patient with triglyceride concentrations greater than 300 mg/dL.[20-22] BAS are associated with elevations in serum triglycerides, with the average elevation observed to be 5%, but larger elevations have been observed when added to other antidiabetic agents (up to 20%).[20-22] This elevation is of greater concern in patients with preexisting high triglycerides and patients with a history of familial hypertriglyceridemia. Serum triglycerides above 500 mg/dL are associated with increased risk of pancreatitis, and levels over 1,000 mg/dL have a 5% risk of pancreatitis.[26] Lipid levels, including triglycerides, LDL, and non-HDL, should be obtained prior to initiating therapy with a BAS, at 3 months after initiation, and then at 6-month intervals thereafter to monitor triglyceride levels. If a patient experiences pancreatitis or serum triglyceride levels exceeding 400 mg/dL, the BAS should be promptly discontinued.[3,20-22]

Gastrointestinal Disorders

BAS can cause gastrointestinal problems, including constipation, so patients with preexisting gastroparesis or motility disorders or a history of gastrointestinal tract surgery may be at risk of bowel obstruction.[20-22] All patients should be instructed to take their BAS with food and plenty of fluid to alleviate the risk of constipation. If a patient reports constipation, treatment with a stool softener may be indicated. In patients with preexisting constipation, the starting dose should be reduced and, if tolerated, the dose may be titrated to the maximum tolerated dose or until constipation is exacerbated. BAS-associated constipation may aggravate preexisting hemorrhoids. Constipation should be avoided in patients with symptomatic coronary artery disease due to the risk of straining with hard stool. These patients will need to be monitored closely and treatment modified if constipation occurs during BAS treatment.[20-22]

Dysphagia

Colesevelam tablets are rather large and should be used with caution in patients with preexisting dysphagia or patients with swallowing disorders, due to risk of new or worsening dysphagia and esophageal obstruction.[20–22]

Phenylketonurics

All marketed BAS contain phenylalanine and so are contraindicated in patients with phenylketonuria.[20–22]

Hypothyroidism

There is a theoretical risk of developing hypothyroidism when taking BAS for patients with a limited thyroid reserve.[12] BAS, specifically cholestyramine and colestipol, have been used off-label for adjunctive treatment of Graves' disease and hyperthyroidism.[12]

SPECIAL POPULATIONS

Pregnancy

BAS as a class are pregnancy category B or C drugs and should be relatively safe since they are not absorbed from the gastrointestinal tract.[20–22] However, because BAS interfere with absorption of fat-soluble vitamins, they should be used with caution in pregnant women.[27] Briggs's *Drugs in Pregnancy and Lactation* rates BAS as *potentially toxic*.[27] This is due to a case report of a vitamin K deficiency-induced hemorrhage in a mother and fetus attributed to use of cholestyramine in pregnancy.[27] If BAS treatment is continued during pregnancy, it is recommended to take all fat-soluble vitamins, including vitamin-K containing supplements, at least 4 h before BAS administration.[27]

Lactation

There are not reports describing the use of BAS in lactation, but as they are not absorbed from the gastrointestinal tract, BAS are classified as *probably compatible*.[20–22,26] Since BAS interfere with the absorption of fat-soluble vitamins, milk produced by women taking BAS may be deficient in these vitamins and supplementation of the woman and infant may be necessary.[20–22,27]

Pediatrics

BAS are not approved to treat diabetes in children and have not been studied in this population.[20–22] However, BAS are used to treat heterozygous familial hypercholesterolemia in children ≥10 years at typical adult dosing and show equivalent safety and efficacy to adult use. Of note, due to the large tablet sizes of colesevelam, it is recommended that children receive the oral suspension or powder formulations of BAS.[20–22]

Geriatrics

In studies, only a small percentage of patients enrolled were over 65 years and very few were over 75 years; among patients that were enrolled, no differences in safety of efficacy were observed between geriatric and younger patients.[20–22] Due to the small sample sizes, greater sensitivity to adverse effects in some individuals cannot be ruled out.[20–22]

Hepatic Impairment

No dosage adjustments are needed as BAS are not absorbed from the gastrointestinal tract.[20–22]

Renal Impairment

No dosage adjustments are needed as BAS are not absorbed from the gastrointestinal tract.[20–22]

PHARMACOGENOMICS

There are no clinically significant pharmacogenomic polymorphisms that lead to altered dosing.[12]

ADVERSE EFFECTS AND MONITORING

BAS are generally well tolerated, and most side effects are mild and subside with continued use or a decrease in dose.[20–22] The most common adverse effect associated with BAS use is constipation, reported by 6–11% of patients. Constipation associated with BAS is typically mild, transient, and easily controlled with a standard regimen of increased fluid and fiber intake and, if necessary, by adding a stool softener. In some patients, the constipation can be severe and lead to fecal impaction or bowel obstruction. Therefore, patients with a history of bowel obstruction or gastrointestinal tract surgery should be treated very cautiously with BAS, and the benefits may not outweigh the risks. For patients with preexisting constipation due to other medical conditions, the use of BAS should be weighed to determine whether the benefits of treatment outweigh the risks. If treatment is initiated, the dose should be decreased and then titrated slowly with frequent monitoring for increased constipation. If constipation presents and does not resolve with increased fluid and fiber, the patient may need to have the dose decreased or to discontinue therapy.

Most of the other frequently reported adverse effects are related to the gastrointestinal tract and include dyspepsia, abdominal discomfort, bloating, flatulence, nausea, and vomiting. These are also generally mild and resolve with continued use or with a decrease in dose.

Rare but serious adverse effects include hypersensitivity reactions (primarily rash and urticaria), cholecystitis, cholelithiasis, and pancreatitis. These effects were noted in less than 2% of patients taking BAS and resolved after discontinuing the BAS.

Patients using BAS should receive the typical monitoring of their diabetes and should be instructed to self-monitor their blood glucose. Other suggested monitoring includes regular (every 3–6 months) monitoring of serum triglycerides and other lipid markers. Patients should also self-monitor for signs and symptoms of pancreatitis (severe abdominal pain with or without nausea and vomiting). Patients with a history of hyper- or hypothyroidism should have their thyroid function monitored before starting BAS treatment and then every 6 months afterward.

BAS have also been associated with transient changes to liver function enzymes (aspartate transaminase [AST], ALT, and alkaline phosphatase), but routine monitoring is not recommended.[20–22]

DRUG INTERACTIONS

BAS are positively charged anion resins that have the potential to bind to any negatively charged oral drug molecules that are coadministered.[20–22] Since there is a potential for many drugs to interact with BAS, the manufacturers recommend administering any drug with a narrow therapeutic window at least 4 h prior to or after BAS administration, and if the coadministered medication has a high risk profile, monitoring therapeutic drug levels is recommended.

Table 15.1—Drug Interactions

Drug/class	Degree of interaction	Interaction type
Cyclosporine	Major	Decreased cyclosporine levels
Deferasirox	Major	Decreased deferasirox levels and corresponding increase in iron levels
Digoxin	Major	Decreased digoxin levels
Mycophenolate	Major	Decreased mycophenolate levels
Pravastatin	Major	Decreased pravastatin levels
Amiodarone	Moderate	Decreased amiodarone levels
Antibiotics (metronidazole, penicillin, cephalexin, tetracycline, etc.)	Moderate	Decreased absorption and decreased efficacy
Oral Contraceptives	Moderate	Decreased contraception efficacy
Diltiazem	Moderate	Decreased diltiazem levels
Levothyroxine	Moderate	Decreased levothyroxine levels and decreased efficacy; may also elevate thyroid-stimulating hormone (TSH) levels
NSAIDs (meloxicam and diclofenac)	Moderate	Decreased efficacy
Phenytoin	Moderate	Decreased phenytoin levels
Propranolol	Moderate	Decreased propranolol levels and decreased efficacy
Sulfonylureas	Moderate	Decreased sulfonylurea levels
Valproic Acid	Moderate	Decreased serum valproic acid levels
Warfarin	Moderate	Variable/reduced INR levels due to changes in vitamin K absorption

INR, international normalized ratios. Source: Micromedex.[10]

DOSAGE AND ADMINISTRATION

The recommended dose of BAS varies by agent, but the dosing required to show benefit in diabetes appears to be the same as the dosing recommended to treat hyperlipidemia.[4,6] Since the primary adverse effect that limits treatment for all agents in the class is constipation, titration of dosing is generally slow, and many patients never reach the maximum dosing for any of the agents.[20-22] All agents need to be taken with food to minimize gastrointestinal upset and should be taken with plenty of fluids to prevent constipation. The powder formulations of BAS need to be mixed with 2–6 ounces of noncarbonated fluid or applesauce and consumed completely.[20-22]

Table 15.2—Doses and Dose Adjustments

Generic (brand)	Form/strength	Dosage
Colesevelam (Welchol)	Oral: 625-mg tablet and 3.75-g powder packet for suspension	■ Once-daily dosing: 3.75 g (6 tablets or 1 packet for suspension); twice-daily dosing: 1.875 g (3 tablets).
Cholestyramine (Questran)	Oral: 4 g powder for suspension (packets and loose powder)	■ Initial: 4 g once or twice daily. Titrate: may increase dose every month to effective or max tolerated dose; maximum dose of 24 g/day.
Colestipol (Colestid)	Oral: 1-g tablets and 5 g powder for suspension (packets and loose granules)	■ Initial (tablets): 2 g (2 tablets) once or twice daily. Titrate: may increase dose every month to effective or max tolerated dose; maximum dose of 16 g/day. ■ Initial (granules): 5 g once or twice daily. Titrate: may increase dose every month to effective or max tolerated dose; maximum dose of 30 g/day.

MONOGRAPHS

Cholestyramine (Questran): https://dailymed.nlm.nih.gov/dailymed/drugInfo. cfm?setid=362ddd91-a63f-4ec6-841a-75785dd208c8

Colestipol (Colestid): https://dailymed.nlm.nih.gov/dailymed/drugInfo. cfm?setid=21b37725-fc0c-4365-a7dc-1a473d42502d

Colesevelam (Welchol): https://dailymed.nlm.nih.gov/dailymed/drugInfo. cfm?setid=fc274f83-4cd6-47bd-b43e-53a0bf345f11

REFERENCES

1. Drugs@FDA. U.S. Food & Drug Administration website. Available from https://www.accessdata.fda.gov/scripts/cder/daf/index.cfm. Accessed 25 April 2020

2. American Diabetes Association. 9. Pharmacologic approaches to glycemic treatment: Standards of Medical Care in Diabetes—2022. *Diabetes Care* 2022;45(Suppl. 1):S125–S143

3. Stone NJ, Robinson JG, Lichtenstein AH, et al. 2013 ACC/AHA Guideline on the treatment of blood cholesterol to reduce atherosclerotic cardiovascular risk in adults. *J Am Coll Cardiol* 2013;63(25PartB):2889–2934

4. Hansen M, Sonne DP, Mikkelsen KH, et al. Bile acid sequestrants for glycemic control in patients with type 2 diabetes: a systematic review with meta-analysis of randomized controlled trials. *J Diabetes Complications* 2017;31(5):918–927

5. Mazidi M, Rezaie P, Karimi E, Kengne AP. The effects of bile acid sequestrants on lipid profile and blood glucose concentrations: a systematic review and meta-analysis of randomized controlled trials. *Int J Cardiol* 2017;15(227):850–857

6. Bays HE, Goldberg RB, Truitt KE, Jones MR. Colesevelam hydrochloride therapy in patients with type 2 diabetes mellitus treated with metformin: glucose and lipid effects. *Arch Intern Med.* 2008;168(18):1975–1983

7. Hansen M, Sonne DP, Knop FK. Bile acid sequestrants: glucose-lowering mechanisms and efficacy in type 2 diabetes. *Curr Diab Rep* 2014;14(5):482

8. Chávez-Talavera O, Tailleux A, Lefebvre P, Staels B. Bile acid control of metabolism and inflammation in obesity, type 2 diabetes, dyslipidemia, and nonalcoholic fatty liver disease. *Gastroenterology* 2017;152(7):1679–1694

9. Sonne DP, Hansen M, Knop FK. Bile acid sequestrants in type 2 diabetes: potential effects on GLP1 secretion. *Eur J Endocrinol* 2014;171(2):R47–65

10. Kårhus ML, Brønden A, Sonne DP, et al. Evidence connecting old, new and neglected glucose-lowering drugs to bile acid-induced GLP-1 secretion: a review. *Diabetes Obes Metab* 2017;19(9):1214–1222

11. Micromedex Healthcare Series. Colesevelam. Greenwood Village, CO, Truven Health Analytics, 2018. Available from www.micromedexsolutions.com. Accessed 25 January 2022

12. Lexicomp Online, Lexi-Drugs Online. Hudson, OH, Lexi-Comp, Inc., 2018. Accessed 16 May 2018.

13. Garber AJ, Abrahamson MJ, Barzilay JI, et al. Consensus statement by the American Association of Clinical Endocrinologists and American College of Endocrinology on the comprehensive type 2 diabetes management algorithm—2018 executive summary. *Endocr Pract* 2018;24(1):91–120

14. Jellinger PS, Handelsman Y, Rosenblit PD, et al. American Association of Clinical Endocrinologists and American College of Endocrinology guidelines for management of dyslipidemia and prevention of cardiovascular disease. *Endocr Pract* 2017;23(Suppl. 2):1–87

15. Garg A, Grundy SM. Cholestyramine therapy for dyslipidemia in non-insulin-dependent diabetes mellitus: a short-term, double-blind, crossover trial. *Ann Intern Med* 1994;121:416–422

16. Zema MJ. Colesevelam hydrochloride: evidence for its use in the treatment of hypercholesterolemia and type 2 diabetes mellitus with insights into mechanism of action. *Core Evid* 2012;7:61–75

17. Ooi CP, Loke SC. Colesevelam for type 2 diabetes mellitus: an abridged Cochrane review. *Diabet Med* 2014;31(1):2–14

18. Brunetti L, Hermes-Desantis ER. The role of colesevelam hydrochloride in hypercholesterolemia and type 2 diabetes mellitus. *Ann Pharmacother* 2010;44(7–8):1196–1206

19. Fonseca VA, Rosenstock J, Wang AC, et al. Colesevelam HCl improves glycemic control and reduces LDL cholesterol in patients with inadequately controlled type 2 diabetes on sulfonylurea-based therapy. *Diabetes Care* 2008;31(8):1479–1484

20. Welchol [package insert]. Basking Ridge, NJ, Daiichi Sankyo, Inc., July 2017

21. Colestid [package insert]. New York, Pfizer, May 2018

22. Questran [package insert]. Spring Valley, NY, Par Pharmaceutical Co., October 2017

23. Ganda OP. The role of bile acid sequestrants in the management of type 2 diabetes mellitus. *Metab Syndr Relat Disord* 2010;8(Suppl. 1):S15–S21

24. Ross S, D'Mello M, Anand SS, et al. Effect of bile acid sequestrants on the risk of cardiovascular events: a mendelian randomization analysis. *Circ Cardiovasc Genet* 2015;8(4):618–627

25. Spinelli V, Chávez-Talavera O, Tailleux A, Staels B. Metabolic effects of bile acid sequestration: impact on cardiovascular risk factors. *Curr Opin Endocrinol Diabetes Obes* 2016;23(2):138–144

26. Scherer J, Singh VP, Pitchumoni CS, Yadav D. Issues in hypertriglyceridemic pancreatitis: an update. *J Clin Gastroenterol* 2014;48(3):195–203

27. Briggs GG, Freeman RK, Yaffe SJ. *Drugs in Pregnancy and Lactation: A Reference Guide to Fetal and Neonatal Risk*, 11th ed. Philadelphia, Lippincott Williams & Wilkins, 2017

Chapter 16
Dopamine-2 Receptor Agonists

Christina R. Buchman, PharmD, BCACP

Bromocriptine is the only dopamine agonist that is approved for treatment of diabetes.[1] Other dopamine agonists include cabergoline, ropinirole, and pramipexole, but their usefulness in diabetes has not been demonstrated. Bromocriptine quick release (QR) was first approved for T2D on 5 May 2009 under the brand name Cycloset.[1] Bromocriptine is not a new drug, and has in fact been used since the late 1970s in the treatment of Parkinson's disease, hyperprolactinemia, and acromegaly. Patients with Parkinson's disease and comorbid diabetes treated with bromocriptine showed decreases in plasma glucose and A1C.[2] This prompted research looking into bromocriptine for diabetes. The new formulation of bromocriptine that was developed and approved for the treatment of diabetes is designed to rapidly release and be absorbed to quickly achieve elevated plasma levels.[3] The absorption timing of this quick-release formulation turns out to be vital for the treatment of diabetes as it is thought that low endogenous levels of dopamine upon waking contribute to insulin resistance.[4,5] Bromocriptine is not indicated for T1D or DKA.[3]

PHARMACOLOGY

MECHANISM OF ACTION

Bromocriptine is a semisynthetic ergot alkaloid derivative and is classified as a sympatholytic, semiselective dopamine-2 (D2) receptor agonist, but its mechanism in diabetes is not thoroughly understood.

Dopamine is an endogenous neurotransmitter that performs many actions in the body and targets many different receptors that potentially play a role in diabetes.[4-7] Dopamine interacts primarily with dopamine receptors, but also with serotonin receptors related to the control of appetite and glucose tolerance. Dopamine's primary actions include control of many physiologic processes, such as motivation, appetite, weight gain, circadian rhythms, and insulin sensitization. These actions are primarily mediated by the D2 receptor pathway, which is the main target of bromocriptine. The majority of D2 receptors involved in processes important for diabetes are in the hypothalamus; these receptors control circadian rhythms and contribute to insulin resistance and dyslipidemia. Persons diagnosed with T2D have been shown to have lower-than-normal hypothalamic dopamine levels upon waking. Low dopamine levels are associated with glucose intolerance, dyslipidemia, increased hepatic gluconeogenesis, and increased risk of CVD.[4-7]

Administration of bromocriptine within 2 h of waking is thought to reset the sympathetic system in the CNS by increasing morning dopamine levels to a point that is similar to the levels in nondiabetic persons.[3,5,6] In studies, the administration of bromocriptine has been associated with decreased fasting and postprandial blood glucose levels without increasing plasma insulin levels. This resulted in modest decreases in A1C (0.6–0.7%). Bromocriptine also decreases plasma free fatty acids and triglycerides. Studies also show that bromocriptine is associated with a decreased risk of cardiovascular events, though the mechanism is unknown.[3,5,6]

PHARMACOKINETICS

Approximately 65–95% of bromocriptine-QR is absorbed, but it undergoes extensive first-pass metabolism, and only 5–10% of the dose reaches the target tissues.[2,5,6] Time to peak concentration is approximately 45–60 min when fasting. Bioavailability is increased by 55–65% and the time to peak concentration is delayed with the intake of food. This pharmacokinetic profile is unique to the QR formulation, and the two formulations are not interchangeable.[2,5,6]

Bromocriptine is highly protein bound with a volume of distribution of 61 L.[2,5,6] It undergoes extensive metabolism in the gastrointestinal tract; CYP3A4 is the primary metabolism pathway through the liver. The metabolites are all inactive and primarily excreted in the bile and feces, with only 2–6% excreted in the urine. The half-life of bromocriptine is approximately 6 h.[2,5,6]

TREATMENT ADVANTAGES/DISADVANTAGES

Per the American Diabetes Association *Standards of Medical Care in Diabetes—2022*, bromocriptine is not recommended as a standard part of therapy in T2D, but may be tried in patients resistant to other treatments or in whom there are other indications for its use.[8] Per the AACE/ACE guidelines, it is an acceptable add-on therapy, but it is the seventh agent in the list in order of preference, falling just behind BAS but ahead of α-glucosidase inhibitors and sulfonylureas.[9]

Bromocriptine should not be used in the treatment of T1D or DKA.[3] It has been studied as monotherapy for the treatment of T2D, showing small decreases in A1C of 0.4–0.6% more than placebo.[10] It has also been studied as add-on therapy with sulfonylureas, with and without metformin, leading to decreases in A1C of 0.4–1.2%.[10] It has been studied in small pilot studies as add-on to insulin therapy with good preliminary results and no increased risk of hypoglycemia.[11] It has not been studied in combination with TZDs, SGLT2 inhibitors, or DPP-4 inhibitors.[3]

One significant advantage of bromocriptine is the cardiovascular risk benefits. Bromocriptine shows a 40% risk reduction of heart attack, stroke, and other major cardiovascular events in patients with preexisting CVD compared to those receiving standard therapy.[12-14] The relative risk reduction was found to be 40%. In this study, the patients were allowed to take no more than two oral antidiabetics, or insulin plus one oral agent, in addition to the bromocriptine and were allowed to change the underlying antidiabetic regimen at the discretion of the study investigators.[12-14] Further studies and observations need to be done to see if this benefit holds true outside of the studies and if the use of bromocriptine is limited by the incidence of side effects.

The barriers to bromocriptine therapy include the high cost of the QR formulation approved for diabetes as well as the relatively high number of tablets that need to be taken to achieve the therapeutic dose.[3] Other barriers include the relatively high incidence of gastrointestinal side effects, leading to discontinuation.[3]

In general, bromocriptine is a useful drug to have in the tool chest of oral antidiabetic agents for T2D and is especially important for patients who have comorbid conditions or cardiovascular risk factors.

THERAPEUTIC CONSIDERATIONS

Patients using bromocriptine need to be instructed to follow the administration timing carefully and to take bromocriptine with food to increase the absorption and half-life, as well as to decrease the incidence of gastrointestinal side effects.

SIGNIFICANT WARNINGS/PRECAUTIONS

Hypotension

In studies, hypotension (including orthostatic hypotension) was reported in patients taking bromocriptine and is particularly seen upon initiation of therapy and with dose increases.[3] Prior to initiation of bromocriptine, patients should be assessed for orthostatic changes and should be advised on the risks of orthostatic hypotension. Caution should be used in patients who are also taking antihypertensives.[3]

Psychiatric Disorders

Patients with severe psychiatric disorders should not receive bromocriptine therapy due to the possibility that bromocriptine may exacerbate the disorder and decrease the efficacy of the neuroleptic treatments they are receiving.[3]

Somnolence

Bromocriptine has been known to cause somnolence, reported as sudden sleep onset, sometimes during activities.[3] This side effect is more common in patients being treated for Parkinson's disease, but was reported in clinical trials for diabetes. Patients should be made aware of the potential for somnolence on bromocriptine therapy and counseled not to drive or operate heavy machinery until they know how the drug affects them.[3]

Syncopal Migraines

Patients who have a known history of syncopal migraines should not take bromocriptine due to an increased risk of syncope.[3] Bromocriptine increases the risk of hypotension among patients with syncopal migraines. Loss of consciousness during a migraine for patients treated with bromocriptine may represent hypersensitivity, and these patients should no longer receive bromocriptine therapy.[3]

SPECIAL POPULATIONS

Pregnancy

Bromocriptine is a pregnancy category B drug, with inadequate studies in humans.[3] Briggs's *Drugs in Pregnancy and Lactation* rates bromocriptine as *compatible*.[15] Observational data from pregnant women who used bromocriptine throughout pregnancy showed safety similar to other medications, and children exposed to intrauterine bromocriptine did not have a higher rate of birth defects than the general population. Because the possibility of harm cannot be ruled out, the use of bromocriptine during pregnancy should be avoided in diabetic patients unless there is a compelling indication without other safer treatment options.[15]

Lactation

Bromocriptine is contraindicated in lactation because it inhibits lactation and decreases levels of prolactin.[3,15]

Pediatrics

Bromocriptine has not been studied in children for the treatment of diabetes.[3] Bromocriptine has been used in children as young as 11 years to treat other conditions and has generally been found to be safe.[16,17]

Geriatrics

No differences in efficacy or safety were noted in geriatric patients taking bromocriptine to treat either diabetes or other approved indications.[3,16,17] Some sensitive populations cannot be ruled out and so use should be monitored in fragile patients.

Sex

Females have an increased plasma exposure of 18–30% compared to males.[3] It is not known if this is clinically relevant.

Hepatic Impairment

Bromocriptine has not been studied in hepatic impairment, but since it primarily undergoes hepatic metabolism, its use is cautioned in hepatic impairment.[3]

Renal Impairment

Bromocriptine has not been studied in renal impairment and has no reported adjustments for impaired renal function.[3]

PHARMACOGENOMICS

There are no known clinically significant pharmacogenomic polymorphisms that lead to altered dosing.[17]

ADVERSE EFFECTS AND MONITORING

Bromocriptine is generally well tolerated, and most side effects are mild and subside with continued use.[3,18–20] The most frequently reported adverse effects associated with bromocriptine are all gastrointestinal related. The most common adverse effect is nausea, affecting 25–30% of patients and lasting for an average of 14 days. In studies, nausea was cited as the primary reason for discontinuing the drug. Other gastrointestinal effects include vomiting (5–8%), constipation (5–11%), diarrhea (8%), dyspepsia (7.5%), and anorexia (5%). Taking bromocriptine with food reduces the incidence of gastrointestinal adverse effects. Other side effects reported in clinical trials that rarely lead to discontinuation include dizziness (14%), drowsiness (6%), fatigue (14%), headache (14%), asthenia (14%), and rhinitis (12%).[3,18–20]

Rare but serious adverse effects include syncope (1.5%) and hypotension (2.2%). Other serious side effects that have been observed with higher doses, but have not been reported with the QR formulation or the doses used to treat diabetes, include hallucinations, fibrotic complications (pulmonary and pleural), stroke, and neuroleptic-like malignant syndrome.[3,18–20] Anaphylaxis has been reported; if a patient has a known reaction to other ergot derivatives, he or she should be cautioned that anaphylaxis is more likely with bromocriptine.[3]

Patients taking bromocriptine should receive the typical monitoring of their diabetes and should be instructed to self-monitor their blood glucose.[3,18–20] Patients should have their blood pressure monitored periodically, with special attention paid during the initiation phase and whenever doses are titrated. Patients should also be evaluated for orthostatic changes prior to initiation and periodically during use. It may also be recommended to monitor serum prolactin levels, although no cases of hypoprolactinemia have been reported with use.[3,18–20]

DRUG INTERACTIONS

Bromocriptine has several clinically relevant drug interactions due to its pharmacology and metabolism by CYP enzymes.[3,16] Bromocriptine is contraindicated with concomitant use of other ergot derivatives, sympathomimetic drugs (e.g., phenylpropanolamine and isometheptene), and selective 5-hydroxytryptamine$_{1B}$ (5-HT$_{1B}$) agonists (e.g., "-triptans"). Bromocriptine is also highly protein-bound, and may increase the unbound fraction of other highly protein-bound drugs (e.g., salicylates, sulfonamides, and probenecid) and alter the efficacy and risk for side effects, so concomitant use is not recommended. Concomitant use of other dopamine agonists is not recommended due to an increased risk for side effects. Bromocriptine is primarily metabolized by CYP3A4, and so it is not recommended for patients to take either strong CYP3A4 inducers or inhibitors while taking bromocriptine due to the potential for changes in efficacy and risk of side effects. Doses should not exceed 1.6 mg daily if used with a moderate inhibitor of CYP3A4 (e.g., erythromycin).[3,16]

DOSAGE AND ADMINISTRATION

The recommended dose of bromocriptine for the treatment of T2D is 1.6–4.8 mg once a day within 2 h of waking.[3] Bromocriptine should be initiated at 0.8 mg (1 tablet) and then titrated slowly by increasing the dose by 0.8 mg (1 tablet) per week until the maximum dose of 4.8 mg (6 tablets) or the maximally tolerated dose is reached. The average dose achieved in clinical trials was 4.0 mg daily, but in postmarketing surveillance, the most common dose used is 3.2 mg daily.[3]

Table 16.1 — Dosage

Generic (brand)	Form/strength	Dosage
Bromocriptine mesylate (Cycloset)	Oral: 0.8-mg tablet	■ Initial: 0.8 mg p.o. daily within 2 h of waking. ■ Titrate: May increase by 0.8 mg every week to a max of 4.8 mg daily, or the maximum tolerated dose.

MONOGRAPHS

Bromocriptine mesylate (Cylcoset): https://dailymed.nlm.nih.gov/dailymed/drugInfo.cfm?setid=3e719d6a-342e-428b-93d3-377d31cb15c7

REFERENCES

1. Drugs@FDA. U.S. Food & Drug Administration website. Available from https://www.accessdata.fda.gov/scripts/cder/daf/index.cfm. Accessed 25 April 2020

2. Valiquette G. Bromocriptine for diabetes mellitus type II. *Cardiol Rev* 2011;19(6):272–275

3. Cycloset (bromocriptine mesylate) [package insert]. Tiverton, RI, Santarus, Inc., February 2017

4. Lopez Vicchi F, Luque GM, Brie B, et al. Dopaminergic drugs in type 2 diabetes and glucose homeostasis. *Pharmacol Res* 2016;109:74–80

5. Holt RI, Barnett AH, Bailey CJ. Bromocriptine: old drug, new formulation and new indication. *Diabetes Obes Metab* 2010;12(12):1048–1057

6. Grunberger, G. Bromocriptine mesylate QR in treatment of type 2 diabetes. *Diabetes Manag* 2014;4(2);203–211

7. Grunberger G. Novel therapies for the management of type 2 diabetes mellitus: part 1. pramlintide and bromocriptine-QR. *J Diabetes* 2013;5(2): 110–117

8. American Diabetes Association. 9. Pharmacologic approaches to glycemic treatment: Standards of Medical Care in Diabetes—2022. *Diabetes Care* 2022;45(Suppl. 1):S125–S143

9. Garber AJ, Abrahamson MJ, Barzilay JI, et al. Consensus statement by the American Association of Clinical Endocrinologists and American College of Endocrinology on the comprehensive type 2 diabetes management algorithm—2018 executive summary. *Endocr Pract* 2018;24(1):91–120

10. DeFronzo RA. Bromocriptine: a sympatholytic, d2-dopamine agonist for the treatment of type 2 diabetes [erratum, *Diabetes Care* 2011;34(6):1442]. *Diabetes Care* 2011;34(4):789–794

11. Roe ED, Chamarthi B, Raskin P. Impact of bromocriptine-QR therapy on glycemic control and daily insulin requirement in type 2 diabetes mellitus subjects whose dysglycemia is poorly controlled on high-dose insulin: a pilot study. *J Diabetes Res* 2015:834903

12. Lamos EM, Levitt DL, Munir KM. A review of dopamine agonist therapy in type 2 diabetes and effects on cardio-metabolic parameters. *Prim Care Diabetes* 2016;10(1):60–65

13. Gaziano JM, Cincotta AH, O'Connor CM, et al. Randomized clinical trial of quick-release bromocriptine among patients with type 2 diabetes on overall safety and cardiovascular outcomes [erratum, *Diabetes Care* 2016;39(10):1846]. *Diabetes Care* 2010;33(7):1503–1508

14. Gaziano JM, Cincotta AH, Vinik A, et al. Effect of bromocriptine-QR (a quick-release formulation of bromocriptine mesylate) on major adverse cardiovascular events in type 2 diabetes subjects [erratum, *J Am Heart Assoc* 2015;4(10)]. *J Am Heart Assoc* 2012;1(5):e002279

15. Briggs GG, Freeman RK, Yaffe SJ. *Drugs in Pregnancy and Lactation: A Reference Guide to Fetal and Neonatal Risk*, 11th ed. Philadelphia, Lippincott Williams & Wilkins, 2017

    Micromedex Healthcare Series. Bromocriptine. Greenwood Village, CO, Truven Health Analytics, 2018. Available from www.micromedexsolutions.com. Accessed 25 January 2022

16. Lexicomp Online, Lexi-Drugs Online. Hudson, OH, Lexi-Comp, Inc., 2018. Accessed 16 May 2018

17. Kerr JL, Timpe EM, Petkewicz KA. Bromocriptine mesylate for glycemic management in type 2 diabetes mellitus. *Ann Pharmacother* 2010;44(11):1777–1785

18. Sando KR, Taylor J. Bromocriptine: its place in type 2 diabetes Tx. *J Fam Pract* 2011;60(11):E1–E5

19. Schwartz SS, Zangeneh F. Evidence-based practice use of quick-release bromocriptine across the natural history of type 2 diabetes mellitus. *Postgrad Med* 2016;128(8):828–838

Chapter 17
Cardiovascular Disease and Risk Management

The American Diabetes Association (ADA) "Standards of Care in Diabetes" includes the ADA's current clinical practice recommendations and is intended to provide the components of diabetes care, general treatment goals and guidelines, and tools to evaluate quality of care. Members of the ADA Professional Practice Committee, a multidisciplinary expert committee, are responsible for updating the Standards of Care annually, or more frequently as warranted. For a detailed description of ADA standards, statements, and reports, as well as the evidence-grading system for ADA's clinical practice recommendations and a full list of Professional Practice Committee members, please refer to Introduction and Methodology. Readers who wish to comment on the Standards of Care are invited to do so at professional.diabetes.org/SOC.

For prevention and management of diabetes complications in children and adolescents, please refer to Section 14, "Children and Adolescents."

Atherosclerotic cardiovascular disease (ASCVD)—defined as coronary heart disease (CHD), cerebrovascular disease, or peripheral arterial disease presumed to be of atherosclerotic origin—is the leading cause of morbidity and mortality for individuals with diabetes and results in an estimated $37.3 billion in cardiovascular-related spending per year associated with diabetes.[1] Common conditions coexisting with type 2 diabetes (e.g., hypertension and dyslipidemia) are clear risk factors for ASCVD, and diabetes itself confers independent risk. Numerous studies have shown the efficacy of controlling individual cardiovascular risk factors in preventing or slowing ASCVD in people with diabetes. Furthermore, large benefits are seen when multiple cardiovascular risk factors are addressed simultaneously. Under the current paradigm of aggressive risk factor modification in people with diabetes, there is evidence that measures of 10-year CHD risk among U.S. adults with diabetes have improved significantly over the past decade[2] and that ASCVD morbidity and mortality have decreased.[3,4]

Heart failure is another major cause of morbidity and mortality from cardiovascular disease. Recent studies have found that rates of incident heart failure

Chapter 17 is an excerpt from ElSayed NA, Aleppo G, Aroda VR, et al., American Diabetes Association. 10. Cardiovascular disease and risk management: Standards of Care in Diabetes—2023. *Diabetes Care* 2023;46(Suppl. 1):S158–S190. This section has received endorsement from the American College of Cardiology.

hospitalization (adjusted for age and sex) were twofold higher in people with diabetes compared with those without.[5,6] People with diabetes may have heart failure with preserved ejection fraction (HFpEF) or with reduced ejection fraction (HFrEF). Hypertension is often a precursor of heart failure of either type, and ASCVD can coexist with either type,[7] whereas prior myocardial infarction (MI) is often a major factor in HFrEF. Rates of heart failure hospitalization have been improved in recent trials including people with type 2 diabetes, most of whom also had ASCVD, with sodium–glucose cotransporter 2 (SGLT2) inhibitors.[8–11]

A recent meta-analysis indicated that SGLT2 inhibitors reduce the risk of heart failure hospitalization, cardiovascular mortality, and all-cause mortality in people with (secondary prevention) and without (primary prevention) cardiovascular disease.[12]

For prevention and management of both ASCVD and heart failure, cardiovascular risk factors should be systematically assessed at least annually in all people with diabetes. These risk factors include duration of diabetes, obesity/overweight, hypertension, dyslipidemia, smoking, a family history of premature coronary dis-

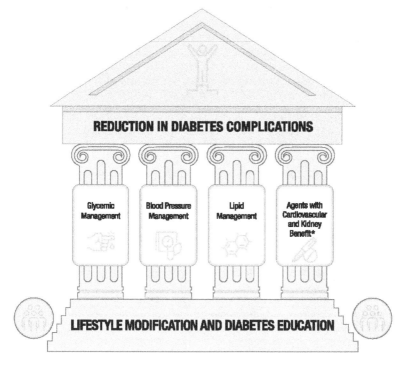

Figure 17.1—Multifactorial approach to reduction in risk of diabetes complications. *Risk reduction interventions to be applied as individually appropriate.

ease, chronic kidney disease (CKD), and the presence of albuminuria. Modifiable abnormal risk factors should be treated as described in these guidelines. Notably, the majority of evidence supporting interventions to reduce cardiovascular risk in diabetes comes from trials of people with type 2 diabetes. No randomized trials have been specifically designed to assess the impact of cardiovascular risk reduction strategies in people with type 1 diabetes. Therefore, the recommendations for cardiovascular risk factor modification for people with type 1 diabetes are extrapolated from data obtained in people with type 2 diabetes and are similar to those for people with type 2 diabetes.

As depicted in Fig. 17.1, a comprehensive approach to the reduction in risk of diabetes-related complications is recommended. Therapy that includes multiple, concurrent evidence-based approaches to care will provide complementary reduction in the risks of microvascular, kidney, neurologic, and cardiovascular complications. Management of glycemia, blood pressure, and lipids and the incorporation of specific therapies with cardiovascular and kidney outcomes benefit (as individually appropriate) are considered fundamental elements of global risk reduction in diabetes.

THE RISK CALCULATOR

The American College of Cardiology/American Heart Association ASCVD risk calculator (Risk Estimator Plus) is generally a useful tool to estimate 10-year risk of a first ASCVD event (available online at tools. acc.org/ASCVD-Risk-Estimator-Plus). The calculator includes diabetes as a risk factor, since diabetes itself confers increased risk for ASCVD, although it should be acknowledged that these risk calculators do not account for the duration of diabetes or the presence of diabetes complications, such as albuminuria. Although some variability in calibration exists in various subgroups, including by sex, race, and diabetes, the overall risk prediction does not differ in those with or without diabetes,[13–16] validating the use of risk calculators in people with diabetes. The 10-year risk of a first ASCVD event should be assessed to better stratify ASCVD risk and help guide therapy, as described below.

Recently, risk scores and other cardiovascular biomarkers have been developed for risk stratification of secondary prevention patients (i.e., those who are already high risk because they have ASCVD) but are not yet in widespread use.[17,18] With newer, more expensive lipid-lowering therapies now available, use of these risk assessments may help target these new therapies to "higher risk" ASCVD patients in the future.

HYPERTENSION/BLOOD PRESSURE CONTROL

Hypertension is defined as a systolic blood pressure ≥130 mmHg or a diastolic blood pressure ≥80 mmHg.[19] This is in agreement with the definition of hypertension by the American College of Cardiology and American Heart Association.[19] Hypertension is common among people with either type 1 or type 2 diabetes. Hypertension is a major risk factor for both ASCVD and microvascular complications. Moreover, numerous studies have shown that antihypertensive therapy reduces ASCVD events, heart failure, and microvascular complications. Please refer to the American Diabetes Association position statement "Diabetes and Hypertension" for a detailed review of the epidemiology, diagnosis, and treatment of hypertension[20] and recent updated hypertension guideline recommendations.[19,21,22]

SCREENING AND DIAGNOSIS

Recommendations

10.1 Blood pressure should be measured at every routine clinical visit. When possible, individuals found to have elevated blood pressure (systolic blood pressure 120–129 mmHg and diastolic <80 mmHg) should have blood pressure confirmed using multiple readings, including measurements on a separate day, to diagnose hypertension. **A** Hypertension is defined as a systolic blood pressure ≥130 mmHg or a diastolic blood pressure ≥80 mmHg based on an average of ≥2 measurements obtained on ≥2 occasions. **A** Individuals with blood pressure ≥180/110 mmHg and cardiovascular disease could be diagnosed with hypertension at a single visit. **E**

10.2 All people with hypertension and diabetes should monitor their blood pressure at home. **A**

Blood pressure should be measured at every routine clinical visit by a trained individual and should follow the guidelines established for the general population: measurement in the seated position, with feet on the floor and arm supported at heart level, after 5 min of rest. Cuff size should be appropriate for the upper-arm circumference. Elevated values should preferably be confirmed on a separate day; however, in individuals with cardiovascular disease and blood pressure ≥180/110 mmHg, it is reasonable to diagnose hypertension at a single visit.[21] Postural changes in blood pressure and pulse may be evidence of autonomic neuropathy and therefore require adjustment of blood pressure targets. Orthostatic blood pressure measurements should be checked on initial visit and as indicated.

Home blood pressure self-monitoring and 24-h ambulatory blood pressure monitoring may provide evidence of white coat hypertension, masked hypertension, or other discrepancies between office and "true" blood pressure.[23,24] In addition to confirming or refuting a diagnosis of hypertension, home blood pressure assessment may be useful to monitor antihypertensive treatment. Studies of individuals without diabetes found that home measurements may better correlate with ASCVD risk than office measurements.[23,24] Moreover, home blood pressure monitoring may improve patient medication taking and thus help reduce cardiovascular risk.[25]

---

* See Table 1.1 (p. 2) for an explanation of the American Diabetes Association evidence-grading system for *Standards of Care in Diabetes*.

TREATMENT GOALS

Recommendations

10.3 For people with diabetes and hypertension, blood pressure targets should be individualized through a shared decision-making process that addresses cardiovascular risk, potential adverse effects of antihypertensive medications, and patient preferences. **B**

10.4 People with diabetes and hypertension qualify for antihypertensive drug therapy when the blood pressure is persistently elevated ≥130/80 mmHg. The on-treatment target blood pressure goal is <130/80 mmHg, if it can be safely attained. **B**

10.5 In pregnant individuals with diabetes and chronic hypertension, a blood pressure threshold of 140/90 mmHg for initiation or titration of therapy is associated with better pregnancy outcomes than reserving treatment for severe hypertension, with no increase in risk of small-for-gestational age birth weight. **A** There are limited data on the optimal lower limit, but therapy should be lessened for blood pressure <90/60 mmHg. **E** A blood pressure target of 110–135/85 mmHg is suggested in the interest of reducing the risk for accelerated maternal hypertension. **A**

Randomized clinical trials have demonstrated unequivocally that treatment of hypertension reduces cardiovascular events as well as microvascular complications.[26–32] There has been controversy on the recommendation of a specific blood pressure goal in people with diabetes. The committee recognizes that there has been no randomized controlled trial to specifically demonstrate a decreased incidence of cardiovascular events in people with diabetes by targeting a blood pressure <130/80 mmHg. The recommendation to support a blood pressure goal of <130/80 mmHg in people with diabetes is consistent with guidelines from the American College of Cardiology and American Heart Association,[20] the International Society of Hypertension,[21] and the European Society of Cardiology.[22] The committee's recommendation for the blood pressure target of <130/80 mmHg derives primarily from the collective evidence of the following randomized controlled trials. The Systolic Blood Pressure Intervention Trial (SPRINT) demonstrated that treatment to a target systolic blood pressure of <120 mmHg decreases cardiovascular event rates by 25% in high-risk patients, although people with diabetes were excluded from this trial.[33] The recently completed Strategy of Blood Pressure Intervention in the Elderly Hypertensive Patients (STEP) trial included nearly 20% of people with diabetes and noted decreased cardiovascular events with treatment of hypertension to a blood pressure target of <130 mmHg.[34] While the ACCORD (Action to Control Cardiovascular Risk in Diabetes) blood pressure trial (ACCORD BP) did not confirm that targeting a systolic blood pressure of <120 mmHg in people with diabetes results in decreased cardiovascular event rates, the prespecified secondary outcome of stroke was reduced by 41% with intensive treatment.[35] The Action in Diabetes and Vascular Disease: Preterax and Diamicron MR Controlled Evaluation (ADVANCE) trial revealed that treatment with perindopril/indapamide to an achieved systolic blood pressure of ~135 mmHg significantly decreased cardiovascular event rates compared with a placebo treatment with an achieved blood pressure of 140 mmHg.[36] Therefore, it is recommended that people with diabetes who have hypertension should be treated to blood pressure targets of <130/80 mmHg. Notably, there is an absence of high-quality data available to guide blood pressure targets in people with type 1 diabetes, but a similar blood pressure target of <130/80 mmHg is recommended in people with type 1 diabetes. As discussed below, treatment should be individualized and treatment should not be targeted to <120/80 mmHg, as a mean achieved blood pressure of <120/80 mmHg is associated with adverse events.

Randomized Controlled Trials of Intensive Versus Standard Blood Pressure Control

SPRINT provides the strongest evidence to support lower blood pressure goals in patients at increased cardiovascular risk, although this trial excluded people with diabetes.[33] The trial enrolled 9,361 patients with a systolic blood pressure of ≥130 mmHg and increased cardiovascular risk and treated to a systolic blood pressure target of <120 mmHg (intensive treatment) versus a target of <140 mmHg (standard treatment). The primary composite outcome of myocardial infarction (MI), coronary syndromes, stroke, heart failure, or death from cardiovascular causes was reduced by 25% in the intensive treatment group. The achieved systolic blood pressures in the trial were 121 mmHg and 136 mmHg in the intensive versus standard treatment group, respectively. Adverse outcomes, including hypotension, syncope, electrolyte abnormality, and acute kidney injury were more common in the intensive treatment arm; risk of adverse outcomes needs to be weighed against the cardiovascular benefit of more intensive blood pressure lowering.

ACCORD BP provides the strongest direct assessment of the benefits and risks of intensive blood pressure control in people with type 2 diabetes.[35] In the study, a total of 4,733 with type 2 diabetes were assigned to intensive therapy (targeting a systolic blood pressure <120 mmHg) or standard therapy (targeting a systolic blood pressure <140 mmHg). The mean achieved systolic blood pressures were 119 mmHg and 133 mmHg in the intensive versus standard group, respectively. The primary composite outcome of nonfatal MI, nonfatal stroke, or death from cardiovascular causes was not significantly reduced in the intensive treatment group. The prespecified secondary outcome of stroke was significantly reduced by 41% in the intensive treatment group. Adverse events attributed to blood pressure treatment, including hypotension, syncope, bradycardia, hyperkalemia, and elevations in serum creatinine occurred more frequently in the intensive treatment arm than in the standard therapy arm (Table 17.1).

Of note, the ACCORD BP and SPRINT trials targeted a similar systolic blood pressure <120 mmHg, but in contrast to SPRINT, the primary composite cardiovascular end point was nonsignificantly reduced in ACCORD BP. The results have been interpreted to be generally consistent between both trials, but ACCORD BP was viewed as underpowered due to the composite primary end point being less sensitive to blood pressure regulation.[33]

The more recent STEP trial assigned 8,511 patients aged 60–80 years with hypertension to a systolic blood pressure target of 110 to <130 mmHg (intensive treatment) or a target of 130 to <150 mmHg.[34] In this trial, the primary composite outcome of stroke, acute coronary syndrome, acute decompensated heart failure, coronary revascularization, atrial fibrillation, or death from cardiovascular causes was reduced by 26% in the intensive treatment group. In this trial, 18.9% of patients in the intensive treatment arm and 19.4% in the standard treatment arm had a diagnosis of type 2 diabetes. Hypotension occurred more frequently in the intensive treatment group (3.4%) compared with the standard treatment group (2.6%), without significant differences in other adverse events, including dizziness, syncope, or fractures.

In ADVANCE, 11,140 people with type 2 diabetes were randomized to receive either treatment with fixed combination perindopril/indapamide or matching placebo.[36] The primary end point, a composite of cardiovascular death, nonfatal stroke infarction, or worsening renal or diabetic eye disease, was reduced by 9% in the combination treatment. The achieved systolic blood pressure was ~135 mmHg in the treatment group and 140 mmHg in the placebo group.

The Hypertension Optimal Treatment (HOT) trial enrolled 18,790 patients and targeted diastolic blood pressure <90 mmHg, <85 mmHg, or <80 mmHg.[37] The cardiovascular event rates, defined as fatal or nonfatal MI, fatal and nonfatal strokes, and all other cardiovascular events, were not significantly different between diastolic blood pressure targets (≤90 mmHg, ≤85 mmHg, and ≤80 mmHg), although the lowest incidence of cardiovascular events occurred with an achieved diastolic blood pressure of 82 mmHg. However, in people with diabetes, there was a significant 51% reduction in the treatment group with a target diastolic blood pressure of <80 mmHg compared with a target diastolic blood pressure of <90 mmHg.

Meta-analyses of Trials

To clarify optimal blood pressure targets in people with diabetes, multiple meta-analyses have been performed. One of the largest meta-analyses included 73,913 people with diabetes. Compared with a less tight blood pressure control, allocation to a tighter blood pressure control significantly reduced the risk of stroke by 31% but did not reduce the risk of MI.[38] Another meta-analysis of 19 trials including 44,989 patients showed that a mean blood pressure of 133/76 mmHg is associated with a 14% risk reduction for major cardiovascular events compared with a mean blood pressure of 140/81 mmHg.[32] This benefit was greatest in people with diabetes. An analysis of trials including people with type 2 diabetes and impaired glucose tolerance with achieved systolic blood pressures of <135 mmHg in the intensive blood pressure treatment group and <140 mmHg in the standard treatment group revealed a 10% reduction in all-cause mortality and a 17% reduction in stroke.[30] More intensive reduction to <130 mmHg was associated with a further reduction in stroke but not other cardiovascular events.

Several meta-analyses stratified clinical trials by mean baseline blood pressure or mean blood pressure attained in the intervention (or intensive treatment) arm. Based on these analyses, antihypertensive treatment appears to be most beneficial when mean baseline blood pressure is ≥140/90 mmHg.[19,26,27,29–31] Among trials with lower baseline or attained blood pressure, antihypertensive treatment reduced the risk of stroke, retinopathy, and albuminuria, but effects on other ASCVD outcomes and heart failure were not evident.

Table 17.1—Randomized controlled trials of intensive versus standard hypertension treatment strategies

Clinical trial	Population	Intensive	Standard	Outcomes
ACCORD BP[35]	4,733 participants with T2D aged 40–79 years with prior evidence of CVD or multiple cardiovascular risk factors	SBP target: <120 mmHg Achieved (mean) SBP/DBP: 119.3/64.4 mmHg	SBP target: 130–140 mmHg Achieved (mean) SBP/DBP: 135/70.5 mmHg	■ No benefit in primary end point: composite of nonfatal MI, nonfatal stroke, and CVD death ■ Stroke risk reduced 41% with intensive control, not sustained through follow-up beyond the period of active treatment ■ Adverse events more common in intensive group, particularly elevated serum creatinine and electrolyte abnormalities
ADVANCE[36]	11,140 participants with T2D aged ≥55 years with prior evidence of CVD or multiple cardiovascular risk factors	Intervention: a single-pill, fixed-dose combination of perindopril and indapamide Achieved (mean) SBP/DBP: 136/73 mmHg	Control: placebo Achieved (mean) SBP/DBP: 141.6/75.2 mmHg	■ Intervention reduced risk of primary composite end point of major macrovascular and microvascular events (9%), death from any cause (14%), and death from CVD (18%) ■ 6-year observational follow-up found reduction in risk of death in intervention group attenuated but still significant[242]
HOT[37]	18,790 participants, including 1,501 with diabetes	DBP target: ≤80 mmHg Achieved (mean): 81.1 mmHg, ≤80 group; 85.2 mmHg, ≤90 group	DBP target: ≤90 mmHg	■ In the overall trial, there was no cardiovascular benefit with more intensive targets ■ In the subpopulation with diabetes, an intensive DBP target was associated with a significantly reduced risk (51%) of CVD events
SPRINT[43]	9,361 participants without diabetes	SBP target: <120 mmHg Achieved (mean): 121.4 mmHg	SBP target: <140 mmHg Achieved (mean): 136.2 mmHg	■ Intensive SBP target lowered risk of the primary composite outcome 25% (MI, ACS, stroke, heart failure, and death due to CVD) ■ Intensive target reduced risk of death 27% ■ Intensive therapy increased risks of electrolyte abnormalities and AKI

(continued)

Table 17.1 (continued)

Clinical trial	Population	Intensive	Standard	Outcomes
STEP[34]	8,511 participants aged 60–80 years, including 1,627 with diabetes	SBP target: <130 mmHg Achieved (mean): 127.5 mmHg	SBP target: <150 mmHg Achieved (mean): 135.3 mmHg	■ Intensive SBP target lowered risk of the primary composite outcome 26% (stroke, ACS [acute MI and hospitalization for unstable angina], acute decompensated heart failure, coronary revascularization, atrial fibrillation, or death from cardiovascular causes) ■ Intensive target reduced risk of cardiovascular death 28% ■ Intensive therapy increased risks of hypotension

ACCORD BP, Action to Control Cardiovascular Risk in Diabetes Blood Pressure trial; ACS, acute coronary syndrome; ADVANCE, Action in Diabetes and Vascular Disease: Preterax and Diamicron MR Controlled Evaluation; AKI, acute kidney injury; CVD, cardiovascular disease; DBP, diastolic blood pressure; HOT, Hypertension Optimal Treatment trial; MI, myocardial infarction; SBP, systolic blood pressure; SPRINT, Systolic Blood Pressure Intervention Trial; STEP, Strategy of Blood Pressure Intervention in the Elderly Hypertensive Patients; T2D, type 2 diabetes.

Individualization of Treatment Targets

Patients and clinicians should engage in a shared decision-making process to determine individual blood pressure targets.[19] This approach acknowledges that the benefits and risks of intensive blood pressure targets are uncertain and may vary across patients and is consistent with a patient-focused approach to care that values patient priorities and health care professional judgment.[39] Secondary analyses of ACCORD BP and SPRINT suggest that clinical factors can help determine individuals more likely to benefit and less likely to be harmed by intensive blood pressure control.[40,41]

Absolute benefit from blood pressure reduction correlated with absolute baseline cardiovascular risk in SPRINT and in earlier clinical trials conducted at higher baseline blood pressure levels.[13,41] Extrapolation of these studies suggests that people with diabetes may also be more likely to benefit from intensive blood pressure control when they have high absolute cardiovascular risk. This approach is consistent with guidelines from the American College of Cardiology and American Heart Association, which also advocate a blood pressure target of <130/80 mmHg for all people, with or without diabetes.[20]

Potential adverse effects of antihypertensive therapy (e.g., hypotension, syncope, falls, acute kidney injury, and electrolyte abnormalities) should also be taken into account.[33,35,42,43] Individuals with older age, CKD, and frailty have been shown to be at higher risk of adverse effects of intensive blood pressure control.[43] In addition, individuals with orthostatic hypotension, substantial comorbidity, functional limitations, or polypharmacy may be at high risk of adverse effects, and some patients may prefer higher blood pressure targets to enhance quality of life. However, in ACCORD BP, it was found that intensive blood pressure lowering decreased the risk of cardiovascular events irrespective of baseline diastolic blood pressure in patients who also received standard glycemic control.[44] Therefore, the presence of low diastolic blood pressure is not necessarily a contraindication to more intensive blood pressure management in the context of otherwise standard care.

Pregnancy and Antihypertensive Medications

There are few randomized controlled trials of antihypertensive therapy in pregnant individuals with diabetes. A 2014 Cochrane systematic review of antihypertensive therapy for mild to moderate chronic hypertension that included 49 trials and over 4,700 women did not find any conclusive evidence for or against blood pressure treatment to reduce the risk of preeclampsia for the mother or effects on perinatal outcomes such as preterm birth, small-for-gestational-age infants, or fetal death.[45] The Control of Hypertension in Pregnancy Study (CHIPS)[46] enrolled mostly women with chronic hypertension. In CHIPS, targeting a diastolic blood pressure of 85 mmHg during pregnancy was associated with reduced likelihood of developing accelerated maternal hypertension and no demonstrable adverse outcome for infants comparezd with targeting a higher diastolic blood pressure. The mean systolic blood pressure achieved in the more intensively treated group was 133.1 ± 0.5 mmHg, and the mean diastolic blood pressure achieved in that group was 85.3 ± 0.3 mmHg. A similar approach is supported by the International Society for the Study of Hypertension in Pregnancy, which specifically recommends use of antihypertensive therapy to maintain systolic blood pressure between 110 and 140 mmHg and diastolic blood pressure between 80 and 85 mmHg.[47]

The more recent Chronic Hypertension and Pregnancy (CHAP) trial assigned pregnant individuals with mild chronic hypertension to antihypertensive medications to target a blood pressure goal of <140/90 mmHg (active treatment group) or to control treatment, in which antihypertensive therapy was withheld unless severe hypertension (systolic pressure ≥160 mmHg or diastolic pressure ≥105 mmHg) developed (control group).[48] The primary outcome, a composite of preeclampsia with severe features, medically indicated preterm birth at <35 weeks of gestation, placental abruption, or fetal/neonatal death, occurred in 30.2% of female participants in the active treatment group vs. 37.0% in the control group ($P < 0.001$). The mean systolic blood pressure between randomization and delivery was 129.5 mmHg in the active treatment group and 132.6 mmHg in the control group.

Current evidence supports controlling blood pressure to 110–135/85 mmHg to reduce the risk xof accelerated maternal hypertension but also to minimize impairment of fetal growth. During pregnancy, treatment with ACE inhibitors, angiotensin receptor blockers (ARBs), and spironolactone are contraindicated as they may cause fetal damage. Special consideration should be taken for individuals of childbearing potential, and people intending to become pregnant should switch from an ACE inhibitor/ARB or spironolactone to an alternative antihypertensive medication approved during pregnancy. Antihypertensive drugs known to be effective and safe in pregnancy include methyldopa, labetalol, and long-acting nifedipine, while hydralzine may be considered in the acute management of hypertension in pregnancy or severe preeclampsia.[49] Diuretics are not recommended for blood pressure control in pregnancy but may be used during late-stage pregnancy if needed for volume control.[49,50] The American College of

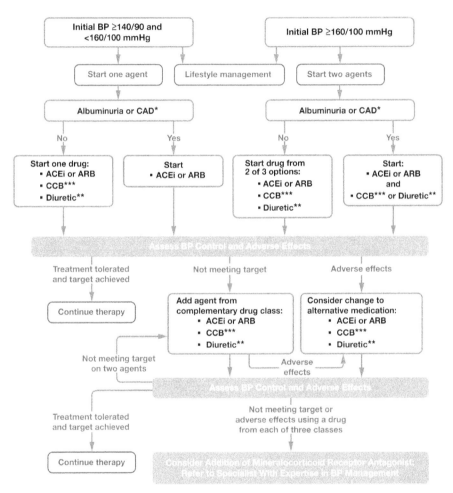

Figure 17.2—Recommendations for the treatment of confirmed hypertension in people with diabetes. *An ACE inhibitor (ACEi) or angiotensin receptor blocker (ARB) is suggested to treat hypertension for people with coronary artery disease (CAD) or urine albumin-to-creatinine ratio 30–299 mg/g creatinine and strongly recommended for individuals with urine albumin-to-creatinine ratio ≥300 mg/g creatinine. **Thiazide-like diuretic; long-acting agents shown to reduce cardiovascular events, such as chlorthalidone and indapamide, are preferred. ***Dihydropyridine calcium channel blocker (CCB). BP, blood pressure. Adapted from de Boer et al.[20]

Obstetricians and Gynecologists also recommends that postpartum individuals with gestational hypertension, preeclampsia, and superimposed preeclampsia have their blood pressures observed for 72 h in the hospital and for 7–10 days postpartum. Long-term follow-up is recommended for these individuals as they have increased lifetime cardiovascular risk.[51] See Section 15, "Management of Diabetes in Pregnancy," for additional information.

TREATMENT STRATEGIES

Lifestyle Intervention

Recommendation

10.6   For people with blood pressure >120/80 mmHg, lifestyle intervention consists of weight loss when indicated, a Dietary Approaches to Stop Hypertension (DASH)-style eating pattern including reducing sodium and increasing potassium intake, moderation of alcohol intake, and increased physical activity. **A**

Lifestyle management is an important component of hypertension treatment because it lowers blood pressure, enhances the effectiveness of some antihypertensive medications, promotes other aspects of metabolic and vascular health, and generally leads to few adverse effects. Lifestyle therapy consists of reducing excess body weight through caloric restriction (see Section 8, "Obesity and Weight Management for the Prevention and Treatment of Type 2 Diabetes"), at least 150 min of moderate-intensity aerobic activity per week (see Section 3, "Prevention or Delay of Type 2 Diabetes and Associated Comorbidities"), restricting sodium intake (<2,300 mg/day), increasing consumption of fruits and vegetables (8–10 servings per day) and low-fat dairy products (2–3 servings per day), avoiding excessive alcohol consumption (no more than 2 servings per day in men and no more than 1 serving per day in women),[52] and increasing activity levels[53] (see Section 5, "Facilitating Positive Health Behaviors and Well-being to Improve Health Outcomes").

These lifestyle interventions are reasonable for individuals with diabetes and mildly elevated blood pressure (systolic >120 mmHg or diastolic >80 mmHg) and should be initiated along with pharmacologic therapy when hypertension is diagnosed (Fig. 17.2).[53] A lifestyle therapy plan should be developed in collaboration with the patient and discussed as part of diabetes management. Use of internet or mobile-based digital platforms to reinforce healthy behaviors may be considered as a component of care, as these interventions have been found to enhance the efficacy of medical therapy for hypertension.[54,55]

Pharmacologic Interventions

Recommendations

10.7   Individuals with confirmed office-based blood pressure ≥130/80 mmHg qualify for initiation and titration of pharmacologic therapy to achieve the recommended blood pressure goal of <130/80 mmHg. **A**

10.8   Individuals with confirmed office-based blood pressure ≥160/100 mmHg should, in addition to lifestyle therapy, have prompt initiation and timely titration of two drugs or a single-pill combination of drugs demonstrated to reduce cardiovascular events in people with diabetes. **A**

10.9   Treatment for hypertension should include drug classes demonstrated to reduce cardiovascular events in people with diabetes. **A** ACE inhibitors or angiotensin receptor blockers are recommended first-line therapy for hypertension in people with diabetes and coronary artery disease. **A**

10.10   Multiple-drug therapy is generally required to achieve blood pressure targets. However, combinations of ACE inhibitors and angiotensin receptor blockers and combinations of ACE inhibitors or angiotensin receptor blockers with direct renin inhibitors should not be used. **A**

10.11   An ACE inhibitor or angiotensin receptor blocker, at the maximum tolerated dose indicated for blood pressure treatment, is the recommended first-line treatment for hypertension in people with diabetes and urinary albumin-to-creatinine ratio ≥300 mg/g creatinine **A** or 30–299 mg/g creatinine. **B** If one class is not tolerated, the other should be substituted. **B**

10.12   For patients treated with an ACE inhibitor, angiotensin receptor blocker, or diuretic, serum creatinine/estimated glomerular filtration rate and serum potassium levels should be monitored at least annually. **B**

Initial Number of Antihypertensive Medications. Initial treatment for people with diabetes depends on the severity of hypertension (Fig. 17.2). Those with blood pressure between 130/80 mmHg and 160/100 mmHg may begin with a single drug. For patients with blood pressure ≥160/100 mmHg, initial pharmacologic treatment with two antihypertensive medications is recommended in order to more effectively achieve adequate blood pressure control.[56–58] Single-pill antihypertensive combinations may improve medication taking in some patients.[59]

Classes of Antihypertensive Medications. Initial treatment for hypertension should include any of the drug classes demonstrated to reduce cardiovascular events in people with diabetes: ACE inhibitors,[60,61] ARBs,[60,61] thiazide-like diuretics,[62] or dihydropyridine calcium channel blockers.[63] In people with diabetes and established coronary artery disease, ACE inhibitors or ARBs are recommended first-line therapy for hypertension.[64–66] For patients with albuminuria (urine albumin-to-creatinine ratio [UACR] ≥30 mg/g), initial treatment should include an ACE inhibitor or ARB to reduce the risk of progressive kidney disease[20] (Fig. 17.2). In patients receiving ACE inhibitor or ARB therapy, continuation of those medications as kidney function declines to estimated glomerular filtration rate (eGFR) <30 mL/min/1.73 m^2 may provide cardiovascular benefit without significantly increasing the risk of end-stage kidney disease.[67] In the absence of albuminuria, risk of progressive kidney disease is low, and ACE inhibitors and ARBs have not been found to afford superior cardioprotection when compared with thiazide-like diuretics or dihydropyridine calcium channel blockers.[68] β-Blockers are indicated in the setting of prior MI, active angina, or HfrEF but have not been shown to reduce mortality as blood pressure-lowering agents in the absence of these conditions.[28,69,70]

Multiple-Drug Therapy. Multiple-drug therapy is often required to achieve blood pressure targets (Fig. 17.2), particularly in the setting of diabetic kidney disease. However, the use of both ACE inhibitors and ARBs in combination, or the combination of an ACE inhibitor or ARB and a direct renin inhibitor, is contraindicated given the lack of added ASCVD benefit and increased rate of adverse events—namely, hyperkalemia, syncope, and acute kidney injury (AKI).[71–73] Titration of and/or addition of further blood pressure medications should be made in a timely fashion to overcome therapeutic inertia in achieving blood pressure targets.

Bedtime Dosing. Although prior analyses of randomized clinical trials found a benefit to evening versus morning dosing of antihypertensive medications,[74,75] these results have not been reproduced in subsequent trials. Therefore, preferential use of antihypertensives at bedtime is not recommended.[76]

Hyperkalemia and Acute Kidney Injury. Treatment with ACE inhibitors or ARBs can cause AKI and hyperkalemia, while diuretics can cause AKI and either hypokalemia or hyperkalemia (depending on mechanism of action).[77,78] Detection and management of these abnormalities is important because AKI and hyperkalemia each increase the risks of cardiovascular events and death.[79] Therefore, serum creatinine and potassium should be monitored during treatment with an ACE inhibitor, ARB, or diuretic, particularly among patients with reduced glomerular filtration who are at increased risk of hyperkalemia and AKI.[77,78,80]

Resistant Hypertension

Recommendation

10.13 Individuals with hypertension who are not meeting blood pressure targets on three classes of antihypertensive medications (including a diuretic) should be considered for mineralocorticoid receptor antagonist therapy. **A**

Resistant hypertension is defined as blood pressure ≥140/90 mmHg despite a therapeutic strategy that includes appropriate lifestyle management plus a diuretic and two other antihypertensive drugs with complementary mechanisms of action at adequate doses. Prior to diagnosing resistant hypertension, a number of other conditions should be excluded, including missed doses of antihypertensive medi-

Table 17.2—High-Intensity and Moderate-Intensity Statin Therapy*

High-intensity statin therapy (lowers LDL cholesterol by ≥50%)	Moderate-intensity statin therapy (lowers LDL cholesterol by 30–49%)
Atorvastatin 40–80 mg	Atorvastatin 10–20 mg
Rosuvastatin 20–40 mg	Rosuvastatin 5–10 mg
	Simvastatin 20–40 mg
	Pravastatin 40–80 mg
	Lovastatin 40 mg
	Fluvastatin XL 80 mg
	Pitavastatin 1–4 mg

*Once-daily dosing. XL, extended release.

cations, white coat hypertension, and secondary hypertension. In general, barriers to medication taking (such as cost and side effects) should be identified and addressed (Fig. 17.2). Mineralocorticoid receptor antagonists, including spirono-lactone and eplerenone, are effective for management of resistant hypertension in people with type 2 diabetes when added to existing treatment with an ACE inhib-itor or ARB, thiazide-like diuretic, or dihydropyridine calcium channel blocker.[81] In addition, mineralocorticoid receptor antagonists reduce albuminuria in people with diabetic nephropathy.[82–84] However, adding a mineralocorticoid receptor antagonist to a regimen including an ACE inhibitor or ARB may increase the risk for hyperkalemia, emphasizing the importance of regular monitoring for serum creatinine and potassium in these patients, and long-term outcome studies are needed to better evaluate the role of mineralocorticoid receptor antagonists in blood pressure management.

LIPID MANAGEMENT

Lifestyle Intervention

Recommendations

10.14 Lifestyle modification focusing on weight loss (if indicated); application of a Mediterranean or Dietary Approaches to Stop Hypertension (DASH) eating pattern; reduction of saturated fat and *trans* fat; increase of dietary n-3 fatty acids, viscous fiber, and plant stanols/sterols intake; and increased physical activity should be recommended to improve the lipid profile and reduce the risk of developing atherosclerotic cardiovascular disease in people with diabetes. **A**

10.15 Intensify lifestyle therapy and optimize glycemic control for patients with elevated triglyceride levels(≥150mg/dL[1.7mmol/L]) and/or low HDL cholesterol (<40 mg/dL [1.0 mmol/L] for men, <50 mg/dL [1.3 mmol/L] for women). **C**

Lifestyle intervention, including weight loss in people with overweight or obesity (when appropriate),[85] increased physical activity, and medical nutrition therapy, allows some patients to reduce ASCVD risk factors. Nutrition interven-tion should be tailored according to each patient's age, pharmacologic treatment, lipid levels, and medical conditions.

Recommendations should focus on application of a Mediterranean[83] or Dietary Approaches to Stop Hypertension (DASH) eating pattern, reducing satu-rated and *trans* fat intake and increasing plant stanols/sterols, n-3 fatty acids, and viscous fiber (such as in oats, legumes, and citrus) intake.[86,87] Glycemic control may also beneficially modify plasma lipid levels, particularly in patients with very high triglycerides and poor glycemic control. See Section 5, "Facilitating Positive Health Behaviors and Well-being to Improve Health Outcomes," for additional nutrition information.

Ongoing Therapy and Monitoring With Lipid Panel

Recommendations

10.16 In adults not taking statins or other lipid-lowering therapy, it is reasonable to obtain a lipid profile at the time of diabetes diagnosis, at an initial medical evaluation, and every 5 years thereafter if under the age of 40 years, or more frequently if indicated. **E**

10.17 Obtain a lipid profile at initiation of statins or other lipid-lowering therapy, 4–12 weeks after initiation or a change in dose, and annually thereafter as it may help to monitor the response to therapy and inform medication taking. **E**

In adults with diabetes, it is reasonable to obtain a lipid profile (total cholesterol, LDL cholesterol, HDL cholesterol, and triglycerides) at the time of diagnosis, at the initial medical evaluation, and at least every 5 years thereafter in patients <40 years of age. In younger people with longer duration of disease (such as those with youth-onset type 1 diabetes), more frequent lipid profiles may be reasonable. A lipid panel should also be obtained immediately before initiating statin therapy. Once a patient is taking a statin, LDL cholesterol levels should be assessed 4–12 weeks after initiation of statin therapy, after any change in dose, and on an individual basis (e.g., to monitor for medication taking and efficacy). If LDL cholesterol levels are not responding in spite of medication taking, clinical judgment is recommended to determine the need for and timing of lipid panels. In individual patients, the highly variable LDL cholesterol–lowering response seen with statins is poorly understood.[88] Clinicians should attempt to find a dose or alternative statin that is tolerable if side effects occur. There is evidence for benefit from even extremely low, less than daily statin doses.[89]

STATIN TREATMENT

Primary Prevention

Recommendations

10.18 For people with diabetes aged 40–75 years without atherosclerotic cardiovascular disease, use moderate-intensity statin therapy in addition to lifestyle therapy. **A**

10.19 For people with diabetes aged 20–39 years with additional atherosclerotic cardiovascular disease risk factors, it may be reasonable to initiate statin therapy in addition to lifestyle therapy. **C**

10.20 For people with diabetes aged 40–75 at higher cardiovascular risk, including those with one or more atherosclerotic cardiovascular disease risk factors, it is recommended to use high-intensity statin therapy to reduce LDL cholesterol by ≥50% of baseline and to target an LDL cholesterol goal of <70 mg/dL. **B**

10.21 For people with diabetes aged 40–75 years at higher cardiovascular risk, especially those with multiple atherosclerotic cardiovascular disease risk factors and an LDL cholesterol ≥70 mg/dL, it may be reasonable to add ezetimibe or a PCSK9 inhibitor to maximum tolerated statin therapy. **C**

10.22 In adults with diabetes aged >75 years already on statin therapy, it is reasonable to continue statin treatment. **B**

10.23 In adults with diabetes aged >75 years, it may be reasonable to initiate moderate-intensity statin therapy after discussion of potential benefits and risks. **C**

10.24 Statin therapy is contraindicated in pregnancy. **B**

Secondary Prevention

Recommendations

10.25 For people of all ages with diabetes and atherosclerotic cardiovascular disease, high-intensity statin therapy should be added to lifestyle therapy. **A**

10.26 For people with diabetes and atherosclerotic cardiovascular disease, treatment with high-intensity statin therapy is recommended to target an LDL cholesterol reduction of ≥50% from baseline and an LDL cholesterol goal of <55 mg/dL. Addition of ezetimibe or a PCSK9 inhibitor with proven benefit in this population is recommended if this goal is not achieved on maximum tolerated statin therapy. **B**

10.27 For individuals who do not tolerate the intended intensity, the maximum tolerated statin dose should be used. **E**

Initiating Statin Therapy Based on Risk

People with type 2 diabetes have an increased prevalence of lipid abnormalities, contributing to their high risk of ASCVD. Multiple clinical trials have demonstrated the beneficial effects of statin therapy on ASCVD outcomes in subjects with and without CHD.[90,91] Subgroup analyses of people with diabetes in larger trials[92–96] and trials in people with diabetes[97,98] showed significant primary and secondary prevention of ASCVD events and CHD death in people with diabetes. Meta-analyses, including data from over 18,000 people with diabetes from 14 randomized trials of statin therapy (mean follow-up 4.3 years), demonstrate a 9% proportional reduction in all-cause mortality and 13% reduction in vascular mortality for each 1 mmol/L (39 mg/dL) reduction in LDL cholesterol.[99] The cardiovascular benefit in this large meta-analysis did not depend on baseline LDL cholesterol levels and was linearly related to the LDL cholesterol reduction without a low threshold beyond which there was no benefit observed.[99]

Accordingly, statins are the drugs of choice for LDL cholesterol lowering and cardioprotection. Table 17.2 shows the two statin dosing intensities that are recommended for use in clinical practice: high-intensity statin therapy will achieve approximately a ≥50% reduction in LDL cholesterol, and moderate-intensity statin regimens achieve 30–49% reductions in LDL cholesterol. Low-dose statin therapy is generally not recommended in people with diabetes but is sometimes the only dose of statin that a patient can tolerate. For patients who do not tolerate the intended intensity of statin, the maximum tolerated statin dose should be used.

As in those without diabetes, absolute reductions in ASCVD outcomes (CHD death and nonfatal MI) are greatest in people with high baseline ASCVD risk (known ASCVD and/or very high LDL cholesterol levels), but the overall benefits of statin therapy in people with diabetes at moderate or even low risk for ASCVD are convincing.[100,101] The relative benefit of lipid-lowering therapy has been uniform across most subgroups tested,[91,99] including subgroups that varied with respect to age and other risk factors.

Primary Prevention (People Without ASCVD)

For primary prevention, moderate-dose statin therapy is recommended for those aged ≥40 years,[93,100,101] although high-intensity therapy should be considered in the context of additional ASCVD risk factors. The evidence is strong for people with diabetes aged 40–75 years, an age-group well represented in statin trials showing benefit. Since cardiovascular risk is enhanced in people with diabetes, as noted above, patients who also have multiple other coronary risk factors have increased risk, equivalent to that of those with ASCVD. Therefore, current guidelines recommend that in people with diabetes who are at higher cardiovascular risk, especially those with one or more ASCVD risk factors, high-intensity statin therapy should be prescribed to reduce LDL cholesterol by ≥50% from baseline and to target an LDL cholesterol of <70 mg/dL.[102–104] Since in clinical practice it is frequently difficult to ascertain the baseline LDL cholesterol level prior to statin therapy initiation, in those individuals, a focus on an LDL cholesterol target level of <70 mg/dL rather than the percent reduction in LDL cholesterol is recommended. In those individuals, it may also be reasonable to add ezetimibe or proprotein convertase subtilisin/kexin type 9 (PCSK9) inhibitor therapy to maximum tolerated statin therapy if needed to reduce LDL cholesterol levels by ≥50% and to achieve the recommended LDL cholesterol target of <70 mg/dL.[14] The evidence is lower for patients aged >75 years; relatively few older people with diabetes have been enrolled in primary prevention trials. However, heterogeneity by age has not been seen in the relative benefit of lipid-lowering therapy in trials that included older participants,[91,98,99] and because older age confers higher risk, the absolute benefits are actually greater.[91,105] Moderate-intensity statin therapy is recommended in people with diabetes who are ≥75 years of age. However, the risk-benefit profile should be routinely evaluated in this population, with downward titration of dose performed as needed. See Section 13, "Older Adults," for more details on clinical considerations for this population.

Age <40 Years and/or Type 1 Diabetes. Very little clinical trial evidence exists for people with type 2 diabetes under the age of 40 years or for people with type diabetes of any age. For pediatric recommendations, see Section 14, "Children and Adolescents." In the Heart Protection Study (lower age limit 40 years), the subgroup of ~600 people with type 1 diabetes had a proportionately similar, although not statistically significant, reduction in risk to that in people with type 2 diabetes.[93] Even though the data are not definitive, similar statin treatment approaches should be considered for people with type 1 or type 2 diabetes, particularly in the presence of other cardiovascular risk factors. Patients <40 years of age have lower risk of developing a cardiovascular event over a 10-year horizon; however, their lifetime risk of developing cardiovascular disease and suffering an MI, stroke, or cardiovascular death is high. For people who are <40 years of age and/or have type 1 diabetes with other ASCVD risk factors, it is recommended that the patient and health care professional discuss the relative benefits and risks and consider the use of moderate-intensity statin therapy. Please refer to "Type 1 Diabetes Mellitus and Cardiovascular Disease: A Scientific Statement From the American Heart Association and American Diabetes Association"[106] for additional discussion.

Secondary Prevention (People With ASCVD)

Because cardiovascular event rates are increased in people with diabetes and established ASCVD, intensive therapy is indicated and has been shown to be of benefit in multiple large meta-analyses and randomized cardiovascular outcomes trials.[91,99,105,107,108] High-intensity statin therapy is recommended for all people with diabetes and ASCVD to target an LDL cholesterol reduction of ≥50% from baseline and an LDL cholesterol goal of <55 mg/dL. Based on the evidence discussed below, addition of ezetimibe or a PCSK9 inhibitor is recommended if this goal is not achieved on maximum tolerated statin therapy. These recommendations are based on the observation that high-intensity versus moderate-intensity statin therapy reduces cardiovascular event rates in high-risk individuals with established cardiovascular disease in randomized trials.[95,107] In addition, the Cholesterol Treatment Trialists' Collaboration involving 26 statin trials, of which 5 compared high-intensity versus moderate-intensity statins,[99] showed a 21% reduction in major cardiovascular events in people with diabetes for every 39 mg/dL of LDL cholesterol lowering, irrespective of baseline LDL cholesterol or patient characteristics.[99] However, the best evidence to support lower LDL cholesterol targets in people with diabetes and established cardiovascular disease derives from multiple large randomized trials investigating the benefits of adding nonstatin agents to statin therapy. As discussed in detail below, these include combination treatment with statins and ezetimibe[105,109] or PCSK9 inhibitors.[108,110–112] Each trial found a significant benefit in the reduction of ASCVD events that was directly related to the degree of further LDL cholesterol lowering. These large trials included a significant number of participants with diabetes and prespecified analyses on cardiovascular outcomes in people with and without diabetes.[109,111,112] The decision to add a nonstatin agent should be made following a clinician-patient discussion about the net benefit, safety, and cost of combination therapy.

Combination Therapy for LDL Cholesterol Lowering

Statins and Ezetimibe

The IMProved Reduction of Outcomes: Vytorin Efficacy International Trial (IMPROVE-IT) was a randomized controlled trial in 18,144 patients comparing the addition of ezetimibe to simvastatin therapy versus simvastatin alone.[105] Individuals were ≥50 years of age, had experienced a recent acute coronary syndrome (ACS) and were treated for an average of 6 years. Overall, the addition of ezetimibe led to a 6.4% relative benefit and a 2% absolute reduction in major adverse cardiovascular events (atherosclerotic cardiovascular events), with the degree of benefit being directly proportional to the change in LDL cholesterol, which was 70 mg/dL in the statin group on average and 54 mg/dL in the combination group.[105] In those with diabetes (27% of participants), the combination of moderate-intensity simvastatin (40 mg) and ezetimibe (10 mg) showed a significant reduction of major adverse cardiovascular events with an absolute risk reduction of 5% (40% vs. 45% cumulative incidence at 7 years) and a relative risk reduction of 14% (hazard ratio [HR] 0.86 [95% CI 0.78–0.94]) over moderate-intensity simvastatin (40 mg) alone.[109]

Statins and PCSK9 Inhibitors

Placebo-controlled trials evaluating the addition of the PCSK9 inhibitors evolocumab and alirocumab to maximum tolerated doses of statin therapy in participants who were at high risk for ASCVD demonstrated an average reduction in LDL cholesterol ranging from 36 to 59%. These agents have been approved as adjunctive therapy for individuals with ASCVD or familial hypercholesterolemia who are receiving maximum tolerated statin therapy but require additional lowering of LDL cholesterol.[113,114] No cardiovascular outcome trials have been performed to assess whether PCSK9 inhibitor therapy reduces ASCVD event rates in individuals without established cardiovascular disease (primary prevention).

The effects of PCSK9 inhibition on ASCVD outcomes was investigated in the Further Cardiovascular Outcomes Research With PCSK9 Inhibition in Subjects With Elevated Risk (FOURIER) trial, which enrolled 27,564 individuals with prior ASCVD and an additional high-risk feature who were receiving their maximum tolerated statin therapy (two-thirds were on high-intensity statin) but who still had LDL cholesterol ≥70 mg/dL or non-HDL cholesterol ≥100 mg/dL.[108] Patients were randomized to receive subcutaneous injections of evolocumab (either 140 mg every 2 weeks or 420 mg every month based on patient preference) versus placebo. Evolocumab reduced LDL cholesterol by 59% from a median of 92 to 30 mg/dL in the treatment arm.

During the median follow-up of 2.2 years, the composite outcome of cardiovascular death, MI, stroke, hospitalization for angina, or revascularization occurred in 11.3% vs. 9.8% of the placebo and evolocumab groups, respectively, representing a 15% relative risk reduction ($P < 0.001$). The combined end point of cardiovascular death, MI, or stroke was reduced by 20%, from 7.4 to 5.9% ($P < 0.001$). Evolocumab therapy also significantly reduced all strokes (1.5% vs. 1.9%; HR 0.79 [95% CI 0.66–0.95]; $P = 0.01$) and ischemic stroke (1.2% vs. 1.6%; HR 0.75 [95% CI 0.62–0.92]; $P = 0.005$) in the total population, with findings being consistent in individuals with or without a history of ischemic stroke at baseline.[115] Importantly, similar benefits were seen in a prespecified subgroup of people with diabetes, comprising 11,031 patients (40% of the trial).[112]

In the ODYSSEY OUTCOMES trial (Evaluation of Cardiovascular Outcomes After an Acute Coronary Syndrome During Treatment With Alirocumab), 18,924 patients (28.8% of whom had diabetes) with recent acute coronary syndrome were randomized to the PCSK9 inhibitor alirocumab or placebo every 2 weeks in addition to maximum tolerated statin therapy, with alirocumab dosing titrated between 75 and 150 mg to achieve LDL cholesterol levels between 25 and 50 mg/dL.[110] Over a median follow-up of 2.8 years, a composite primary end point (comprising death from CHD, nonfatal MI, fatal or nonfatal ischemic stroke, or unstable angina requiring hospital admission) occurred in 903 patients (9.5%) in the alirocumab group and in 1,052 patients (11.1%) in the placebo group (HR 0.85 [95% CI 0.78–0.93]; $P < 0.001$). Combination therapy with alirocumab plus statin therapy resulted in a greater absolute reduction in the incidence of the primary end point in people with diabetes (2.3% [95% CI 0.4–4.2]) than in those with prediabetes (1.2% [0.0–2.4]) or normoglycemia (1.2% [–0.3 to 2.7]).[111]

In addition to monoclonal antibodies targeting PCSK9, the siRNA inclisiran has been developed and has recently become available in the U.S. In the Inclisiran for Participants With Atherosclerotic Cardiovascular Disease and Elevated Low-density Lipoprotein Cholesterol (ORION-10) and Inclisiran for Subjects With ASCVD or ASCVD-Risk Equivalents and Elevated Low-density Lipoprotein Cholesterol (ORION-11) trials,[116] individuals with established cardiovascular disease or ASCVD risk equivalent were randomized to receive inclisiran or placebo. Inclisiran allows less frequent administration compared with monoclonal antibodies and was administered on day 1, on day 90, and every 6 months in these trials. In the ORION-10 trial, 47.5% of patients in the inclisiran group and 42.4% in the placebo group had diabetes; in the ORION-11 trial, 36.5% of patients in the inclisiran group and 33.7% in the placebo group had diabetes. The coprimary end point of placebo-corrected percentage change in LDL cholesterol level from baseline to day 510 was 52.3% in the ORION-10 trial and 49.9% in the ORION-11 trial. In an exploratory analysis, the prespecified cardiovascular end point, defined as a cardiovascular basket of nonadjudicated terms, including those classified within cardiac death, and any signs or symptoms of cardiac arrest, nonfatal MI, or stroke, occurred in 7.4% of the inclisiran group and 10.2% of the placebo group in the ORION-10 trial and in 7.8% of the inclisiran group and 10.3% of the placebo group in the ORION-11 trial. A cardiovascular outcome trial using inclisiran in people with established cardiovascular disease is currently ongoing.[117]

Statins and Bempedoic Acid

Bempedoic acid is a novel LDL cholesterol–lowering agent that is indicated as an adjunct to diet and maximum tolerated statin therapy for the treatment of adults with heterozygous familial hypercholesterolemia or established ASCVD who require additional lowering of LDL cholesterol. A pooled analysis suggests that bempedoic acid therapy lowers LDL cholesterol levels by about 23% compared with placebo.[118] At this time, there are no completed trials demonstrating a cardiovascular outcomes benefit to use of this medication; however, this agent may be considered for patients who cannot use or tolerate other evidence-based LDL cholesterol-lowering approaches, or for whom those other therapies are inadequately effective.[119]

Treatment of Other Lipoprotein Fractions or Targets

Recommendations

10.28 For individuals with fasting triglyceride levels ≥500 mg/dL, evaluate for secondary causes of hypertriglyceridemia and consider medical therapy to reduce the risk of pancreatitis. **C**

10.29 In adults with moderate hypertriglyceridemia (fasting or nonfasting triglycerides 175–499 mg/dL), clinicians should address and treat lifestyle factors (obesity and metabolic syndrome), secondary factors (diabetes, chronic liver or kidney disease and/or nephrotic syndrome, hypothyroidism), and medications that raise triglycerides. **C**

10.30 In individuals with atherosclerotic cardiovascular disease or other cardiovascular risk factors on a statin with controlled LDL cholesterol but elevated triglycerides (135–499 mg/dL), the addition of icosapent ethyl can be considered to reduce cardiovascular risk. **A**

Hypertriglyceridemia should be addressed with dietary and lifestyle changes including weight loss and abstinence from alcohol.[120] Severe hypertriglyceridemia (fasting triglycerides ≥500 mg/dL and especially >1,000 mg/dL) may warrant pharmacologic therapy (fibric acid derivatives and/or fish oil) and reduction in dietary fat to reduce the risk of acute pancreatitis. Moderate- or high-intensity statin therapy should also be used as indicated to reduce risk of cardiovascular events (see statin treatment). In people with moderate hypertriglyceridemia, lifestyle interventions, treatment of secondary factors, and avoidance of medications that might raise triglycerides are recommended.

The Reduction of Cardiovascular Events with Icosapent Ethyl-Intervention Trial (REDUCE-IT) enrolled 8,179 adults receiving statin therapy with moderately elevated triglycerides (135–499 mg/dL, median baseline of 216 mg/dL) who had either established cardiovascular disease (secondary prevention cohort) or diabetes plus at least one other cardiovascular risk factor (primary prevention cohort).[121] Patients were randomized to icosapent ethyl 4 g/day (2 g twice daily with food) versus placebo. The trial met its primary end point, demonstrating a 25% relative risk reduction (*P* < 0.001) for the primary end point composite of cardiovascular death, nonfatal MI, nonfatal stroke, coronary revascularization, or unstable angina. This reduction in risk was seen in people with or without diabetes at baseline. The composite of cardiovascular death, nonfatal MI, or nonfatal stroke was reduced by 26% (*P* < 0.001). Additional ischemic end points were significantly lower in the icosapent ethyl group than in the placebo group, including cardiovascular death, which was reduced by 20% (*P* = 0.03). The proportions of patients experiencing adverse events and serious adverse events were similar between the active and placebo treatment groups. It should be noted that data are lacking with other n-3 fatty acids, and results of the REDUCE-IT trial should not be extrapolated to other products.[121] As an example, the addition of 4 g per day of a carboxylic acid formulation of the n-3 fatty acids eicosapentaenoic acid (EPA) and docosahexaenoic acid (DHA) (n-3 carboxylic acid) to statin therapy in patients with atherogenic dyslipidemia and high cardiovascular risk, 70% of whom had diabetes, did not reduce the risk of major adverse cardiovascular events compared with the inert comparator of corn oil.[122]

Low levels of HDL cholesterol, often associated with elevated triglyceride levels, are the most prevalent pattern of dyslipidemia in people with type 2 diabetes. However, the evidence for the use of drugs that target these lipid fractions is substantially less robust than that for statin therapy.[123] In a large trial in people with diabetes, fenofibrate failed to reduce overall cardiovascular outcomes.[124]

Other Combination Therapy

Recommendations

10.31 Statin plus fibrate combination therapy has not been shown to improve atherosclerotic cardiovascular disease outcomes and is generally not recommended. **A**

10.32 Statin plus niacin combination therapy has not been shown to provide additional cardiovascular benefit above statin therapy alone, may increase the risk of stroke with additional side effects, and is generally not recommended. **A**

Statin and Fibrate Combination Therapy

Combination therapy (statin and fibrate) is associated with an increased risk for abnormal transaminase levels, myositis, and rhabdomyolysis. The risk of rhabdomyolysis is more common with higher doses of statins and renal insufficiency and appears to be higher when statins are combined with gemfibrozil (compared with fenofibrate).[125]

In the ACCORD study, in people with type 2 diabetes who were at high risk for ASCVD, the combination of fenofibrate and simvastatin did not reduce the rate of fatal cardiovascular events, nonfatal MI, or nonfatal stroke compared with simvastatin alone. Prespecified subgroup analyses suggested heterogeneity in treatment effects with possible benefit for men with both a triglyceride level ≥204 mg/dL (2.3 mmol/L) and an HDL cholesterol level ≤34 mg/dL (0.9 mmol/L).[126]

Statin and Niacin Combination Therapy

The Atherothrombosis Intervention in Metabolic Syndrome With Low HDL/High Triglycerides: Impact on Global Health Outcomes (AIM-HIGH) trial randomized over 3,000 people (about one-third with diabetes) with established ASCVD, LDL cholesterol levels <180 mg/dL [4.7 mmol/L], low HDL cholesterol levels (men <40 mg/dL [1.0 mmol/L] and women <50 mg/dL [1.3 mmol/L]), and triglyceride levels of 150–400 mg/dL (1.7–4.5 mmol/L) to statin therapy plus extended-release niacin or placebo. The trial was halted early due to lack of efficacy on the primary ASCVD outcome (first event of the composite of death from CHD, nonfatal MI, ischemic stroke, hospitalization for an ACS, or symptom-driven coronary or cerebral revascularization) and a possible increase in ischemic stroke in those on combination therapy.[127]

The much larger Heart Protection Study 2–Treatment of HDL to Reduce the Incidence of Vascular Events (HPS2-THRIVE) trial also failed to show a benefit of adding niacin to background statin therapy.[128] A total of 25,673 individuals with prior vascular disease were randomized to receive 2 g of extended-release niacin and 40 mg of laropiprant (an antagonist of the prostaglandin D2 receptor DP1 that has been shown to improve participation in niacin therapy) versus a matching placebo daily and followed for a median follow-up period of 3.9 years. There was no significant difference in the rate of coronary death, MI, stroke, or coronary revascularization with the addition of niacin–laropiprant versus placebo (13.2% vs. 13.7%; rate ratio 0.96; $P = 0.29$). Niacin–laropiprant was associated with an increased incidence of new-onset diabetes (absolute excess, 1.3 percentage points; $P < 0.001$) and disturbances in diabetes management among those with diabetes. In addition, there was an increase in serious adverse events associated with the gastrointestinal system, musculoskeletal system, skin, and, unexpectedly, infection and bleeding.

Therefore, combination therapy with a statin and niacin is not recommended given the lack of efficacy on major ASCVD outcomes and increased side effects.

Diabetes Risk With Statin Use

Several studies have reported a modestly increased risk of incident diabetes with statin use,[129,130] which may be limited to those with diabetes risk factors. An analysis of one of the initial studies suggested that although statin use was associated with diabetes risk, the cardiovascular event rate reduction with statins far outweighed the risk of incident diabetes even for patients at highest risk for diabetes.[131] The absolute risk increase was small (over 5 years of follow-up, 1.2% of participants on placebo developed diabetes and 1.5% on rosuvastatin developed diabetes).[131] A meta-analysis of 13 randomized statin trials with 91,140 participants showed an odds ratio of 1.09 for a new diagnosis of diabetes, so that (on average) treatment of 255 patients with statins for 4 years resulted in one additional case of diabetes while simultaneously preventing 5.4 vascular events among those 255 patients.[130]

Lipid-Lowering Agents and Cognitive Function

Although concerns regarding a potential adverse impact of lipid-lowering agents on cognitive function have been raised, several lines of evidence point against this association, as detailed in a 2018 European Atherosclerosis Society Consensus Panel statement.[132] First, there are three large randomized trials of statin versus placebo where specific cognitive tests were performed, and no differences were seen between statin and placebo.[133-136] In addition, no change in cognitive function has been reported in studies with the addition of ezetimibe[105] or PCSK9 inhibitors[108,137] to statin therapy, including among patients treated to very low LDL cholesterol levels. In addition, the most recent systematic review of the U.S. Food and Drug Administration's (FDA's) postmarketing surveillance databases, randomized controlled trials, and cohort, case-control, and cross-sectional studies evaluating cognition in patients receiving statins found that published data do not reveal an adverse effect of statins on cognition.[138] Therefore, a concern that statins or other lipid-lowering agents might cause cognitive dysfunction or dementia is not currently supported by evidence and should not deter their use in individuals with diabetes at high risk for ASCVD.[138]

ANTIPLATELET AGENTS

Recommendations

10.33 Use aspirin therapy (75–162 mg/day) as a secondary prevention strategy in those with diabetes and a history of atherosclerotic cardiovascular disease. **A**

10.34 For individuals with atherosclerotic cardiovascular disease and documented aspirin allergy, clopidogrel (75 mg/day) should be used. **B**

10.35 Dual antiplatelet therapy (with low-dose aspirin and a P2Y12 inhibitor) is reasonable for a year after an acute coronary syndrome and may have benefits beyond this period. **A**

10.36 Long-term treatment with dual antiplatelet therapy should be considered for individuals with prior coronary intervention, high ischemic risk, and low bleeding risk to prevent major adverse cardiovascular events. **A**

10.37 Combination therapy with aspirin plus low-dose rivaroxaban should be considered for individuals with stable coronary and/or peripheral artery disease and low bleeding risk to prevent major adverse limb and cardiovascular events. **A**

10.38 Aspirin therapy (75–162 mg/day) may be considered as a primary prevention strategy in those with diabetes who are at increased cardiovascular risk, after a comprehensive discussion with the patient on the benefits versus the comparable increased risk of bleeding. **A**

Risk Reduction

Aspirin has been shown to be effective in reducing cardiovascular morbidity and mortality in high-risk patients with previous MI or stroke (secondary prevention) and is strongly recommended. In primary prevention, however, among patients with no previous cardiovascular events, its net benefit is more controversial.[129,140]

Previous randomized controlled trials of aspirin specifically in people with diabetes failed to consistently show a significant reduction in overall ASCVD end points, raising questions about the efficacy of aspirin for primary prevention in people with diabetes, although some sex differences were suggested.[141–143]

The Antithrombotic Trialists' Collaboration published an individual patient–level meta-analysis[139] of the six large trials of aspirin for primary prevention in the general population. These trials collectively enrolled over 95,000 participants, including almost 4,000 with diabetes. Overall, they found that aspirin reduced the risk of serious vascular events by 12% (relative risk 0.88 [95% CI 0.82–0.94]). The largest reduction was for nonfatal MI, with little effect on CHD death (relative risk 0.95 [95% CI 0.78–1.15]) or total stroke.

Most recently, the ASCEND (A Study of Cardiovascular Events iN Diabetes) trial randomized 15,480 people with diabetes but no evident cardiovascular disease to aspirin 100 mg daily or placebo.[144] The primary efficacy end point was vascular death, MI, or stroke or transient ischemic attack. The primary safety outcome was major bleeding (i.e., intracranial hemorrhage, sight-threatening bleeding in the eye, gastrointestinal bleeding, or other serious bleeding). During a mean follow-up of 7.4 years, there was a significant 12% reduction in the primary efficacy end point (8.5% vs. 9.6%; $P = 0.01$). In contrast, major bleeding was significantly increased from 3.2 to 4.1% in the aspirin group (rate ratio 1.29; $P = 0.003$), with most of the excess being gastrointestinal bleeding and other extracranial bleeding. There were no significant differences by sex, weight, or duration of diabetes or other baseline factors including ASCVD risk score.

Two other large, randomized trials of aspirin for primary prevention, in people without diabetes (ARRIVE [Aspirin to Reduce Risk of Initial Vascular Events])[145] and in the elderly (ASPREE [Aspirin in Reducing Events in the Elderly]),[146] which included 11% with diabetes, found no benefit of aspirin on the primary efficacy end point and an increased risk of bleeding. In ARRIVE, with 12,546 patients over a period of 60 months follow-up, the primary end point occurred in 4.29% vs. 4.48% of patients in the aspirin versus placebo groups (HR 0.96 [95% CI 0.81–1.13]; $P = 0.60$). Gastrointestinal bleeding events (characterized as mild) occurred in 0.97% of patients in the aspirin group vs. 0.46% in the placebo group (HR 2.11 [95% CI 1.36–3.28]; $P = 0.0007$). In ASPREE, including 19,114 individuals, for cardiovascular disease (fatal CHD, MI, stroke, or hospitalization for heart failure) after a median of 4.7 years of follow-up, the rates per 1,000 person-years were 10.7 vs. 11.3 events in aspirin vs. placebo groups (HR 0.95 [95% CI 0.83–1.08]). The rate of major hemorrhage per 1,000 person-years was 8.6 events vs. 6.2 events, respectively (HR 1.38 [95% CI 1.18–1.62]; $P < 0.001$).

Thus, aspirin appears to have a modest effect on ischemic vascular events, with the absolute decrease in events depending on the underlying ASCVD risk. The main adverse effect is an increased risk of gastrointestinal bleeding. The excess risk may be as high as 5 per 1,000 per year in real-world settings. However, for adults with ASCVD risk >1% per year, the number of ASCVD events prevented will be similar to the number of episodes of bleeding induced, although these complications do not have equal effects on long-term health.[147]

Recommendations for using aspirin as primary prevention include both men and women aged ≥50 years with diabetes and at least one additional major risk factor (family history of premature ASCVD, hypertension, dyslipidemia, smoking, or CKD/albuminuria) who are not at increased risk of bleeding (e.g., older age, anemia, renal disease).[148–151] Noninvasive imaging techniques such as coronary calcium scoring may potentially help further tailor aspirin therapy, particularly in those at low risk.[152,153] For people >70 years of age (with or without diabetes), the balance appears to have greater risk than benefit.[144,146] Thus, for primary prevention, the use of aspirin needs to be carefully considered and may generally not be recommended. Aspirin may be considered in the context of high cardiovascular risk with low bleeding risk, but generally not in older adults. Aspirin therapy for primary prevention may be considered in the context of shared decision-making, which carefully weighs the cardiovascular benefits with the fairly comparable increase in risk of bleeding.

For people with documented ASCVD, use of aspirin for secondary prevention has far greater benefit than risk; for this indication, aspirin is still recommended.[139]

Aspirin Use in People <50 Years of Age

Aspirin is not recommended for those at low risk of ASCVD (such as men and women aged <50 years with diabetes with no other major ASCVD risk factors) as the low benefit is likely to be outweighed by the risks of bleeding. Clinical judgment should be used for those at intermediate risk (younger patients with one or more risk factors or older patients with no risk factors) until further research is available. Patients' willingness to undergo long-term aspirin therapy should also be considered.[154] Aspirin use in patients aged <21 years is generally contraindicated due to the associated risk of Reye syndrome.

Aspirin Dosing

Average daily dosages used in most clinical trials involving people with diabetes ranged from 50 mg to 650 mg but were mostly in the range of 100–325 mg/day. There is little evidence to support any specific dose but using the lowest possible dose may help to reduce side effects.[155] In the ADAPTABLE (Aspirin Dosing: A Patient-Centric Trial Assessing Benefits and Long-term Effectiveness) trial of individuals with established cardiovascular disease, 38% of whom had diabetes, there were no significant differences in cardiovascular events or major bleeding between patients assigned to 81 mg and those assigned to 325 mg of aspirin daily.[156] In the U.S., the most common low-dose tablet is 81 mg. Although platelets from people with diabetes have altered function, it is unclear what, if any, effect that finding has on the required dose of aspirin for cardioprotective effects in people with diabetes. Many alternate pathways for platelet activation exist that are independent of thromboxane A_2 and thus are not sensitive to the effects of aspirin.[157] "Aspirin resistance" has been described in people with diabetes when measured by a variety of ex vivo and in vitro methods (platelet aggregometry, measurement of thromboxane B_2),[158] but other studies suggest no impairment in aspirin response among people with diabetes.[159] A trial suggested that more frequent dosing regimens of aspirin may reduce platelet reactivity in individuals with diabetes;[160] however, these observations alone are insufficient to empirically recommend that higher doses of aspirin be used in this group at this time. Another meta-analysis raised the hypothesis that low-dose aspirin efficacy is reduced in those weighing >70 kg;[161] however, the ASCEND trial found benefit of low-dose aspirin in those in this weight range, which would thus not validate this suggested hypothesis.[144] It appears that 75–162 mg/day is optimal.

Indications for P2Y12 Receptor Antagonist Use

A P2Y12 receptor antagonist in combination with aspirin is reasonable for at least 1 year in patients following an ACS and may have benefits beyond this period. Evidence supports use of either ticagrelor or clopidogrel if no percutaneous coronary intervention was performed and clopidogrel, ticagrelor, or prasugrel if a percutaneous coronary intervention was performed.[162] In people with diabetes and prior MI (1–3 years before), adding ticagrelor to aspirin significantly reduces the risk of recurrent ischemic events including cardiovascular and CHD death.[163] Similarly, the addition of ticagrelor to aspirin reduced the risk of ischemic cardiovascular events compared with aspirin alone in people with diabetes and stable coronary artery disease.[164,165] However, a higher incidence of major bleeding, including intracranial hemorrhage, was noted with dual antiplatelet therapy. The net clinical benefit (ischemic benefit vs. bleeding risk) was improved with ticagrelor therapy in the large prespecified subgroup of patients with history of percutaneous coronary intervention, while no net benefit was seen in patients without prior percutaneous coronary intervention.[165] However, early aspirin discontinuation compared with continued dual antiplatelet therapy after coronary stenting may reduce the risk of bleeding without a corresponding increase in the risks of mortality and ischemic events, as shown in a prespecified analysis of people with diabetes enrolled in the TWILIGHT (Ticagrelor With Aspirin or Alone in High-Risk Patients After Coronary Intervention) trial and a recent meta-analysis.[166,167]

Combination Antiplatelet and Anticoagulation Therapy

Combination therapy with aspirin plus low dose rivaroxaban may be considered for people with stable coronary and/or peripheral artery disease to prevent major adverse limb and cardiovascular complications. In the COMPASS (Cardiovascular Outcomes for People Using Anticoagulation Strategies) trial of 27,395 individuals with established coronary artery disease and/or peripheral artery disease, aspirin plus rivaroxaban 2.5 mg twice daily was superior to aspirin plus placebo in the reduction of cardiovascular ischemic events including major adverse limb events. The absolute benefits of combination therapy appeared larger in people with diabetes, who comprised 10,341 of the trial participants.[168,169] A similar treatment strategy was evaluated in the Vascular Outcomes Study of ASA (acetylsalicylic acid) Along with Rivaroxaban in Endovascular or Surgical Limb Revascularization for Peripheral Artery Disease (VOYAGER PAD) trial,[170] in which 6,564 individuals with peripheral artery disease who had undergone revascularization were randomly assigned to receive rivaroxaban 2.5 mg twice daily plus aspirin or placebo plus aspirin. Rivaroxaban treatment in this group of patients was also associated with a significantly lower incidence of ischemic cardiovascular events, including major adverse limb events. However, an increased risk of major bleeding was noted with rivaroxaban added to aspirin treatment in both COMPASS and VOYAGER PAD.

The risks and benefits of dual antiplatelet or antiplatelet plus anticoagulant treatment strategies should be thoroughly discussed with eligible patients, and shared decision-making should be used to determine an individually appropriate treatment approach. This field of cardiovascular risk reduction is evolving rapidly, as are the definitions of optimal care for patients with differing types and circumstances of cardiovascular complications.

CARDIOVASCULAR DISEASE

SCREENING

Recommendations

10.39 In asymptomatic individuals, routine screening for coronary artery disease is not recommended as it does not improve outcomes as long as atherosclerotic cardiovascular disease risk factors are treated. **A**

10.40 Consider investigations for coronary artery disease in the presence of any of the following: atypical cardiac symptoms (e.g., unexplained dyspnea, chest discomfort); signs or symptoms of associated vascular disease including carotid bruits, transient ischemic attack, stroke, claudication, or peripheral arterial disease; or electrocardiogram abnormalities (e.g., Q waves). **E**

TREATMENT

Recommendations

10.41 Among people with type 2 diabetes who have established atherosclerotic cardiovascular disease or established kidney disease, a sodium–glucose cotransporter 2 inhibitor or glucagon-like peptide 1 receptor agonist with demonstrated cardiovascular disease benefit (Table 17.3b and Table 17.3c) is recommended as part of the comprehensive cardiovascular risk reduction and/or glucose-lowering regimens. **A**

10.41a In people with type 2 diabetes and established atherosclerotic cardiovascular disease, multiple atherosclerotic cardiovascular disease risk factors, or diabetic kidney disease, a sodium–glucose cotransporter 2 inhibitor with demonstrated cardiovascular benefit is recommended to reduce the risk of major adverse cardiovascular events and/or heart failure hospitalization. **A**

10.41b In people with type 2 diabetes and established atherosclerotic cardiovascular disease or multiple risk factors for atherosclerotic cardiovascular disease, a glucagon-like peptide 1 receptor agonist with demonstrated cardiovascular benefit is recommended to reduce the risk of major adverse cardiovascular events. **A**

10.41c In people with type 2 diabetes and established atherosclerotic cardiovascular disease or multiple risk factors for atherosclerotic cardiovascular disease, combined therapy with a sodium–glucose cotransporter 2 inhibitor with demonstrated cardiovascular benefit and a glucagon-like peptide 1 receptor agonist with demonstrated cardiovascular benefit may be considered for additive reduction in the risk of adverse cardiovascular and kidney events. **A**

10.42a In people with type 2 diabetes and established heart failure with either preserved or reduced ejection fraction, a sodium–glucose cotransporter 2 inhibitor with proven benefit in this patient population is recommended to reduce risk of worsening heart failure and cardiovascular death. **A**

10.42b In people with type 2 diabetes and established heart failure with either preserved or reduced ejection fraction, a sodium–glucose cotransporter 2 inhibitor with proven benefit in this patient population is recommended to improve symptoms, physical limitations, and quality of life. **A**

10.43 For people with type 2 diabetes and chronic kidney disease with albuminuria treated with maximum tolerated doses of ACE inhibitor or angiotensin receptor blocker, addition of finerenone is recommended to improve cardiovascular outcomes and reduce the risk of chronic kidney disease progression. **A**

10.44 In people with known atherosclerotic cardiovascular disease, particularly coronary artery disease, ACE inhibitor or angiotensin receptor blocker therapy is recommended to reduce the risk of cardiovascular events. **A**

10.45 In people with prior myocardial infarction, β-blockers should be continued for 3 years after the event. **B**

10.46 Treatment of individuals with heart failure with reduced ejection fraction should include a β-blocker with proven cardiovascular outcomes benefit, unless otherwise contraindicated. **A**

10.47 In people with type 2 diabetes with stable heart failure, metformin may be continued for glucose lowering if estimated glomerular filtration rate remains >30 mL/min/1.73 m^2 but should be avoided in unstable or hospitalized individuals with heart failure. **B**

CARDIAC TESTING

Candidates for advanced or invasive cardiac testing include those with *1*) typical or atypical cardiac symptoms and *2*) an abnormal resting electrocardiogram (ECG). Exercise ECG testing without or with echocardiography may be used as the initial test. In adults with diabetes ≥40 years of age, measurement of coronary artery calcium is also reasonable for cardiovascular risk assessment. Pharmacologic stress echocardiography or nuclear imaging should be considered in individuals with diabetes in whom resting ECG abnormalities preclude exercise stress testing (e.g., left bundle branch block or ST-T abnormalities). In addition, individuals who require stress testing and are unable to exercise should undergo pharmacologic stress echocardiography or nuclear imaging.

SCREENING ASYMPTOMATIC PATIENTS

The screening of asymptomatic patients with high ASCVD risk is not recommended,[171] in part because these high-risk patients should already be receiving intensive medical therapy—an approach that provides benefit similar to invasive revascularization.[172,173] There is also some evidence that silent ischemia may reverse over time, adding to the controversy concerning aggressive screening strategies.[174] In prospective studies, coronary artery calcium has been established as an independent predictor of future ASCVD events in people with diabetes and is consistently superior to both the UK Prospective Diabetes Study (UKPDS) risk engine and the Framingham Risk Score in predicting risk in this population.[175–177]

Table 17.3a—Cardiovascular and Cardiorenal Outcomes Trials of Available Antihyperglycemic Medications Completed After the Issuance of the FDA 2008 Guidelines: DPP-4 Inhibitors

	SAVOR-TIMI 53[224] (n = 16,492)	EXAMINE[235] (n = 5,380)	TECOS[226] (n = 14,671)	CARMELINA[193,236] (n = 6,979)	CAROLINA[193,237] (n = 6,042)
Intervention	Saxagliptin/placebo	Alogliptin/placebo	Sitagliptin/placebo	Linagliptin/placebo	Linagliptin/glimepiride
Main inclusion criteria	Type 2 diabetes and history of or multiple risk factors for CVD	Type 2 diabetes and ACS within 15–90 days before randomization	Type 2 diabetes and preexisting CVD	Type 2 diabetes and high CV and renal risk	Type 2 diabetes and high CV risk
A1C inclusion criteria (%)	≥6.5	6.5–11.0	6.5–8.0	6.5–10.0	6.5–8.5
Age (years)[†]	65.1	61.0	65.4	65.8	64.0
Race (% white)	75.2	72.7	67.9	80.2	73.0
Sex (% male)	66.9	67.9	70.7	62.9	60.0
Diabetes duration (years)[†]	10.3	7.1	11.6	14.7	6.2
Median follow-up (years)	2.1	1.5	3.0	2.2	6.3
Statin use (%)	78	91	80	71.8	64.1
Metformin use (%)	70	66	82	54.8	82.5
Prior CVD/CHF (%)	78/13	100/28	74/18	57/26.8	34.5/4.5
Mean baseline A1C (%)	8.0	8.0	7.2	7.9	7.2
Mean difference in A1C between groups at end of treatment (%)	−0.3‡	−0.3‡	−0.3‡	−0.36‡	0
Year started/reported	2010/2013	2009/2013	2008/2015	2013/2018	2010/2019

(continued)

Table 17.3a (continued)

	SAVOR-TIMI 53[224] (n = 16,492)	EXAMINE[235] (n = 5,380)	TECOS[226] (n = 14,671)	CARMELINA[193,236] (n = 6,979)	CAROLINA[193,237] (n = 6,042)
Primary outcome§	3-point MACE 1.00 (0.89–1.12)	3-point MACE 0.96 (95% UL ≤1.16)	4-point MACE 0.98 (0.89–1.08)	3-point MACE 1.02 (0.89–1.17)	3-point MACE 0.98 (0.84–1.14)
Key secondary outcome§	Expanded MACE 1.02 (0.94–1.11)	4-point MACE 0.95 (95% UL ≤1.14)	3-point MACE 0.99 (0.89–1.10)	Kidney composite (ESRD, sustained ≥40% decrease in eGFR, or renal death) 1.04 (0.89–1.22)	4-point MACE 0.99 (0.86–1.14)
Cardiovascular death§	1.03 (0.87–1.22)	0.85 (0.66–1.10)	1.03 (0.89–1.19)	0.96 (0.81–1.14)	1.00 (0.81–1.24)
MI§	0.95 (0.80–1.12)	1.08 (0.88–1.33)	0.95 (0.81–1.11)	1.12 (0.90–1.40)	1.03 (0.82–1.29)
Stroke§	1.11 (0.88–1.39)	0.91 (0.55–1.50)	0.97 (0.79–1.19)	0.91 (0.67–1.23)	0.86 (0.66–1.12)
HF hospitalization§	1.27 (1.07–1.51)	1.19 (0.90–1.58)	1.00 (0.83–1.20)	0.90 (0.74–1.08)	1.21 (0.92–1.59)
Unstable angina hospitalization§	1.19 (0.89–1.60)	0.90 (0.60–1.37)	0.90 (0.70–1.16)	0.87 (0.57–1.31)	1.07 (0.74–1.54)
All-cause mortality§	1.11 (0.96–1.27)	0.88 (0.71–1.09)	1.01 (0.90–1.14)	0.98 (0.84–1.13)	0.91 (0.78–1.06)
Worsening nephropathy§‖	1.08 (0.88–1.32)	—	—	Kidney composite (see above)	—

—, not assessed/reported; ACS, acute coronary syndrome; CHF, congestive heart failure; CV, cardiovascular; CVD, cardiovascular disease; DPP-4, dipeptidyl peptidase 4; eGFR, estimated glomerular filtration rate; ESRD, end-stage renal disease; GLP-1, glucagon-like peptide 1; HF, heart failure; MACE, major adverse cardiovascular event; MI, myocardial infarction; UL, upper limit. Data from this table was adapted from Cefalu et al.[238] in the January 2018 issue of Diabetes Care. †Age was reported as means in all trials except EXAMINE, which reported medians; diabetes duration was reported as means in all trials except SAVOR-TIMI 53 and EXAMINE, which reported medians. ‡Significant difference in A1C between groups (P < 0.05). §Outcomes reported as hazard ratio (95% CI). ‖ Worsening nephropathy is defined as a doubling of creatinine level, initiation of dialysis, renal transplantation, or creatinine >6.0 mg/dL (530 mmol/L) in SAVOR-TIMI 53. Worsening nephropathy was a prespecified exploratory adjudicated outcome in SAVOR-TIMI 53.

Table 17.3b—Cardiovascular and Cardiorenal Outcomes Trials of Available Antihyperglycemic Medications Completed After the Issuance of the FDA 2008 Guidelines: GLP-1 Receptor Agonists

	ELIXA[208] (n = 6,068)	LEADER[203] (n = 9,340)	SUSTAIN-6[204]* (n = 3,297)	EXSCEL[209] (n = 14,752)	REWIND[207] (n = 9,901)	PIONEER-6[205] (n = 3,183)
Intervention	Lixisenatide/placebo	Liraglutide/placebo	Semaglutide s.c. injection/placebo	Exenatide QW/placebo	Dulaglutide/placebo	Semaglutide oral/placebo
Main inclusion criteria	Type 2 diabetes and history of ACS (<180 days)	Type 2 diabetes and preexisting CVD, CKD, or HF at ≥50 years of age or CV risk at ≥60 years of age	Type 2 diabetes and preexisting CVD, HF, or CKD at ≥50 years of age or CV risk at ≥60 years of age	Type 2 diabetes with or without preexisting CVD	Type 2 diabetes and prior ASCVD event or risk factors for ASCVD	Type 2 diabetes and high CV risk (age of ≥50 years with established CVD or CKD, or age of ≥60 years with CV risk factors only)
A1C inclusion criteria (%)	5.5–11.0	≥7.0	≥7.0	6.5–10.0	≤9.5	None
Age (years)†	60.3	64.3	64.6	62	66.2	66
Race (% white)	75.2	77.5	83.0	75.8	75.7	72.3
Sex (% male)	69.3	64.3	60.7	62	53.7	68.4
Diabetes duration (years)†	9.3	12.8	13.9	12	10.5	14.9
Median follow-up (years)	2.1	3.8	2.1	3.2	5.4	1.3
Statin use (%)	93	72	73	74	66	85.2 (all lipid-lowering)
Metformin use (%)	66	76	73	77	81	77.4
Prior CVD/CHF (%)	100/22	81/18	60/24	73.1/16.2	32/9	84.7/12.2
Mean baseline A1C (%)	7.7	8.7	8.7	8.0	7.4	8.2

(continued)

Table 17.3b (continued)

	ELIXA[208] (n = 6,068)	LEADER[203] (n = 9,340)	SUSTAIN-6[204*] (n = 3,297)	EXSCEL[209] (n = 14,752)	REWIND[207] (n = 9,901)	PIONEER-6[205] (n = 3,183)
Mean difference in A1C between groups at end of treatment (%)	−0.3‡^	−0.4‡	−0.7 or −1.0^	−0.53‡^	−0.61	−0.7
Year started/reported	2010/2015	2010/2016	2013/2016	2010/2017	2011/2019	2017/2019
Primary outcome§	4-point MACE 1.02 (0.89–1.17)	3-point MACE 0.87 (0.78–0.97)	3-point MACE 0.74 (0.58–0.95)	3-point MACE 0.91 (0.83–1.00)	3-point MACE 0.88 (0.79–0.99)	3-point MACE 0.79 (0.57–1.11)
Key secondary outcomes§	Expanded MACE 1.02 (0.90–1.11)	Expanded MACE 0.88 (0.81–0.96)	Expanded MACE 0.74 (0.62–0.89)	Individual components of MACE (see below)	Composite microvascular outcome (eye or renal outcome) 0.87 (0.79–0.95)	Expanded MACE or HF hospitalization 0.82 (0.61–1.10)
Cardiovascular death§	0.98 (0.78–1.22)	0.78 (0.66–0.93)	0.98 (0.65–1.48)	0.88 (0.76–1.02)	0.91 (0.78–1.06)	0.49 (0.27–0.92)
MI§	1.03 (0.87–1.22)	0.86 (0.73–1.00)	0.74 (0.51–1.08)	0.97 (0.85–1.10)	0.96 (0.79–1.15)	1.18 (0.73–1.90)
Stroke§	1.12 (0.79–1.58)	0.86 (0.71–1.06)	0.61 (0.38–0.99)	0.85 (0.70–1.03)	0.76 (0.61–0.95)	0.74 (0.35–1.57)
HF hospitalization§	0.96 (0.75–1.23)	0.87 (0.73–1.05)	1.11 (0.77–1.61)	0.94 (0.78–1.13)	0.93 (0.77–1.12)	0.86 (0.48–1.55)
Unstable angina hospitalization§	1.11 (0.47–2.62)	0.98 (0.76–1.26)	0.82 (0.47–1.44)	1.05 (0.94–1.18)	1.14 (0.84–1.54)	1.56 (0.60–4.01)
All-cause mortality§	0.94 (0.78–1.13)	0.85 (0.74–0.97)	1.05 (0.74–1.50)	0.86 (0.77–0.97)	0.90 (0.80–1.01)	0.51 (0.31–0.84)
Worsening nephropathy§||	—	0.78 (0.67–0.92)	0.64 (0.46–0.88)	—	0.85 (0.77–0.93)	—

—, not assessed/reported; ACS, acute coronary syndrome; ASCVD, atherosclerotic cardiovascular disease; CHF, congestive heart failure; CV, cardiovascular; CVD, cardiovascular disease; GLP-1, glucagon-like peptide 1; HF, heart failure; MACE, major adverse cardiovascular event; MI, myocardial infarction. Data from this table was adapted from Cefalu et al.[238] in the January 2018 issue of Diabetes Care. *Powered to rule out a hazard ratio of 1.8; superiority hypothesis not prespecified. †Age was reported as means in all trials; diabetes duration was reported as means in all trials except EXSCEL, which reported medians. ‡Significant difference in A1C between groups (P < 0.05). ^A1C change of 0.66% with 0.5 mg and 1.05% with 1 mg dose of semaglutide. §Outcomes reported as hazard ratio (95% CI). ||Worsening nephropathy is defined as the new onset of urine albumin-to-creatinine ratio >300 mg/g creatinine or a doubling of the serum creatinine level and an estimated glomerular filtration rate of <45 mL/min/1.73 m², the need for continuous renal replacement therapy, or death from renal disease in LEADER and SUSTAIN-6 and as new macroalbuminuria, a sustained decline in estimated glomerular filtration rate of 30% or more from baseline, or chronic renal replacement therapy in REWIND. Worsening nephropathy was a prespecified exploratory adjudicated outcome in LEADER, SUSTAIN-6, and REWIND.

However, a randomized observational trial demonstrated no clinical benefit to routine screening of asymptomatic people with type 2 diabetes and normal ECGs.[178] Despite abnormal myocardial perfusion imaging in more than one in five patients, cardiac outcomes were essentially equal (and very low) in screened versus unscreened patients. Accordingly, indiscriminate screening is not considered cost-effective. Studies have found that a risk factor-based approach to the initial diagnostic evaluation and subsequent follow-up for coronary artery disease fails to identify which people with type 2 diabetes will have silent ischemia on screening tests.[179,180]

Any benefit of newer noninvasive coronary artery disease screening methods, such as computed tomography calcium scoring and computed tomography angiography, to identify patient subgroups for different treatment strategies remains unproven in asymptomatic people with diabetes, though research is ongoing. Since asymptomatic people with diabetes with higher coronary disease burden have more future cardiac events,[175,181,182] these additional imaging tests may provide reasoning for treatment intensification and/or guide informed patient decision-making and willingness for medication initiation and participation.

While coronary artery screening methods, such as calcium scoring, may improve cardiovascular risk assessment in people with type 2 diabetes,[183] their routine use leads to radiation exposure and may result in unnecessary invasive testing such as coronary angiography and revascularization procedures. The ultimate balance of benefit, cost, and risks of such an approach in asymptomatic patients remains controversial, particularly in the modern setting of aggressive ASCVD risk factor control.

LIFESTYLE AND PHARMACOLOGIC INTERVENTIONS

Intensive lifestyle intervention focusing on weight loss through decreased caloric intake and increased physical activity as performed in the Action for Health in Diabetes (Look AHEAD) trial may be considered for improving glucose control, fitness, and some ASCVD risk factors.[184] Patients at increased ASCVD risk should receive statin, ACE inhibitor, or ARB therapy if the patient has hypertension, and possibly aspirin, unless there are contraindications to a particular drug class. Clear benefit exists for ACE inhibitor or ARB therapy in people with diabetic kidney disease or hypertension, and these agents are recommended for hypertension management in people with known ASCVD (particularly coronary artery disease).[65,66,185] People with type 2 diabetes and CKD should be considered for treatment with finerenone to reduce cardiovascular outcomes and the risk of CKD progression.[186–189] β-Blockers should be used in individuals with active angina or HFrEF and for 3 years after Ml in those with preserved left ventricular function.[190,191]

GLUCOSE-LOWERING THERAPIES AND CARDIOVASCULAR OUTCOMES

In 2008, the FDA issued a guidance for industry to perform cardiovascular outcomes trials for all new medications for the treatment for type 2 diabetes amid concerns of increased cardiovascular risk.[192] Previously approved diabetes medications were not subject to the guidance. Recently published cardiovascular outcomes trials have provided additional data on cardiovascular and renal outcomes in people with type 2 diabetes with cardiovascular disease or at high risk for cardiovascular disease (Table 17.3a, Table 17.3b, and Table 17.3c). An expanded review of the effects of glucose-lowering and other therapies in people with CKD is included in Section 11, "Chronic Kidney Disease and Risk Management."

Cardiovascular outcomes trials of dipeptidyl peptidase 4 (DPP-4) inhibitors have all, so far, not shown cardiovascular benefits relative to placebo. In addition, the CAROLINA (Cardiovascular Outcome Study of Linagliptin Versus Glimepiride in Type 2 Diabetes) study demonstrated noninferiority between a DPP-4 inhibitor, linagliptin, and a sulfonylurea, glimepiride, on cardiovascular outcomes despite lower rates of hypoglycemia in the linagliptin treatment group.[193] However, results from other new agents have provided a mix of results.

SGLT2 Inhibitor Trials

The BI 10773 (Empagliflozin) Cardiovascular Outcome Event Trial in Type 2 Diabetes Mellitus Patients (EMPA-REG OUTCOME) was a randomized, doubleblind trial that assessed the effect of empagliflozin, an SGLT2 inhibitor, versus placebo on cardiovascular outcomes in 7,020 people with type 2 diabetes and existing cardiovascular disease. Study participants had a mean age of 63 years, 57% had diabetes for more than 10 years, and 99% had established cardiovascular disease. EMPA-REG OUTCOME showed that over a median follow-up of 3.1 years, treatment reduced the composite outcome of MI, stroke, and cardiovascular death by 14% (absolute rate 10.5% vs. 12.1% in the placebo group, HR in the empagliflozin group 0.86 [95% CI 0.74–0.99]; $P = 0.04$ for superiority) and cardiovascular death by 38% (absolute rate 3.7% vs. 5.9%, HR 0.62 [95% CI 0.49–0.77]; $P < 0.001$).[8]

Two large outcomes trials of the SGLT2 inhibitor canagliflozin have been conducted that separately assessed *1)* the cardiovascular effects of treatment in patients at high risk for major adverse cardiovascular events[9] and *2)* the impact of canagliflozin therapy on cardiorenal outcomes in people with diabetes-related CKD.[194] First, the Canagliflozin Cardiovascular Assessment Study (CANVAS) Program integrated data from two trials. The CANVAS trial that started in 2009 was partially unblinded prior to completion because of the need to file interim cardiovascular outcomes data for regulatory approval of the drug.[195] Thereafter, the post approval CANVAS-Renal (CANVAS-R) trial was started in 2014. Combining both trials, 10,142 participants with type 2 diabetes were randomized to canagliflozin or placebo and were followed for an average 3.6 years. The mean age of patients was 63 years, and 66% had a history of cardiovascular disease. The combined analysis of the two trials found that canagliflozin significantly reduced the composite outcome of cardiovascular death, MI, or stroke versus placebo (occurring in 26.9 vs. 31.5 participants per 1,000 patient-years; HR 0.86 [95% CI 0.75–0.97]). The specific estimates for canagliflozin versus placebo on the primary composite cardiovascular outcome were HR 0.88 (95% CI 0.75–1.03) for the CANVAS trial and 0.82 (0.66–1.01) for CANVAS-R, with no heterogeneity found between trials. Of note, there was an increased risk of lower-limb amputation with canagliflozin (6.3 vs. 3.4 participants per 1,000 patient-years; HR 1.97 [95% CI 1.41–2.75]).[9] Second, the Canagliflozin and Renal Events in Diabetes with Established Nephropathy Clinical Evaluation (CREDENCE) trial randomized 4,401 people with type 2 diabetes and chronic diabetes-related kidney disease (UACR >300 mg/g and eGFR 30 to <90 mL/min/1.73 m^2) to canagliflozin 100 mg daily or placebo.[194] The primary outcome was a composite of end-stage kidney disease, doubling of serum creatinine, or death from renal or cardiovascular causes. The trial was stopped early due to conclusive evidence of efficacy identified during a prespecified interim analysis with no unexpected safety signals. The risk of the primary composite outcome was 30% lower with canagliflozin treatment when compared with placebo (HR 0.70 [95% CI 0.59–0.82]). Moreover, it reduced the prespecified end point of end-stage kidney disease alone by 32% (HR 0.68 [95% CI 0.54–0.86]). Canagliflozin was additionally found to have a lower risk of the composite of cardiovascular death, MI, or stroke (HR 0.80 [95% CI 0.67–0.95]), as well as lower risk of hospitalizations for heart failure (HR 0.61 [95% CI 0.47–0.80]) and of the composite of cardiovascular death or hospitalization for heart failure (HR 0.69 [95% CI 0.57–0.83]). In terms of safety, no significant increase in lower-limb amputations, fractures, acute kidney injury, or hyperkalemia was noted for canagliflozin relative to placebo in CREDENCE. An increased risk for diabetic ketoacidosis was noted, however, with 2.2 and 0.2 events per 1,000 patient-years noted in the canagliflozin and placebo groups, respectively (HR 10.80 [95% CI 1.39–83.65]).[194]

The Dapagliflozin Effect on Cardiovascular Events-Thrombosis in Myocardial Infarction 58 (DECLARE-TIMI 58) trial was another randomized, double-blind trial that assessed the effects of dapagliflozin versus placebo on cardiovascular and renal outcomes in 17,160 people with type 2 diabetes and established ASCVD or multiple risk factors for ASCVD.[196] Study participants had a mean age of 64 years, with ~40% of study participants having established ASCVD at baseline—a characteristic of this trial that differs from other large cardiovascular trials where a majority of participants had established cardiovascular disease. DECLARE-TIMI 58 met the prespecified criteria for noninferiority to placebo with respect to major adverse cardiovascular events but did not show a lower rate of major adverse cardiovascular events when compared with placebo (8.8% in the dapagliflozin group and 9.4% in the placebo group; HR 0.93 [95% CI 0.84–1.03]; P = 0.17). A lower rate of cardiovascular death or hospitalization for heart failure was noted (4.9% vs. 5.8%; HR 0.83 [95% CI 0.73–0.95]; P = 0.005), which reflected a lower rate of hospitalization for heart failure (HR 0.73 [95% CI 0.61–0.88]). No difference was seen in cardiovascular death between groups.

In the Dapagliflozin and Prevention of Adverse Outcomes in Chronic Kidney Disease (DAPA-CKD) trial,[197] 4,304 individuals with CKD (UACR 200–5,000 mg/g and eGFR 25–75 mL/min/1.73 m^2), with or without diabetes, were randomized to dapagliflozin 10 mg daily or placebo. The primary outcome was a composite of sustained decline in eGFR of at least 50%, end-stage kidney disease, or death from renal or cardiovascular causes. Over a median follow-up period of 2.4 years, a primary outcome event occurred in 9.2% of participants in the dapagliflozin group and 14.5% of those in the placebo group. The risk of the primary composite outcome was significantly lower with dapagliflozin therapy compared with placebo (HR 0.61 [95% CI 0.51–0.72]), as were the risks for a renal composite outcome of sustained decline in eGFR of at least 50%, endstage kidney disease, or death from renal causes (HR 0.56 [95% CI 0.45–0.68]), and a composite of cardiovascular death or hospitalization for heart failure (HR 0.71 [95% CI 0.55–0.92]). The effects of dapagliflozin therapy were similar in individuals with and without type 2 diabetes.

Results of the Dapagliflozin and Prevention of Adverse Outcomes in Heart Failure (DAPA-HF) trial, the Empagliflozin Outcome Trial in Patients With Chronic Heart Failure and a Reduced Ejection Fraction (EMPEROR-Reduced), Empagliflozin Outcome Trial in Patients With Chronic Heart Failure With Preserved Ejection Fraction (EMPEROR-Preserved), Effects of Dapagliflozin on Biomarkers, Symptoms and Functional Status in Patients With PRESERVED Ejection Fraction Heart Failure (PRESERVED-HF), and Dapagliflozin Evaluation to Improve the Lives of Patients with Preserved Ejection Fraction Heart Failure (DELIVER), which assessed the effects of dapagliflozin and empagliflozin in individuals with established heart failure,[11,189,198,199,200] are described below in GLUCOSE-LOWERING THERAPIES AND HEART FAILURE.

The Evaluation of Ertugliflozin Efficacy and Safety Cardiovascular Outcomes Trial (VERTIS CV)[201] was a randomized, double-blind trial that established the effects of ertugliflozin versus placebo on cardiovascular outcomes in 8,246 people with type 2 diabetes and established ASCVD. Participants were assigned to the addition of 5 mg or 15 mg of ertugliflozin or to placebo once daily to background standard care. Study participants had a mean age of 64.4 years and a mean duration of diabetes of 13 years at baseline and were followed for a median of 3.0 years. VERTIS CV met the prespecified criteria for noninferiority of ertugliflozin to placebo with respect to the primary outcome of major adverse cardiovascular events (11.9% in the pooled ertugliflozin group and 11.9% in the placebo group; HR 0.97 [95% CI 0.85–1.11]; $P < 0.001$). Ertugliflozin was not superior to placebo for the key secondary outcomes of death from cardiovascular causes or hospitalization for heart failure; death from cardiovascular causes; or the composite of death from renal causes, renal replacement therapy, or doubling of the serum creatinine level. The HR for a secondary outcome of hospitalization for heart failure (ertugliflozin vs. placebo) was 0.70 [95% CI 0.54–0.90], consistent with findings from other SGLT2 inhibitor cardiovascular outcomes trials.

Sotagliflozin, an SGLT1 and SGLT2 inhibitor not currently approved by the FDA in the U.S., lowers glucose via delayed glucose absorption in the gut in addition to increasing urinary glucose excretion and has been evaluated in the Effect of Sotagliflozin on Cardiovascular and Renal Events in Patients With Type 2 Diabetes and Moderate Renal Impairment Who Are at Cardiovascular Risk (SCORED) trial.[202] A total of 10,584 people with type 2 diabetes, CKD, and additional cardiovascular risk were enrolled in SCORED and randomized to sotagliflozin 200 mg once daily (uptitrated to 400 mg once daily if tolerated) or placebo. SCORED ended early due to a lack of funding; thus, changes to the prespecified primary end points were made prior to unblinding to accommodate a lower than anticipated number of end point events. The primary end point of the trial was the total number of deaths from cardiovascular causes, hospitalizations for heart failure, and urgent visits for heart failure. After a median of 16 months of follow-up, the rate of primary end point events was reduced with sotagliflozin (5.6 events per 100 patient-years in the sotagliflozin group and 7.5 events per 100 patient-years in the placebo group [HR 0.74 (95% CI 0.63–0.88); $P < 0.001$]). Sotagliflozin also reduced the risk of the secondary end point of

Table 17.3c—Cardiovascular and cardiorenal outcomes trials of available antihyperglycemic medications completed after the issuance of the FDA 2008 guidelines: SGLT2 inhibitors

	EMPA-REG OUTCOME[8] (n = 7,020)	CANVAS Program[9] (n = 10,142)	DECLARE-TIMI 58[196] (n = 17,160)	CREDENCE[194] (n = 4,401)	DAPA-CKD[197,239] (n = 4,304; 2,906 with diabetes)	VERTIS CV[201,240] (n = 8,246)	DAPA-HF[1] (n = 4,744; 1,983 with diabetes)	EMPEROR-Reduced[200] (n = 3,730; 1,856 with diabetes)	EMPEROR-Preserved[189,241] (n = 5,988; 2,938 with diabetes)	DELIVER[199] (n = 6,263; 2,807 with diabetes)
Intervention	Empagliflozin/placebo	Canagliflozin/placebo	Dapagliflozin/placebo	Canagliflozin/placebo	Dapagliflozin/placebo	Ertugliflozin/placebo	Dapagliflozin/placebo	Empagliflozin/placebo*	Empagliflozin/placebo	Dapagliflozin/placebo
Main inclusion criteria	Type 2 diabetes and preexisting CVD	Type 2 diabetes and preexisting CVD at ≥30 years of age or ≥2 CV risk factors at ≥50 years of age	Type 2 diabetes and established ASCVD or multiple risk factors for ASCVD	Type 2 diabetes and albuminuric kidney disease	Albuminuric kidney disease, with or without diabetes	Type 2 diabetes and ASCVD	NYHA class II, III, or IV heart failure and an ejection fraction ≤40%, with or without diabetes	NYHA class II, III, or IV heart failure and an ejection fraction ≤40%, with or without diabetes	NYHA class II, III, or IV heart failure and an ejection fraction >40%	NYHA class II, III, or IV heart failure and an ejection fraction >40% with or without diabetes
A1C inclusion criteria (%)	7.0–10.0	7.0–10.5	≥6.5	6.5–12	—	7.0–10.5	—	—	—	—
Age (years)†	63.1	63.3	64.0	63	61.8	64.4	66	67.2, 66.5	71.8, 71.9	71.7
Race (% White)	72.4	78.3	79.6	66.6	53.2	87.8	70.3	71.1, 69.8	76.3, 75.4	71.2
Sex (% male)	71.5	64.2	62.6	66.1	66.9	70	76.6	76.5, 75.6	55.4, 55.3	56.1
Diabetes duration (years)†	57% >10	13.5	11.0	15.8		12.9				

(continued)

Table 17.3c (continued)

	EMPA-REG OUTCOME[8] (n = 7,020)	CANVAS Program[9] (n = 10,142)	DECLARE-TIMI 58[196] (n = 17,160)	CREDENCE[194] (n = 4,401)	DAPA-CKD[197,239] (n = 4,304; 2,906 with diabetes)	VERTIS CV[201,240] (n = 8,246)	DAPA-HF[11] (n = 4,744; 1,983 with diabetes)	EMPEROR-Reduced[200] (n = 3,730; 1,856 with diabetes)	EMPEROR-Preserved[189,241] (n = 5,988; 2,938 with diabetes)	DELIVER[199] (n = 6,263; 2,807 with diabetes)
Median follow-up (years)	3.1	3.6	4.2	2.6	2.4	3.5	1.5	1.3	2.2	2.3
Statin use (%)	77	75	75 (statin or ezetimibe use)	69	64.9	—	—	—	68.1, 68.8	—
Metformin use (%)	74	77	82	57.8	29		51.2% (of people with diabetes)	—	—	—
Prior CVD/CHF (%)	99/10	65.6/14.4	40/10	50.4/14.8	37.4/10.9	99.9/23.1	100% with CHF	100% with CHF	100% with CHF	100% with CHF
Mean baseline A1C (%)	8.1	8.2	8.3	8.3	7.1% (7.8% in those with diabetes)	8.2	—	—	—	6.6
Mean difference in A1C between groups at end of treatment (%)	−0.3^	−0.58‡	−0.43‡	−0.31	—	−0.48 to −0.5	—	—	—	—
Year started/reported	2010/2015	2009/2017	2013/2018	2017/2019	2017/2020	2013/2020	2017/2019	2017/2020	2017/2020	2018/2022

(continued)

Table 17.3c (continued)

	EMPA-REG OUTCOME[8] (n = 7,020)	CANVAS Program[9] (n = 10,142)	DECLARE-TIMI 58[196] (n = 17,160)	CREDENCE[194] (n = 4,401)	DAPA-CKD[197,239] (n = 4,304; 2,906 with diabetes)	VERTIS CV[201,240] (n = 8,246)	DAPA-HF[11] (n = 4,744; 1,983 with diabetes)	EMPEROR-Reduced[200] (n = 3,730; 1,856 with diabetes)	EMPEROR-Preserved[189,241] (n = 5,988; 2,938 with diabetes)	DELIVER[199] (n = 6,263; 2,807 with diabetes)
Primary outcome§	3-point MACE 0.86 (0.74–0.99)	3-point MACE 0.86 (0.75–0.97)	3-point MACE 0.93 (0.84–1.03) CV death or HF hospitalization 0.83 (0.73–0.95)	ESRD, doubling of creatinine, or death from renal or CV cause 0.70 (0.59–0.82)	≥50% decline in eGFR, ESKD, or death from renal or CV cause 0.61 (0.51–0.72)	3-point MACE 0.97 (0.85–1.11)	Worsening heart failure or death from CV causes 0.74 (0.65–0.85) Results did not differ by diabetes status	CV death or HF hospitalization 0.75 (0.65–0.86)	CV death or HF hospitalization 0.79 (0.69–0.90)	Worsening HF or CV death 0.82 (0.73–0.92)
Key secondary outcome§	4-point MACE 0.89 (0.78–1.01)	All-cause and CV mortality (see below)	Death from any cause 0.93 (0.82–1.04) Renal composite (≥40% decrease in eGFR rate to <60 mL/min/1.73 m², new ESRD, or death from renal or CV causes 0.76 (0.67–0.87)	CV death or HF hospitalization 0.69 (0.57–0.83) 3-point MACE 0.80 (0.67–0.95)	≥50% decline in eGFR, ESKD, or death from renal cause 0.56 (0.45–0.68) CV death or HF hospitalization 0.71 (0.55–0.92) Death from any cause 0.69 (0.53–0.88)	CV death or HF hospitalization 0.88 (0.75–1.03) CV death 0.92 (0.77–1.11) Renal death, renal replacement therapy, or doubling of creatinine 0.81 (0.63–1.04)	CV death or HF hospitalization 0.75 (0.65–0.85)	Total HF hospitalizations 0.70 (0.58–0.85) Mean slope of change in eGFR 1.73 (1.10–2.37)	All HF hospitalizations (first and recurrent) 0.73 (0.61–0.88) Rate of decline in eGFR (−1.25 vs. −2.62 mL/min/1.73 m²; P < 0.001)	Total number worsening HF and CV deaths 0.77 (0.67–0.89) Change in KCCQ TSS at month 8 1.11 (1.03–1.21) Mean change in KCCQ TSS 2.4 (1.5–3.4) All-cause mortality 0.94 (0.83–1.07)
Cardiovascular death§	0.62 (0.49–0.77)	0.87 (0.72–1.06)	0.98 (0.82–1.17)	0.78 (0.61–1.00)	0.81 (0.58–1.12)	0.92 (0.77–1.11)	0.82 (0.69–0.98)	0.92 (0.75–1.12)	0.91 (0.76–1.09)	0.88 (0.74–1.05)

(continued)

Table 17.3c (continued)

	EMPA-REG OUTCOME[6] (n = 7,020)	CANVAS Program[9] (n = 10,142)	DECLARE-TIMI 58[196] (n = 17,160)	CREDENCE[194] (n = 4,401)	DAPA-CKD[197,239] (n = 4,304; 2,906 with diabetes)	VERTIS CV[201,240] (n = 8,246)	DAPA-HF[11] (n = 4,744; 1,983 with diabetes)	EMPEROR-Reduced[200] (n = 3,730; 1,856 with diabetes)	EMPEROR-Preserved[189,241] (n = 5,988; 2,938 with diabetes)	DELIVER[199] (n = 6,263; 2,807 with diabetes)
MI§	0.87 (0.70–1.09)	0.89 (0.73–1.09)	0.89 (0.77–1.01)	—	—	1.04 (0.86–1.26)	—	—	—	—
Stroke§	1.18 (0.89–1.56)	0.87 (0.69–1.09)	1.01 (0.84–1.21)	—	—	1.06 (0.82–1.37)	—	—	—	—
HF hospitalization§	0.65 (0.50–0.85)	0.67 (0.52–0.87)	0.73 (0.61–0.88)	0.61 (0.47–0.80)	—	0.70 (0.54–0.90)	0.70 (0.59–0.83)	0.69 (0.59–0.81)	0.73 (0.61–0.88)	0.77 (0.67–0.89)
Unstable angina hospitalization§	0.99 (0.74–1.34)	—	—	—	—	—	—	—	—	—
All-cause mortality§	0.68 (0.57–0.82)	0.87 (0.74–1.01)	0.93 (0.82–1.04)	0.83 (0.68–1.02)	0.69 (0.53–0.88)	0.93 (0.80–1.08)	0.83 (0.71–0.97)	0.92 (0.77–1.10)	1.00 (0.87–1.15)	0.94 (0.83–1.07)
Worsening nephropathy§||	0.61 (0.53–0.70)	0.60 (0.47–0.77)	0.53 (0.43–0.66)	(See primary outcome)	(See primary outcome)	(See secondary outcomes)	0.71 (0.44–1.16)	Composite renal outcome 0.50 (0.32–0.77)	Composite renal outcome** 0.95 (0.73–1.24)	—

—, not assessed/reported; CHF, congestive heart failure; CV, cardiovascular; CVD, cardiovascular disease; eGFR, estimated glomerular filtration rate; ESRD, end-stage renal disease; HF, heart failure; KCCQ TSS, Kansas City Cardiomyopathy Questionnaire Total Symptom Score; MACE, major adverse cardiovascular event; MI, myocardial infarction; SGLT2, sodium–glucose cotransporter 2; NYFIA, New York Fleart Association. Data from this table was adapted from Cefalu et al.[238] in the January 2018 issue of Diabetes Care. *Baseline characteristics for EMPEROR-Reduced displayed as empagliflozin, placebo. †Age was reported as means in all trials; diabetes duration was reported as means in all trials except EMPA-REG OUTCOME, which reported as percentage of population with diabetes duration >10 years, and DECLARE-TIMI 58, which reported median. ‡Significant difference in A1C between groups (P < 0.05). ^A1C change of 0.30 in EMPA-REG OUTCOME is based on pooled results for both doses (i.e., 0.24% for 10 mg and 0.36% for 25 mg of empagliflozin). §Outcomes reported as hazard ratio (95% CI). ||Definitions of worsening nephropathy differed between trials. **Composite outcome in EMPEROR-Preserved: time to first occurrence of chronic dialysis, renal transplantation; sustained reduction of ≥40% in eGFR, sustained eGFR <15 mL/min/1.73 m² for individuals with baseline eGFR ≥30 mL/min/1.73 m².

total number of hospitalizations for heart failure and urgent visits for heart failure (3.5% in the sotagliflozin group and 5.1% in the placebo group; HR 0.67 [95% CI 0.55–0.82]; $P < 0.001$) but not the secondary end point of deaths from cardiovascular causes. No significant between-group differences were found for the outcome of all-cause mortality or for a composite renal outcome comprising the first occurrence of long-term dialysis, renal transplantation, or a sustained reduction in eGFR. In general, the adverse effects of sotagliflozin were similar to those seen with use of SGLT2 inhibitors, but they also included an increased rate of diarrhea potentially related to the inhibition of SGLT1.

GLP-1 Receptor Agonist Trials

The Liraglutide Effect and Action in Diabetes: Evaluation of Cardiovascular Outcome Results (LEADER) trial was a randomized, double-blind trial that assessed the effect of liraglutide, a glucagon-like peptide 1 (GLP-1) receptor agonist, versus placebo on cardiovascular outcomes in 9,340 people with type 2 diabetes at high risk for cardiovascular disease or with cardiovascular disease.[203] Study participants had a mean age of 64 years and a mean duration of diabetes of nearly 13 years. Over 80% of study participants had established cardiovascular disease. After a median follow-up of 3.8 years, LEADER showed that the primary composite outcome (MI, stroke, or cardiovascular death) occurred in fewer participants in the treatment group (13.0%) when compared with the placebo group (14.9%) (HR 0.87 [95% CI 0.78–0.97]; $P < 0.001$ for noninferiority; $P = 0.01$ for superiority). Deaths from cardiovascular causes were significantly reduced in the liraglutide group (4.7%) compared with the placebo group (6.0%) (HR 0.78 [95% CI 0.66–0.93]; $P = 0.007$).[203]

Results from a moderate-sized trial of another GLP-1 receptor agonist, semaglutide, were consistent with the LEADER trial.[204] Semaglutide is a once-weekly GLP-1 receptor agonist approved by the FDA for the treatment of type 2 diabetes. The Trial to Evaluate Cardiovascular and Other Long-term Outcomes With Semaglutide in Subjects With Type 2 Diabetes (SUSTAIN-6) was the initial randomized trial powered to test noninferiority of semaglutide for the purpose of regulatory approval.[204] In this study, 3,297 people with type 2 diabetes were randomized to receive once-weekly semaglutide (0.5 mg or 1.0 mg) or placebo for 2 years. The primary outcome (the first occurrence of cardiovascular death, nonfatal MI, or nonfatal stroke) occurred in 108 patients (6.6%) in the semaglutide group vs. 146 patients (8.9%) in the placebo group (HR 0.74 [95% CI 0.58–0.95]; $P < 0.001$). More patients discontinued treatment in the semaglutide group because of adverse events, mainly gastrointestinal. The cardiovascular effects of the oral formulation of semaglutide compared with placebo have been assessed in Peptide Innovation for Early Diabetes Treatment (PIONEER) 6, a preapproval trial designed to rule out an unacceptable increase in cardiovascular risk.[205] In this trial of 3,183 people with type 2 diabetes and high cardiovascular risk followed for a median of 15.9 months, oral semaglutide was noninferior to placebo for the primary composite outcome of cardiovascular death, nonfatal MI, or nonfatal stroke (HR 0.79 [95% CI 0.57–1.11]; $P < 0.001$ for noninferiority).[205] The cardiovascular effects of this formulation of semaglutide will be further tested in a large, longer-term outcomes trial.

The Harmony Outcomes trial randomized 9,463 people with type 2 diabetes and cardiovascular disease to once-weekly subcutaneous albiglutide or matching placebo, in addition to their standard care.[206] Over a median duration of 1.6 years, the GLP-1 receptor agonist reduced the risk of cardiovascular death, MI, or stroke to an incidence rate of 4.6 events per 100 person-years in the albiglutide group vs. 5.9 events in the placebo group (HR ratio 0.78, $P = 0.0006$ for superiority).[206] This agent is not currently available for clinical use.

The Researching Cardiovascular Events With a Weekly Incretin in Diabetes (REWIND) trial was a randomized, double-blind, placebo-controlled trial that assessed the effect of the once-weekly GLP-1 receptor agonist dulaglutide versus placebo on major adverse cardiovascular events in ~9,990 people with type 2 diabetes at risk for cardiovascular events or with a history of cardiovascular disease.[207] Study participants had a mean age of 66 years and a mean duration of diabetes of ~10 years. Approximately 32% of participants had history of atherosclerotic cardiovascular events at baseline. After a median follow-up of 5.4 years, the primary composite outcome of nonfatal MI, nonfatal stroke, or death from cardiovascular causes occurred in 12.0% and 13.4% of participants in the dulaglutide and placebo treatment groups, respectively (HR 0.88 [95% CI 0.79–0.99]; $P = 0.026$). These findings equated to incidence rates of 2.4 and 2.7 events per 100 person-years, respectively. The results were consistent across the subgroups of patients with and without history of CV events. Allcause mortality did not differ between groups ($P = 0.067$).

The Evaluation of Lixisenatide in Acute Coronary Syndrome (ELIXA) trial studied the once-daily GLP-1 receptor agonist lixisenatide on cardiovascular outcomes in people with type 2 diabetes who had had a recent acute coronary event.[208] A total of 6,068 people with type 2 diabetes with a recent hospitalization for MI or unstable angina within the previous 180 days were randomized to receive lixisenatide or placebo in addition to standard care and were followed for a median of ~2.1 years. The primary outcome of cardiovascular death, MI, stroke, or hospitalization for unstable angina occurred in 406 patients (13.4%) in the lixisenatide group vs. 399 (13.2%) in the placebo group (HR 1.2 [95% CI 0.89–1.17]), which demonstrated the noninferiority of lixisenatide to placebo ($P < 0.001$) but did not show superiority ($P = 0.81$).

The Exenatide Study of Cardiovascular Event Lowering (EXSCEL) trial also reported results with the once-weekly GLP-1 receptor agonist extended-release exenatide and found that major adverse cardiovascular events were numerically lower with use of extended-release exenatide compared with placebo, although this difference was not statistically significant.[209] A total of 14,752 people with type 2 diabetes (of whom 10,782 [73.1%] had previous cardiovascular disease) were randomized to receive extended-release exenatide 2 mg or placebo and followed for a median of 3.2 years. The primary end point of cardiovascular death, MI, or stroke occurred in 839 patients (11.4%; 3.7 events per 100 person-years) in the exenatide group and in 905 patients (12.2%; 4.0 events per 100 person-years) in the placebo group (HR 0.91 [95% CI 0.83–1.00]; $P < 0.001$ for noninferiority), but exenatide was not superior to placebo with respect to the primary end point ($P = 0.06$ for superiority). However, all-cause mortality was lower in the exenatide group (HR 0.86 [95% CI 0.77–0.97]). The incidence of acute pancreatitis, pancreatic cancer, medullary thyroid carcinoma, and serious adverse events did not differ significantly between the two groups.

In summary, there are now numerous large randomized controlled trials reporting statistically significant reductions in cardiovascular events for three of the FDA-approved SGLT2 inhibitors (empagliflozin, canagliflozin, dapagliflozin, with lesser benefits seen with ertugliflozin) and four FDA-approved GLP-1 receptor agonists (liraglutide, albiglutide [although that agent was removed from the market for business reasons], semaglutide [lower risk of cardiovascular events in a moderate-sized clinical trial but one not powered as a cardiovascular outcomes trial], and dulaglutide). Meta-analyses of the trials reported to date suggest that GLP-1 receptor agonists and SGLT2 inhibitors reduce risk of atherosclerotic major adverse cardiovascular events to a comparable degree in people with type 2 diabetes and established ASCVD.[210,211] SGLT2 inhibitors also reduce risk of heart failure hospitalization and progression of kidney disease in people with established ASCVD, multiple risk factors for ASCVD, or albuminuric kidney disease.[212,213] In people with type 2 diabetes and established ASCVD, multiple ASCVD risk factors, or diabetic kidney disease, an SGLT2 inhibitor with demonstrated cardiovascular benefit is recommended to reduce the risk of major adverse cardiovascular events and/or heart failure hospitalization. In people with type 2 diabetes and established ASCVD or multiple risk factors for ASCVD, a glucagon-like peptide 1 receptor agonist with demonstrated cardiovascular benefit is recommended to reduce the risk of major adverse cardiovascular events. For many patients, use of either an SGLT2 inhibitor or a GLP-1 receptor agonist to reduce cardiovascular risk is appropriate. Emerging data suggest that use of both classes of drugs will provide an additive cardiovascular and kidney outcomes benefit; thus, combination therapy with an SGLT2 inhibitor and a GLP-1 receptor agonist may be considered to provide the complementary outcomes benefits associated with these classes of medication. Evidence to support such an approach includes findings from AMPLITUDE-O (Effect of Efpeglenatide on Cardiovascular Outcomes), an outcomes trial of people with type 2 diabetes and either cardiovascular or kidney disease plus at least one other risk factor randomized to the investigational GLP-1 receptor agonist efpeglenatide or placebo.[214] Randomization was stratified by current or potential use of SGLT2 inhibitor therapy, a class ultimately used by >15% of the trial participants. Over a median follow-up of 1.8 years, efpeglenatide therapy reduced the risk of incident major adverse cardiovascular events by 27% and of a composite renal outcome event by 32%. Importantly, the effects of efpeglenatide did not vary by use of SGLT2 inhibitors, suggesting that the beneficial effects of the GLP-1 receptor agonist were independent of those provided by SGLT2 inhibitor therapy.[215] Efpeglenatide is currently not approved by the FDA for use in the U.S.

Glucose-Lowering Therapies and Heart Failure

As many as 50% of people with type 2 diabetes may develop heart failure.[216] These conditions, which are each associated with increased morbidity and mortality, commonly coincide, and independently contribute to adverse outcomes.[217] Strategies to mitigate these risks are needed, and the heart failure-related risks and benefits of glucose-lowering medications should be considered carefully when determining a regimen of care for people with diabetes and either established heart failure or high risk for the development of heart failure.

Data on the effects of glucose-lowering agents on heart failure outcomes have demonstrated that thiazolidinediones have a strong and consistent relationship with increased risk of heart failure.[218–220] Therefore, thiazolidinedione use should be avoided in people with symptomatic heart failure. Restrictions to use of metformin in people with medically treated heart failure were removed by the FDA in 2006.[221] Observational studies of people with type 2 diabetes and heart failure suggest that metformin users have better outcomes than individuals treated with other anti-hyperglycemic agents;[222] however, no randomized trial of metformin therapy has been conducted in people with heart failure. Metformin may be used for the management of hyperglycemia in people with stable heart failure as long as kidney function remains within the recommended range for use.[223]

Recent studies examining the relationship between DPP-4 inhibitors and heart failure have had mixed results. The Saxagliptin Assessment of Vascular Outcomes Recorded in Patients with Diabetes Mellitus – Thrombolysis in Myocardial Infarction 53 (SAVOR-TIMI 53) study showed that patients treated with the DPP-4 inhibitor saxagliptin were more likely to be hospitalized for heart failure than those given placebo (3.5% vs. 2.8%, respectively).[224] However, three other cardiovascular outcomes trials—Examination of Cardiovascular Outcomes with Alogliptin versus Standard of Care (EXAMINE),[225] Trial Evaluating Cardiovascular Outcomes with Sitagliptin (TECOS),[226] and the Cardiovascular and Renal Microvascular Outcome Study With Linagliptin (CARMELINA)[193]—did not find a significant increase in risk of heart failure hospitalization with DPP-4 inhibitor use compared with placebo. No increased risk of heart failure hospitalization has been identified in the cardiovascular outcomes trials of the GLP-1 receptor agonists lixisenatide, liraglutide, sema--glutide, exenatide once-weekly, albiglutide, or dulaglutide compared with placebo (Table 17.3b).[203,204,207–209]

Reduced incidence of heart failure has been observed with the use of SGLT2 inhibitors.[8,194,196] In EMPAREG OUTCOME, the addition of empagliflozin to standard care led to a significant 35% reduction in hospitalization for heart failure compared with placebo.[8] Although the majority of patients in the study did not have heart failure at baseline, this benefit was consistent in patients with and without a history of heart failure.[10] Similarly, in CANVAS and DECLARE-TIMI 58, there were 33% and 27% reductions in hospitalization for heart failure, respectively, with SGLT2 inhibitor use versus placebo.[9,196] Additional data from the CREDENCE trial with canagliflozin showed a 39% reduction in hospitalization for heart failure, and 31% reduction in the composite of cardiovascular death or hospitalization for heart failure, in a diabetic kidney disease population with albuminuria (UACR >300 to 5,000 mg/g).[194] These combined findings from four large outcomes trials of three different SGLT2 inhibitors are highly consistent and clearly indicate robust benefits of SGLT2 inhibitors in the prevention of heart failure hospitalizations. The EMPA-REG OUTCOME, CANVAS, DECLARE-TIMI 58, and CREDENCE trials suggested, but did not prove, that SGLT2 inhibitors would be beneficial in the treatment of people with established heart failure. More recently, the placebo-controlled DAPA-HF trial evaluated the effects of dapagliflozin on the primary outcome of a composite of worsening heart failure or cardiovascular death in patients with New York Heart Association

(NYHA) class II, III, or IV heart failure and an ejection fraction of 40% or less. Of the 4,744 trial participants, 45% had a history of type 2 diabetes. Over a median of 18.2 months, the group assigned to dapagliflozin treatment had a lower risk of the primary outcome (HR 0.74 [95% CI 0.65–0.85]), lower risk of first worsening heart failure event (HR 0.70 [95% CI 0.59–0.83]), and lower risk of cardiovascular death (HR 0.82 [95% CI 0.69–0.98]) compared with placebo. The effect of dapagliflozin on the primary outcome was consistent regardless of the presence or absence of type 2 diabetes.[11]

EMPEROR-Reduced assessed the effects of empagliflozin 10 mg once daily versus placebo on a primary composite outcome of cardiovascular death or hospitalization for worsening heart failure in a population of 3,730 patients with NYHA class II, III, or IV heart failure and an ejection fraction of 40% or less.[200] At baseline, 49.8% of participants had a history of diabetes. Over a median follow-up of 16 months, those in the empagliflozin-treated group had a reduced risk of the primary outcome (HR 0.75 [95% CI 0.65–0.86]; $P < 0.001$) and fewer total hospitalizations for heart failure (HR 0.70 [95% CI 0.58–0.85]; $P < 0.001$). The effect of empagliflozin on the primary outcome was consistent irrespective of diabetes diagnosis at baseline. The risk of a prespecified renal composite outcome (chronic dialysis, renal transplantation, or a sustained reduction in eGFR) was lower in the empagliflozin group than in the placebo group (1.6% in the empagliflozin group vs. 3.1% in the placebo group; HR 0.50 [95% CI 0.32–0.77]).

EMPEROR-Preserved, a randomized double-blinded placebo-controlled trial of 5,988 adults with NYHA functional class I–IV chronic HFpEF (left ventricular ejection fraction >40%), evaluated the efficacy of empagliflozin 10 mg daily versus placebo on top of standard of care on the primary outcome of composite cardiovascular death or hospitalization for heart failure.[189] Approximately 50% of subjects had type 2 diabetes at baseline. Over a median of 26.2 months, there was a 21% reduction (HR 0.79 [95% CI 0.69–0.90]; $P < 0.001$) of the primary outcome. The effects of empagliflozin were consistent in people with or without diabetes.[189]

In the DELIVER trial, 6,263 individuals with heart failure and an ejection fraction >40% were randomized to receive either dapagliflozin or placebo.[199] The primary outcome of a composite of worsening heart failure, defined as hospitalization or urgent visit for heart failure, or cardiovascular death was reduced by 18% in patients treated with dapagliflozin compared with placebo (HR 0.82 [95% CI 0.73–0.92]; $P < 0.001$). Approximately 44% of patients randomized to either dapagliflozin or placebo had type 2 diabetes, and results were consistent regardless of the presence of type 2 diabetes.

A large recent meta-analysis[227] including data from EMPEROR-Reduced, EMPEROR-Preserved, DAPA-HF, DELIVER, and Effect of Sotagliflozin on Cardiovascular Events in Patients With Type 2 Diabetes Post Worsening Heart Failure (SOLOIST-WHF) included 21,947 patients and demonstrated reduced risk for the composite of cardiovascular death or hospitalization for heart failure, cardiovascular death, first hospitalization for heart failure, and all-cause mortality. The findings on the studied end points were consistent in both trials of heart failure with mildly reduced or preserved ejection fraction and in all five trials combined. Collectively, these studies indicate that SGLT2 inhibitors reduce the risk for heart failure hospitalization and cardiovascular death in a wide range of people with heart failure.

Additional data are accumulating regarding the effects of SGLT inhibition in people hospitalized for acute decompensated heart failure and in people with heart failure and HFpEF. As an example, the investigational SGLT1 and SGLT2 inhibitor sotagliflozin has also been studied in the SOLOIST-WHF trial.[228] In SOLOIST-WHF, 1,222 people with type 2 diabetes who were recently hospitalized for worsening heart failure were randomized to sotagliflozin 200 mg once daily (with uptitration to 400 mg once daily if tolerated) or placebo either before or within 3 days after hospital discharge. Patients were eligible if hospitalized for signs and symptoms of heart failure (including elevated natriuretic peptide levels) requiring treatment with intravenous diuretic therapy. Exclusion criteria included end-stage heart failure or recent acute coronary syndrome or intervention, or an eGFR <30 mL/min/1.73 m^2). Patients were required to be clinically stable prior to randomization, defined as no use of supplemental oxygen, a systolic blood pressure ≥100 mmHg, and no need for intravenous inotropic or vasodilator therapy other than nitrates. Similar to SCORED, SOLOIST-WHF ended early due to a lack of funding, resulting in a change to the prespecified primary end point prior to unblinding to accommodate a lower than anticipated number of end point events. At a median follow-up of 9 months, the rate of primary end point events (the total number of cardiovascular deaths and hospitalizations and urgent visits for heart failure) was lower in the sotagliflozin group than in the placebo group (51.0 vs. 76.3; HR 0.67 [95% CI 0.52–0.85]; *P* < 0.001). No significant between-group differences were found in the rates of cardiovascular death or all-cause mortality. Both diarrhea (6.1% vs. 3.4%) and severe hypoglycemia (1.5% vs. 0.3%) were more common with sotagliflozin than with placebo. The trial was originally also intended to evaluate the effects of SGLT inhibition in people with HFpEF, and ultimately no evidence of heterogeneity of treatment effect by ejection fraction was noted. However, the relatively small percentage of such patients enrolled (only 21% of participants had ejection fraction >50%) and the early termination of the trial limited the ability to determine the effects of sotagliflozin in HFpEF specifically.

In addition to the hospitalization and mortality benefit in people with heart failure, several recent analyses have addressed whether SGLT2 inhibitor treatment improves clinical stability and functional status in individuals with heart failure. In 3,730 patients with NYHA class II–IV heart failure with an ejection fraction of ≤40%, treatment with empagliflozin reduced the combined risk of death, hospitalization for heart failure, or an emergent/urgent heart failure visit requiring intravenous treatment and reduced the total number of hospitalizations for heart failure requiring intensive care, a vasopressor or positive inotropic drug, or mechanical or surgical intervention.[229] In addition, patients treated with empagliflozin were more likely to experience an improvement in NYHA functional class.[229] In people hospitalized for acute de novo or decompensated chronic heart failure, initiation of empagliflozin treatment during hospitalization reduced the primary outcome of a composite of death from any cause, number of heart failure events and time to first heart failure event, or a 5-point or greater difference in change from baseline in the Kansas City Cardiomyopathy Questionnaire Total Symptom Score.[230] Furthermore, PRESERVED-HF, a multicenter study (26 sites in the U.S.) showed that dapagliflozin treatment leads to significant improvement in both symptoms and physical limitation, as well as objective measures of exercise function in people with chronic HFpEF, regardless of diabetes status.[198] Finally, canagliflozin improved heart failure symptoms assessed using the Kansas City Cardiomyopathy Questionnaire Total Symptom Score, irrespective of left ventricular ejection fraction or the presence of diabetes.[231] Therefore, in people with type 2 diabetes and established HFpEF or HFrEF, an SGLT2 inhibitor with proven benefit in this patient population is recommended to reduce the risk of worsening heart failure and cardiovascular death. In addition, an SGLT2 inhibitor is recommended in this patient population to improve symptoms, physical limitations, and quality of life. The benefits seen in this patient population likely represent a class effect, and they appear unrelated to glucose lowering given comparable outcomes in people with heart failure with and without diabetes.

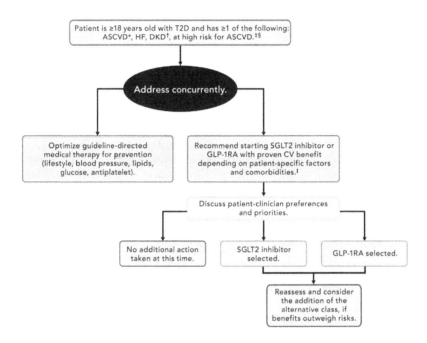

*ASCVD is defined as a history of an acute coronary syndrome or MI, stable or unstable angina, coronary heart disease with or without revascularization, other arterial revascularization, stroke, or peripheral artery disease assumed to be atherosclerotic in origin.

†DKD is a clinical diagnosis marked by reduced eGFR, the presence of albuminuria, or both.

‡ Consider an SGLT2 inhibitor when your patient has established ASCVD, HF, DKD or is at high risk for ASCVD. Consider a GLP-1RA when your patient has established ASCVD or is at high risk for ASCVD.

§Patients at high risk for ASCVD include those with end organ damage such as left ventricular hypertrophy or retinopathy or with multiple CV risk factors (e.g., age, hypertension, smoking, dyslipidemia, obesity).

∥ Most patients enrolled in the relevant trials were on metformin at baseline as glucose-lowering therapy.

ASCVD = atherosclerotic cardiovascular disease; CV = cardiovascular; DKD = diabetic kidney disease; eGFR = estimated glomerular filtration rate; GLP-1RA = glucagon-like peptide-1 receptor agonist; HF = heart failure; MI = myocardial infarction; SGLT2 = sodium-glucose cotransporter-2; T2D = type 2 diabetes

Figure 17.3—Approach to risk reduction with SGLT2 inhibitor or GLP-1 receptor agonist therapy in conjunction with other traditional, guideline-based preventive medical therapies for blood pressure, lipids, and glycemia and antiplatelet therapy. Reprinted with permission from Das et al.[234]

Finerenone in People With Type 2 Diabetes and Chronic Kidney Disease

As discussed in detail in Section 11, "Chronic Kidney Disease and Risk Management," people with diabetes are at an increased risk for CKD, which increases cardiovascular risk.[232] Finerenone, a selective nonsteroidal mineralocorticoid antagonist, has been shown in the Finerenone in Reducing Kidney Failure and Disease Progression in Diabetic Kidney Disease (FIDELIO-DKD) trial to improve CKD outcomes in people with type 2 diabetes with stage 3 or 4 CKD and severe albuminuria.[233] In the Finerenone in Reducing Cardiovascular Mortality and Morbidity in Diabetic Kidney Disease (FIGARO-DKD) trial, 7,437 patients with UACR 30–300 mg/g and eGFR 25–90 mL/min/1.73 m^2 or UACR 300–5,000 and eGFR ≥60 mL/min/1.73 m^2 on maximum dose of renin-angiotensin system blockade were randomized to receive finerenone or placebo.[186] The HR of the primary outcome of cardiovascular death, nonfatal MI, nonfatal stroke, or hospitalization from heart failure was reduced by 13% in patients treated with finerenone. A prespecified subgroup analysis from FIGARO-DKD further revealed that in patients without symptomatic HFrEF, finerenone reduces the risk for new-onset heart failure and improves heart failure outcomes in people with type 2 diabetes and CKD.[187] Finally, in the pooled analysis of 13,026 people with type 2 diabetes and CKD from both FIDELIO-DKD and FIGARO-DKD, the HRs for the composite of cardiovascular death, nonfatal MI, nonfatal stroke, or hospitalization for heart failure as well as a composite of kidney failure, a sustained ≥57% decrease in eGFR from baseline over ≥4 weeks, or renal death were 0.86 and 0.77, respectively.[188] These collective studies indicate that finerenone improves cardiovascular and renal outcomes in people with type 2 diabetes. Therefore, in people with type 2 diabetes and CKD with albuminuria treated with maximum tolerated doses of ACE inhibitor or ARB, addition of finernone should be considered to improve cardiovascular outcomes and reduce the risk of CKD progression.

Clinical Approach

As has been carefully outlined in Fig. 9.3 in the preceding Section 9, "Pharmacologic Approaches to Glycemic Treatment," people with type 2 diabetes with or at high risk for ASCVD, heart failure, or CKD should be treated with a cardioprotective SGLT2 inhibitor and/or GLP-1 receptor agonist as part of the comprehensive approach to cardiovascular and kidney risk reduction. Importantly, these agents should be included in the regimen of care irrespective of the need for additional glucose lowering, and irrespective of metformin use. Such an approach has also been described in the American Diabetes Association–endorsed American College of Cardiology "2020 Expert Consensus Decision Pathway on Novel Therapies for Cardiovascular Risk Reduction in Patients With Type 2 Diabetes".[234] Figure 17.3, reproduced from that decision pathway, outlines the approach to risk reduction with SGLT2 inhibitor or GLP-1 receptor agonist therapy in conjunction with other traditional, guideline-based preventive medical therapies for blood pressure, lipids, and glycemia and antiplatelet therapy.

Adoption of these agents should be reasonably straightforward in people with established cardiovascular or kidney disease who are later diagnosed with diabetes, as the cardioprotective agents can be used from the outset of diabetes management. On the other hand, incorporation of SGLT2 inhibitor or GLP-1 receptor agonist therapy in the care of individuals with more long-standing diabetes may be more challenging, particularly if patients are using an already complex glucose-lowering regimen. In such patients, SGLT2 inhibitor or GLP-1 receptor agonist therapy may need to replace some or all of their existing medications to minimize risks of hypoglycemia and adverse side effects, and potentially to minimize medication costs. Close collaboration between primary and specialty care professionals can help to facilitate these transitions in clinical care and, in turn, improve outcomes for highrisk people with type 2 diabetes.

REFERENCES

1. American Diabetes Association. Economic costs of diabetes in the U.S. in 2017. Diabetes Care 2018;41:917–928

2. Ali MK, Bullard KM, Saaddine JB, Cowie CC, Imperatore G, Gregg EW. Achievement of goals in U.S. diabetes care, 1999-2010. N Engl J Med 2013;368:1613–1624

3. Buse JB, Ginsberg HN, Bakris GL, et al.; American Heart Association; American Diabetes Association. Primary prevention of cardiovascular diseases in people with diabetes mellitus: a scientific statement from the American Heart Association and the American Diabetes Association. Diabetes Care 2007;30:162–172

4. Gaede P, Lund-Andersen H, Parving HH, Pedersen O. Effect of a multifactorial intervention on mortality in type 2 diabetes. N Engl J Med 2008;358:580–591

5. Cavender MA, Steg PG, Smith SC Jr, et al.; REACH Registry Investigators. Impact of diabetes mellitus on hospitalization for heart failure, cardiovascular events, and death: outcomes at 4 years from the Reduction of Atherothrombosis for Continued Health (REACH) Registry. Circulation 2015;132:923–931

6. McAllister DA, Read SH, Kerssens J, et al. Incidence of hospitalization for heart failure and case-fatality among 3.25 million people with and without diabetes mellitus. Circulation 2018;138:2774–2786

7. Lam CSP, Voors AA, de Boer RA, Solomon SD, van Veldhuisen DJ. Heart failure with preserved ejection fraction: from mechanisms to therapies. Eur Heart J 2018;39:2780–2792

8. Zinman B, Wanner C, Lachin JM, et al.; EMPA-REG OUTCOME Investigators. Empagliflozin, cardiovascular outcomes, and mortality in type 2 diabetes. N Engl J Med 2015;373:2117–2128

9. Neal B, Perkovic V, Mahaffey KW, et al.; CANVAS Program Collaborative Group. Canagliflozin and cardiovascular and renal events in type 2 diabetes. N Engl J Med 2017;377:644–657

10. Fitchett D, Butler J, van de Borne P, et al.; EMPA-REG OUTCOME trial investigators. Effects of empagliflozin on risk for cardiovascular death and heart failure hospitalization across the spectrum of heart failure risk in the EMPA-REG OUTCOME trial. Eur Heart J 2018;39:363–370

11. McMurray JJV, Solomon SD, Inzucchi SE, et al.; DAPA-HF Trial Committees and Investigators. Dapagliflozin in patients with heart failure and reduced ejection fraction. N Engl J Med 2019; 381:1995–2008

12. Arnott C, Li Q, Kang A, et al. Sodium-glucose cotransporter 2 inhibition for the prevention of cardiovascular events in patients with type 2 diabetes mellitus: a systematic review and metaanalysis. J Am Heart Assoc 2020;9:e014908

13. Blood Pressure Lowering Treatment Trialists' Collaboration. Blood pressure-lowering treatment based on cardiovascular risk: a meta-analysis of individual patient data. Lancet 2014;384:591–598

14. Grundy SM, Stone NJ, Bailey AL, et al. 2018 AHA/ACC/AACVPR/AAPA/ ABC/ACPM/ADA/AGS/APhA/ASPC/NLA/PCNA guideline on the management of blood cholesterol: executive summary: a report of the American College of Cardiology/American Heart Association Task Force on Clinical Practice Guidelines. J Am Coll Cardiol 2019;73:3168–3209

15. Muntner P, Colantonio LD, Cushman M, et al. Validation of the atherosclerotic cardiovascular disease Pooled Cohort risk equations. JAMA 2014;311:1406–1415

16. DeFilippis AP, Young R, McEvoy JW, et al. Risk score overestimation: the impact of individual cardiovascular risk factors and preventive therapies on the performance of the American Heart Association-American College of Cardiology-Atherosclerotic Cardiovascular Disease risk score in a modern multi-ethnic cohort. Eur Heart J 2017;38:598–608

17. Bohula EA, Morrow DA, Giugliano RP, et al. Atherothrombotic risk stratification and ezetimibe for secondary prevention. J Am Coll Cardiol 2017;69:911–921

18. Bohula EA, Bonaca MP, Braunwald E, et al. Atherothrombotic risk stratification and the efficacy and safety of vorapaxar in patients with stable ischemic heart disease and previous myocardial infarction. Circulation 2016;134:304–313

19. Whelton PK, Carey RM, Aronow WS, et al. 2017 ACC/AHA/AAPA/ABC/ ACPM/AGS/APhA/ASH/ASPC/NMA/PCNA guideline for the prevention, detection, evaluation, and management of high blood pressure in adults: a report of the American College of Cardiology/American Heart Association Task Force on Clinical Practice Guidelines. J Am Coll Cardiol 2018;71:e127–e248

20. de Boer IH, Bangalore S, Benetos A, et al. Diabetes and hypertension: a position statement by the American Diabetes Association. Diabetes Care 2017;40:1273–1284

21. Unger T, Borghi C, Charchar F, et al. 2020 International Society of Hypertension Global Hypertension Practice Guidelines. Hypertension 2020;75:1334–1357

22. Williams B, Mancia G, Spiering W, et al.; ESC Scientific Document Group. 2018 ESC/ESH guidelines for the management of arterial hypertension. Eur Heart J 2018;39:3021–3104

23. Bobrie G, Genés N, Vaur L, et al. Is "isolated home" hypertension as opposed to "isolated office" hypertension a sign of greater cardiovascular risk? Arch Intern Med 2001;161:2205–2211

24. Sega R, Facchetti R, Bombelli M, et al. Prognostic value of ambulatory and home blood pressures compared with office blood pressure in the general population: follow-up results from the Pressioni Arteriose Monitorate e Loro Associazioni (PAMELA) study. Circulation 2005;111:1777–1783

25. Omboni S, Gazzola T, Carabelli G, Parati G. Clinical usefulness and cost effectiveness of home blood pressure telemonitoring: meta-analysis of randomized controlled studies. J Hypertens 2013; 31:455–467; discussion 467–468

26. Emdin CA, Rahimi K, Neal B, Callender T, Perkovic V, Patel A. Blood pressure lowering in type 2 diabetes: a systematic review and metaanalysis. JAMA 2015;313:603–615

27. Arguedas JA, Leiva V, Wright JM. Blood pressure targets for hypertension in people with diabetes mellitus. Cochrane Database Syst Rev 2013;10:CD008277

28. Ettehad D, Emdin CA, Kiran A, et al. Blood pressure lowering for prevention of cardiovascular disease and death: a systematic review and metaanalysis. Lancet 2016;387:957–967

29. Brunström M, Carlberg B. Effect of antihypertensive treatment at different blood pressure levels in patients with diabetes mellitus: systematic review and meta-analyses. BMJ 2016; 352:i717

30. Bangalore S, Kumar S, Lobach I, Messerli FH. Blood pressure targets in subjects with type 2 diabetes mellitus/impaired fasting glucose: observations from traditional and bayesian random-effects meta-analyses of randomized trials. Circulation 2011;123:2799–2810

31. Thomopoulos C, Parati G, Zanchetti A. Effects of blood-pressure-lowering treatment on outcome incidence in hypertension: 10 - Should blood pressure management differ in hypertensive patients with and without diabetes mellitus? Overview and meta-analyses of randomized trials. J Hypertens 2017;35:922–944

32. Xie X, Atkins E, Lv J, et al. Effects of intensive blood pressure lowering on cardiovascular and renal outcomes: updated systematic review and meta-analysis. Lancet 2016;387:435–443

33. Wright JT Jr, Williamson JD, Whelton PK, et al.; SPRINT Research Group. A randomized trial of intensive versus standard blood-pressure control. N Engl J Med 2015;373:2103–2116

34. Zhang W, Zhang S, Deng Y, et al.; STEP Study Group. Trial of intensive blood-pressure control in older patients with hypertension. N Engl J Med 2021;385:1268–1279

35. Cushman WC, Evans GW, Byington RP, et al.; ACCORD Study Group. Effects of intensive blood-pressure control in type 2 diabetes mellitus. N Engl J Med 2010;362:1575–1585

36. Patel A, MacMahon S, Chalmers J, et al.; ADVANCE Collaborative Group. Effects of a fixed combination of perindopril and indapamide on macrovascular and microvascular outcomes in patients with type 2 diabetes mellitus (the ADVANCE trial): a randomised controlled trial. Lancet 2007;370:829–840

37. Hansson L, Zanchetti A, Carruthers SG, et al.; HOT Study Group. Effects of intensive blood-pressure lowering and low-dose aspirin in patients with hypertension: principal results of the Hypertension Optimal Treatment (HOT) randomised trial. Lancet 1998;351:1755–1762

38. Reboldi G, Gentile G, Angeli F, Ambrosio G, Mancia G, Verdecchia P. Effects of intensive blood pressure reduction on myocardial infarction and stroke in diabetes: a meta-analysis in 73,913 patients. J Hypertens 2011;29:1253–1269

39. de Boer IH, Bakris G, Cannon CP. Individualizing blood pressure targets for people with diabetes and hypertension: comparing the ADA and the ACC/AHA recommendations. JAMA 2018;319:1319–1320

40. Basu S, Sussman JB, Rigdon J, Steimle L, Denton BT, Hayward RA. Benefit and harm of intensive blood pressure treatment: derivation and validation of risk models using data from the SPRINT and ACCORD trials. PLoS Med 2017;14: e1002410

41. Phillips RA, Xu J, Peterson LE, Arnold RM, Diamond JA, Schussheim AE. Impact of cardiovascular risk on the relative benefit and harm of intensive treatment of hypertension. J Am Coll Cardiol 2018;71:1601–1610

42. Beddhu S, Greene T, Boucher R, et al. Intensive systolic blood pressure control and incident chronic kidney disease in people with and without diabetes mellitus: secondary analyses of two randomised controlled trials. Lancet Diabetes Endocrinol 2018;6:555–563

43. Sink KM, Evans GW, Shorr RI, et al. Syncope, hypotension, and falls in the treatment of hypertension: results from the randomized clinical systolic blood pressure intervention trial. J Am Geriatr Soc 2018;66:679–686

44. Ilkun OL, Greene T, Cheung AK, et al. The influence of baseline diastolic blood pressure on the effects of intensive blood pressure lowering on car-

diovascular outcomes and all-cause mortality in type 2 diabetes. Diabetes Care 2020;43:1878–1884

45. Abalos E, Duley L, Steyn DW. Antihypertensive drug therapy for mild to moderate hypertension during pregnancy. Cochrane Database Syst Rev 2014;2:CD002252

46. Magee LA, von Dadelszen P, Rey E, et al. Less-tight versus tight control of hypertension in pregnancy. N Engl J Med 2015;372:407–417

47. Brown MA, Magee LA, Kenny LC, et al.; International Society for the Study of Hypertension in Pregnancy (ISSHP). Hypertensive disorders of pregnancy: ISSHP classification, diagnosis, and management recommendations for international practice. Hypertension 2018;72:24–43

48. Tita AT, Szychowski JM, Boggess K, et al.; Chronic Hypertension and Pregnancy (CHAP) Trial Consortium. Treatment for mild chronic hypertension during pregnancy. N Engl J Med 2022;386:1781–1792

49. American College of Obstetricians and Gynecologists, Task Force on Hypertension in Pregnancy. Hypertension in pregnancy. Report of the American College of Obstetricians and Gynecologists' Task Force on Hypertension in Pregnancy. Obstet Gynecol 2013;122:1122–1131

50. Al-Balas M, Bozzo P, Einarson A. Use of diuretics during pregnancy. Can Fam Physician 2009;55:44–45

51. Irgens HU, Reisaeter L, Irgens LM, Lie RT. Long term mortality of mothers and fathers after pre-eclampsia: population based cohort study. BMJ 2001;323:1213–1217

52. Sacks FM, Svetkey LP, Vollmer WM, et al.; DASH-Sodium Collaborative Research Group. Effects on blood pressure of reduced dietary sodium and the Dietary Approaches to Stop Hypertension (DASH) diet. N Engl J Med 2001;344:3–10

53. James PA, Oparil S, Carter BL, et al. 2014 evidence-based guideline for the management of high blood pressure in adults: report from the panel members appointed to the Eighth Joint National Committee (JNC 8). JAMA 2014;311:507–520

54. Mao Y, Lin W, Wen J, Chen G. Impact and efficacy of mobile health intervention in the management of diabetes and hypertension: a systematic review and meta-analysis. BMJ Open Diabetes Res Care 2020;8:e001225

55. Stogios N, Kaur B, Huszti E, Vasanthan J, Nolan RP. Advancing digital health interventions as a clinically applied science for blood pressure reduction: a systematic review and meta-analysis. Can J Cardiol 2020;36:764–774

56. Bakris GL; Weir MR; Study of Hypertension and the Efficacy of Lotrel in Diabetes (SHIELD) Investigators. Achieving goal blood pressure in patients with type 2 diabetes: conventional versus fixed-dose combination approaches. J Clin Hypertens (Greenwich) 2003;5:202–209

57. Feldman RD, Zou GY, Vandervoort MK, Wong CJ, Nelson SAE, Feagan BG. A simplified approach to the treatment of uncomplicated hypertension: a cluster randomized, controlled trial. Hypertension 2009;53:646–653

58. Webster R, Salam A, de Silva HA, et al.; TRIUMPH Study Group. Fixed low-dose triple combination antihypertensive medication vs usual care for blood pressure control in patients with mild to moderate hypertension in Sri Lanka: a randomized clinical trial. JAMA 2018;320:566–579

59. Bangalore S, Kamalakkannan G, Parkar S, Messerli FH. Fixed-dose combinations improve medication compliance: a meta-analysis. Am J Med 2007;120:713–719

60. Catalá-López F, Macías Saint-Gerons D, González-Bermejo D, et al. Cardiovascular and renal outcomes of renin-angiotensin system blockade in adult patients with diabetes mellitus: a systematic review with network meta-analyses. PLoS Med 2016;13:e1001971

61. Palmer SC, Mavridis D, Navarese E, et al. Comparative efficacy and safety of blood pressure-lowering agents in adults with diabetes and kidney disease: a network meta-analysis. Lancet 2015;385:2047–2056

62. Barzilay JI, Davis BR, Bettencourt J, et al.; ALLHAT Collaborative Research Group. Cardiovascular outcomes using doxazosin vs. chlorthalidone for the treatment of hypertension in older adults with and without glucose disorders: a report from the ALLHAT study. J Clin Hypertens (Greenwich) 2004;6:116–125

63. Weber MA, Bakris GL, Jamerson K, et al.; ACCOMPLISH Investigators. Cardiovascular events during differing hypertension therapies in patients with diabetes. J Am Coll Cardiol 2010;56:77–85

64. Heart Outcomes Prevention Evaluation Study Investigators. Effects of ramipril on cardiovascular and microvascular outcomes in people with diabetes mellitus: results of the HOPE study and MICRO-HOPE substudy. Lancet 2000;355:253–259

65. Arnold SV, Bhatt DL, Barsness GW, et al.; American Heart Association Council on Lifestyle and Cardiometabolic Health and Council on Clinical Cardiology. Clinical management of stable coronary artery disease in patients with type 2 diabetes mellitus: a scientific statement from the American Heart Association. Circulation 2020; 141:e779–e806

66. Yusuf S, Teo K, Anderson C, et al.; Telmisartan Randomised AssessmeNt Study in ACE iNtolerant subjects with cardiovascular Disease (TRANSCEND) Investigators. Effects of the angiotensin-receptor blocker telmisartan on cardiovascular events in high-risk patients intolerant to angiotensin-converting enzyme inhibitors: a randomised controlled trial. Lancet 2008;372:1174–1183

67. Qiao Y, Shin JI, Chen TK, et al. Association between renin-angiotensin system blockade discontinuation and all-cause mortality among persons with

low estimated glomerular filtration rate. JAMA Intern Med 2020;180:718–726

68. Bangalore S, Fakheri R, Toklu B, Messerli FH. Diabetes mellitus as a compelling indication for use of renin angiotensin system blockers: systematic review and meta-analysis of randomized trials. BMJ 2016;352:i438

69. Carlberg B, Samuelsson O, Lindholm LH. Atenolol in hypertension: is it a wise choice? Lancet 2004;364:1684–1689

70. Murphy SP, Ibrahim NE, Januzzi JL Jr. Heart failure with reduced ejection fraction: a review. JAMA 2020;324:488–504

71. Yusuf S, Teo KK, Pogue J, et al.; ONTARGET Investigators. Telmisartan, ramipril, or both in patients at high risk for vascular events. N Engl J Med 2008;358:1547–1559

72. Fried LF, Emanuele N, Zhang JH, et al.; VA NEPHRON-D Investigators. Combined angiotensin inhibition for the treatment of diabetic nephropathy. N Engl J Med 2013;369:1892–1903

73. Makani H, Bangalore S, Desouza KA, Shah A, Messerli FH. Efficacy and safety of dual blockade of the renin-angiotensin system: meta-analysis of randomised trials. BMJ 2013;346:f360

74. Zhao P, Xu P, Wan C, Wang Z. Evening versus morning dosing regimen drug therapy for hypertension. Cochrane Database Syst Rev 2011 (10):CD004184

75. Hermida RC, Ayala DE, Mojón A, Fernández JR. Influence of time of day of blood pressure-lowering treatment on cardiovascular risk in hypertensive patients with type 2 diabetes. Diabetes Care 2011;34:1270–1276

76. Rahman M, Greene T, Phillips RA, et al. A trial of 2 strategies to reduce nocturnal blood pressure in Blacks with chronic kidney disease. Hypertension 2013;61:82–88

77. Nilsson E, Gasparini A, Ärnlöv J, et al. Incidence and determinants of hyperkalemia and hypokalemia in a large healthcare system. Int J Cardiol 2017;245:277–284

78. Bandak G, Sang Y, Gasparini A, et al. Hyperkalemia after initiating renin-angiotensin system blockade: the Stockholm Creatinine Measurements (SCREAM) project. J Am Heart Assoc 2017;6:e005428

79. Hughes-Austin JM, Rifkin DE, Beben T, et al. The relation of serum potassium concentration with cardiovascular events and mortality in community-living individuals. Clin J Am Soc Nephrol 2017;12:245–252

80. James MT, Grams ME, Woodward M, et al.; CKD Prognosis Consortium. A meta-analysis of the association of estimated GFR, albuminuria, diabetes mellitus, and hypertension with acute kidney injury. Am J Kidney Dis 2015;66:602–612

81. Williams B, MacDonald TM, Morant S, et al.; British Hypertension Society's PATHWAY Studies Group. Spironolactone versus placebo, bisoprolol, and doxazosin to determine the optimal treatment for drug-resistant hypertension (PATHWAY-2): a randomised, double-blind, crossover trial. Lancet 2015;386:2059–2068

82. Sato A, Hayashi K, Naruse M, Saruta T. Effectiveness of aldosterone blockade in patients with diabetic nephropathy. Hypertension 2003;41: 64–68

83. Mehdi UF, Adams-Huet B, Raskin P, Vega GL, Toto RD. Addition of angiotensin receptor blockade or mineralocorticoid antagonism to maximal angiotensin-converting enzyme inhibition in diabetic nephropathy. J Am Soc Nephrol 2009;20:2641–2650

84. Bakris GL, Agarwal R, Chan JC, et al.; Mineralocorticoid Receptor Antagonist Tolerability Study–Diabetic Nephropathy (ARTS-DN) Study Group. Effect of finerenone on albuminuria in patients with diabetic nephropathy: a randomized clinical trial. JAMA 2015;314:884–894

85. Jensen MD, Ryan DH, Apovian CM, et al.; American College of Cardiology/American Heart Association Task Force on Practice Guidelines; Obesity Society. 2013 AHA/ACC/TOS guideline for the management of overweight and obesity in adults: a report of the American College of Cardiology/American Heart Association Task Force on Practice Guidelines and The Obesity Society. J Am Coll Cardiol 2014;63(25 Pt B): 2985–3023

86. Eckel RH, Jakicic JM, Ard JD, et al.; 2013 AHA/ACC guideline on lifestyle management to reduce cardiovascular risk: a report of the American College of Cardiology/American Heart Association Task Force on Practice Guidelines. Circulation 2013;129:S76–S99

87. Arnett DK, Blumenthal RS, Albert MA, et al. 2019 ACC/AHA guideline on the primary prevention of cardiovascular disease: a report of the American College of Cardiology/American Heart Association Task Force on Clinical Practice Guidelines. Circulation 2019;140:e596–e646

88. Chasman DI, Posada D, Subrahmanyan L, Cook NR, Stanton VP Jr, Ridker PM. Pharmacogenetic study of statin therapy and cholesterol reduction. JAMA 2004;291:2821–2827

89. Meek C, Wierzbicki AS, Jewkes C, et al. Daily and intermittent rosuvastatin 5 mg therapy in statin intolerant patients: an observational study. Curr Med Res Opin 2012;28:371–378

90. Mihaylova B, Emberson J, Blackwell L, et al.; Cholesterol Treatment Trialists' (CTT) Collaborators. The effects of lowering LDL cholesterol with statin therapy in people at low risk of vascular disease: meta-analysis of individual data from 27 randomised trials. Lancet 2012;380:581–590

91. Baigent C, Keech A, Kearney PM, et al.; Cholesterol Treatment Trialists' (CTT) Collaborators. Efficacy and safety of cholesterol-lowering treatment: prospective meta-analysis of data from 90,056 participants in 14 randomised trials of statins. Lancet 2005;366:1267–1278

92. Pyörälä K, Pedersen TR, Kjekshus J, Faergeman O, Olsson AG, Thorgeirs-son G. Cholesterol lowering with simvastatin improves prognosis of diabetic patients with coronary heart disease. A subgroup analysis of the Scandinavian Simvastatin Survival Study (4S). Diabetes Care 1997;20:614–620

93. Collins R, Armitage J, Parish S, Sleigh P; Heart Protection Study Collaborative Group. MRC/BHF Heart Protection Study of cholesterol-lowering with simvastatin in 5963 people with diabetes: a randomised placebo-controlled trial. Lancet 2003; 361:2005–2016

94. Goldberg RB, Mellies MJ, Sacks FM, et al.; The Care Investigators. Cardiovascular events and their reduction with pravastatin in diabetic and glucose-intolerant myocardial infarction survivors with average cholesterol levels: subgroup analyses in the Cholesterol and Recurrent Events (CARE) trial. Circulation 1998;98:2513–2519

95. Shepherd J, Barter P, Carmena R, et al. Effect of lowering LDL cholesterol substantially below currently recommended levels in patients with coronary heart disease and diabetes: the Treating to New Targets (TNT) study. Diabetes Care 2006;29:1220–1226

96. Sever PS, Poulter NR, Dahlöf B, et al. Reduction in cardiovascular events with atorvastatin in 2,532 patients with type 2 diabetes: Anglo-Scandinavian Cardiac Outcomes Trial–lipid-lowering arm (ASCOT-LLA). Diabetes Care 2005;28:1151–1157

97. Knopp RH, d'Emden M, Smilde JG, Pocock SJ. Efficacy and safety of atorvastatin in the prevention of cardiovascular end points in subjects with type 2 diabetes: the Atorvastatin Study for Prevention of Coronary Heart Disease Endpoints in non-insulin-dependent diabetes mellitus (ASPEN). Diabetes Care 2006;29:1478–1485

98. Colhoun HM, Betteridge DJ, Durrington PN, et al.; CARDS investigators. Primary prevention of cardiovascular disease with atorvastatin in type 2 diabetes in the Collaborative Atorvastatin Diabetes Study (CARDS): multicentre randomised placebo-controlled trial. Lancet 2004;364:685–696

99. Kearney PM, Blackwell L, Collins R, et al.; Cholesterol Treatment Trialists' (CTT) Collaborators. Efficacy of cholesterol-lowering therapy in 18,686 people with diabetes in 14 randomised trials of statins: a meta-analysis. Lancet 2008;371:117–125

100. Taylor F, Huffman MD, Macedo AF, et al. Statins for the primary prevention of cardiovascular disease. Cochrane Database Syst Rev 2013;1: CD004816

101. Carter AA, Gomes T, Camacho X, Juurlink DN, Shah BR, Mamdani MM. Risk of incident diabetes among patients treated with statins: population based study. BMJ 2013;346:f2610–f2610

102. Jellinger PS, Handelsman Y, Rosenblit PD, et al. American Association of Clinical Endocrinologists and American College of Endocrinology guide-

lines for management of dyslipidemia and prevention of cardiovascular disease. Endocr Pract 2017;23(Suppl. 2):1–87

103. Goldberg RB, Stone NJ, Grundy SM. The 2018 AHA/ACC/AACVPR/AAPA/ABC/ACPM/ADA/AGS/APhA/ASPC/NLA/PCNA guidelines on the management of blood cholesterol in diabetes. Diabetes Care 2020;43:1673–1678

104. Mach F, Baigent C, Catapano AL, et al.; ESC Scientific Document Group. 2019 ESC/EAS guidelines for the management of dyslipidaemias: lipid modification to reduce cardiovascular risk. Eur Heart J 2020;41:111–188

105. Cannon CP, Blazing MA, Giugliano RP, et al.; IMPROVE-IT Investigators. Ezetimibe added to statin therapy after acute coronary syndromes. N Engl J Med 2015;372:2387–2397

106. de Ferranti SD, de Boer IH, Fonseca V, et al. Type 1 diabetes mellitus and cardiovascular disease: a scientific statement from the American Heart Association and American Diabetes Association. Diabetes Care 2014;37:2843–2863

107. Cannon CP, Braunwald E, McCabe CH, et al.; Pravastatin or Atorvastatin Evaluation and Infection Therapy-Thrombolysis in Myocardial Infarction 22 Investigators. Intensive versus moderate lipid lowering with statins after acute coronary syndromes. N Engl J Med 2004;350:1495–1504

108. Sabatine MS, Giugliano RP, Keech AC, et al.; FOURIER Steering Committee and Investigators. Evolocumab and clinical outcomes in patients with cardiovascular disease. N Engl J Med 2017; 376:1713–1722

109. Giugliano RP, Cannon CP, Blazing MA, et al.; IMPROVE-IT (Improved Reduction of Outcomes: Vytorin Efficacy International Trial) Investigators. Benefit of adding ezetimibe to statin therapy on cardiovascular outcomes and safety in patients with versus without diabetes mellitus: results from IMPROVE-IT (Improved Reduction of Outcomes: Vytorin Efficacy International Trial). Circulation 2018;137:1571–1582

110. Schwartz GG, Steg PG, Szarek M, et al.; ODYSSEY OUTCOMES Committees and Investigators. Alirocumab and cardiovascular outcomes after acute coronary syndrome. N Engl J Med 2018;379: 2097–2107

111. Ray KK, Colhoun HM, Szarek M, et al.; ODYSSEY OUTCOMES Committees and Investigators. Effects of alirocumab on cardiovascular and metabolic outcomes after acute coronary syndrome in patients with or without diabetes: a prespecified analysis of the ODYSSEY OUTCOMES randomised controlled trial. Lancet Diabetes Endocrinol 2019; 7:618–628

112. Sabatine MS, Leiter LA, Wiviott SD, et al. Cardiovascular safety and efficacy of the PCSK9 inhibitor evolocumab in patients with and without diabetes and the effect of evolocumab on glycaemia and risk of new-onset diabetes: a prespecified analysis of the FOURIER randomised controlled trial. Lancet Diabetes Endocrinol 2017; 5:941–950

113. Moriarty PM, Jacobson TA, Bruckert E, et al. Efficacy and safety of ali-rocumab, a monoclonal antibody to PCSK9, in statin-intolerant patients: design and rationale of ODYSSEY ALTERNATIVE, a randomized phase 3 trial. J Clin Lipidol 2014;8:554–561

114. Zhang XL, Zhu QQ, Zhu L, et al. Safety and efficacy of anti-PCSK9 anti-bodies: a meta-analysis of 25 randomized, controlled trials. BMC Med 2015;13:123

115. Giugliano RP, Pedersen TR, Saver JL, et al.; FOURIER Investigators. Stroke prevention with the PCSK9 (proprotein convertase subtilisin-kexin type 9) inhibitor evolocumab added to statin in high-risk patients with sta-ble atherosclerosis. Stroke 2020;51:1546–1554

116. Ray KK, Wright RS, Kallend D, et al.; ORION-10 and ORION-11 Inves-tigators. Two phase 3 trials of inclisiran in patients with elevated LDL cho-lesterol. N Engl J Med 2020;382:1507–1519

117. University of Oxford. A Randomized Trial Assessing the Effects of Inclisiran on Clinical Outcomes Among People With Cardiovascular Disease (ORION-4). In: ClinicalTrials.gov. Bethesda, MD, National Library of Medicine. NLM Identifier: NCT03705234. Accessed 15 October 2022. Available from https://clinicaltrials.gov/ct2/show/NCT03705234

118. Dai L, Zuo Y, You Q, Zeng H, Cao S. Efficacy and safety of bempedoic acid in patients with hypercholesterolemia: a systematic review and meta-analy-sis of randomized controlled trials. Eur J Prev Cardiol 2021;28:825–83

119. Di Minno A, Lupoli R, Calcaterra I, et al. Efficacy and safety of bempedoic acid in patients with hypercholesterolemia: systematic review and meta-analysis of randomized controlled trials. J Am Heart Assoc 2020;9:e016262

120. Berglund L, Brunzell JD, Goldberg AC, et al.; Endocrine society. Evalua-tion and treatment of hypertriglyceridemia: an Endocrine Society clinical practice guideline. J Clin Endocrinol Metab 2012; 97:2969–2989

121. Bhatt DL, Steg PG, Miller M, et al.; REDUCE-IT Investigators. Cardio-vascular risk reduction with icosapent ethyl for hypertriglyceridemia. N Engl J Med 2019;380:11–22

122. Nicholls SJ, Lincoff AM, Garcia M, et al. Effect of high-dose omega-3 fatty acids vs corn oil on major adverse cardiovascular events in patients at high cardiovascular risk: the STRENGTH randomized clinical trial. JAMA 2020;324:2268–2280

123. Singh IM, Shishehbor MH, Ansell BJ. High-density lipoprotein as a thera-peutic target: a systematic review. JAMA 2007;298:786–798

124. Keech A, Simes RJ, Barter P, et al.; FIELD study investigators. Effects of long-term feno-fibrate therapy on cardiovascular events in 9795 people with type 2 diabetes mellitus (the FIELD study): randomised controlled trial. Lancet 2005;366:1849–1861

125. Jones PH, Davidson MH. Reporting rate of rhabdomyolysis with fenofibrate + statin versus gemfibrozil + any statin. Am J Cardiol 2005;95: 120–122

126. Ginsberg HN, Elam MB, Lovato LC, et al.; ACCORD Study Group. Effects of combination lipid therapy in type 2 diabetes mellitus. N Engl J Med 2010;362:1563–1574

127. Boden WE, Probstfield JL, Anderson T, et al.; AIM-HIGH Investigators. Niacin in patients with low HDL cholesterol levels receiving intensive statin therapy. N Engl J Med 2011;365:2255–2267

128. Landray MJ, Haynes R, Hopewell JC, et al.; HPS2-THRIVE Collaborative Group. Effects of extended-release niacin with laropiprant in high-risk patients. N Engl J Med 2014;371:203–212

129. Rajpathak SN, Kumbhani DJ, Crandall J, Barzilai N, Alderman M, Ridker PM. Statin therapy and risk of developing type 2 diabetes: a metaanalysis. Diabetes Care 2009;32:1924–1929

130. Sattar N, Preiss D, Murray HM, et al. Statins and risk of incident diabetes: a collaborative meta-analysis of randomised statin trials. Lancet 2010;375:735–742

131. Ridker PM, Pradhan A, MacFadyen JG, Libby P, Glynn RJ. Cardiovascular benefits and diabetes risks of statin therapy in primary prevention: an analysis from the JUPITER trial. Lancet 2012;380:565–571

132. Mach F, Ray KK, Wiklund O, et al.; European Atherosclerosis Society Consensus Panel. Adverse effects of statin therapy: perception vs. the evidence - focus on glucose homeostasis, cognitive, renal and hepatic function, haemorrhagic stroke and cataract. Eur Heart J 2018;39:2526–2539

133. Heart Protection Study Collaborative Group. MRC/BHF Heart Protection Study of cholesterol lowering with simvastatin in 20,536 high-risk individuals: a randomised placebo-controlled trial. Lancet 2002;360:7–22

134. Shepherd J, Blauw GJ, Murphy MB, et al.; PROSPER study group. PROspective Study of Pravastatin in the Elderly at Risk. Pravastatin in elderly individuals at risk of vascular disease (PROSPER): a randomised controlled trial. Lancet 2002;360:1623–1630

135. Trompet S, van Vliet P, de Craen AJM, et al. Pravastatin and cognitive function in the elderly. Results of the PROSPER study. J Neurol 2010; 257:85–90

136. Yusuf S, Bosch J, Dagenais G, et al.; HOPE-3 Investigators. Cholesterol lowering in intermediate-risk persons without cardiovascular disease. N Engl J Med 2016;374:2021–2031

137. Giugliano RP, Mach F, Zavitz K, et al.; EBBINGHAUS Investigators. Cognitive function in a randomized trial of evolocumab. N Engl J Med 2017;377:633–643

138. Richardson K, Schoen M, French B, et al. Statins and cognitive function: a systematic review. Ann Intern Med 2013;159:688–697

139. Baigent C, Blackwell L, Collins R, et al.; Antithrombotic Trialists' (ATT) Collaboration. Aspirin in the primary and secondary prevention of vascular disease: collaborative meta-analysis of individual participant data from randomised trials. Lancet 2009;373:1849–1860

140. Perk J, De Backer G, Gohlke H, et al.; European Association for Cardiovascular Prevention & Rehabilitation (EACPR); ESC Committee for Practice Guidelines (CPG). European Guidelines on cardiovascular disease prevention in clinical practice (version 2012). The Fifth Joint Task Force of the European Society of Cardiology and Other Societies on Cardiovascular Disease Prevention in Clinical Practice (constituted by representatives of nine societies and by invited experts). Eur Heart J 2012; 33:1635–1701

141. Belch J, MacCuish A, Campbell I, et al.; Prevention of Progression of Arterial Disease and Diabetes Study Group; Diabetes Registry Group; Royal College of Physicians Edinburgh. The prevention of progression of arterial disease and diabetes (POPADAD) trial: factorial randomised placebo controlled trial of aspirin and antioxidants in patients with diabetes and asymptomatic peripheral arterial disease. BMJ 2008;337:a1840–a1840

142. Zhang C, Sun A, Zhang P, et al. Aspirin for primary prevention of cardiovascular events in patients with diabetes: A meta-analysis. Diabetes Res Clin Pract 2010;87:211–218

143. De Berardis G, Sacco M, Strippoli GFM, et al. Aspirin for primary prevention of cardiovascular events in people with diabetes: meta-analysis of randomised controlled trials. BMJ 2009;339:b4531

144. ASCEND Study Collaborative Group. Effects of aspirin for primary prevention in persons with diabetes mellitus. N Engl J Med 2018;379:1529–1539

145. Gaziano JM, Brotons C, Coppolecchia R, et al.; ARRIVE Executive Committee. Use of aspirin to reduce risk of initial vascular events in patients at moderate risk of cardiovascular disease (ARRIVE): a randomised, double-blind, placebo-controlled trial. Lancet 2018;392:1036–1046

146. McNeil JJ, Wolfe R, Woods RL, et al.; ASPREE Investigator Group. Effect of aspirin on cardiovascular events and bleeding in the healthy elderly. N Engl J Med 2018;379:1509–1518

147. Pignone M, Earnshaw S, Tice JA, Pletcher MJ. Aspirin, statins, or both drugs for the primary prevention of coronary heart disease events in men: a cost-utility analysis. Ann Intern Med 2006;144:326–336

148. Huxley RR, Peters SAE, Mishra GD, Woodward M. Risk of all-cause mortality and vascular events in women versus men with type 1 diabetes: a systematic review and meta-analysis. Lancet Diabetes Endocrinol 2015;3:198–206

149. Peters SAE, Huxley RR, Woodward M. Diabetes as risk factor for incident coronary heart disease in women compared with men: a systematic review and meta-analysis of 64 cohorts including 858,507 individuals and 28,203 coronary events. Diabetologia 2014;57:1542–1551

150. Kalyani RR, Lazo M, Ouyang P, et al. Sex differences in diabetes and risk of incident coronary artery disease in healthy young and middle-aged adults. Diabetes Care 2014;37:830–838

151. Peters SAE, Huxley RR, Woodward M. Diabetes as a risk factor for stroke in women compared with men: a systematic review and metaanalysis of 64 cohorts, including 775,385 individuals and 12,539 strokes. Lancet 2014;383:1973–1980

152. Miedema MD, Duprez DA, Misialek JR, et al. Use of coronary artery calcium testing to guide aspirin utilization for primary prevention: estimates from the multi-ethnic study of atherosclerosis. Circ Cardiovasc Qual Outcomes 2014;7:453–460

153. Dimitriu-Leen AC, Scholte AJHA, van Rosendael AR, et al. Value of coronary computed tomography angiography in tailoring aspirin therapy for primary prevention of atherosclerotic events in patients at high risk with diabetes mellitus. Am J Cardiol 2016;117:887–893

154. Mora S, Ames JM, Manson JE. Low-dose aspirin in the primary prevention of cardiovascular disease: shared decision making in clinical practice. JAMA 2016;316:709–710

155. Campbell CL, Smyth S, Montalescot G, Steinhubl SR. Aspirin dose for the prevention of cardiovascular disease: a systematic review. JAMA 2007;297:2018–2024

156. Jones WS, Mulder H, Wruck LM, et al.; ADAPTABLE Team. Comparative effectiveness of aspirin dosing in cardiovascular disease. N Engl J Med 2021;384:1981–1990

157. Daví G, Patrono C. Platelet activation and atherothrombosis. N Engl J Med 2007;357:2482–2494

158. Larsen SB, Grove EL, Neergaard-Petersen S, Würtz M, Hvas AM, Kristensen SD. Determinants of reduced antiplatelet effect of aspirin in patients with stable coronary artery disease. PLoS One 2015;10:e0126767

159. Zaccardi F, Rizzi A, Petrucci G, et al. In vivo platelet activation and aspirin responsiveness in type 1 diabetes. Diabetes 2016;65:503–509

160. Bethel MA, Harrison P, Sourij H, et al. Randomized controlled trial comparing impact on platelet reactivity of twice-daily with once-daily aspirin in people with type 2 diabetes. Diabet Med 2016;33:224–230

161. Rothwell PM, Cook NR, Gaziano JM, et al. Effects of aspirin on risks of vascular events and cancer according to bodyweight and dose: analysis of individual patient data from randomised trials. Lancet 2018;392:387–399

162. Vandvik PO, Lincoff AM, Gore JM, et al. Primary and secondary prevention of cardiovascular disease: Antithrombotic Therapy and Prevention of Thrombosis, 9th ed: American College of Chest Physicians Evidence-Based Clinical Practice Guidelines. Chest 2012;141(Suppl.):e637S–e668S

163. Bhatt DL, Bonaca MP, Bansilal S, et al. Reduction in ischemic events with ticagrelor in diabetic patients with prior myocardial infarction in PEGA-SUS-TIMI 54. J Am Coll Cardiol 2016;67: 2732–2740

164. Steg PG, Bhatt DL, Simon T, et al.; THEMIS Steering Committee and Investigators. Ticagrelor in patients with stable coronary disease and diabetes. N Engl J Med 2019;381:1309–1320

165. Bhatt DL, Steg PG, Mehta SR, et al.; THEMIS Steering Committee and Investigators. Ticagrelor in patients with diabetes and stable coronary artery disease with a history of previous percutaneous coronary intervention (THEMIS-PCI): a phase 3, placebo-controlled, randomised trial. Lancet 2019;394:1169–1180

166. Angiolillo DJ, Baber U, Sartori S, et al. Ticagrelor with or without aspirin in high-risk patients with diabetes mellitus undergoing percutaneous coronary intervention. J Am Coll Cardiol 2020;75:2403–2413

167. Wiebe J, Ndrepepa G, Kufner S, et al. Early aspirin discontinuation after coronary stenting: a systematic review and meta-analysis. J Am Heart Assoc 2021;10:e018304

168. Bhatt DL, Eikelboom JW, Connolly SJ, et al.; COMPASS Steering Committee and Investigators. Role of combination antiplatelet and anticoagulation therapy in diabetes mellitus and cardiovascular disease: insights from the COMPASS trial. Circulation 2020;141:1841–1854

169. Connolly SJ, Eikelboom JW, Bosch J, et al.; COMPASS investigators. Rivaroxaban with or without aspirin in patients with stable coronary artery disease: an international, randomised, double-blind, placebo-controlled trial. Lancet 2018;391:205–218

170. Bonaca MP, Bauersachs RM, Anand SS, et al. Rivaroxaban in peripheral artery disease after revascularization. N Engl J Med 2020;382:1994–2004

171. Bax JJ, Young LH, Frye RL, Bonow RO, Steinberg HO; ADA. Screening for coronary artery disease in patients with diabetes. Diabetes Care 2007;30:2729–2736

172. Boden WE, O'Rourke RA, Teo KK, et al.; COURAGE Trial Research Group. Optimal medical therapy with or without PCI for stable coronary disease. N Engl J Med 2007;356:1503–1516

173. Frye RL, August P, Brooks MM, et al.; BARI 2D Study Group. A randomized trial of therapies for type 2 diabetes and coronary artery disease. N Engl J Med 2009;360:2503–2515

174. Wackers FJT, Chyun DA, Young LH, et al.; Detection of Ischemia in Asymptomatic Diabetics (DIAD) Investigators. Resolution of asymptomatic

myocardial ischemia in patients with type 2 diabetes in the Detection of Ischemia in Asymptomatic Diabetics (DIAD) study. Diabetes Care 2007;30:2892–2898

175. Elkeles RS, Godsland IF, Feher MD, et al.; PREDICT Study Group. Coronary calcium measurement improves prediction of cardiovascular events in asymptomatic patients with type 2 diabetes: the PREDICT study. Eur Heart J 2008;29:2244–2251

176. Raggi P, Shaw LJ, Berman DS, Callister TQ. Prognostic value of coronary artery calcium screening in subjects with and without diabetes. J Am Coll Cardiol 2004;43:1663–1669

177. Anand DV, Lim E, Hopkins D, et al. Risk stratification in uncomplicated type 2 diabetes: prospective evaluation of the combined use of coronary artery calcium imaging and selective myocardial perfusion scintigraphy. Eur Heart J 2006;27:713–721

178. Young LH, Wackers FJT, Chyun DA, et al.; DIAD Investigators. Cardiac outcomes after screening for asymptomatic coronary artery disease in patients with type 2 diabetes: the DIAD study: a randomized controlled trial. JAMA 2009; 301:1547–1555

179. Wackers FJT, Young LH, Inzucchi SE, et al.; Detection of Ischemia in Asymptomatic Diabetics Investigators. Detection of silent myocardial ischemia in asymptomatic diabetic subjects: the DIAD study. Diabetes Care 2004;27:1954–1961

180. Scognamiglio R, Negut C, Ramondo A, Tiengo A, Avogaro A. Detection of coronary artery disease in asymptomatic patients with type 2 diabetes mellitus. J Am Coll Cardiol 2006;47:65–71

181. Hadamitzky M, Hein F, Meyer T, et al. Prognostic value of coronary computed tomographic angiography in diabetic patients without known coronary artery disease. Diabetes Care 2010; 33:1358–1363

182. Choi EK, Chun EJ, Choi SI, et al. Assessment of subclinical coronary atherosclerosis in asymptomatic patients with type 2 diabetes mellitus with single photon emission computed tomography and coronary computed tomography angiography. Am J Cardiol 2009;104:890–896

183. Malik S, Zhao Y, Budoff M, et al. Coronary artery calcium score for long-term risk classification in individuals with type 2 diabetes and metabolic syndrome from the Multi-Ethnic Study of Atherosclerosis. JAMA Cardiol 2017;2:1332–1340

184. Wing RR, Bolin P, Brancati FL, et al.; Look AHEAD Research Group. Cardiovascular effects of intensive lifestyle intervention in type 2 diabetes. N Engl J Med 2013;369:145–154

185. Braunwald E, Domanski MJ, Fowler SE, et al.; PEACE Trial Investigators. Angiotensin-converting-enzyme inhibition in stable coronary artery disease. N Engl J Med 2004;351:2058–2068

186. Pitt B, Filippatos G, Agarwal R, et al.; FIGARO-DKD Investigators. Cardiovascular events with finerenone in kidney disease and type 2 diabetes. N Engl J Med 2021;385:2252–2263

187. Filippatos G, Anker SD, Agarwal R, et al.; FIGARO-DKD Investigators. Finerenone reduces risk of incident heart failure in patients with chronic kidney disease and type 2 diabetes: analyses from the FIGARO-DKD trial. Circulation 2022;145:437–447

188. Agarwal R, Filippatos G, Pitt B, et al.; FIDELIO-DKD and FIGARO-DKD investigators. Cardiovascular and kidney outcomes with finerenone in patients with type 2 diabetes and chronic kidney disease: the FIDELITY pooled analysis. Eur Heart J 2022; 43:474–484

189. Anker SD, Butler J, Filippatos G, et al.; EMPEROR-Preserved Trial Investigators. Empagliflozin in heart failure with a preserved ejection fraction. N Engl J Med 2021;385:1451–1461

190. Kezerashvili A, Marzo K, De Leon J. Beta blocker use after acute myocardial infarction in the patient with normal systolic function: when is it "ok" to discontinue? Curr Cardiol Rev 2012; 8:77–84

191. Fihn SD, Gardin JM, Abrams J, et al.; American College of Cardiology Foundation; American Heart Association Task Force on Practice Guidelines; American College of Physicians; American Association for Thoracic Surgery; Preventive Cardiovascular Nurses Association; Society for Cardiovascular Angiography and Interventions; Society of Thoracic Surgeons. 2012 ACCF/AHA/ACP/AATS/PCNA/SCAI/STS Guideline for the diagnosis and management of patients with stable ischemic heart disease: a report of the American College of Cardiology Foundation/American Heart Association Task Force on Practice Guidelines, and the American College of Physicians, American Association for Thoracic Surgery, Preventive Cardiovascular Nurses Association, Society for Cardiovascular Angiography and Interventions, and Society of Thoracic Surgeons. J Am Coll Cardiol 2012;60:e44–e164

192. U.S. Food and Drug Administration. Guidance for industry. Diabetes mellitus— evaluating cardiovascular risk in new antidiabetic therapies to treat type 2 diabetes. Silver Spring, MD, 2008. Accessed 21 October 2022. Available from https://www.federalregister.gov/documents/2008/12/19/E8-30086/guidance-for-industry-on-diabetes-mellitus-evaluating-cardiovascular-risk-in-new-antidiabetic

193. Rosenstock J, Perkovic V, Johansen OE, et al.; CARMELINA Investigators. Effect of linagliptin vs placebo on major cardiovascular events in adults with type 2 diabetes and high cardiovascular and renal risk: the CARMELINA randomized clinical trial. JAMA 2019;321:69–79

194. Perkovic V, Jardine MJ, Neal B, et al.; CREDENCE Trial Investigators. Canagliflozin and renal outcomes in type 2 diabetes and nephropathy. N Engl J Med 2019;380:2295–2306

195. Neal B, Perkovic V, Matthews DR, et al.; CANVAS-R Trial Collaborative Group. Rationale, design and baseline characteristics of the CANagliflozin cardioVascular Assessment Study-Renal (CANVAS-R): A randomized, placebo-controlled trial. Diabetes Obes Metab 2017;19: 387–393

196. Wiviott SD, Raz I, Bonaca MP, et al.; DECLARE–TIMI 58 Investigators. Dapagliflozin and cardiovascular outcomes in type 2 diabetes. N Engl J Med 2019;380:347–357

197. Heerspink HJL, Stefánsson BV, Correa-Rotter R, et al.; DAPA-CKD Trial Committees and Investigators. Dapagliflozin in patients with chronic kidney disease. N Engl J Med 2020;383:1436–1446

198. Nassif ME, Windsor SL, Borlaug BA, et al. The SGLT2 inhibitor dapagliflozin in heart failure with preserved ejection fraction: a multicenter randomized trial. Nat Med 2021;27:1954–1960

199. Solomon SD, McMurray JJV, Claggett B, et al.; DELIVER Trial Committees and Investigators. Dapagliflozin in heart failure with mildly reduced or preserved ejection fraction. N Engl J Med 2022;387:1089–1098

200. Packer M, Anker SD, Butler J, et al.; EMPEROR Reduced Trial Investigators. Cardiovascular and renal outcomes with empagliflozin in heart failure. N Engl J Med 2020;383:1413–1424

201. Cannon CP, Pratley R, Dagogo-Jack S, et al.; VERTIS CV Investigators. Cardiovascular outcomes with ertugliflozin in type 2 diabetes. N Engl J Med 2020;383:1425–1435

202. Bhatt DL, Szarek M, Pitt B, et al.; SCORED Investigators. Sotagliflozin in patients with diabetes and chronic kidney disease. N Engl J Med 2021;384:129–139

203. Marso SP, Daniels GH, Brown-Frandsen K, et al.; LEADER Steering Committee; LEADER Trial Investigators. Liraglutide and cardiovascular outcomes in type 2 diabetes. N Engl J Med 2016; 375:311–322

204. Marso SP, Bain SC, Consoli A, et al.; SUSTAIN-6 Investigators. Semaglutide and cardiovascular outcomes in patients with type 2 diabetes. N Engl J Med 2016;375:1834–1844

205. Husain M, Birkenfeld AL, Donsmark M, et al. Oral semaglutide and cardiovascular outcomes in patients with type 2 diabetes. N Engl J Med 2019;381:841–851

206. Hernandez AF, Green JB, Janmohamed S, et al.; Harmony Outcomes committees and investigators. Albiglutide and cardiovascular outcomes in patients with type 2 diabetes and cardiovascular disease (Harmony Outcomes): a double-blind, randomised placebo-controlled trial. Lancet 2018;392:1519–1529

207. Gerstein HC, Colhoun HM, Dagenais GR, et al.; REWIND Investigators. Dulaglutide and cardiovascular outcomes in type 2 diabetes (REWIND): a

double-blind, randomised placebo-controlled trial. Lancet 2019;394:121–130

208. Pfeffer MA, Claggett B, Diaz R, et al.; ELIXA Investigators. Lixisenatide in patients with type 2 diabetes and acute coronary syndrome. N Engl J Med 2015;373:2247–2257

209. Holman RR, Bethel MA, Mentz RJ, et al.; EXSCEL Study Group. Effects of once-weekly exenatide on cardiovascular outcomes in type 2 diabetes. N Engl J Med 2017;377:1228–1239

210. Zelniker TA, Wiviott SD, Raz I, et al. Comparison of the effects of glucagon-like peptide receptor agonists and sodium-glucose cotransporter 2 inhibitors for prevention of major adverse cardiovascular and renal outcomes in type 2 diabetes mellitus. Circulation 2019;139:2022–2031

211. Palmer SC, Tendal B, Mustafa RA, et al. Sodium-glucose cotransporter protein-2 (SGLT-2) inhibitors and glucagon-like peptide-1 (GLP-1) receptor agonists for type 2 diabetes: systematic review and network meta-analysis of randomised controlled trials. BMJ 2021;372:m4573

212. Zelniker TA, Wiviott SD, Raz I, et al. SGLT2 inhibitors for primary and secondary prevention of cardiovascular and renal outcomes in type 2 diabetes: a systematic review and meta-analysis of cardiovascular outcome trials. Lancet 2019; 393:31–39

213. McGuire DK, Shih WJ, Cosentino F, et al. Association of SGLT2 inhibitors with cardiovascular and kidney outcomes in patients with type 2 diabetes: a meta-analysis. JAMA Cardiol 2021;6: 148–158

214. Gerstein HC, Sattar N, Rosenstock J, et al. Cardiovascular and renal outcomes with efpeglenatide in type 2 diabetes. N Engl J Med 2021;385:896–907

215. Lam CSP, Ramasundarahettige C, Branch KRH, et al. Efpeglenatide and clinical outcomes with and without concomitant sodium-glucose cotransporter-2 inhibition use in type 2 diabetes: exploratory analysis of the AMPLITUDE-O Trial. Circulation 2022;145:565–574

216. Kannel WB, Hjortland M, Castelli WP. Role of diabetes in congestive heart failure: the Framingham study. Am J Cardiol 1974;34:29–34

217. Dunlay SM, Givertz MM, Aguilar D, et al.; American Heart Association Heart Failure and Transplantation Committee of the Council on Clinical Cardiology; Council on Cardiovascular and Stroke Nursing; Heart Failure Society of America. Type 2 diabetes mellitus and heart failure, a scientific statement from the American Heart Association and Heart Failure Society of America. J Card Fail 2019;25:584–619

218. Dormandy JA, Charbonnel B, Eckland DJA, et al.; PROactive Investigators. Secondary prevention of macrovascular events in patients with type 2 diabetes in the PROactive Study (PROspective pioglitAzone Clinical Trial In

macroVascular Events): a randomised controlled trial. Lancet 2005;366: 1279–1289

219. Singh S, Loke YK, Furberg CD. Long-term risk of cardiovascular events with rosiglitazone: a meta-analysis. JAMA 2007;298:1189–1195

220. Lincoff AM, Wolski K, Nicholls SJ, Nissen SE. Pioglitazone and risk of cardiovascular events in patients with type 2 diabetes mellitus: a metaanalysis of randomized trials. JAMA 2007;298: 1180–1188

221. Inzucchi SE, Masoudi FA, McGuire DK. Metformin in heart failure. Diabetes Care 2007; 30:e129–e129

222. Eurich DT, Majumdar SR, McAlister FA, Tsuyuki RT, Johnson JA. Improved clinical outcomes associated with metformin in patients with diabetes and heart failure. Diabetes Care 2005;28:2345–2351

223. U.S. Food and Drug Administration. FDA drug safety communication: FDA revises warnings regarding use of the diabetes medicine metformin in certain patients with reduced kidney function, 2016. Accessed 21 October 2022. Available from https://www.fda.gov/drugs/drug-safety-and-availability/fda-drug-safety-communication-fda-revises-warnings-regarding-use-diabetes-medicine-metformin-certain

224. Scirica BM, Bhatt DL, Braunwald E, et al.; SAVOR-TIMI 53 Steering Committee and Investigators. Saxagliptin and cardiovascular outcomes in patients with type 2 diabetes mellitus. N Engl J Med 2013;369:1317–1326

225. Zannad F, Cannon CP, Cushman WC, et al.; EXAMINE Investigators. Heart failure and mortality outcomes in patients with type 2 diabetes taking alogliptin versus placebo in EXAMINE: a multicentre, randomised, double-blind trial. Lancet 2015;385:2067–2076

226. Green JB, Bethel MA, Armstrong PW, et al.; TECOS Study Group. Effect of sitagliptin on cardiovascular outcomes in type 2 diabetes. N Engl J Med 2015;373:232–242

227. Vaduganathan M, Docherty KF, Claggett BL, et al.; SGLT-2 inhibitors in patients with heart failure: a comprehensive meta-analysis of five randomised controlled trials. Lancet 2022;400: 757–767

228. Bhatt DL, Szarek M, Steg PG, et al.; SOLOIST-WHF Trial Investigators. Sotagliflozin in patients with diabetes and recent worsening heart failure. N Engl J Med 2021;384:117–128

229. Packer M, Anker SD, Butler J, et al. Effect of empagliflozin on the clinical stability of patients with heart failure and a reduced ejection fraction: the EMPEROR-Reduced trial. Circulation 2021;143:326–336

230. Voors AA, Angermann CE, Teerlink JR, et al. The SGLT2 inhibitor empagliflozin in patients hospitalized for acute heart failure: a multinational randomized trial. Nat Med 2022;28:568–574

231. Spertus JA, Birmingham MC, Nassif M, et al. The SGLT2 inhibitor cana-gliflozin in heart failure: the CHIEF-HF remote, patient-centered random-ized trial. Nat Med 2022;28:809–813

232. Gansevoort RT, Correa-Rotter R, Hemmelgarn BR, et al. Chronic kidney disease and cardiovascular risk: epidemiology, mechanisms, and prevention. Lancet 2013;382:339–352

233. Bakris GL, Agarwal R, Anker SD, et al.; FIDELIO-DKD Investigators. Effect of finerenone on chronic kidney disease outcomes in type 2 diabetes. N Engl J Med 2020;383:2219–2229

234. Das SR, Everett BM, Birtcher KK, et al. 2020 expert consensus decision pathway on novel therapies for cardiovascular risk reduction in patients with type 2 diabetes: a report of the American College of Cardiology Solu-tion Set Oversight Committee. J Am Coll Cardiol 2020;76: 1117–1145

235. White WB, Cannon CP, Heller SR, et al.; EXAMINE Investigators. Alo-gliptin after acute coronary syndrome in patients with type 2 diabetes. N Engl J Med 2013;369:1327–1335

236. Rosenstock J, Perkovic V, Alexander JH, et al.; CARMELINA investigators. Rationale, design, and baseline characteristics of the CArdiovascular safety and Renal Microvascular outcomE study with LINAgliptin (CARME-LINA): a randomized, double-blind, placebo-controlled clinical trial in patients with type 2 diabetes and high cardio-renal risk. Cardiovasc Diabe-tol 2018; 17:39

237. Marx N, Rosenstock J, Kahn SE, et al. Design and baseline characteristics of the CARdiovascular Outcome Trial of LINAgliptin Versus Glimepiride in Type 2 Diabetes (CAROLINA®). Diab Vasc Dis Res 2015;12:164–174

238. Cefalu WT, Kaul S, Gerstein HC, et al. Cardiovascular outcomes trials in type 2 diabetes: where do we go from here? Reflections from a *Diabetes Care* Editors' Expert Forum. Diabetes Care 2018;41:14–31

239. Wheeler DC, Stefansson BV, Batiushin M, et al. The dapagliflozin and pre-vention of adverse outcomes in chronic kidney disease (DAPA-CKD) trial: baseline characteristics. Nephrol Dial Transplant 2020;35:1700–1711

240. Cannon CP, McGuire DK, Pratley R, et al.; VERTIS-CV Investigators. Design and baseline characteristics of the eValuation of ERTugliflozin effI-cacy and Safety CardioVascular outcomes trial (VERTIS-CV). Am Heart J 2018;206:11–23

241. Anker SD, Butler J, Filippatos G, et al.; EMPEROR-Preserved Trial Com-mittees and Investigators. Baseline characteristics of patients with heart fail-ure with preserved ejection fraction in the EMPEROR-Preserved trial. Eur J Heart Fail 2020;22:2383–2392

242. Zoungas S, Chalmers J, Neal B, et al.; ADVANCE-ON Collaborative Group. Follow-up of blood-pressure lowering and glucose control in type 2 diabetes. N Engl J Med 2014;371:1392–1406

Chapter 18
Chronic Kidney Disease and Risk Management

The American Diabetes Association (ADA) "Standards of Care in Diabetes" includes the ADA's current clinical practice recommendations and is intended to provide the components of diabetes care, general treatment goals and guidelines, and tools to evaluate quality of care. Members of the ADA Professional Practice Committee, a multidisciplinary expert committee, are responsible for updating the Standards of Care annually, or more frequently as warranted. For a detailed description of ADA standards, statements, and reports, as well as the evidence-grading system for ADA's clinical practice recommendations and a full list of Professional Practice Committee members, please refer to Introduction and Methodology. Readers who wish to comment on the Standards of Care are invited to do so at professional.diabetes.org/SOC.

For prevention and management of diabetes complications in children and adolescents, please refer to Section 14, "Children and Adolescents."

CHRONIC KIDNEY DISEASE

SCREENING

Recommendations

11.1a At least annually, urinary albumin (e.g., spot urinary albumin-to-creatinine ratio) and estimated glomerular filtration rate should be assessed in people with type 1 diabetes with duration of ≥5 years and in all people with type 2 diabetes regardless of treatment. **B**

11.1b In people with established diabetic kidney disease, urinary albumin (e.g., spot urinary albumin-to-creatinine ratio) and estimated glomerular filtration rate should be monitored 1–4 times per year depending on the stage of the disease (Fig. 18.1). **B**

Chapter 18 is an excerpt from ElSayed NA, Aleppo G, Aroda VR, et al., American Diabetes Association. 11. Chronic kidney disease and risk management: Standards of Care in Diabetes—2023. *Diabetes Care* 2023;46(Suppl. 1):S191–S202

* See Table 1.1 (p. 2) for an explanation of the American Diabetes Association evidence-grading system for *Standards of Care in Diabetes*.

TREATMENT

Recommendations

11.2   Optimize glucose control to reduce the risk or slow the progression of chronic kidney disease. **A**

11.3   Optimize blood pressure control and reduce blood pressure variability to reduce the risk or slow the progression of chronic kidney disease. **A**

					Albuminuria categories Description and range		
CKD is classified based on: • Cause (C) • GFR (G) • Albuminuria (A)					A1	A2	A3
					Normal to mildly increased	Moderately increased	Severely increased
					<30 mg/g <3 mg/mmol	30-299 mg/g 3-29 mg/mmol	≥300 mg/g ≥30 mg/mmol
	G1	Normal to high	≥90		1 if CKD	Treat 1	Refer* 2
	G2	Mildly decreased	60-89		1 if CKD	Treat 1	Refer* 2
GFR categories (mL/min/1.73 m²) Description and range	G3a	Mildly to moderately decreased	45-59		Treat 1	Treat 2	Refer 3
	G3b	Moderately to severely decreased	30-44		Treat 2	Treat 3	Refer 3
	G4	Severely decreased	15-29		Refer* 3	Refer* 3	Refer 4+
	G5	Kidney failure	<15		Refer 4+	Refer 4+	Refer 4+

Figure 18.1—Risk of chronic kidney disease (CKD) progression, frequency of visits, and referral to a nephrologist according to glomerular filtration rate (GFR) and albuminuria. The GFR and albuminuria grid depicts the risk of progression, morbidity, and mortality by color, from best to worst (green, yellow, orange, red, dark red). The numbers in the boxes are a guide to the frequency of visits (number of times per year). Green can reflect CKD with normal estimated GFR and albumin-to-creatinine ratio only in the presence of other markers of kidney damage, such as imaging showing polycystic kidney disease or kidney biopsy abnormalities, with follow-up measurements annually; yellow requires caution and measurements at least once per year; orange requires measurements twice per year; red requires measurements three times per year; and dark red requires measurements four times per year. These are general parameters only, based on expert opinion, and underlying comorbid conditions and disease state, as well as the likelihood of impacting a change in management for any individual patient, must be taken into account. "Refer" indicates that nephrology services are recommended. *Referring clinicians may wish to discuss with their nephrology service, depending on local arrangements regarding treating or referring. Reprinted with permission from Vassalotti et al.[121]

11.4a In nonpregnant people with diabetes and hypertension, either an ACE inhibitor or an angiotensin receptor blocker is recommended for those with moderately increased albuminuria (urinary albumin-to-creatinine ratio 30–299 mg/g creatinine) **B** and is strongly recommended for those with severely increased albuminuria (urinary albumin-to-creatinine ratio ≥300 mg/g creatinine) and/or estimated glomerular filtration rate <60 mL/min/1.73 m². **A**

11.4b Periodically monitor serum creatinine and potassium levels for the development of increased creatinine and hyperkalemia when ACE inhibitors, angiotensin receptor blockers, and mineralocorticoid receptor antagonists are used, or hypokalemia when diuretics are used. **B**

11.4c An ACE inhibitor or an angiotensin receptor blocker is not recommended for the primary prevention of chronic kidney disease in people with diabetes who have normal blood pressure, normal urinary albumin-to-creatinine ratio (<30 mg/g creatinine), and normal estimated glomerular filtration rate. **A**

11.4d Do not discontinue renin-angiotensin system blockade for increases in serum creatinine (≤30%) in the absence of volume depletion. **A**

11.5a For people with type 2 diabetes and diabetic kidney disease, use of a sodium–glucose cotransporter 2 inhibitor is recommended to reduce chronic kidney disease progression and cardiovascular events in patients with an estimated glomerular filtration rate ≥20 mL/min/1.73 m² and urinary albumin ≥200 mg/g creatinine. **A**

11.5b For people with type 2 diabetes and diabetic kidney disease, use of a sodium–glucose cotransporter 2 inhibitor is recommended to reduce chronic kidney disease progression and cardiovascular events in patients with an estimated glomerular filtration rate ≥20 mL/min/1.73 m² and urinary albumin ranging from normal to 200 mg/g creatinine. **B**

11.5c In people with type 2 diabetes and diabetic kidney disease, consider use of sodium–glucose cotransporter 2 inhibitors (if estimated glomerular filtration rate is ≥20 mL/min/1.73 m²), a glucagon-like peptide 1 agonist, or a nonsteroidal mineralocorticoid receptor antagonist (if estimated glomerular filtration rate is ≥25 mL/min/1.73 m²) additionally for cardiovascular risk reduction. **A**

11.5d In people with chronic kidney disease and albuminuria who are at increased risk for cardiovascular events or chronic kidney disease progression, a nonsteroidal mineralocorticoid receptor antagonist shown to be effective in clinical trials is recommended to reduce chronic kidney disease progression and cardiovascular events. **A**

11.6 In people with chronic kidney disease who have ≥300 mg/g urinary albumin, a reduction of 30% or greater in mg/g urinary albumin is recommended to slow chronic kidney disease progression. **B**

11.7 For people with non–dialysis-dependent stage 3 or higher chronic kidney disease, dietary protein intake should be aimed to a target level of 0.8 g/kg body weight per day. **A** For patients on dialysis, higher levels of dietary protein intake should be considered since protein energy wasting is a major problem in some individuals on dialysis. **B**

11.8   Patients should be referred for evaluation by a nephrologist if they have continuously increasing urinary albumin levels and/or continuously decreasing estimated glomerular filtration rate and if the estimated glomerular filtration rate is <30 mL/min/1.73 m². **A**

11.9   Promptly refer to a nephrologist for uncertainty about the etiology of kidney disease, difficult management issues, and rapidly progressing kidney disease. **A**

Epidemiology of Diabetes and Chronic Kidney Disease

Chronic kidney disease (CKD) is diagnosed by the persistent elevation of urinary albumin excretion (albuminuria), low estimated glomerular filtration rate (eGFR), or other manifestations of kidney damage.[1,2] In this section, the focus is on CKD attributed to diabetes (diabetic kidney disease) in adults, which occurs in 20–40% of people with diabetes.[1,3–5] Diabetic kidney disease typically develops after a diabetes duration of 10 years in type 1 diabetes (the most common presentation is 5–15 years after the diagnosis of type 1 diabetes) but may be present at diagnosis of type 2 diabetes. CKD can progress to end-stage renal disease (ESRD) requiring dialysis or kidney transplantation and is the leading cause of ESRD in the U.S.[6] In addition, among people with type 1 or type 2 diabetes, the presence of CKD markedly increases cardiovascular risk and health care costs.[7] For details on the management of diabetic kidney disease in children, please see section 14, "Children and Adolescents."

Assessment of Albuminuria and Estimated Glomerular Filtration Rate

Screening for albuminuria can be most easily performed by urinary albumin-to-creatinine ratio (UACR) in a random spot urine collection.[1,2] Timed or 24-h collections are more burdensome and add little to prediction or accuracy. Measurement of a spot urine sample for albumin alone (whether by immunoassay or by using a sensitive dipstick test specific for albuminuria) without simultaneously measuring urine creatinine is less expensive but susceptible to false-negative and false-positive determinations as a result of variation in urine concentration due to hydration.[8] Thus, to be useful for patient screening, semiquantitative or qualitative (dipstick) screening tests should be >85% positive in those with moderately increased albuminuria (≥30 mg/g) and confirmed by albumin-to-creatinine values in an accredited laboratory.[9,10] Hence, it is better to simply collect a spot urine sample for albumin-to-creatinine ratio because it will ultimately need to be done.

Normal albuminuria is defined as <30 mg/g creatinine, moderately elevated albuminuria is defined as ≥30–300 mg/g creatinine, and severely elevated albuminuria is defined as ≥300 mg/g creatinine. However, UACR is a continuous measurement, and differences within the normal and abnormal ranges are associated with renal and cardiovascular outcomes.[7,11,12] Furthermore, because of high biological variability of >20% between measurements in urinary albumin excretion, two of three specimens of UACR collected within a 3- to 6-month period should be abnormal before considering a patient to have moderately or severely elevated albuminuria.[1,2,13,14] Exercise within 24 h, infection, fever, congestive heart failure, marked hyperglycemia, menstruation, and marked hypertension may elevate UACR independently of kidney damage.[15]

Traditionally, eGFR is calculated from serum creatinine using a validated formula.[16] The Chronic Kidney Disease Epidemiology Collaboration (CKD-EPI) equation is preferred.[2] eGFR is routinely reported by laboratories along with serum creatinine, and eGFR calculators are available online at nkdep.nih.gov. An eGFR persistently <60 mL/min/1.73 m^2 in concert with a urinary albumin value of >30 mg/g creatinine is considered abnormal, though optimal thresholds for clinical diagnosis are debated in older adults over age 70 years.[2,17] Historically, a correction factor for muscle mass was included in a modified equation for African American people; however, race is a social and not a biologic construct, making it problematic to apply race to clinical algorithms, and the need to advance health equity and social justice is clear. Thus, it was decided that the equation should be altered such that it applies to all.[16] Hence, a committee was convened, resulting in the recommendation for immediate implementation of the CKD-EPI creatinine equation refit without the race variable in all laboratories in the U.S. Additionally, increased use of cystatin C (another marker of eGFR) is suggested in combination with the serum creatinine because combining filtration markers (creatinine and cystatin C) is more accurate and would support better clinical decisions than either marker alone.

Diagnosis of Diabetic Kidney Disease

Diabetic kidney disease is usually a clinical diagnosis made based on the presence of albuminuria and/or reduced eGFR in the absence of signs or symptoms of other primary causes of kidney damage. The typical presentation of diabetic kidney disease is considered to include a long-standing duration of diabetes, retinopathy, albuminuria without gross hematuria, and gradually progressive loss of eGFR. However, signs of diabetic kidney disease may be present at diagnosis or without retinopathy in type 2 diabetes. Reduced eGFR without albuminuria has been frequently reported in type 1 and type 2 diabetes and is becoming more common over time as the prevalence of diabetes increases in the U.S.[3,4,18,19]

An active urinary sediment (containing red or white blood cells or cellular casts), rapidly increasing albuminuria or total proteinuria, the presence of nephrotic syndrome, rapidly decreasing eGFR, or the absence of retinopathy (in type 1 diabetes) suggests alternative or additional causes of kidney disease. For patients with these features, referral to a nephrologist for further diagnosis, including the possibility of kidney biopsy, should be considered. It is rare for people with type 1 diabetes to develop kidney disease without retinopathy. In type 2 diabetes, retinopathy is only moderately sensitive and specific for CKD caused by diabetes, as confirmed by kidney biopsy.[20]

Staging of Chronic Kidney Disease

Stage 1 and stage 2 CKD are defined by evidence of high albuminuria with eGFR ≥60 mL/min/1.73 m^2, and stages 3–5 CKD are defined by progressively lower ranges of eGFR[21] (Fig. 18.1). At any eGFR, the degree of albuminuria is associated with risk of cardiovascular disease (CVD), CKD progression, and mortality.[7] Therefore, Kidney Disease: Improving Global Outcomes (KDIGO) recommends a more comprehensive CKD staging that incorporates albuminuria at all stages of eGFR; this system is more closely associated with risk but is also more complex and does not translate directly to treatment decisions.[2] Thus, based on the current classification system, both eGFR and albuminuria must be quantified to guide treatment decisions. This is also important because eGFR levels are essential for modifications of drug dosages or restrictions of use (Fig. 18.1).[22,23] The degree of albuminuria should influence the choice of antihypertensive medications (see Section 10, "Cardiovascular Disease and Risk Management") or glucose-lowering medications (see below). Observed history of eGFR loss (which is also associated with risk of CKD progression and other adverse health outcomes) and cause of kidney damage (including possible causes other than diabetes) may also affect these decisions.[24]

Acute Kidney Injury

Acute kidney injury (AKI) is diagnosed by a 50% or greater sustained increase in serum creatinine over a short period of time, which is also reflected as a rapid decrease in eGFR.[25,26] People with diabetes are at higher risk of AKI than those without diabetes.[27] Other risk factors for AKI include preexisting CKD, the use of medications that cause kidney injury (e.g., nonsteroidal anti-inflammatory drugs), and the use of medications that alter renal blood flow and intrarenal hemodynamics. In particular, many antihypertensive medications (e.g., diuretics, ACE inhibitors, and angiotensin receptor blockers [ARBs]) can reduce intravascular volume, renal blood flow, and/or glomerular filtration. There was concern that sodium–glucose cotransporter 2 (SGLT2) inhibitors may promote AKI through volume depletion, particularly when combined with diuretics or other medications that reduce glomerular filtration; however, this has not been found to be true in randomized clinical outcome trials of advanced kidney disease[28] or high CVD risk with normal kidney function.[29–31] It is also noteworthy that the nonsteroidal mineralocorticoid receptor antagonists (MRAs) do not increase the risk of AKI when used to slow kidney disease progression.[32] Timely identification and treatment of AKI is important because AKI is associated with increased risks of progressive CKD and other poor health outcomes.[33]

Elevations in serum creatinine (up to 30% from baseline) with renin-angiotensin system (RAS) blockers (such as ACE inhibitors and ARBs) must not be confused with AKI.[34] An analysis of the Action to Control Cardiovascular Risk in Diabetes Blood Pressure (ACCORD BP) trial demonstrates that participants randomized to intensive blood pressure lowering with up to a 30% increase in serum creatinine did not have any increase in mortality or progressive kidney disease.[35–38] Moreover, a measure of markers for AKI showed no significant increase of any markers with increased creatinine.[37] Accordingly, ACE inhibitors and ARBs should not be discontinued for increases in serum creatinine (<30%) in the absence of volume depletion.

Lastly, it should be noted that ACE inhibitors and ARBs are commonly not dosed at maximum tolerated doses because of fear that serum creatinine will rise. As noted above, this is an error. Note that in all clinical trials demonstrating efficacy of ACE inhibitors and ARBs in slowing kidney disease progression, the maximum tolerated doses were used—not very low doses that do not provide benefit. Moreover, there are now studies demonstrating outcome benefits on both mortality and slowed CKD progression in people with diabetes who have an eGFR <30 mL/min/1.73 m^2.[38] Additionally, when increases in serum creatinine reach 30% without associated hyperkalemia, RAS blockade should be continued.[36,39]

Surveillance

Both albuminuria and eGFR should be monitored annually to enable timely diagnosis of CKD, monitor progression of CKD, detect superimposed kidney diseases including AKI, assess risk of CKD complications, dose drugs appropriately, and determine whether nephrology referral is needed. Among people with existing kidney disease, albuminuria and eGFR may change due to progression of CKD, development of a separate superimposed cause of kidney disease, AKI, or other effects of medications, as noted above. Serum potassium should also be monitored in patients treated with diuretics because these medications can cause hypokalemia, which is associated with cardiovascular risk and mortality.[40–42] Patients with eGFR <60 mL/min/1.73 m² receiving ACE inhibitors, ARBs, or MRAs should have serum potassium measured periodically. Additionally, people with this lower range of eGFR should have their medication dosing verified, their exposure to nephrotoxins (e.g., nonsteroidal antiinflammatory drugs and iodinated contrast) should be minimized, and they should be evaluated for potential CKD complications (Table 18.1).

There is a clear need for annual quantitative assessment of urinary albumin excretion. This is especially true after a diagnosis of albuminuria, institution of ACE inhibitors or ARB therapy to maximum tolerated doses, and achievement of blood pressure targets. Early changes in kidney function may be detected by increases in albuminuria before changes in eGFR,[43] and this also significantly affects cardiovascular risk. Moreover, an initial reduction of >30% from baseline, subsequently maintained over at least 2 years, is considered a valid surrogate for renal benefit by the Division of Cardiology and Nephrology of the U.S. Food and Drug Administration (FDA).[10] Continued surveillance can assess both response to therapy and disease progression and may aid in assessing participation in ACE inhibitor or ARB therapy. In addition, in clinical trials of ACE inhibitors or ARB therapy in type 2 diabetes, reducing albuminuria to levels <300 mg/g creatinine or by >30% from baseline has been associated with improved renal and cardiovascular outcomes, leading some to suggest that medications should be titrated to maximize reduction in UACR. Data from post hoc analyses demonstrate less benefit on cardiorenal outcomes at half doses of RAS blockade.[44] In type 1 diabetes, remission of albuminuria may occur spontaneously, and cohort studies evaluating associations of change in albuminuria with clinical outcomes have reported inconsistent results.[45,46]

The prevalence of CKD complications correlates with eGFR.[42] When eGFR is <60 mL/min/1.73 m², screening for complications of CKD is indicated (Table 18.1). Early vaccination against hepatitis B virus is indicated in individuals likely to progress to ESRD (see Section 4, "Comprehensive Medical Evaluation and Assessment of Comorbidities," for further information on immunization).

Prevention

The only proven primary prevention interventions for CKD are blood glucose and blood pressure control. There is no evidence that renin-angiotensin-aldosterone system (RAAS) inhibitors or any other interventions prevent the development of diabetic kidney disease. Thus, the American Diabetes Association

Table 18.1—Selected complications of chronic kidney disease

Complication	Physical and laboratory evaluation
Blood pressure >130/80 mmHg	Blood pressure, weight
Volume overload	History, physical examination, weight
Electrolyte abnormalities	Serum electrolytes
Metabolic acidosis	Serum electrolytes
Anemia	Hemoglobin; iron testing if indicated
Metabolic bone disease	Serum calcium, phosphate, PTH, vitamin 25(OH)D

Complications of chronic kidney disease (CKD) generally become prevalent when estimated glomerular filtration rate falls below 60 mL/min/1.73 m2 (stage 3 CKD or greater) and become more common and severe as CKD progresses. Evaluation of elevated blood pressure and volume overload should occur at every clinical contact possible; laboratory evaluations are generally indicated every 6–12 months for stage 3 CKD, every 3–5 months for stage 4 CKD, and every 1–3 months for stage 5 CKD, or as indicated to evaluate symptoms or changes in therapy. PTH, parathyroid hormone; 25(OH)D, 25-hydroxyvitamin D.

does not recommend routine use of these medications solely for the purpose of prevention of the development of diabetic kidney disease.

Interventions

Nutrition

For people with non-dialysis-dependent CKD, dietary protein intake should be ~0.8 g/kg body weight per day (the recommended daily allowance).[1] Compared with higher levels of dietary protein intake, this level slowed GFR decline with evidence of a greater effect over time. Higher levels of dietary protein intake (>20% of daily calories from protein or >1.3 g/kg/day) have been associated with increased albuminuria, more rapid kidney function loss, and CVD mortality and therefore should be avoided. Reducing the amount of dietary protein below the recommended daily allowance of 0.8 g/kg/day is not recommended because it does not alter blood glucose levels, cardiovascular risk measures, or the course of GFR decline.[47]

Restriction of dietary sodium (to <2,300 mg/day) may be useful to control blood pressure and reduce cardiovascular risk,[48,49] and individualization of dietary potassium may be necessary to control serum potassium concentrations.[27,40–42] These interventions may be most important for individuals with reduced eGFR, for whom urinary excretion of sodium and potassium may be impaired. For patients on dialysis, higher levels of dietary protein intake should be considered since malnutrition is a major problem for some patients on dialysis.[50] Recommendations for dietary sodium and potassium intake should be individualized based on comorbid conditions, medication use, blood pressure, and laboratory data.

Glycemic Targets

Intensive lowering of blood glucose with the goal of achieving near-normoglycemia has been shown in large randomized studies to delay the onset and progression of albuminuria and reduce eGFR in people with type 1 diabetes[51,52] and type 2 diabetes.[1,53–58] Insulin alone was used to lower blood glucose in the Diabetes Control and Complications Trial (DCCT)/Epidemiology of Diabetes Interventions and Complications (EDIC) study of type 1 diabetes, while a variety of agents were used in clinical trials of type 2 diabetes, supporting the conclusion that lowering blood glucose itself helps prevent CKD and its progression. The effects of glucose-lowering therapies on CKD have helped define A1C targets (see Table 6.2).

The presence of CKD affects the risks and benefits of intensive lowering of blood glucose and a number of specific glucose-lowering medications. In the Action to Control Cardiovascular Risk in Diabetes (ACCORD) trial of type 2 diabetes, adverse effects of intensive management of blood glucose levels (hypoglycemia and mortality) were increased among people with kidney disease at baseline.[59,60] Moreover, there is a lag time of at least 2 years in type 2 diabetes to over 10 years in type 1 diabetes for the effects of intensive glucose control to manifest as improved eGFR outcomes.[56,60,61] Therefore, in some people with prevalent CKD and substantial comorbidity, target A1C levels may be less intensive.[1,62]

Blood Pressure and Use of RAAS Inhibitors

RAAS inhibition remains a mainstay of management for people with diabetic kidney disease with albuminuria and for the treatment of hypertension in people with diabetes (with or without diabetic kidney disease). Indeed, all the trials that evaluated the benefits of SGLT2 inhibition or nonsteroidal mineralocorticoid receptor antagonist effects were done in individuals who were being treated with an ACE inhibitor or ARB, in some trials up to maximum tolerated doses.

Hypertension is a strong risk factor for the development and progression of CKD.[63] Antihypertensive therapy reduces the risk of albuminuria,[64–67] and among people with type 1 or 2 diabetes with established CKD (eGFR <60 mL/min/1.73 m^2 and UACR ≥300 mg/g creatinine), ACE inhibitor or ARB therapy reduces the risk of progression to ESRD.[68–70,74–80] Moreover, antihypertensive therapy reduces the risk of cardiovascular events.[64]

A blood pressure level <130/80 mmHg is recommended to reduce CVD mortality and slow CKD progression among all people with diabetes. Lower blood pressure targets (e.g., <130/80 mmHg) should be considered for patients based on individual anticipated benefits and risks. People with CKD are at increased risk of CKD progression (particularly those with albuminuria) and CVD; therefore, lower blood pressure targets may be suitable in some cases, especially in individuals with severely elevated albuminuria (≥300 mg/g creatinine).

ACE inhibitors or ARBs are the preferred first-line agents for blood pressure treatment among people with diabetes, hypertension, eGFR <60 mL/min/1.73 m^2, and UACR ≥300 mg/g creatinine because of their proven benefits for prevention of CKD progression.[68,69,74] ACE inhibitors and ARBs are considered to have similar benefits[75,76] and risks. In the setting of lower levels of albuminuria (30–299 mg/g creatinine), ACE inhibitor or ARB therapy at maximum tolerated doses in trials has reduced progression to more advanced albuminuria (≥300 mg/g creatinine), slowed CKD progression, and reduced cardiovascular events but has not reduced progression to ESRD.[74,77] While ACE inhibitors or ARBs are often prescribed for moderately increased albuminuria without hypertension, outcome trials have not been performed in this setting to determine whether they improve renal outcomes. Moreover, two long-term, double-blind studies demonstrated no renoprotective effect of either ACE inhibitors or ARBs in type 1 and type 2 diabetes among those who were normotensive with or without high albuminuria (formerly microalbuminuria).[78,79]

Absent kidney disease, ACE inhibitors or ARBs are useful to manage blood pressure but have not proven superior to alternative classes of antihypertensive therapy, including thiazide-like diuretics and dihydropyridine calcium channel blockers.[80] In a trial of people with type 2 diabetes and normal urinary albumin excretion, an ARB reduced or suppressed the development of albuminuria but increased the rate of cardiovascular events.[81] In a trial of people with type 1 diabetes exhibiting neither albuminuria nor hypertension, ACE inhibitors or ARBs did not prevent the development of diabetic glomerulopathy assessed by kidney biopsy.[78] This was further supported by a similar trial in people with type 2 diabetes.[79]

Two clinical trials studied the combinations of ACE inhibitors and ARBs and found no benefits on CVD or CKD, and the drug combination had higher adverse event rates (hyperkalemia and/or AKI).[82,83] Therefore, the combined use of ACE inhibitors and ARBs should be avoided.

Direct Renal Effects of Glucose-Lowering Medications

Some glucose-lowering medications also have effects on the kidney that are direct, i.e., not mediated through glycemia. For example, SGLT2 inhibitors reduce renal tubular glucose reabsorption, weight, systemic blood pressure, intraglomerular pressure, and albuminuria and slow GFR loss through mechanisms that appear independent of glycemia.[30,84–87] Moreover, recent data support the notion that SGLT2 inhibitors reduce oxidative stress in the kidney by >50% and blunt increases in angiotensinogen as well as reduce NLRP3 inflammasome activity.[88–90] Glucagon-like peptide 1 receptor agonists (GLP-1 RAs) also have direct effects on the kidney and have been reported to improve renal outcomes compared with placebo.[91–95] Renal effects should be considered when selecting antihyperglycemia agents (see Section 9, "Pharmacologic Approaches to Glycemic Treatment").

Selection of Glucose-Lowering Medications for People With Chronic Kidney Disease

For people with type 2 diabetes and established CKD, special considerations for the selection of glucose-lowering medications include limitations to available medications when eGFR is diminished and a desire to mitigate risks of CKD progression, CVD, and hypoglycemia.[96,97] Drug dosing may require modification with eGFR <60 mL/min/1.73 m^2.[1]

The FDA revised its guidance for the use of metformin in CKD in 2016,[98] recommending use of eGFR instead of serum creatinine to guide treatment and expanding the pool of people with kidney disease for whom metformin treatment should be considered. The revised FDA guidance states that *1)* metformin is contraindicated in patients with an eGFR <30 mL/min/1.73 m^2, *2)* eGFR should be monitored while taking metformin, *3)* the benefits and risks of continuing treatment should be reassessed when eGFR falls to <45 mL/min/1.73 m^2,[99,100] *4)* metformin should not be initiated for patients with an eGFR <45 mL/min/1.73 m^2, and *5)* metformin should be temporarily discontinued at the time of or before iodinated contrast imaging procedures in patients with eGFR 30–60 mL/min/1.73 m^2.

A number of recent studies have shown cardiovascular protection from SGLT2 inhibitors and GLP-1 RAs as well as renal protection from SGLT2 inhibitors and possibly from GLP-1 RAs. Selection of which glucose-lowering medications to use should be based on the usual criteria of an individual patient's risks (cardiovascular and renal in addition to glucose control) as well as convenience and cost.

SGLT2 inhibitors are recommended for people with stage 3 CKD or higher and type 2 diabetes, as they slow CKD progression and reduce heart failure risk independent of glucose management.[101] GLP-1 RAs are suggested for cardiovascular risk reduction if such risk is a predominant problem, as they reduce risks of CVD events and hypoglycemia and appear to possibly slow CKD progression.[102–105]

A number of large cardiovascular outcomes trials in people with type 2 diabetes at high risk for CVD or with existing CVD examined kidney effects as secondary outcomes. These trials include EMPA-REG OUTCOME [BI 10773 (Empagliflozin) Cardiovascular Outcome Event Trial in Type 2 Diabetes Mellitus Patients], CANVAS (Canagliflozin Cardiovascular Assessment Study), LEADER (Liraglutide Effect and Action in Diabetes: Evaluation of Cardiovascular Outcome Results), and SUSTAIN-6 (Trial to Evaluate Cardiovascular and Other Long-term Outcomes With Semaglutide in Subjects With Type 2 Diabetes).[71,86,91,94,102] Specifically, compared with placebo, empagliflozin reduced the risk of incident or worsening nephropathy (a composite of progression to UACR >300 mg/g creatinine, doubling of serum creatinine, ESRD, or death from ESRD) by 39% and the risk of doubling of serum creatinine accompanied by eGFR ≤45 mL/min/1.73 m² by 44%; canagliflozin reduced the risk of progression of albuminuria by 27% and the risk of reduction in eGFR, ESRD, or death from ESRD by 40%; liraglutide reduced the risk of new or worsening nephropathy (a composite of persistent macroalbuminuria, doubling of serum creatinine, ESRD, or death from ESRD) by 22%; and semaglutide reduced the risk of new or worsening nephropathy (a composite of persistent UACR >300 mg/g creatinine, doubling of serum creatinine, or ESRD) by 36% (each $P < 0.01$). These analyses were limited by evaluation of study populations not selected primarily for CKD and examination of renal effects as secondary outcomes.

Some large clinical trials of SGLT2 inhibitors have focused on people with advanced CKD, and assessment of primary renal outcomes is either completed or ongoing. Canagliflozin and Renal Events in Diabetes with Established Nephropathy Clinical Evaluation (CREDENCE), a placebo-controlled trial of canagliflozin among 4,401 adults with type 2 diabetes, UACR ≥300–5,000 mg/g creatinine, and eGFR range 30–90 mL/min/1.73 m² (mean eGFR 56 mL/min/1.73 m² with a mean albuminuria level of >900 mg/day), had a primary composite end point of ESRD, doubling of serum creatinine, or renal or cardiovascular death.[28,72] It was stopped early due to positive efficacy and showed a 32% risk reduction for development of ESRD over control.[28] Additionally, the development of the primary end point, which included chronic dialysis for ≥30 days, kidney transplantation or eGFR <15 mL/min/1.73 m² sustained for ≥30 days by central laboratory assessment, doubling from the baseline serum creatinine average sustained for ≥30 days by central laboratory assessment, or renal death or cardiovascular death, was reduced by 30%. This benefit was on background ACE inhibitor or ARB therapy in >99% of the patients.[28] Moreover, in this advanced CKD group, there were clear benefits on cardiovascular outcomes demonstrating a 31% reduction in cardiovascular death or heart failure hospitalization and a 20% reduction in cardiovascular death, nonfatal myocardial infarction, or nonfatal stroke.[28,73,105]

A second trial in advanced diabetic kidney disease was the Dapagliflozin and Prevention of Adverse Outcomes in Chronic Kidney Disease (DAPA-CKD) study.[106] This trial examined a cohort similar to that in CREDENCE except 67.5% of the participants had type 2 diabetes and CKD (the other one-third had CKD without type 2 diabetes), and the end points were slightly different. The primary outcome was time to the first occurrence of any of the components of the composite, including ≥50% sustained decline in eGFR or reaching ESRD or cardiovascular death, or renal death. Secondary outcome measures included time to the first occurrence of any of the components of the composite kidney outcome (≥50% sustained decline in eGFR or reaching ESRD or renal death), time to the first occurrence of either of the components of the cardiovascular composite (cardiovascular death or hospitalization for heart failure), and time to death from any cause. The trial had 4,304 participants with a mean eGFR at baseline of 43.1 ± 12.4 mL/min/1.73 m^2 (range 25–75 mL/min/1.73 m^2) and a median UACR of 949 mg/g (range 200–5,000 mg/g). There was a significant benefit by dapagliflozin for the primary end point (hazard ratio [HR] 0.61 [95% CI 0.51–0.72]; $P < 0.001$).[106]

The HR for the kidney composite of a sustained decline in eGFR of ≥50%, ESRD, or death from renal causes was 0.56 (95% CI 0.45–0.68; $P < 0.001$). The HR for the composite of death from cardiovascular causes or hospitalization for heart failure was 0.71 (95% CI 0.55–0.92; $P = 0.009$). Finally, all-cause mortality was decreased in the dapagliflozin group compared with the placebo group ($P < 0.004$).

In addition to renal effects, while SGLT2 inhibitors demonstrated reduced risk of heart failure hospitalizations, some also demonstrated cardiovascular risk reduction. GLP-1 RAs clearly demonstrated cardiovascular benefits. Namely, in the EMPA-REG OUTCOME, CANVAS, Dapagliflozin Effect on Cardiovascular Events–Thrombolysis in Myocardial Infarction 58 (DECLARE-TIMI 58), LEADER, and SUSTAIN-6 trials, empagliflozin, canagliflozin, dapagliflozin, liraglutide, and semaglutide, respectively, each reduced cardiovascular events, evaluated as primary outcomes, compared with placebo (see Section 10, "Cardiovascular Disease and Risk Management," for further discussion). While the glucose-lowering effects of SGLT2 inhibitors are blunted with eGFRq <45 mL/min/1.73 m^2, the renal and cardiovascular benefits were still seen at eGFR levels of 25 mL/min/1.73 m^2 with no significant change in glucose.[28,30,51,62,71,94,106,107] Most participants with CKD in these trials also had diagnosed atherosclerotic cardiovascular disease (ASCVD) at baseline, although ~28% of CANVAS participants with CKD did not have diagnosed ASCVD.[31]

Based on evidence from the CREDENCE and DAPA-CKD trials, as well as secondary analyses of cardiovascular outcomes trials with SGLT2 inhibitors, cardio-vascular and renal events are reduced with SGLT2 inhibitor use in patients with an eGFR of 20 mL/min/1.73 m^2, independent of glucose-lowering effects.[73,105]

While there is clear cardiovascular risk reduction associated with GLP-1 RA use in people with type 2 diabetes and CKD, the proof of benefit on renal outcomes will come with the results of the ongoing FLOW (A Research Study to See How Semaglutide Works Compared with Placebo in People With Type 2 Diabetes and Chronic Kidney Disease) trial with injectable semaglutide.[108] As noted above, published data address a limited group of people with CKD, mostly with coexisting ASCVD. Renal events, however, have been examined as both primary and secondary outcomes in large published trials. Adverse event profiles of these agents also must be considered. Please refer to Table 9.2 for drug-specific factors, including adverse event information, for these agents. Additional clinical trials focusing on CKD and cardiovascular outcomes in people with CKD are ongoing and will be reported in the next few years.

For people with type 2 diabetes and CKD, the selection of specific agents may depend on comorbidity and CKD stage. SGLT2 inhibitors may be more useful for individuals at high risk of CKD progression (i.e., with albuminuria or a history of documented eGFR loss) (Fig. 9.3) due to an apparent large beneficial effect on CKD incidence. However, for people with type 2 diabetes and diabetic kidney disease, use of an SGLT2 inhibitor in individuals with eGFR $\geq$20 mL/min/1.73 m^2 and UACR $\geq$200 mg/g creatinine is recommended to reduce CKD progression and cardiovascular events. This is a change in eGFR from previous recommendations that suggested an eGFR level >25 mL/min/1.73 m^2. The reason for the lower limit of eGFR is as follows. The major clinical trials for SGLT2 inhibitors that showed benefit for people with diabetic kidney disease are CREDENCE and DAPA-CKD.[28,105] CREDENCE enrollment criteria included an eGFR >30 mL/min/1.73 m^2 and UACR >300 mg/g.[28,105] DAPA-CKD enrolled individuals with eGFR >25 mL/min/1.73 m^2 and UACR >200 mg/g. Subgroup analyses from DAPA-CKD[109] and analyses from the EMPEROR heart failure trials suggest that SGLT2 inhibitors are safe and effective at eGFR levels of >20 mL/min/1.73 m^2. The Empagliflozin Outcome Trial in Patients With Chronic Heart Failure With Preserved Ejection Fraction (EMPEROR-Preserved) enrolled 5,998 participants,[110] and the Empagliflozin Outcome Trial in Patients With Chronic Heart Failure and a Reduced Ejection Fraction (EMPEROR-Reduced) enrolled 3,730 participants;[111] enrollment criteria included eGFR >60 mL/min/1.73 m^2, but efficacy was seen at eGFR >20 mL/min/1.73 m^2 in people with heart failure. Hence, the new recommendation is to use SGLT2 inhibitors in individuals with eGFR as low as 20 mL/min/1.73 m^2. In addition, the DECLARE-TIMI 58 trial suggested effectiveness in participants with normal urinary albumin levels.[112] In sum, for people with type 2 diabetes and diabetic kidney disease, use of an SGLT2 inhibitor is recommended to reduce CKD progression and cardiovascular events in people with an eGFR $\geq$20 mL/min/1.73 m^2.

Of note, GLP-1 RAs may also be used at low eGFR for cardiovascular protection but may require dose adjustment.[113]

Renal and Cardiovascular Outcomes of Mineralocorticoid Receptor Antagonists in Chronic Kidney Disease

MRAs historically have not been well studied in diabetic kidney disease because of the risk of hyperkalemia.[114,115] However, data that do exist suggest sustained benefit on albuminuria reduction. There are two different classes of MRAs, steroidal and nonsteroidal, with one group not extrapolatable to the other.[116] Late in 2020, the results of the first of two trials, the Finerenone in Reducing Kidney Failure and Disease Progression in Diabetic Kidney Disease (FIDELIO-DKD) trial, which examined the renal effects of finerenone, demonstrated a significant reduction in diabetic kidney disease progression and cardiovascular events in people with advanced diabetic kidney disease.[32,117] This trial had a primary end point of time to first occurrence of the composite end point of onset of kidney failure, a sustained decrease of eGFR >40% from baseline over at least 4 weeks, or renal death. A prespecified secondary outcome was time to first occurrence of the composite end point cardiovascular death or nonfatal cardiovascular events (myocardial infarction, stroke, or hospitalization for heart failure). Other secondary outcomes included all-cause mortality, time to all-cause hospitalizations, and change in UACR from baseline to month 4, and time to first occurrence of the following composite end point: onset of kidney failure, a sustained decrease in eGFR of ≥57% from baseline over at least 4 weeks, or renal death.

The double-blind, placebo-controlled trial randomized 5,734 people with CKD and type 2 diabetes to receive finerenone, a novel nonsteroidal MRA, or placebo. Eligible participants had a UACR of 30 to <300 mg/g, an eGFR of 25 to <60 mL/min/1.73 m², and diabetic retinopathy, or a UACR of 300–5,000 mg/g and an eGFR of 25 to <75 mL/min/1.73 m². The mean age of participants was 65.6 years, and 30% were female. The mean eGFR was 44.3 mL/min/1.73 m², and the mean albuminuria was 852 mg/g (interquartile range 446–1,634 mg/g). The primary end point was reduced with finerenone compared with placebo (HR 0.82 [95% CI 0.73–0.93]; $P = 0.001$), as was the key secondary composite of cardiovascular outcome (HR 0.86 [95% CI 0.75–0.99]; $P = 0.03$). Hyperkalemia resulted in 2.3% discontinuation in the study group compared with 0.9% in the placebo group. However, the study was completed, and there were no deaths related to hyperkalemia. Of note, 4.5% of the total group were being treated with SGLT2 inhibitors.

The Finerenone in Reducing Cardiovascular Mortality and Morbidity in Diabetic Kidney Disease (FIGARO-DKD) trial assessed the safety and efficacy of finerenone in reducing cardiovascular events among people with type 2 diabetes and CKD with elevated UACR (30 to <300 mg/g creatinine) and eGFR 25–90 mL/min/1.73 m².[118] The study randomized eligible subjects to either finerenone ($n = 3,686$) or placebo ($n = 3,666$). Participants with an eGFR of 25–60 mL/min/1.73 m² at the screening visit received an initial dose at baseline of 10 mg once daily, and if eGFR at screening was ≥60 mL/min/1.73 m², the initial dose was 20 mg once daily. An increase in the dose from 10 to 20 mg once daily was encouraged after 1 month, provided the serum potassium level was ≤4.8 mmol/L and eGFR was stable. The mean age of participants was 64.1 years (31% were female), and the median follow-up duration was 3.4 years. The median A1C was 7.7%, the mean systolic blood pressure was 136 mmHg, and the mean GFR was 67.8 mL/min/1.73 m². People with heart failure with a reduced ejection fraction and uncontrolled hypertension were excluded.

The primary composite outcome was cardiovascular death, myocardial infarction, stroke, and hospitalization for heart failure. The finerenone group showed a 13% reduction in the primary end point compared with the placebo group (12.4% vs. 14.2%; HR 0.87 [95% CI 0.76–0.98]; $P = 0.03$). This benefit was primarily driven by a reduction in heart failure hospitalizations: 3.2% vs. 4.4% in the placebo group (HR 0.71 [95% CI 0.56–0.90]).

Of the secondary outcomes, the most noteworthy was a 36% reduction in end-stage kidney disease: 0.9% vs. 1.3% in the placebo group (HR 0.64 [95% CI 0.41–0.995]). There was a higher incidence of hyperkalemia in the finerenone group, 10.8% vs. 5.3%, although only 1.2% of the 3,686 individuals on finerenone stopped the study due to hyperkalemia (0.6% vs. 0.4% of the placebo group).

The FIDELITY prespecified pooled efficacy and safety analysis incorporated individuals from both the FIGARO-DKD and FIDELIO-DKD trials (*n* = 13,171) to allow for evaluation across the spectrum of severity of CKD, since the populations were different (with a slight overlap) and the study designs were similar.[119] The analysis showed a 14% reduction in composite cardiovascular death, nonfatal myocardial infarction, nonfatal stroke, and hospitalization for heart failure for finerenone vs. placebo (12.7% vs. 14.4%; HR 0.86 [95% CI 0.78–0.95]; *P* = 0.0018).

It also demonstrated a 23% reduction in the composite kidney outcome, consisting of sustained ≥57% decrease in eGFR from baseline over ≥4 weeks, or renal death, for finerenone vs. placebo (5.5% vs. 7.1%; HR 0.77 [95% CI 0.67–0.88]; *P* = 0.0002).

The pooled FIDELITY trial analysis confirms and strengthens the positive cardiovascular and renal outcomes with finerenone across the spectrum of CKD, irrespective of baseline ASCVD history (with the exclusion of those with heart failure with reduced ejection fraction).

Referral to a Nephrologist

Health care professionals should consider referral to a nephrologist if the patient has continuously rising UACR levels and/or continuously declining eGFR, if there is uncertainty about the etiology of kidney disease, for difficult management issues (anemia, secondary hyperparathyroidism, significant increases in albuminuria in spite of good blood pressure management, metabolic bone disease, resistant hypertension, or electrolyte disturbances), or when there is advanced kidney disease (eGFR <30 mL/min/1.73 m²) requiring discussion of renal replacement therapy for ESRD.[2] The threshold for referral may vary depending on the frequency with which a health care professional encounters people with diabetes and kidney disease. Consultation with a nephrologist when stage 4 CKD develops (eGFR <30 mL/min/1.73 m²) has been found to reduce cost, improve quality of care, and delay dialysis.[120] However, other specialists and health care professionals should also educate their patients about the progressive nature of CKD, the kidney preservation benefits of proactive treatment of blood pressure and blood glucose, and the potential need for renal replacement therapy.

REFERENCES

1. Tuttle KR, Bakris GL, Bilous RW, et al. Diabetic kidney disease: a report from an ADA Consensus Conference. Diabetes Care 2014;37:2864–2883

2. National Kidney Foundation. KDIGO 2012 clinical practice guideline for the evaluation and management of chronic kidney disease. Kidney Int Suppl 2013;3:1–150

3. Afkarian M, Zelnick LR, Hall YN, et al. Clinical manifestations of kidney disease among US adults with diabetes, 1988-2014. JAMA 2016;316: 602–610

4. de Boer IH, Rue TC, Hall YN, Heagerty PJ, Weiss NS, Himmelfarb J. Temporal trends in the prevalence of diabetic kidney disease in the United States. JAMA 2011;305:2532–2539

5. de Boer IH; DCCT/EDIC Research Group. Kidney disease and related findings in the Diabetes Control and Complications Trial/Epidemiology of Diabetes Interventions and Complications study. Diabetes Care 2014;37:24–30

6. Johansen KL, Chertow GM, Foley RN, et al. US Renal Data System 2020 annual data report: epidemiology of kidney disease in the United States. Am J Kidney Dis 2021;77(Suppl. 1): A7–A8

7. Fox CS, Matsushita K, Woodward M, et al.; Chronic Kidney Disease Prognosis Consortium. Associations of kidney disease measures with mortality and end-stage renal disease in individuals with and without diabetes: a meta-analysis. Lancet 2012;380:1662–1673

8. Yarnoff BO, Hoerger TJ, Simpson SK, et al.; Centers for Disease Control and Prevention CKD Initiative. The cost-effectiveness of using chronic kidney disease risk scores to screen for early-stage chronic kidney disease. BMC Nephrol 2017; 18:85

9. Coresh J, Heerspink HJL, Sang Y, et al.; Chronic Kidney Disease Prognosis Consortium and Chronic Kidney Disease Epidemiology Collaboration. Change in albuminuria and subsequent risk of end-stage kidney disease: an individual participant-level consortium meta-analysis of observational studies. Lancet Diabetes Endocrinol 2019;7:115–127

10. Levey AS, Gansevoort RT, Coresh J, et al. Change in albuminuria and GFR as end points for clinical trials in early stages of CKD: a scientific workshop sponsored by the National Kidney Foundation in collaboration with the US Food and Drug Administration and European Medicines Agency. Am J Kidney Dis 2020;75:84–104

11. Afkarian M, Sachs MC, Kestenbaum B, et al. Kidney disease and increased mortality risk in type 2 diabetes. J Am Soc Nephrol 2013;24: 302–308

12. Groop P-H, Thomas MC, Moran JL, et al.; FinnDiane Study Group. The presence and severity of chronic kidney disease predicts allcause mortality in type 1 diabetes. Diabetes 2009;58:1651–1658

13. Gomes MB, Gonçalves MF. Is there a physiological variability for albumin excretion rate? Study in patients with diabetes type 1 and non-diabetic individuals. Clin Chim Acta 2001;304: 117–123

14. Naresh CN, Hayen A, Weening A, Craig JC, Chadban SJ. Day-to-day variability in spot urine albumin-creatinine ratio. Am J Kidney Dis 2013; 62:1095–1101

15. Tankeu AT, Kaze FF, Noubiap JJ, Chelo D, Dehayem MY, Sobngwi E. Exercise-induced albuminuria and circadian blood pressure abnormalities in type 2 diabetes. World J Nephrol 2017;6:209–216

16. Delanaye P, Glassock RJ, Pottel H, Rule AD. An age-calibrated definition of chronic kidney disease: rationale and benefits. Clin Biochem Rev 2016;37:17–26

17. Kramer HJ, Nguyen QD, Curhan G, Hsu C-Y. Renal insufficiency in the absence of albuminuria and retinopathy among adults with type 2 diabetes mellitus. JAMA 2003;289:3273–3277

18. Molitch ME, Steffes M, Sun W, et al.; Epidemiology of Diabetes Interventions and Complications Study Group. Development and progression of renal insufficiency with and without albuminuria in adults with type 1 diabetes in the Diabetes Control and Complications Trial and the Epidemiology of Diabetes Interventions and Complications study. Diabetes Care 2010;33:1536–1543

19. He F, Xia X, Wu XF, Yu XQ, Huang FX. Diabetic retinopathy in predicting diabetic nephropathy in patients with type 2 diabetes and renal disease: a meta-analysis. Diabetologia 2013;56:457–466

20. Levey AS, Coresh J, Balk E, et al.; National Kidney Foundation. National Kidney Foundation practice guidelines for chronic kidney disease: evaluation, classification, and stratification. Ann Intern Med 2003;139:137–147

21. Flynn C, Bakris GL. Noninsulin glucose-lowering agents for the treatment of patients on dialysis. Nat Rev Nephrol 2013;9:147–153

22. Matzke GR, Aronoff GR, Atkinson AJ Jr, et al. Drug dosing consideration in patients with acute and chronic kidney disease—a clinical update from Kidney Disease: Improving Global Outcomes (KDIGO). Kidney Int 2011;80:1122–1137

23. Coresh J, Turin TC, Matsushita K, et al. Decline in estimated glomerular filtration rate and subsequent risk of end-stage renal disease and mortality. JAMA 2014;311:2518–2531

24. Vassalotti JA, Centor R, Turner BJ, Greer RC, Choi M; National Kidney Foundation Kidney Disease Outcomes Quality Initiative. Practical approach to detection and management of chronic kidney disease for the primary care clinician. Am J Med 2016;129:153–162.e7

25. Zhou J, Liu Y, Tang Y, et al. A comparison of RIFLE, AKIN, KDIGO, and Cys-C criteria for the definition of acute kidney injury in critically ill patients. Int Urol Nephrol 2016;48:125–132

26. Hoste EAJ, Kellum JA, Selby NM, et al. Global epidemiology and outcomes of acute kidney injury. Nat Rev Nephrol 2018;14:607–625

27. James MT, Grams ME, Woodward M, et al.; CKD Prognosis Consortium. A meta-analysis of the association of estimated GFR, albuminuria, diabetes

mellitus, and hypertension with acute kidney injury. Am J Kidney Dis 2015;66:602–612

28. Perkovic V, Jardine MJ, Neal B, et al. Canagliflozin and renal outcomes in type 2 diabetes and nephropathy. N Engl J Med 2019; 380:2295–2306

29. Nadkarni GN, Ferrandino R, Chang A, et al. Acute kidney injury in patients on SGLT2 inhibitors: a propensity-matched analysis. Diabetes Care 2017;40:1479–1485

30. Wanner C, Inzucchi SE, Lachin JM, et al.; EMPA-REG OUTCOME Investigators. Empagliflozin and progression of kidney disease in type 2 diabetes. N Engl J Med 2016;375:323–334

31. Neuen BL, Ohkuma T, Neal B, et al. Cardiovascular and renal outcomes with canagliflozin according to baseline kidney function: data from the CANVAS Program. Circulation 2018;138:1537–1550

32. Bakris GL, Agarwal R, Anker SD, et al.; FIDELIO-DKD Investigators. Effect of finerenone on chronic kidney disease outcomes in type 2 diabetes. N Engl J Med 2020;383:2219–2229

33. Thakar CV, Christianson A, Himmelfarb J, Leonard AC. Acute kidney injury episodes and chronic kidney disease risk in diabetes mellitus. Clin J Am Soc Nephrol 2011;6:2567–2572

34. Bakris GL, Weir MR. Angiotensin-converting enzyme inhibitor-associated elevations in serum creatinine: is this a cause for concern? Arch Intern Med 2000;160:685–693

35. Beddhu S, Greene T, Boucher R, et al. Intensive systolic blood pressure control and incident chronic kidney disease in people with and without diabetes mellitus: secondary analyses of two randomised controlled trials. Lancet Diabetes Endocrinol 2018;6:555–563

36. Collard D, Brouwer TF, Peters RJG, Vogt L, van den Born BH. Creatinine rise during blood pressure therapy and the risk of adverse clinical outcomes in patients with type 2 diabetes mellitus. Hypertension 2018;72:1337–1344

37. Malhotra R, Craven T, Ambrosius WT, et al.; SPRINT Research Group. Effects of intensive blood pressure lowering on kidney tubule injury in CKD: a longitudinal subgroup analysis in SPRINT. Am J Kidney Dis 2019;73:21–30

38. Qiao Y, Shin J-I, Chen TK, et al. Association between renin-angiotensin system blockade discontinuation and all-cause mortality among persons with low estimated glomerular filtration rate. JAMA Intern Med 2020;180:718–726

39. Ohkuma T, Jun M, Rodgers A, et al.; ADVANCE Collaborative Group. Acute increases in serum creatinine after starting angiotensin-converting enzyme inhibitor-based therapy and effects of its continuation on major clinical outcomes in type 2 diabetes mellitus. Hypertension 2019;73:84–91

40. Hughes-Austin JM, Rifkin DE, Beben T, et al. The relation of serum potassium concentration with cardiovascular events and mortality in community-living individuals. Clin J Am Soc Nephrol 2017;12:245–252

41. Bandak G, Sang Y, Gasparini A, et al. Hyperkalemia after initiating renin-angiotensin system blockade: the Stockholm Creatinine Measurements (SCREAM) project. J Am Heart Assoc 2017;6:e005428

42. Nilsson E, Gasparini A, Ärnlöv J, et al. Incidence and determinants of hyperkalemia and hypokalemia in a large healthcare system. Int J Cardiol 2017;245:277–284

43. Zelniker TA, Raz I, Mosenzon O, et al. Effect of dapagliflozin on cardiovascular outcomes according to baseline kidney function and albuminuria status in patients with type 2 diabetes: a prespecified secondary analysis of a randomized clinical trial. JAMA Cardiol 2021;6:801–810

44. Epstein M, Reaven NL, Funk SE, McGaughey KJ, Oestreicher N, Knispel J. Evaluation of the treatment gap between clinical guidelines and the utilization of renin-angiotensin-aldosterone system inhibitors. Am J Manag Care 2015;21(Suppl.): S212–S220

45. de Boer IH, Gao X, Cleary PA, et al.; Diabetes Control and Complications Trial/Epidemiology of Diabetes Interventions and Complications (DCCT/EDIC) Research Group. Albuminuria changes and cardiovascular and renal outcomes in type 1 diabetes: the DCCT/EDIC study. Clin J Am Soc Nephrol 2016;11:1969–1977

46. Sumida K, Molnar MZ, Potukuchi PK, et al. Changes in albuminuria and subsequent risk of incident kidney disease. Clin J Am Soc Nephrol 2017;12:1941–1949

47. Klahr S, Levey AS, Beck GJ, et al.; Modification of Diet in Renal Disease Study Group. The effects of dietary protein restriction and blood-pressure control on the progression of chronic renal disease. N Engl J Med 1994;330: 877–884

48. Mills KT, Chen J, Yang W, et al.; Chronic Renal Insufficiency Cohort (CRIC) Study Investigators. Sodium excretion and the risk of cardiovascular disease in patients with chronic kidney disease. JAMA 2016;315:2200–2210

49. Whelton PK, Carey RM, Aronow WS, et al. 2017 ACC/AHA/AAPA/ABC/ACPM/AGS/ APhA/ASH/ASPC/NMA/PCNA guideline for the prevention, detection, evaluation, and management of high blood pressure in adults: executive summary: a report of the American College of Cardiology/American Heart Association Task Force on Clinical Practice Guidelines. Hypertension 2018;71:1269–1324

50. Murray DP, Young L, Waller J, et al. Is dietary protein intake predictive of 1-year mortality in dialysis patients? Am J Med Sci 2018;356:234–243

51. DCCT/EDIC Research Group. Effect of intensive diabetes treatment on albuminuria in type 1 diabetes: long-term follow-up of the Diabetes Con-

trol and Complications Trial and Epidemiology of Diabetes Interventions and Complications study. Lancet Diabetes Endocrinol 2014;2:793–800

52. de Boer IH, Sun W, Cleary PA, et al.; DCCT/EDIC Research Group. Intensive diabetes therapy and glomerular filtration rate in type 1 diabetes. N Engl J Med 2011;365:2366–2376

53. UK Prospective Diabetes Study (UKPDS) Group. Intensive blood-glucose control with sulphonylureas or insulin compared with conventional treatment and risk of complications in patients with type 2 diabetes (UKPDS 33). Lancet 1998;352:837–853

54. Patel A, MacMahon S, Chalmers J, et al.; ADVANCE Collaborative Group. Intensive blood glucose control and vascular outcomes in patients with type 2 diabetes. N Engl J Med 2008; 358:2560–2572

55. Ismail-Beigi F, Craven T, Banerji MA, et al.; ACCORD trial group. Effect of intensive treatment of hyperglycaemia on microvascular outcomes in type 2 diabetes: an analysis of the ACCORD randomised trial. Lancet 2010;376:419–430

56. Zoungas S, Chalmers J, Neal B, et al.; ADVANCE-ON Collaborative Group. Follow-up of blood-pressure lowering and glucose control in type 2 diabetes. N Engl J Med 2014;371:1392–1406

57. Zoungas S, Arima H, Gerstein HC, et al.; Collaborators on Trials of Lowering Glucose (CONTROL) group. Effects of intensive glucose control on microvascular outcomes in patients with type 2 diabetes: a meta-analysis of individual participant data from randomised controlled trials. Lancet Diabetes Endocrinol 2017;5:431–437

58. Agrawal L, Azad N, Bahn GD, et al.; VADT Study Group. Long-term follow-up of intensive glycaemic control on renal outcomes in the Veterans Affairs Diabetes Trial (VADT). Diabetologia 2018;61:295–299

59. Papademetriou V, Lovato L, Doumas M, et al.; ACCORD Study Group. Chronic kidney disease and intensive glycemic control increase cardiovascular risk in patients with type 2 diabetes. Kidney Int 2015;87:649–659

60. Perkovic V, Heerspink HL, Chalmers J, et al.; ADVANCE Collaborative Group. Intensive glucose control improves kidney outcomes in patients with type 2 diabetes. Kidney Int 2013;83: 517–523

61. Wong MG, Perkovic V, Chalmers J, et al.; ADVANCE-ON Collaborative Group. Longterm benefits of intensive glucose control for preventing endstage kidney disease: ADVANCE-ON. Diabetes Care 2016;39:694–700

62. National Kidney Foundation. KDOQI clinical practice guideline for diabetes and CKD: 2012 update. Am J Kidney Dis 2012;60:850–886

63. Leehey DJ, Zhang JH, Emanuele NV, et al.; VA NEPHRON-D Study Group. BP and renal outcomes in diabetic kidney disease: the Veterans Affairs Nephropathy in Diabetes Trial. Clin J Am Soc Nephrol 2015;10:2159–2169

64. Emdin CA, Rahimi K, Neal B, Callender T, Perkovic V, Patel A. Blood pressure lowering in type 2 diabetes: a systematic review and metaanalysis. JAMA 2015;313:603–615

65. Cushman WC, Evans GW, Byington RP, et al.; ACCORD Study Group. Effects of intensive blood-pressure control in type 2 diabetes mellitus. N Engl J Med 2010;362:1575–1585

66. UK Prospective Diabetes Study Group. Tight blood pressure control and risk of macrovascular and microvascular complications in type 2 diabetes: UKPDS 38. BMJ 1998;317:703–713

67. de Boer IH, Bangalore S, Benetos A, et al. Diabetes and hypertension: a position statement by the American Diabetes Association. Diabetes Care 2017;40:1273–1284

68. Brenner BM, Cooper ME, de Zeeuw D, et al.; RENAAL Study Investigators. Effects of losartan on renal and cardiovascular outcomes in patients with type 2 diabetes and nephropathy. N Engl J Med 2001;345:861–869

69. Lewis EJ, Hunsicker LG, Bain RP; The Collaborative Study Group. The effect of angiotensin-converting-enzyme inhibition on diabetic nephropathy. N Engl J Med 1993;329:1456–1462

70. Lewis EJ, Hunsicker LG, Clarke WR, et al.; Collaborative Study Group. Renoprotective effect of the angiotensin-receptor antagonist irbesartan in patients with nephropathy due to type 2 diabetes. N Engl J Med 2001;345:851–860

71. Zinman B, Wanner C, Lachin JM, et al.; EMPA-REG OUTCOME Investigators. Empagliflozin, cardiovascular outcomes, and mortality in type 2 diabetes. N Engl J Med 2015;373:2117–2128

72. Jardine MJ, Mahaffey KW, Neal B, et al.; CREDENCE study investigators. The Canagliflozin and Renal Endpoints in Diabetes with Established Nephropathy Clinical Evaluation (CREDENCE) study rationale, design, and baseline characteristics. Am J Nephrol 2017;46:462–472

73. Mahaffey KW, Jardine MJ, Bompoint S, et al. Canagliflozin and cardiovascular and renal outcomes in type 2 diabetes mellitus and chronic kidney disease in primary and secondary cardiovascular prevention groups. Circulation 2019;140: 739–750

74. Heart Outcomes Prevention Evaluation Study Investigators. Effects of ramipril on cardiovascular and microvascular outcomes in people with diabetes mellitus: results of the HOPE study and MICRO-HOPE substudy. Lancet 2000;355: 253–259

75. Barnett AH, Bain SC, Bouter P, et al.; Diabetics Exposed to Telmisartan and Enalapril Study Group. Angiotensin-receptor blockade versus converting-enzyme inhibition in type 2 diabetes and nephropathy. N Engl J Med 2004; 351:1952–1961

76. Wu HY, Peng CL, Chen PC, et al. Comparative effectiveness of angiotensin-converting enzyme inhibitors versus angiotensin II receptor blockers for major renal outcomes in patients with diabetes: a 15-year cohort study. PLoS One 2017; 12:e0177654

77. Parving HH, Lehnert H, Bröchner-Mortensen J, Gomis R, Andersen S; Irbesartan in Patients with Type 2 Diabetes and Microalbuminuria Study Group. The effect of irbesartan on the development of diabetic nephropathy in patients with type 2 diabetes. N Engl J Med 2001;345: 870–878

78. Mauer M, Zinman B, Gardiner R, et al. Renal and retinal effects of enalapril and losartan in type 1 diabetes. N Engl J Med 2009;361:40–51

79. Weil EJ, Fufaa G, Jones LI, et al. Effect of losartan on prevention and progression of early diabetic nephropathy in American Indians with type 2 diabetes. Diabetes 2013;62:3224–3231

80. Bangalore S, Fakheri R, Toklu B, Messerli FH. Diabetes mellitus as a compelling indication for use of renin angiotensin system blockers: systematic review and meta-analysis of randomized trials. BMJ 2016;352:i438

81. Haller H, Ito S, Izzo JL Jr, et al.; ROADMAP Trial Investigators. Olmesartan for the delay or prevention of microalbuminuria in type 2 diabetes. N Engl J Med 2011;364:907–917

82. Yusuf S, Teo KK, Pogue J, et al.; ONTARGET Investigators. Telmisartan, ramipril, or both in patients at high risk for vascular events. N Engl J Med 2008;358:1547–1559

83. Fried LF, Emanuele N, Zhang JH, et al.; VA NEPHRON-D Investigators. Combined angiotensin inhibition for the treatment of diabetic nephropathy. N Engl J Med 2013;369:1892–1903

84. Cherney DZI, Perkins BA, Soleymanlou N, et al. Renal hemodynamic effect of sodium-glucose cotransporter 2 inhibition in patients with type 1 diabetes mellitus. Circulation 2014; 129:587–597

85. Heerspink HJL, Desai M, Jardine M, Balis D, Meininger G, Perkovic V. Canagliflozin slows progression of renal function decline independently of glycemic effects. J Am Soc Nephrol 2017;28:368–375

86. Neal B, Perkovic V, Mahaffey KW, et al.; CANVAS Program Collaborative Group. Canagliflozin and cardiovascular and renal events in type 2 diabetes. N Engl J Med 2017;377:644–657

87. Zelniker TA, Braunwald E. Cardiac and renal effects of sodium-glucose cotransporter 2 inhibitors in diabetes: JACC state-of-the-art review. J Am Coll Cardiol 2018;72:1845–1855

88. Woods TC, Satou R, Miyata K, et al. Canagliflozin prevents intrarenal angiotensinogen augmentation and mitigates kidney injury and hypertension in mouse model of type 2 diabetes mellitus. Am J Nephrol 2019;49:331–342

89. Heerspink HJL, Perco P, Mulder S, et al. Canagliflozin reduces inflammation and fibrosis biomarkers: a potential mechanism of action for beneficial effects of SGLT2 inhibitors in diabetic kidney disease. Diabetologia 2019;62: 1154–1166

90. Yaribeygi H, Butler AE, Atkin SL, Katsiki N, Sahebkar A. Sodium-glucose cotransporter 2 inhibitors and inflammation in chronic kidney disease: possible molecular pathways. J Cell Physiol 2018;234:223–230

91. Marso SP, Daniels GH, Brown-Frandsen K, et al.; LEADER Steering Committee; LEADER Trial Investigators. Liraglutide and cardiovascular outcomes in type 2 diabetes. N Engl J Med 2016;375:311–322

92. Cooper ME, Perkovic V, McGill JB, et al. Kidney disease end points in a pooled analysis of individual patient-level data from a large clinical trials program of the dipeptidyl peptidase 4 inhibitor linagliptin in type 2 diabetes. Am J Kidney Dis 2015;66:441–449

93. Mann JFE, Ørsted DD, Brown-Frandsen K, Marso SP, Poulter NR, Rasmussen S, et al. Liraglutide and renal outcomes in type 2 diabetes. N Engl J Med. 2017;377:839–848

94. Marso SP, Bain SC, Consoli A, et al.; SUSTAIN-6 Investigators. Semaglutide and cardiovascular outcomes in patients with type 2 diabetes. N Engl J Med 2016;375:1834–1844

95. Shaman AM, Bain SC, Bakris GL, et al. Effect of the glucagon-like peptide-1 receptor agonists semaglutide and liraglutide on kidney outcomes in patients with type 2 diabetes: pooled analysis of SUSTAIN 6 and LEADER. Circulation 2022;145: 575–585

96. Karter AJ, Warton EM, Lipska KJ, et al. Development and validation of a tool to identify patients with type 2 diabetes at high risk of hypoglycemia-related emergency department or hospital use. JAMA Intern Med 2017;177: 1461–1470

97. Moen MF, Zhan M, Hsu VD, et al. Frequency of hypoglycemia and its significance in chronic kidney disease. Clin J Am Soc Nephrol 2009;4: 1121–1127

98. U.S. Food and Drug Administration. FDA drug safety communication: FDA revises warnings regarding use of the diabetes medicine metformin in certain patients with reduced kidney function, 2017. Accessed 20 October 2022. Available from https://www.fda.gov/drugs/drug-safety-and-availability/fda-drug-safety-communication-fda-revises-warnings-regarding-use-diabetes-medicine-metformin-certain

99. Lalau JD, Kajbaf F, Bennis Y, Hurtel-Lemaire AS, Belpaire F, De Broe ME. Metformin treatment in patients with type 2 diabetes and chronic kidney disease stages 3A, 3B, or 4. Diabetes Care 2018;41:547–553

100. Chu PY, Hackstadt AJ, Chipman J, et al. Hospitalization for lactic acidosis among patients with reduced kidney function treated with metformin or sulfonylureas. Diabetes Care 2020; 43:1462–1470

101. McGuire DK, Shih WJ, Cosentino F, et al. Association of SGLT2 inhibitors with cardiovascular and kidney outcomes in patients with type 2 diabetes: a meta-analysis. JAMA Cardiol 2021;6: 148–158

102. Zelniker TA, Wiviott SD, Raz I, et al. Comparison of the effects of glucagon-like peptide receptor agonists and sodium-glucose cotransporter 2 inhibitors for prevention of major adverse cardiovascular and renal outcomes in type 2 diabetes mellitus. Circulation 2019;139: 2022–2031

103. Mann JFE, Hansen T, Idorn T, et al. Effects of once-weekly subcutaneous semaglutide on kidney function and safety in patients with type 2 diabetes: a post-hoc analysis of the SUSTAIN 1-7 randomised controlled trials. Lancet Diabetes Endocrinol 2020;8:880–893

104. Mann JFE, Muskiet MHA. Incretin-based drugs and the kidney in type 2 diabetes: choosing between DPP-4 inhibitors and GLP-1 receptor agonists. Kidney Int 2021;99:314–318

105. Bakris GL. Major advancements in slowing diabetic kidney disease progression: focus on SGLT2 inhibitors. Am J Kidney Dis 2019;74: 573–575

106. 106 Heerspink HJL, Stefánsson BV, Correa-Rotter R, et al.; DAPA-CKD Trial Committees and Investigators. Dapagliflozin in patients with chronic kidney disease. N Engl J Med 2020;383: 1436–1446

107. Wiviott SD, Raz I, Bonaca MP, Mosenzon O, Kato ET, Cahn A, et al. Dapagliflozin and cardiovascular outcomes in type 2 diabetes. N Engl J Med 2019;380:347–357

108. Novo Nordisk A/S. A research study to see how semaglutide works compared to placebo in people with type 2 diabetes and chronic kidney disease (FLOW). In: ClinicalTrials.gov. Bethesda, MD, National Library of Medicine, 2019. Accessed 20 October 2022. Available from https://clinicaltrials.gov/ct2/show/NCT03819153

109. Chertow GM, Vart P, Jongs N, et al.; DAPA-CKD Trial Committees and Investigators. Effects of dapagliflozin in stage 4 chronic kidney disease. J Am Soc Nephrol 2021;32:2352–2361

110. Anker SD, Butler J, Filippatos G, et al.; EMPEROR-Preserved Trial Investigators. Empag-liflozin in heart failure with a preserved ejection fraction. N Engl J Med 2021;385:1451–1461

111. Packer M, Anker SD, Butler J, et al.; EMPEROR-Reduced Trial Investigators. Cardiovascular and renal outcomes with empagliflozin in heart failure. N Engl J Med 2020;383: 1413–1424

112. Mosenzon O, Wiviott SD, Heerspink HJL, et al. The effect of dapagliflozin on albuminuria in DECLARE-TIMI 58. Diabetes Care 2021;44: 1805–1815

113. Romera I, Cebrín-Cuenca A, Álvarez-Guisasola F, Gomez-Peralta F, Reviriego J. A review of practical issues on the use of glucagon-like peptide-1 receptor agonists for the management of type 2 diabetes. Diabetes Ther 2019;10:5–19

114. Bomback AS, Kshirsagar AV, Amamoo MA, Klemmer PJ. Change in proteinuria after adding aldosterone blockers to ACE inhibitors or angiotensin receptor blockers in CKD: a systematic review. Am J Kidney Dis 2008;51:199–211

115. Sarafidis P, Papadopoulos CE, Kamperidis V, Giannakoulas G, Doumas M. Cardiovascular protection with sodium-glucose cotransporter-2 inhibitors and mineralocorticoid receptor an-tagonists in chronic kidney disease: a milestone achieved. Hypertension 2021;77: 1442–1455

116. Agarwal R, Kolkhof P, Bakris G, et al. Steroidal and non-steroidal mineralocorticoid receptor antagonists in cardiorenal medicine. Eur Heart J 2021;42:152–161

117. Filippatos G, Anker SD, Agarwal R, et al.; FIDELIO-DKD Investigators. Finerenone and cardiovascular outcomes in patients with chronic kidney disease and type 2 diabetes. Circulation 2021;143:540–552

118. Pitt B, Filippatos G, Agarwal R, et al.; FIGARO-DKD Investigators. Cardiovascular events with finerenone in kidney disease and type 2 diabetes. N Engl J Med 2021;385:2252–2263

119. Agarwal R, Filippatos G, Pitt B, et al.; FIDELIO-DKD and FIGARO-DKD investigators. Cardiovascular and kidney outcomes with finerenone in patients with type 2 diabetes and chronic kidney disease: the FIDELITY pooled analysis. Eur Heart J 2022;43:474–484

120. Smart NA, Dieberg G, Ladhani M, Titus T. Early referral to specialist nephrology services for preventing the progression to end-stage kidney disease. Cochrane Database Syst Rev 2014;6:CD007333

121. Vassalotti JA, Centor R, Turner BJ, Greer RC, Choi M; National Kidney Foundation Kidney Disease Outcomes Quality Initiative. Practical approach to detection and management of chronic kidney disease for the primary care clinician. Am J Med 2016;129:153–162.e7

Chapter 19
Retinopathy, Neuropathy, and Foot Care

The American Diabetes Association (ADA) "Standards of Care in Diabetes" includes the ADA's current clinical practice recommendations and is intended to provide the components of diabetes care, general treatment goals and guidelines, and tools to evaluate quality of care. Members of the ADA Professional Practice Committee, a multidisciplinary expert committee, are responsible for updating the Standards of Care annually, or more frequently as warranted. For a detailed description of ADA standards, statements, and reports, as well as the evidence-grading system for ADA's clinical practice recommendations and a full list of Professional Practice Committee members, please refer to Introduction and Methodology. Readers who wish to comment on the Standards of Care are invited to do so at professional.diabetes.org/SOC.

For prevention and management of diabetes complications in children and adolescents, please refer to Section 14, "Children and Adolescents."

DIABETIC RETINOPATHY

Recommendations
12.1   Optimize glycemic control to reduce the risk or slow the progression of diabetic retinopathy. **A**
12.2   Optimize blood pressure and serum lipid control to reduce the risk or slow the progression of diabetic retinopathy. **A**

Diabetic retinopathy is a highly specific vascular complication of both type 1 and type 2 diabetes, with prevalence strongly related to both the duration of diabetes and the level of glycemic control.[1] Diabetic retinopathy is the most frequent cause of new cases of blindness among adults aged 20–74 years in developed countries. Glaucoma, cataracts, and other eye disorders occur earlier and more frequently in people with diabetes.

Chapter 19 is an excerpt from ElSayed NA, Aleppo G, Aroda VR, et al., American Diabetes Association. 12. Retinopathy, neuropathy, and foot care: Standards of Care in Diabetes—2023. *Diabetes Care* 2023; 46(Suppl. 1):S203–S215

* See Table 1.1 (p. 2) for an explanation of the American Diabetes Association evidence-grading system for *Standards of Care in Diabetes*.

In addition to diabetes duration, factors that increase the risk of, or are associated with, retinopathy include chronic hyperglycemia[2,3], nephropathy[4], hypertension[5], and dyslipidemia.[6] Intensive diabetes management with the goal of achieving near-normoglycemia has been shown in large prospective randomized studies to prevent and/or delay the onset and progression of diabetic retinopathy, reduce the need for future ocular surgical procedures, and potentially improve patient-reported visual function.[2,7–10] A meta-analysis of data from cardiovascular outcomes studies showed no association between glucagon-like peptide 1 receptor agonist (GLP-1 RA) treatment and retinopathy per se, except through the association between retinopathy and average A1C reduction at the 3-month and 1-year follow-up. Long-term impact of improved glycemic control on retinopathy was not studied in these trials. Retinopathy status should be assessed when intensifying glucose-lowering therapies such as those using GLP-1 RAs, since rapid reductions in A1C can be associated with initial worsening of retinopathy.[11]

SCREENING

Recommendations

12.3   Adults with type 1 diabetes should have an initial dilated and comprehensive eye examination by an ophthalmologist or optometrist within 5 years after the onset of diabetes. **B**

12.4   People with type 2 diabetes should have an initial dilated and comprehensive eye examination by an ophthalmologist or optometrist at the time of the diabetes diagnosis. **B**

12.5   If there is no evidence of retinopathy for one or more annual eye exams and glycemia is well controlled, then screening every 1–2 years may be considered. If any level of diabetic retinopathy is present, subsequent dilated retinal examinations should be repeated at least annually by an ophthalmologist or optometrist. If retinopathy is progressing or sight-threatening, then examinations will be required more frequently. **B**

12.6   Programs that use retinal photography (with remote reading or use of a validated assessment tool) to improve access to diabetic retinopathy screening can be appropriate screening strategies for diabetic retinopathy. Such programs need to provide pathways for timely referral for a comprehensive eye examination when indicated. **B**

12.7   Individuals of childbearing potential with preexisting type 1 or type 2 diabetes who are planning pregnancy or who are pregnant should be counseled on the risk of development and/or progression of diabetic retinopathy. **B**

12.8   Individuals with preexisting type 1 or type 2 diabetes should receive an eye exam before pregnancy and in the first trimester and should be monitored every trimester and for 1 year postpartum as indicated by the degree of retinopathy. **B**

The preventive effects of therapy and the fact that individuals with proliferative diabetic retinopathy (PDR) or macular edema may be asymptomatic provide strong support for screening to detect diabetic retinopathy. Prompt diagnosis allows triage of patients and timely intervention that may prevent vision loss in individuals who are asymptomatic despite advanced diabetic eye disease.

Diabetic retinopathy screening should be performed using validated approaches and methodologies. Youth with type 1 or type 2 diabetes are also at risk for complications and need to be screened for diabetic retinopathy[12] (see Section 14, "Children and Adolescents"). If diabetic retinopathy is evident on screening, prompt referral to an ophthalmologist is recommended. Subsequent examinations for individuals with type 1 or type 2 diabetes are generally repeated annually for individuals with minimal to no retinopathy. Exams every 1–2 years may be cost-effective after one or more normal eye exams. In a population with well-controlled type 2 diabetes, there was little risk of development of significant retinopathy within a 3-year interval after a normal examination[13], and less frequent intervals have been found in simulated modeling to be potentially effective in screening for diabetic retinopathy in individuals without diabetic retinopathy.[14] However, it is important to adjust screening intervals based on the presence of specific risk factors for retinopathy onset and worsening retinopathy. More frequent examinations by the ophthalmologist will be required if retinopathy is progressing or risk factors such as uncontrolled hyperglycemia, advanced baseline retinopathy, or diabetic macular edema are present.

Retinal photography with remote reading by experts has great potential to provide screening services in areas where qualified eye care professionals are not readily available.[15-17] High-quality fundus photographs can detect most clinically significant diabetic retinopathy. Interpretation of the images should be performed by a trained eye care professional. Retinal photography may also enhance efficiency and reduce costs when the expertise of ophthalmologists can be used for more complex examinations and for therapy.[15,18,19] In-person exams are still necessary when the retinal photos are of unacceptable quality and for follow-up if abnormalities are detected. Retinal photos are not a substitute for dilated comprehensive eye exams, which should be performed at least initially and at yearly intervals thereafter or more frequently as recommended by an eye care professional. Artificial intelligence systems that detect more than mild diabetic retinopathy and diabetic macular edema, authorized for use by the U.S. Food and Drug Administration (FDA), represent an alternative to traditional screening approaches.[20] However, the benefits and optimal utilization of this type of screening have yet to be fully determined. Results of all screening eye examinations should be documented and transmitted to the referring health care professional.

Type 1 Diabetes

Because retinopathy is estimated to take at least 5 years to develop after the onset of hyperglycemia, people with type 1 diabetes should have an initial dilated and comprehensive eye examination within 5 years after the diagnosis of diabetes.[21]

Type 2 Diabetes

People with type 2 diabetes who may have had years of undiagnosed diabetes and have a significant risk of prevalent diabetic retinopathy at the time of diagnosis should have an initial dilated and comprehensive eye examination at the time of diagnosis.

Pregnancy

Individuals who develop gestational diabetes mellitus do not require eye examinations during pregnancy since they do not appear to be at increased risk of developing diabetic retinopathy during pregnancy.[22] However, individuals of childbearing potential with preexisting type 1 or type 2 diabetes who are planning pregnancy or who have become pregnant should be counseled on the baseline prevalence and risk of development and/or progression of diabetic retinopathy. In a systematic review and meta-analysis of 18 observational studies of pregnant individuals with preexisting type 1 or type 2 diabetes, the prevalence of any diabetic retinopathy and PDR in early pregnancy was 52.3% and 6.1%, respectively. The pooled progression rate per 100 pregnancies for new diabetic retinopathy development was 15.0 (95% CI 9.9–20.8), worsened nonproliferative diabetic retinopathy was 31.0 (95% CI 23.2–39.2), pooled sight-threatening progression rate from nonproliferative diabetic retinopathy to PDR was 6.3 (95% CI 3.3–10.0), and worsened PDR was 37.0 (95% CI 21.2–54.0), demonstrating that close follow-up should be maintained during pregnancy to prevent vision loss.[23] In addition, rapid implementation of intensive glycemic management in the setting of retinopathy is associated with early worsening of retinopathy.[24]

A systematic review and meta-analysis and a controlled prospective study demonstrate that pregnancy in individuals with type 1 diabetes may aggravate retinopathy and threaten vision, especially when glycemic control is poor or retinopathy severity is advanced at the time of conception.[23,24] Laser photocoagulation surgery can minimize the risk of vision loss during pregnancy for individuals with high-risk PDR or center-involved diabetic macular edema.[24] Anti–vascular endothelial growth factor (anti-VEGF) medications should not be used in pregnant individuals with diabetes because of theoretical risks to the vasculature of the developing fetus.

TREATMENT

Recommendations

12.9 Promptly refer individuals with any level of diabetic macular edema, moderate or worse nonproliferative diabetic retinopathy (a precursor of proliferative diabetic retinopathy), or any proliferative diabetic retinopathy to an ophthalmologist who is knowledgeable and experienced in the management of diabetic retinopathy. **A**

12.10 Panretinal laser photocoagulation therapy is indicated to reduce the risk of vision loss in individuals with high-risk proliferative diabetic retinopathy and, in some cases, severe nonproliferative diabetic retinopathy. **A**

12.11 Intravitreous injections of anti–vascular endothelial growth factor are a reasonable alternative to traditional panretinal laser photocoagulation for some individuals with proliferative diabetic retinopathy and also reduce the risk of vision loss in these individuals. **A**

12.12 Intravitreous injections of anti–vascular endothelial growth factor are indicated as first-line treatment for most eyes with diabetic macular edema that involves the foveal center and impairs vision acuity. **A**

12.13 Macular focal/grid photocoagulation and intravitreal injections of corticosteroid are reasonable treatments in eyes with persistent diabetic macular edema despite previous anti–vascular endothelial growth factor therapy or eyes that are not candidates for this first-line approach. **A**

12.14 The presence of retinopathy is not a contraindication to aspirin therapy for cardioprotection, as aspirin does not increase the risk of retinal hemorrhage. **A**

Two of the main motivations for screening for diabetic retinopathy are to prevent loss of vision and to intervene with treatment when vision loss can be prevented or reversed.

Photocoagulation Surgery

Two large trials, the Diabetic Retinopathy Study (DRS) in individuals with PDR and the Early Treatment Diabetic Retinopathy Study (ETDRS) in individuals with macular edema, provide the strongest support for the therapeutic benefits of photocoagulation surgery. The DRS[25] showed in 1978 that panretinal photocoagulation surgery reduced the risk of severe vision loss from PDR from 15.9% in untreated eyes to 6.4% in treated eyes with the greatest benefit ratio in those with more advanced baseline disease (disc neovascularization or vitreous hemorrhage). In 1985, the ETDRS also verified the benefits of panretinal photocoagulation for high-risk PDR and in older-onset individuals with severe nonproliferative diabetic retinopathy or less-than-high-risk PDR. Panretinal laser photocoagulation is still commonly used to manage complications of diabetic retinopathy that involve retinal neovascularization and its complications. A more gentle, macular focal/grid laser photocoagulation technique was shown in the ETDRS to be effective in treating eyes with clinically significant macular edema from diabetes[26], but this is now largely considered to be second-line treatment for diabetic macular edema.

Anti–Vascular Endothelial Growth Factor Treatment

Data from the DRCR Retina Network (formerly the Diabetic Retinopathy Clinical Research Network) and others demonstrate that intravitreal injections of anti-VEGF agents are effective at regressing proliferative disease and lead to noninferior or superior visual acuity outcomes compared with panretinal laser over 2 years of follow-up.[27,28] In addition, it was observed that individuals treated with ranibizumab tended to have less peripheral visual field loss, fewer vitrectomy surgeries for secondary complications from their proliferative disease, and a lower risk of developing diabetic macular edema. However, a potential drawback in using anti-VEGF therapy to manage proliferative disease is that patients were required to have a greater number of visits and received a greater number of treatments than is typically required for management with panretinal laser, which may not be optimal for some individuals. The FDA has approved aflibercept and ranibizumab for the treatment of eyes with diabetic retinopathy. Other emerging therapies for retinopathy that may use sustained intravitreal delivery of pharmacologic agents are currently under investigation. Anti-VEGF treatment of eyes with nonproliferative diabetic retinopathy has been demonstrated to reduce subsequent development of retinal neovascularization and diabetic macular edema but has not been shown to improve visual outcomes over 2 years of therapy and therefore is not routinely recommended for this indication.[29]

While the ETDRS[26] established the benefit of focal laser photocoagulation surgery in eyes with clinically significant macular edema (defined as retinal edema located at or threatening the macular center), current data from well-designed clinical trials demonstrate that intravitreal anti-VEGF agents provide a more effective treatment plan for center-involved diabetic macular edema than mono-therapy with laser.[30,31] Most patients require near-monthly administration of intra-vitreal therapy with anti-VEGF agents during the first 12 months of treatment, with fewer injections needed in subsequent years to maintain remission from central-involved diabetic macular edema. There are currently three anti-VEGF agents commonly used to treat eyes with central-involved diabetic macular edema—bevacizumab, ranibizumab, and aflibercept[1]—and a comparative effec-tiveness study demonstrated that aflibercept provides vision outcomes superior to those of bevacizumab when eyes have moderate visual impairment (vision of 20/50 or worse) from diabetic macular edema.[32] For eyes that have good vision (20/25 or better) despite diabetic macular edema, close monitoring with initiation of anti-VEGF therapy if vision worsens provides similar 2-year vision outcomes compared with immediate initiation of anti-VEGF therapy.[33]

Eyes that have persistent diabetic macular edema despite anti-VEGF treat-ment may benefit from macular laser photocoagulation or intravitreal therapy with corticosteroids. Both of these therapies are also reasonable first-line approaches for individuals who are not candidates for anti-VEGF treatment due to systemic considerations such as pregnancy.

Adjunctive Therapy

Lowering blood pressure has been shown to decrease retinopathy progression, although tight targets (systolic blood pressure <120 mmHg) do not impart addi-tional benefit.[8] In individuals with dyslipidemia, retinopathy progression may be slowed by the addition of fenofibrate, particularly with very mild nonproliferative diabetic retinopathy at baseline.[34,35]

NEUROPATHY

SCREENING

Recommendations

12.15 All people with diabetes should be assessed for diabetic peripheral neuropathy starting at diagnosis of type 2 diabetes and 5 years after the diagnosis of type 1 diabetes and at least annually thereafter. **B**

12.16 Assessment for distal symmetric polyneuropathy should include a careful history and assessment of either temperature or pinprick sensation (small-fiber function) and vibration sensation using a 128-Hz tuning fork (for large-fiber function). All people with diabetes should have annual 10-g monofilament testing to identify feet at risk for ulceration and amputation. **B**

12.17 Symptoms and signs of autonomic neuropathy should be assessed in people with diabetes starting at diagnosis of type 2 diabetes and 5 years after the diagnosis of type 1 diabetes and at least annually thereafter and with evidence of other microvascular complications, particularly kidney disease and diabetic peripheral neuropathy. Screening can include asking about orthostatic dizziness, syncope, or dry cracked skin in the extremities. Signs of autonomic neuropathy include orthostatic hypotension, a resting tachy-cardia, or evidence of peripheral dryness or cracking of skin. **E**

Diabetic neuropathies are a heterogeneous group of disorders with diverse clinical manifestations. The early recognition and appropriate management of neuropathy in people with diabetes is important. Points to be aware of include the following:

1. Diabetic neuropathy is a diagnosis of exclusion. Nondiabetic neuropathies may be present in people with diabetes and may be treatable.
2. Up to 50% of diabetic peripheral neuropathy may be asymptomatic. If not recognized and if preventive foot care is not implemented, people with diabetes are at risk for injuries as well as diabetic foot ulcers and amputations.
3. Recognition and treatment of autonomic neuropathy may improve symptoms, reduce sequelae, and improve quality of life.

Specific treatment to reverse the underlying nerve damage is currently not available. Glycemic control can effectively prevent diabetic peripheral neuropathy (DPN) and cardiac autonomic neuropathy (CAN) in type 1 diabetes[36,37] and may modestly slow their progression in type 2 diabetes[38], but it does not reverse neuronal loss. Treatments of other modifiable risk factors (including lipids and blood pressure) can aid in prevention of DPN progression in type 2 diabetes and may reduce disease progression in type 1 diabetes.[39-41] Therapeutic strategies (pharmacologic and nonpharmacologic) for the relief of painful DPN and symptoms of autonomic neuropathy can potentially reduce pain[42] and improve quality of life.

Diagnosis

Diabetic Peripheral Neuropathy
Individuals with a type 1 diabetes duration ≥5 years and all individuals with type 2 diabetes should be assessed annually for DPN using the medical history and simple clinical tests.[42] Symptoms vary according to the class of sensory fibers involved. The most common early symptoms are induced by the involvement of small fibers and include pain and dysesthesia (unpleasant sensations of burning and tingling). The involvement of large fibers may cause numbness and loss of protective sensation (LOPS). LOPS indicates the presence of distal sensorimotor polyneuropathy and is a risk factor for diabetic foot ulceration. The following clinical tests may be used to assess small- and large-fiber function and protective sensation:

1. Small-fiber function: pinprick and temperature sensation.
2. Large-fiber function: lower-extremity reflexes, vibration perception, and 10-g monofilament.
3. Protective sensation: 10-g monofilament.

These tests not only screen for the presence of dysfunction but also predict future risk of complications. Electrophysiological testing or referral to a neurologist is rarely needed, except in situations where the clinical features are atypical or the diagnosis is unclear.

In all people with diabetes and DPN, causes of neuropathy other than diabetes should be considered, including toxins (e.g., alcohol), neurotoxic medications (e.g., chemotherapy), vitamin B12 deficiency, hypothyroidism, renal disease, malignancies (e.g., multiple myeloma, bronchogenic carcinoma), infections (e.g., HIV), chronic inflammatory demyelinating neuropathy, inherited neuropathies, and vasculitis.[43] See the American Diabetes Association position statement "Diabetic Neuropathy" for more details.[42]

Diabetic Autonomic Neuropathy

Individuals who have had type 1 diabetes for ≥5 years and all individuals with type 2 diabetes should be assessed annually for autonomic neuropathy.[42] The symptoms and signs of autonomic neuropathy should be elicited carefully during the history and physical examination. Major clinical manifestations of diabetic autonomic neuropathy include resting tachycardia, orthostatic hypotension, gastroparesis, constipation, diarrhea, fecal incontinence, erectile dysfunction, neurogenic bladder, and sudomotor dysfunction with either increased or decreased sweating. Screening for symptoms of autonomic neuropathy includes asking about symptoms of orthostatic intolerance (dizziness, lightheadedness, or weakness with standing), syncope, exercise intolerance, constipation, diarrhea, urinary retention, urinary incontinence, or changes in sweat function. Further testing can be considered if symptoms are present and will depend on the end organ involved but might include cardiovascular autonomic testing, sweat testing, urodynamic studies, gastric emptying, or endoscopy/colonoscopy. Impaired counterregulatory responses to hypoglycemia in type 1 and type 2 diabetes can lead to hypoglycemia unawareness but are not directly linked to autonomic neuropathy.

Cardiovascular Autonomic Neuropathy. CAN is associated with mortality independently of other cardiovascular risk factors.[44,45] In its early stages, CAN may be completely asymptomatic and detected only by decreased heart rate variability with deep breathing. Advanced disease may be associated with resting tachycardia (>100 bpm) and orthostatic hypotension (a fall in systolic or diastolic blood pressure by >20 mmHg or >10 mmHg, respectively, upon standing without an appropriate increase in heart rate). CAN treatment is generally focused on alleviating symptoms.

Gastrointestinal Neuropathies. Gastrointestinal neuropathies may involve any portion of the gastrointestinal tract, with manifestations including esophageal dysmotility, gastroparesis, constipation, diarrhea, and fecal incontinence. Gastroparesis should be suspected in individuals with erratic glycemic control or with upper gastrointestinal symptoms without another identified cause. Exclusion of reversible/iatrogenic causes such as medications or organic causes of gastric outlet obstruction or peptic ulcer disease (with esophagogastroduodenoscopy or a barium study of the stomach) is needed before considering a diagnosis of or specialized testing for gastroparesis. The diagnostic gold standard for gastroparesis is the measurement of gastric emptying with scintigraphy of digestible solids at 15-min intervals for 4 h after food intake. The use of ^{13}C octanoic acid breath test is an approved alternative.

Genitourinary Disturbances. Diabetic autonomic neuropathy may also cause genitourinary disturbances, including sexual dysfunction and bladder dysfunction. In men, diabetic autonomic neuropathy may cause erectile dysfunction and/or retrograde ejaculation.[42] Female sexual dysfunction occurs more frequently in those with diabetes and presents as decreased sexual desire, increased pain during intercourse, decreased sexual arousal, and inadequate lubrication.[46] Lower urinary tract symptoms manifest as urinary incontinence and bladder dysfunction (nocturia, frequent urination, urination urgency, and weak urinary stream). Evaluation of bladder function should be performed for individuals with diabetes who have recurrent urinary tract infections, pyelonephritis, incontinence, or a palpable bladder.

Treatment

Recommendations

12.18 Optimize glucose control to prevent or delay the development of neuropathy in people with type 1 diabetes **A** and to slow the progression of neuropathy in people with type 2 diabetes. **C** Optimize blood pressure and serum lipid control to reduce the risk or slow the progression of diabetic neuropathy. **B**

12.19 Assess and treat pain related to diabetic peripheral neuropathy **B** and symptoms of autonomic neuropathy to improve quality of life. **E**

12.20 Gabapentinoids, serotonin-norepinephrine reuptake inhibitors, tricyclic antidepressants, and sodium channel blockers are recommended as initial pharmacologic treatments for neuropathic pain in diabetes. **A** Refer to neurologist or pain specialist when pain control is not achieved within the scope of practice of the treating physician. **E**

Glycemic Control

Near-normal glycemic control, implemented early in the course of diabetes, has been shown to effectively delay or prevent the development of DPN and CAN in people with type 1 diabetes.[47-50] Although the evidence for the benefit of near-normal glycemic control is not as strong that for type 2 diabetes, some studies have demonstrated a modest slowing of progression without reversal of neuronal loss.[38,51] Specific glucose-lowering strategies may have different effects. In a post hoc analysis, participants, particularly men, in the Bypass Angioplasty Revascularization Investigation in Type 2 Diabetes (BARI 2D) trial treated with insulin sensitizers had a lower incidence of distal symmetric polyneuropathy over 4 years than those treated with insulin/sulfonylurea.[52] Additionally, recent evidence from the Action to Control Cardiovascular Risk in Diabetes (ACCORD) trial showed clear benefit of intensive glucose and blood pressure control on the prevention of CAN in type 2 diabetes.[53]

Lipid Control

Dyslipidemia is a key factor in the development of neuropathy in people with type 2 diabetes and may contribute to neuropathy risk in people with type 1 diabetes.[54,55] Although the evidence for a relationship between lipids and neuropathy development has become increasingly clear in type 2 diabetes, the optimal therapeutic intervention has not been identified. Positive effects of physical activity, weight loss, and bariatric surgery have been reported in individuals with DPN, but use of conventional lipid-lowering pharmacotherapy (such as statins or fenofibrates) does not appear to be effective in treating or preventing DPN development.[56]

Blood Pressure Control

There are multiple reasons for blood pressure control in people with diabetes, but neuropathy progression (especially in type 2 diabetes) has now been added to this list. Although data from many studies have supported the role of hypertension in risk of neuropathy development, a recent meta-analysis of data from 14 countries in the International Prevalence and Treatment of Diabetes and Depression (INTERPRET-DD) study revealed hypertension as an independent risk of DPN development with an odds ratio of 1.58.[57] In the ACCORD trial, intensive blood pressure intervention decreased CAN risk by 25%.[53]

Neuropathic Pain

Neuropathic pain can be severe and can impact quality of life, limit mobility, and contribute to depression and social dysfunction.[58] No compelling evidence exists in support of glycemic control or lifestyle management as therapies for neuropathic pain in diabetes or prediabetes, which leaves only pharmaceutical interventions.[59] A recent guideline by the American Academy of Neurology recommends that the initial treatment of pain should also focus on the concurrent treatment of both sleep and mood disorders because of increased frequency of these problems in individuals with DPN.[60]

A number of pharmacologic therapies exist for treatment of pain in diabetes. The American Academy of Neurology update suggested that gabapentinoids, serotonin-norepinephrine reuptake inhibitors (SNRIs), sodium channel blockers, tricyclic antidepressants (TCAs), and SNRI/opioid dual-mechanism agents could all be considered in the treatment of pain in DPN.[60] These American Academy of Neurology recommendations offer a supplement to a recent American Diabetes Association pain monograph, although some areas of disagreement exist, particularly around SNRI/opioid dual-mechanism agents.[61] A recent head-to-head trial suggested therapeutic equivalency for TCAs, SNRIs, and gabapentinoids in the treatment of pain in DPN.[62] The trial also supported the role of combination therapy over monotherapy for the treatment of pain in DPN.

Gabapentinoids. Gabapentinoids include several calcium channel $\alpha2$-δ subunit ligands. Eight high-quality studies and seven medium-quality studies support the role of pregabalin in treatment of pain in DPN. One high-quality study and many small studies support the role of gabapentin in the treatment of pain in DPN. Two medium-quality studies suggest that micro-gabalin has a small effect on pain in DPN.[60] Adverse effects may be more severe in older individuals[63] and may be attenuated by lower starting doses and more gradual titration.

SNRIs. SNRIs include duloxetine, venla-faxine, and desvenlafaxine, all selective SNRIs. Two high-quality studies and five medium-quality studies support the role of duloxetine in the treatment of pain in DPN. A high-quality study supports the role of venlafaxine in the treatment of pain in DPN. Only one medium-quality study supports a possible role for desvenlafaxine for treatment of pain in DPN.[60] Adverse events may be more severe in older people but may be attenuated with lower doses and slower titration of duloxetine.

Tapentadol and Tramadol. Tapentadol and tramadol are centrally acting opioid analgesics that exert their analgesic effects through both m-opioid receptor agonism and norepinephrine and serotonin reuptake inhibition. SNRI/opioid agents are probably effective in the treatment of pain in DPN. However, the use of any opioids for management of chronic neuropathic pain carries the risk of addiction and should be avoided.

Tricyclic Antidepressants. Tricyclic antidepressants have been studied for treatment of pain, and most of the relevant data was acquired from trials of amitriptyline and include two high-quality studies and two medium-quality studies supporting the treatment of pain in DPN.[60,62] Anticholinergic side effects may be dose limiting and restrict use in individuals ≥65 years of age.

Sodium Channel Blockers. Sodium channel blockers include lamotrigine, lacosamide, oxcarbazepine, and valproic acid. Five medium-quality studies support the role of sodium channel blockers in treating pain in DPN.[60]

Capsaicin. Capsaicin has received FDA approval for treatment of pain in DPN using an 8% patch, with one high-quality study reported. One medium-quality study of 0.075% capsaicin cream has been reported. In patients with contraindications to oral pharmacotherapy or who prefer topical treatments, the use of topical capsaicin can be considered.

Carbamazepine and α-Lipoic Acid. Carbamazepine and α-lipoic acid, although not approved for the treatment of painful DPN, may be effective and considered for the treatment of painful DPN.[41,54,56]

Orthostatic Hypotension

Treating orthostatic hypotension is challenging. The therapeutic goal is to minimize postural symptoms rather than to restore normotension. Most patients require both nonpharmacologic measures (e.g., ensuring adequate salt intake, avoiding medications that aggravate hypotension, or using compressive garments over the legs and abdomen) and pharmacologic measures. Physical activity and exercise should be encouraged to avoid deconditioning, which is known to exacerbate orthostatic intolerance, and volume repletion with fluids and salt is critical. There have been clinical studies that assessed the impact of an approach incorporating the aforementioned non-pharmacologic measures. Additionally, supine blood pressure tends to be much higher in these individuals, often requiring treatment of blood pressure at bedtime with shorter-acting drugs that also affect baroreceptor activity such as guanfacine or clonidine, shorter-acting calcium blockers (e.g., isradipine), or shorter-acting β-blockers such as atenolol or metoprolol tartrate. Alternatives can include enalapril if an individual is unable to tolerate preferred agents.[64-66] Midodrine and droxidopa are approved by the FDA for the treatment of orthostatic hypotension.

Gastroparesis

Treatment for diabetic gastroparesis may be very challenging. A low-fiber, low-fat eating plan provided in small frequent meals with a greater proportion of liquid calories may be useful.[67-69] In addition, foods with small particle size may improve key symptoms.[70] Withdrawing drugs with adverse effects on gastrointestinal motility, including opioids, anticholinergics, tricyclic antidepressants, GLP-1 RAs, and pramlintide, may also improve intestinal motility.[67,71] However, the risk of removal of GLP-1 RAs should be balanced against their potential benefits. In cases of severe gastroparesis, pharmacologic interventions are needed. Only metoclopramide, a prokinetic agent, is approved by the FDA for the treatment of gastroparesis. However, the level of evidence regarding the benefits of metoclopramide for the management of gastroparesis is weak, and given the risk for serious adverse effects (extrapyramidal signs such as acute dystonic reactions, drug-induced parkinsonism, akathisia, and tardive dyskinesia), its use in the treatment of gastroparesis beyond 12 weeks is no longer recommended by the FDA. It should be reserved for severe cases that are unresponsive to other therapies.[71] Other treatment options include domperidone (available outside the U.S.) and erythromycin, which is only effective for short-term use due to tachyphylaxis.[72,73] Gastric electrical stimulation using a surgically implantable device has received approval from the FDA, although its efficacy is variable and use is limited to individuals with severe symptoms that are refractory to other treatments.[74]

Erectile Dysfunction

In addition to treatment of hypogonadism if present, treatments for erectile dysfunction may include phosphodiesterase type 5 inhibitors, intracorporeal or intraurethral prostaglandins, vacuum devices, or penile prostheses. As with DPN treatments, these interventions do not change the underlying pathology and natural history of the disease process but may improve a person's quality of life.

FOOT CARE

Recommendations

12.21 Perform a comprehensive foot evaluation at least annually to identify risk factors for ulcers and amputations. **A**

12.22 The examination should include inspection of the skin, assessment of foot deformities, neurological assessment (10-g monofilament testing with at least one other assessment: pinprick, temperature, vibration), and vascular assessment, including pulses in the legs and feet. **B**

12.23 Individuals with evidence of sensory loss or prior ulceration or amputation should have their feet inspected at every visit. **A**

12.24 Obtain a prior history of ulceration, amputation, Charcot foot, angioplasty or vascular surgery, cigarette smoking, retinopathy, and renal disease and assess current symptoms of neuropathy (pain, burning, numbness) and vascular disease (leg fatigue, claudication). **B**

12.25 Initial screening for peripheral arterial disease should include assessment of lower-extremity pulses, capillary refill time, rubor on dependency, pallor on elevation, and venous filling time. Individuals with a history of leg fatigue, claudication, and rest pain relieved with dependency or decreased or absent pedal pulses should be referred for ankle–brachial index and for further vascular assessment as appropriate. **B**

12.26 A multidisciplinary approach is recommended for individuals with foot ulcers and high-risk feet (e.g., those on dialysis, those with Charcot foot, those with a history of prior ulcers or amputation, and those with peripheral arterial disease). **B**

12.27 Refer individuals who smoke and have a history of prior lower-extremity complications, loss of protective sensation, structural abnormalities, or peripheral arterial disease to foot care specialists for ongoing preventive care and lifelong surveillance. **B**

12.28 Provide general preventive foot self-care education to all people with diabetes, including those with loss of protective sensation, on appropriate ways to examine their feet (palpation or visual inspection with an unbreakable mirror) for daily surveillance of early foot problems. **B**

12.29 The use of specialized therapeutic footwear is recommended for people with diabetes at high risk for ulceration, including those with loss of protective sensation, foot deformities, ulcers, callous formation, poor peripheral circulation, or history of amputation. **B**

12.30 For chronic diabetic foot ulcers that have failed to heal with optimal standard care alone, adjunctive treatment with randomized controlled trial–proven advanced agents should be considered. Considerations might include negative-pressure wound therapy, placental membranes, bioengineered skin substitutes, several acellular matrices, autologous fibrin and leukocyte platelet patches, and topical oxygen therapy. **A**

Foot ulcerations and amputations are common complications associated with diabetes. These may be the consequences of several factors, including peripheral neuropathy, peripheral arterial disease (PAD), and foot deformities. They represent major causes of morbidity and mortality in people with diabetes. Early recognition of at-risk feet, preulcerative lesions, and prompt treatment of ulcerations and other lower-extremity complications can delay or prevent adverse outcomes.

Early recognition requires an understanding of those factors that put people with diabetes at increased risk for ulcerations and amputations. Factors that are associated with the at-risk foot include the following:

- Poor glycemic control
- Peripheral neuropathy/LOPS
- PAD
- Foot deformities (bunions, hammertoes, Charcot joint, etc.)
- Preulcerative corns or calluses
- Prior ulceration
- Prior amputation
- Smoking
- Retinopathy
- Nephropathy (particularly individuals on dialysis or posttransplant)

Identifying the at-risk foot begins with a detailed history documenting diabetes control, smoking history, exercise tolerance, history of claudication or rest pain, and prior ulcerations or amputations. A thorough examination of the feet should be performed annually in all people with diabetes and more frequently in at-risk individuals.[75] The examination should include assessment of skin integrity, assessment for LOPS using the 10-g monofilament along with at least one other neurological assessment tool, pulse examination of the dorsalis pedis and posterior tibial arteries, and assessment for foot deformities such as bunions, hammertoes, and prominent metatarsals, which increase plantar foot pressures and increase risk for ulcerations. At-risk individuals should be assessed at each visit and should be referred to foot care specialists for ongoing preventive care and surveillance. The physical examination can stratify patients into different categories and determine the frequency of these visits[76] (Table 19.1).

EVALUATION FOR LOSS OF PROTECTIVE SENSATION

The presence of peripheral sensory neuropathy is the single most common component cause for foot ulceration. In a multicenter trial, peripheral neuropathy was found to be a component cause in 78% of people with diabetes with ulcerations and that the triad of peripheral sensory neuropathy, minor trauma, and foot deformity was present in >63% of participants.[77] All people with diabetes should undergo a comprehensive foot examination at least annually, or more frequently for those in higher-risk categories.[75,76]

LOPS is vital to risk assessment. One of the most useful tests to determine LOPS is the 10-g monofilament test. Studies have shown that clinical examination and the 10-g monofilament test are the two most sensitive tests in identifying the foot at risk for ulceration.[78] The monofilament test should be performed with at least one other neurologic assessment tool (e.g., pinprick, temperature perception, ankle reflexes, or vibratory perception with a 128-Hz tuning fork or similar device). Absent monofilament sensation and one other abnormal test confirms the presence of LOPS. Further neurological testing, such as nerve conduction, electromyography, nerve biopsy, or intraepidermal nerve fiber density biopsies, are rarely indicated for the diagnosis of peripheral sensory neuropathy.[42]

EVALUATION FOR PERIPHERAL ARTERIAL DISEASE

Initial screening for PAD should include a history of leg fatigue, claudication, and rest pain relieved with dependency. Physical examination for PAD should include assessment of lower-extremity pulses, capillary refill time, rubor on dependency, pallor on elevation, and venous filling time.[75,79] Any patient exhibiting signs and symptoms of PAD should be referred for noninvasive arterial studies in the form of Doppler ultrasound with pulse volume recordings. While ankle–brachial indices will be calculated, they should be interpreted carefully, as they are known to be inaccurate in people with diabetes due to noncompressible vessels. Toe systolic blood pressure tends to be more accurate. Toe systolic blood pressures <30 mmHg are suggestive of PAD and an inability to heal foot ulcerations.[80] Individuals with abnormal pulse volume recording tracings and toe pressures <30 mmHg with foot ulcers should be referred for immediate vascular evaluation. Due to the high prevalence of PAD in people with diabetes, it has been recommended by the Society for Vascular Surgery and the American Podiatric Medical Association in their 2016 guidelines that all people with diabetes >50 years of age should undergo screening via noninvasive arterial studies.[79,81] If normal, these should be repeated every 5 years.[79]

PATIENT EDUCATION

All people with diabetes (and their families), particularly those with the aforementioned high-risk conditions, should receive general foot care education, including appropriate management strategies.[82–84] This education should be provided to all newly diagnosed people with diabetes as part of an annual comprehensive examination and to individuals with high-risk conditions at every visit. Recent studies have shown that while education improves knowledge of diabetic foot

Table 19.1—International Working Group on the Diabetic Foot risk stratification system and corresponding foot screening frequency

Category	Ulcer risk	Characteristics	Examination frequency*
0	Very low	No LOPS and No PAD	Annually
1	Low	LOPS or PAD	Every 6–12 months
2	Moderate	LOPS + PAD, or LOPS + foot deformity, or PAD + foot deformity	Every 3–6 months
3	High	LOPS or PAD and one or more of the following: • History of foot ulcer • Amputation (minor or major) • End-stage renal disease	Every 1–3 months

Adapted with permission from Schaper et al.[76] LOPS, loss of protective sensation; PAD, peripheral artery disease. *Examination frequency suggestions are based on expert opinion and patient-centered requirements.

problems and self-care of the foot, it does not improve behaviors associated with active participation in their overall diabetes care and to achieve personal health goals.[85] Evidence also suggests that while patient and family education are important, the knowledge is quickly forgotten and needs to be reinforced regularly.[86]

Individuals considered at risk should understand the implications of foot deformities, LOPS, and PAD; the proper care of the foot, including nail and skin care; and the importance of foot inspections on a daily basis. Individuals with LOPS should be educated on appropriate ways to examine their feet (palpation or visual inspection with an unbreakable mirror) for daily surveillance of early foot problems. Patients should also be educated on the importance of referrals to foot care specialists. A recent study showed that people with diabetes and foot disease lacked awareness of their risk status and why they were being referred to a multidisciplinary team of foot care specialists. Further, they exhibited a variable degree of interest in learning further about foot complications.[87]

Patients' understanding of these issues and their physical ability to conduct proper foot surveillance and care should be assessed. Those with visual difficulties, physical constraints preventing movement, or cognitive problems that impair their ability to assess the condition of the foot and to institute appropriate responses will need other people, such as family members, to assist with their care.

The selection of appropriate footwear and footwear behaviors at home should also be discussed (e.g., no walking barefoot, avoiding open-toed shoes). Therapeutic footwear with custom-made orthotic devices have been shown to reduce peak plantar pressures.[84] Most studies use reduction in peak plantar pressures as an outcome as opposed to ulcer prevention. Certain design features of the orthoses, such as rocker soles and metatarsal accommodations, can reduce peak plantar pressures more significantly than insoles alone. A systematic review, however, showed there was no significant reduction in ulcer incidence after 18 months compared with standard insoles and extra-depth shoes. Further, it was also noted that evidence to prevent first ulcerations was nonexistent.[88]

TREATMENT

Treatment recommendations for people with diabetes will be determined by their risk category. No-risk or low-risk individuals can often be managed with education and self-care. People in the moderate- to high-risk category should be referred to foot care specialists for further evaluation and regular surveillance as outlined in Table 19.1. This includes individuals with LOPS, PAD, and/or structural foot deformities, such as Charcot foot, bunions, or hammertoes. Individuals with any open ulceration or unexplained swelling, erythema, or increased skin temperature should be referred urgently to a foot care specialist or multidisciplinary team.

Initial treatment recommendations should include daily foot inspection, use of moisturizers for dry, scaly skin, and avoidance of self-care of ingrown nails and calluses. Well-fitted athletic or walking shoes with customized pressure-relieving orthoses should be part of initial recommendations for people with increased plantar pressures (as demonstrated by plantar calluses). Individuals with deformities such as bunions or hammertoes may require specialized footwear such as extra-depth shoes. Those with even more significant deformities, as in Charcot joint disease, may require custom-made footwear.

Special consideration should be given to individuals with neuropathy who present with a warm, swollen, red foot with or without a history of trauma and without an open ulceration. These individuals require a thorough workup for possible Charcot neuroarthropathy.[89] Early diagnosis and treatment of this condition is of paramount importance in preventing deformities and instability that can lead to ulceration and amputation. These individuals require total non–weight-bearing and urgent referral to a foot care specialist for further management. Foot and ankle X-rays should be performed in all individuals presenting with the above clinical findings.

There have been a number of developments in the treatment of ulcerations over the years.[90] These include negative-pressure therapy, growth factors, bioengineered tissue, acellular matrix tissue, stem cell therapy, hyperbaric oxygen therapy, and, most recently, topical oxygen therapy.[91–93] While there is literature to support many modalities currently used to treat diabetic foot wounds, robust randomized controlled trials (RCTs) are often lacking. However, it is agreed that the initial treatment and evaluation of ulcerations include the following five basic principles of ulcer treatment:

- Offloading of plantar ulcerations
- Debridement of necrotic, nonviable tissue
- Revascularization of ischemic wounds when necessary
- Management of infection: soft tissue or bone
- Use of physiologic, topical dressings

However, despite following the above principles, some ulcerations will become chronic and fail to heal. In those situations, advanced wound therapy can play a role. When to employ advanced wound therapy has been the subject of much discussion, as the therapy is often quite expensive. It has been determined that if a wound fails to show a reduction of 50% or more after 4 weeks of appropriate wound management (i.e., the five basic principles above), consideration should be given to the use of advanced wound therapy.[94] Treatment of these chronic wounds is best managed in a multidisciplinary setting.

Evidence to support advanced wound therapy is challenging to produce and to assess. Randomization of trial participants is difficult, as there are many variables that can affect wound healing. In addition, many RCTs exclude certain cohorts of people, e.g., individuals with chronic renal disease or those on dialysis. Finally, blinding of participants and clinicians is not always possible. Meta-analyses and systematic reviews of observational studies are used to determine the clinical effectiveness of these modalities. Such studies can augment formal RCTs by including a greater variety of participants in various clinical settings who are typically excluded from the more rigidly structured clinical trials.

Advanced wound therapy can be categorized into nine broad categories[90] (Table 19.2). Topical growth factors, acellular matrix tissues, and bioengineered cellular therapies are commonly employed in offices and wound care centers to expedite healing of chronic, more superficial ulcerations. Numerous clinical reports and retrospective studies have demonstrated the clinical effectiveness of each of these modalities. Over the years, there has been increased evidence to support the use of these modalities. Nonetheless, use of those products or agents with robust RCTs or systematic reviews should generally be preferred over those without level 1 evidence (Table 19.2).

Negative-pressure wound therapy was first introduced in the early to mid-1990s. It has become especially useful in wound preparation for skin grafts and flaps and assists in the closure of deep, large wounds.[95,96] A variety of types exist in the marketplace and range from electrically powered to mechanically powered in different sizes depending upon the specific wound requirements.

Electrical stimulation, pulsed radiofrequency energy, and extracorporeal shockwave therapy are biophysical modalities that are believed to upregulate growth factors or cytokines to stimulate wound healing, while low-frequency non-contact ultrasound is used to debride wounds. However, most of the studies advocating the use of these modalities have been retrospective observational or poor-quality RCTs.

Hyperbaric oxygen therapy is the delivery of oxygen through a chamber, either individual or multiperson, with the intention of increasing tissue oxygenation to increase tissue perfusion and neovascularization, combat resistant bacteria, and stimulate wound healing. While there had been great interest in this modality being able to expedite healing of chronic diabetic foot ulcers (DFUs), there has only been one positive RCT published in the last decade that reported increased healing rates at 9 and 12 months compared with control subjects.[97] More recent studies with significant design deficiencies and participant dropouts have failed to provide corroborating evidence that hyperbaric oxygen therapy should be widely used for managing nonhealing DFUs.[98,99] While there may be some benefit in prevention of amputation in selected chronic neuroischemic ulcers, recent studies have shown no benefit in healing DFUs in the absence of ischemia and/or infection.[93,100]

Table 19.2—Categories of advanced wound therapies

Negative-pressure wound therapy
■ Standard electrically powered
■ Mechanically powered
Oxygen therapies
■ Hyperbaric oxygen therapy
■ Topical oxygen therapy
■ Oxygen-releasing sprays, dressings
Biophysical
■ Electrical stimulation, diathermy
■ Pulsed electromagnetic fields, pulsed radiofrequency energy
■ Low-frequency noncontact ultrasound
■ Extracorporeal shock wave therapy
Growth factors
■ Becaplermin: platelet-derived growth factor
■ Fibroblast growth factor
■ Epidermal growth factor
Autologous blood products
■ Platelet-rich plasma
■ Leukocyte, platelet, fibrin multilayered patches
■ Whole blood clot
Acellular matrix tissues
■ Xenograft dermis
– Bovine dermis
■ Xenograft acellular matrices
– Small intestine submucosa
– Porcine urinary bladder matrix
– Ovine forestomach
– Equine pericardium
– Bovine collagen
– Bilayered dermal regeneration matrix
■ Human dermis products
■ Human pericardium
■ Placental tissues
– Amniotic tissues/amniotic fluid
– Umbilical cord
Bioengineered allogeneic cellular therapies
■ Bilayered skin equivalent (human keratinocytes and fibroblasts)
■ Dermal replacement therapy (human fibroblasts)
Stem cell therapies
■ Autogenous: bone marrow–derived stem cells
■ Allogeneic: amniotic matrix with mesenchymal stem cells
Miscellaneous active dressings
■ Hyaluronic acid, honey dressings, etc.
■ Sucrose octasulfate dressing

Adapted with permission from Frykberg and Banks.[90]

Topical oxygen therapy has been studied rather vigorously in recent years, with several high-quality RCTs and at least five systematic reviews and meta-analyses all supporting its efficacy in healing chronic DFUs at 12 weeks.[19,20,30–34,91,92,101–105] Three types of topical oxygen devices are available, including continuous-delivery, low-constant-pressure, and cyclical-pressure modalities. Importantly, topical oxygen therapy devices provide for home-based therapy rather than the need for daily visits to specialized centers. Very high participation with very few reported adverse events combined with improved healing rates makes this therapy another attractive option for advanced wound care.

If DFUs fail to heal despite appropriate wound care, adjunctive advanced therapies should be instituted and are best managed in a multidisciplinary manner. Once healed, all individuals should be enrolled in a formal comprehensive prevention program focused on reducing the incidence of recurrent ulcerations and subsequent amputations.[75,106,107]

REFERENCES

1. Solomon SD, Chew E, Duh EJ, et al. Diabetic retinopathy: a position statement by the American Diabetes Association. Diabetes Care 2017;40:412–418

2. Diabetes Control and Complications Trial Research Group; Nathan DM, Genuth S, Lachin J, et al. The effect of intensive treatment of diabetes on the development and progression of longterm complications in insulin-dependent diabetes mellitus. N Engl J Med 1993;329:977–986

3. Stratton IM, Kohner EM, Aldington SJ, et al. UKPDS 50: risk factors for incidence and progression of retinopathy in type II diabetes over 6 years from diagnosis. Diabetologia 2001;44:156–163

4. Estacio RO, McFarling E, Biggerstaff S, Jeffers BW, Johnson D, Schrier RW. Overt albuminuria predicts diabetic retinopathy in Hispanics with NIDDM. Am J Kidney Dis 1998;31:947–953

5. Yau JWY, Rogers SL, Kawasaki R, et al.; Meta-Analysis for Eye Disease (META-EYE) Study Group. Global prevalence and major risk factors of diabetic retinopathy. Diabetes Care 2012;35: 556–564

6. Eid S, Sas KM, Abcouwer SF, et al. New insights into the mechanisms of diabetic complications: role of lipids and lipid metabolism. Diabetologia 2019;62:1539–1549

7. UK Prospective Diabetes Study (UKPDS) Group. Intensive blood-glucose control with sulphonylureas or insulin compared with conventional treatment and risk of complications in patients with type 2 diabetes (UKPDS 33). Lancet 1998;352:837–853

8. Chew EY, Ambrosius WT, Davis MD, et al.; ACCORD Study Group; ACCORD Eye Study Group. Effects of medical therapies on retinopathy progression in type 2 diabetes. N Engl J Med 2010;363:233–244

9. Writing Team for the DCCT/EDIC Research Group; Gubitosi-Klug RA, Sun W, Cleary PA, et al. Effects of prior intensive insulin therapy and risk factors on patient-reported visual function outcomes in the Diabetes Control and Complications Trial/Epidemiology of Diabetes Interventions and Complications (DCCT/EDIC) cohort. JAMA Ophthalmol 2016;134:137–145

10. Aiello LP, Sun W, Das A, et al.; DCCT/EDIC Research Group. Intensive diabetes therapy and ocular surgery in type 1 diabetes. N Engl J Med 2015;372:1722–1733

11. Bethel MA, Diaz R, Castellana N, Bhattacharya I, Gerstein HC, Lakshmanan MC. HbA1c change and diabetic retinopathy during GLP-1 receptor agonist cardiovascular outcome trials: a meta-analysis and meta-regression. Diabetes Care 2021;44:290–296

12. Dabelea D, Stafford JM, Mayer-Davis EJ, D'Agostino R, Dolan L, Imperatore G, et al. Association of type 1 diabetes vs type 2 diabetes diagnosed during childhood and adolescence with complications during teenage years and young adulthood. JAMA 2017;317:825–835

13. Agardh E, Tababat-Khani P. Adopting 3-year screening intervals for sight-threatening retinal vascular lesions in type 2 diabetic subjects without retinopathy. Diabetes Care 2011;34: 1318–1319

14. Nathan DM, Bebu I, Hainsworth D, et al.; DCCT/EDIC Research Group. Frequency of evidence-based screening for retinopathy in type 1 diabetes. N Engl J Med 2017;376:1507–1516

15. Silva PS, Horton MB, Clary D, et al. Identification of diabetic retinopathy and ungradable image rate with ultrawide field imaging in a national teleophthalmology program. Ophthalmology 2016; 123:1360–1367

16. Bragge P, Gruen RL, Chau M, Forbes A, Taylor HR. Screening for presence or absence of diabetic retinopathy: a meta-analysis. Arch Ophthalmol 2011;129:435–444

17. Walton OB 4th, Garoon RB, Weng CY, et al. Evaluation of automated teleretinal screening program for diabetic retinopathy. JAMA Ophthalmol 2016;134:204–209

18. Daskivich LP, Vasquez C, Martinez C Jr, Tseng CH, Mangione CM. Implementation and evaluation of a large-scale teleretinal diabetic retinopathy screening program in the Los Angeles County Department of Health Services. JAMA Intern Med 2017;177:642–649

19. Sim DA, Mitry D, Alexander P, et al. The evolution of teleophthalmology programs in the United Kingdom: beyond diabetic retinopathy screening. J Diabetes Sci Technol 2016;10: 308–317

20. Abràmoff MD, Lavin PT, Birch M, Shah N, Folk JC. Pivotal trial of an autonomous AI-based diagnostic system for detection of diabetic retinopathy in primary care offices. NPJ Digit Med 2018;1:1–8

21. Hooper P, Boucher MC, Cruess A, Dawson KG, Delpero W, Greve M, et al. Canadian Ophthalmological Society evidence-based clinical practice guidelines for the management of diabetic retinopathy. Can J Ophthalmol 2012; 47(2 Suppl):S1–S54

22. Gunderson EP, Lewis CE, Tsai AL, et al. A 20-year prospective study of childbearing and incidence of diabetes in young women, controlling for glycemia before conception: the Coronary Artery Risk Development in Young Adults (CARDIA) study. Diabetes 2007;56:2990–2996

23. Widyaputri F, Rogers SL, Kandasamy R, Shub A, Symons RCA, Lim LL. Global estimates of diabetic retinopathy prevalence and progression in pregnant women with preexisting diabetes: a systematic review and meta-analysis. JAMA Ophthalmol 2022;140:486–494

24. Diabetes Control and Complications Trial Research Group. Effect of pregnancy on micro-vascular complications in the diabetes control and complications trial. Diabetes Care 2000;23: 1084–1091

25. The Diabetic Retinopathy Study Research Group. Preliminary report on effects of photocoagulation therapy. Am J Ophthalmol 1976;81: 383–396

26. Early Treatment Diabetic Retinopathy Study research group. Photocoagulation for diabetic macular edema. Early Treatment Diabetic Retinopathy Study report number 1. Arch Ophthalmol 1985;103:1796–1806

27. Gross JG, Glassman AR, Jampol LM, et al.; Writing Committee for the Diabetic Retinopathy Clinical Research Network. Panretinal photocoagulation vs intravitreous ranibizumab for proliferative diabetic retinopathy: a randomized clinical trial. JAMA 2015;314:2137–2146

28. Sivaprasad S, Prevost AT, Vasconcelos JC, et al.; CLARITY Study Group. Clinical efficacy of intravitreal aflibercept versus panretinal photocoagulation for best corrected visual acuity in patients with proliferative diabetic retinopathy at 52 weeks (CLARITY): a multicentre, single-blinded, randomised, controlled, phase 2b, non-inferiority trial. Lancet 2017;389:2193–2203

29. Maturi RK, Glassman AR, Josic K, et al.; DRCR Retina Network. Effect of intravitreous anti-vascular endothelial growth factor vs sham treatment for prevention of vision-threatening complications of diabetic retinopathy: the Protocol W randomized clinical trial. JAMA Ophthalmol 2021;139:701–712

30. Elman MJ, Bressler NM, Qin H, et al.; Diabetic Retinopathy Clinical Research Network. Expanded 2-year follow-up of ranibizumab plus prompt or deferred laser or triamcinolone plus prompt laser for diabetic macular edema. Ophthalmology 2011;118:609–614

31. Mitchell P, Bandello F, Schmidt-Erfurth U, et al.; RESTORE study group. The RESTORE study: ranibizumab monotherapy or combined with laser versus laser monotherapy for diabetic macular edema. Ophthalmology 2011;118:615–625

32. Wells JA, Glassman AR, Ayala AR, et al.; Diabetic Retinopathy Clinical Research Network. Aflibercept, bevacizumab, or ranibizumab for diabetic macular edema. N Engl J Med 2015; 372:1193–1203

33. Baker CW, Glassman AR, Beaulieu WT, et al.; DRCR Retina Network. Effect of initial management with aflibercept vs laser photocoagulation vs observation on vision loss among patients with diabetic macular edema involving the center of the macula and good visual acuity: a randomized clinical trial. JAMA 2019;321:1880–1894

34. Chew EY, Davis MD, Danis RP, et al.; Action to Control Cardiovascular Risk in Diabetes Eye Study Research Group. The effects of medical management on the progression of diabetic retinopathy in persons with type 2 diabetes: the Action to Control Cardiovascular Risk in Diabetes (ACCORD) eye study. Ophthalmology 2014;121:2443–2451

35. Shi R, Zhao L, Wang F, et al. Effects of lipid-lowering agents on diabetic retinopathy: a Metaanalysis and systematic review. Int J Ophthalmol 2018;11:287–295

36. Ang L, Jaiswal M, Martin C, Pop-Busui R. Glucose control and diabetic neuropathy: lessons from recent large clinical trials. Curr Diab Rep 2014;14:528

37. Martin CL, Albers JW; DCCT/EDIC Research Group. Neuropathy and related findings in the diabetes control and complications trial/epidemiology of diabetes interventions and complications study. Diabetes Care 2014;37:31–38

38. Ismail-Beigi F, Craven T, Banerji MA, et al.; ACCORD trial group. Effect of intensive treatment of hyperglycaemia on microvascular outcomes in type 2 diabetes: an analysis of the ACCORD randomised trial. Lancet 2010;376:419–430

39. Bashir M, Elhadd T, Dabbous Z, et al. Optimal glycaemic and blood pressure but not lipid targets are related to a lower prevalence of diabetic microvascular complications. Diabetes Metab Syndr 2021;15:102241

40. Look AHEAD Research Group. Effects of a long-term lifestyle modification programme on peripheral neuropathy in overweight or obese adults with type 2 diabetes: the Look AHEAD study. Diabetologia 2017;60:980–988

41. Callaghan BC, Reynolds EL, Banerjee M, et al. Dietary weight loss in people with severe obesity stabilizes neuropathy and improves symptomatology. Obesity (Silver Spring) 2021;29: 2108–2118

42. Pop-Busui R, Boulton AJM, Feldman EL, et al. Diabetic neuropathy: a position statement by the American Diabetes Association. Diabetes Care 2017;40:136–154

43. Freeman R. Not all neuropathy in diabetes is of diabetic etiology: differential diagnosis of diabetic neuropathy. Curr Diab Rep 2009;9:423–431

44. Pop-Busui R, Evans GW, Gerstein HC, et al.; Action to Control Cardiovascular Risk in Diabetes Study Group. Effects of cardiac autonomic dysfunction on mortality risk in the Action to Control Cardiovascular Risk in Diabetes (ACCORD) trial. Diabetes Care 2010;33:1578–1584

45. Pop-Busui R, Cleary PA, Braffett BH, et al.; DCCT/EDIC Research Group. Association between cardiovascular autonomic neuropathy and left ventricular dysfunction: DCCT/EDIC study (Diabetes Control and Complications Trial/Epidemiology of Diabetes Interventions and Complications). J Am Coll Cardiol 2013;61:447–454

46. Smith AG, Lessard M, Reyna S, Doudova M, Singleton JR. The diagnostic utility of Sudoscan for distal symmetric peripheral neuropathy. J Diabetes Complications 2014;28: 511–516

47. Diabetes Control and Complications Trial (DCCT) Research Group. Effect of intensive diabetes treatment on nerve conduction in the Diabetes Control and Complications Trial. Ann Neurol 1995;38:869–880

48. CDC Study Group. The effect of intensive diabetes therapy on measures of autonomic nervous system function in the Diabetes Control and Complications Trial (DCCT). Diabetologia 1998; 41:416–423

49. Albers JW, Herman WH, Pop-Busui R, et al.; Diabetes Control and Complications Trial/Epidemiology of Diabetes Interventions and Complications Research Group. Effect of prior intensive insulin treatment during the Diabetes Control and Complications Trial (DCCT) on peripheral neuropathy in type 1 diabetes during the Epidemiology of Diabetes Interventions and Complications (EDIC) study. Diabetes Care 2010; 33:1090–1096

50. Pop-Busui R, Low PA, Waberski BH, et al.; DCCT/EDIC Research Group. Effects of prior intensive insulin therapy on cardiac autonomic nervous system function in type 1 diabetes mellitus: the Diabetes Control and Complications Trial/Epidemiology of Diabetes Interventions and Complications study (DCCT/EDIC). Circulation 2009;119:2886–2893

51. Callaghan BC, Little AA, Feldman EL, Hughes RAC. Enhanced glucose control for preventing and treating diabetic neuropathy. Cochrane Database Syst Rev 2012;6:CD007543

52. Pop-Busui R, Lu J, Brooks MM, et al.; BARI 2D Study Group. Impact of glycemic control strategies on the progression of diabetic peripheral neuropathy in the Bypass Angioplasty Revascularization Investigation 2 Diabetes (BARI 2D) cohort. Diabetes Care 2013;36:3208–3215

53. Tang Y, Shah H, Bueno Junior CR, et al. Intensive risk factor management and cardiovascular autonomic neuropathy in type 2 diabetes: the ACCORD trial. Diabetes Care 2021;44:164–173

54. Callaghan BC, Xia R, Banerjee M, et al.; Health ABC Study. Metabolic syndrome components are associated with symptomatic polyneuropathy independent of glycemic status. Diabetes Care 2016;39:801–807

55. Andersen ST, Witte DR, Dalsgaard EM, et al. Risk factors for incident diabetic polyneuropathy in a cohort with screen-detected type 2 diabetes followed for 13 years: ADDITION-Denmark. Diabetes Care 2018;41:1068–1075

56. Afshinnia F, Reynolds EL, Rajendiran TM, et al. Serum lipidomic determinants of human diabetic neuropathy in type 2 diabetes. Ann Clin Transl Neurol 2022;9:1392–1404

57. Lu Y, Xing P, Cai X, et al. Prevalence and risk factors for diabetic peripheral neuropathy in type 2 diabetic patients from 14 countries: estimates of the INTERPRET-DD study. Front Public Health 2020;8:534372

58. Sadosky A, Schaefer C, Mann R, et al. Burden of illness associated with painful diabetic peripheral neuropathy among adults seeking treatment in the US: results from a retrospective chart review and cross-sectional survey. Diabetes Metab Syndr Obes 2013;6:79–92

59. Waldfogel JM, Nesbit SA, Dy SM, et al. Pharmacotherapy for diabetic peripheral neuropathy pain and quality of life: a systematic review. Neurology 2017;88:1958–1967

60. Price R, Smith D, Franklin G, et al. Oral and topical treatment of painful diabetic polyneuropathy: practice guideline update summary: report of the AAN Guideline Subcommittee. Neurology 2022;98:31–43

61. Pop-Busui R, Ang L, Boulton AJM, et al. Diagnosis and Treatment of Painful Diabetic Peripheral Neuropathy. Arlington, VA, American Diabetes Association, 2022

62. Tesfaye S, Sloan G, Petrie J, et al.; OPTION-DM trial group. Comparison of amitriptyline supplemented with pregabalin, pregabalin supplemented with amitriptyline, and duloxetine supplemented with pregabalin for the treatment of diabetic peripheral neuropathic pain (OPTION-DM): a multicentre, double-blind, randomised crossover trial. Lancet 2022;400: 680–690

63. Dworkin RH, Jensen MP, Gammaitoni AR, Olaleye DO, Galer BS. Symptom profiles differ in patients with neuropathic versus non-neuropathic pain. J Pain 2007;8:118–126

64. Briasoulis A, Silver A, Yano Y, Bakris GL. Orthostatic hypotension associated with baro-receptor dysfunction: treatment approaches. J Clin Hypertens (Greenwich) 2014;16:141–148

65. Figueroa JJ, Basford JR, Low PA. Preventing and treating orthostatic hypotension: as easy as A, B, C. Cleve Clin J Med 2010;77:298–306

66. Jordan J, Fanciulli A, Tank J, et al. Management of supine hypertension in patients with neurogenic orthostatic hypotension: scientific statement of the American Autonomic Society, European Federation of Autonomic Societies, and the European Society of Hypertension. J Hypertens 2019;37:1541–1546

67. Camilleri M, Parkman HP, Shafi MA, Abell TL; American College of Gastroenterology. Clinical guideline: management of gastroparesis. Am J Gastroenterol 2013;108:18–37

68. Parrish CR, Pastors JG. Nutritional management of gastroparesis in people with diabetes. Diabetes Spectr 2007;20:231–234

69. Parkman HP, Yates KP, Hasler WL, et al.; NIDDK Gastroparesis Clinical Research Consortium. Dietary intake and nutritional deficiencies in patients with diabetic or idiopathic gastroparesis. Gastroenterology 2011;141:486–498, 498.e1–498.e7

70. Olausson EA, Störsrud S, Grundin H, Isaksson M, Attvall S, Simrén M. A small particle size diet reduces upper gastrointestinal symptoms in patients with diabetic gastroparesis: a randomized controlled trial. Am J Gastroenterol 2014;109: 375–385

71. Umpierrez GE (Ed.) Therapy for Diabetes Mellitus and Related Disorders. 6th ed. Arlington, VA, American Diabetes Association; 2014

72. Sugumar A, Singh A, Pasricha PJ. A systematic review of the efficacy of domperidone for the treatment of diabetic gastroparesis. Clin Gastroenterol Hepatol 2008;6:726–733

73. Maganti K, Onyemere K, Jones MP. Oral erythromycin and symptomatic relief of gastroparesis: a systematic review. Am J Gastroenterol 2003;98:259–263

74. McCallum RW, Snape W, Brody F, Wo J, Parkman HP, Nowak T. Gastric electrical stimulation with Enterra therapy improves symptoms from diabetic gastroparesis in a prospective study. Clin Gastroenterol Hepatol 2010;8:947–954; quiz e116

75. Boulton AJM, Armstrong DG, Albert SF, et al.; American Diabetes Association; American Association of Clinical Endocrinologists. Comprehensive foot examination and risk assessment: a report of the task force of the foot care interest group of the American Diabetes Association, with endorsement by the American Association of Clinical Endocrinologists. Diabetes Care 2008;31: 1679–1685

76. Schaper NC, van Netten JJ, Apelqvist J, Bus SA, Hinchliffe RJ; IWGDF Editorial Board. Practical guidelines on the prevention and management of diabetic foot disease (IWGDF 2019 update). Diabetes Metab Res Rev 2020;36(Suppl. 1):e3266

77. Reiber GE, Vileikyte L, Boyko EJ, et al. Causal pathways for incident lower-extremity ulcers in patients with diabetes from two settings. Diabetes Care 1999;22:157–162

78. Pham H, Armstrong DG, Harvey C, Harkless LB, Giurini JM, Veves A. Screening techniques to identify people at high risk for diabetic foot ulceration: a prospective multicenter trial. Diabetes Care 2000;23:606–611

79. Hingorani A, LaMuraglia GM, Henke P, et al. The management of diabetic foot: a clinical practice guideline by the Society for Vascular Surgery in collaboration with the American Podiatric Medical Association and the Society for Vascular Medicine. J Vasc Surg 2016;63(Suppl.): 3S–21S

80. Conte MS, Bradbury AW, Kolh P, White JV, Dick F, Fitridge R, et al. Global vascular guidelines on the management of chronic limb-threatening ischemia. Eur J Vasc Endovasc Surg 2019;58(1S): S1–S109.e33

81. American Diabetes Association. Peripheral arterial disease in people with diabetes. Diabetes Care 2003;26:3333–3341

82. Reaney M, Gladwin T, Churchill S. Information about foot care provided to people with diabetes with or without their partners: Impact on recommended foot care behavior. Appl Psychol Health Well-Being 2022;14:465–482

83. Heng ML, Kwan YH, Ilya N, et al. A collaborative approach in patient education for diabetes foot and wound care: A pragmatic randomised controlled trial. Int Wound J 2020; 17:1678–1686

84. Bus SA, Lavery LA, Monteiro-Soares M, et al.; International Working Group on the Diabetic Foot. Guidelines on the prevention of foot ulcers in persons with diabetes (IWGDF 2019 update). Diabetes Metab Res Rev 2020;36(Suppl. 1):e3269

85. Goodall RJ, Ellauzi J, Tan MKH, Onida S, Davies AH, Shalhoub J. A systematic review of the impact of foot care education on self efficacy and self care in patients with diabetes. Eur J Vasc Endovasc Surg 2020;60:282–292

86. Yuncken J, Williams CM, Stolwyk RJ, Haines TP. People with diabetes do not learn and recall their diabetes foot education: a cohort study. Endocrine 2018;62:250–258

87. Walton DV, Edmonds ME, Bates M, Vas PRJ, Petrova NL, Manu CA. People living with diabetes are unaware of their foot risk status or why they are referred to a multidisciplinary foot team. J Wound Care 2021;30:598–603

88. Bus SA, van Deursen RW, Armstrong DG, Lewis JE, Caravaggi CF; International Working Group on the Diabetic Foot. Footwear and offloading interventions to prevent and heal foot ulcers and reduce plantar pressure in patients with diabetes: a systematic review. Diabetes Metab Res Rev 2016;32(Suppl. 1):99–118

89. Rogers LC, Frykberg RG, Armstrong DG, et al. The Charcot foot in diabetes. Diabetes Care 2011; 34:2123–2129

90. Frykberg RG, Banks J. Challenges in the treatment of chronic wounds. Adv Wound Care (New Rochelle) 2015;4:560–582

91. Carter MJ, Frykberg RG, Oropallo A, Sen CK, Armstrong DG, Nair HKR, et al. Efficacy of topical wound oxygen therapy in healing chronic diabetic foot ulcers: systematic review and meta-analysis. Adv Wound Care (New

Rochelle). 21 June 2022 [Epub ahead of print]. DOI: 10.1089/wound .2022.0041

92. Frykberg RG, Franks PJ, Edmonds M, et al.; TWO2 Study Group. A multinational, multicenter, randomized, double-blinded, placebo-controlled trial to evaluate the efficacy of cyclical topical wound oxygen (TWO2) therapy in the treatment of chronic diabetic foot ulcers: the TWO2 study. Diabetes Care 2020;43:616–624

93. Boulton AJM, Armstrong DG, Löndahl M, et al. New Evidence-Based Therapies for Complex Diabetic Foot Wounds. Arlington, VA, American Diabetes Association, 2022

94. Sheehan P, Jones P, Caselli A, Giurini JM, Veves A. Percent change in wound area of diabetic foot ulcers over a 4-week period is a robust predictor of complete healing in a 12-week prospective trial. Diabetes Care 2003;26:1879–1882

95. Blume PA, Walters J, Payne W, Ayala J, Lantis J. Comparison of negative pressure wound therapy using vacuum-assisted closure with advanced moist wound therapy in the treatment of diabetic foot ulcers: a multicenter randomized controlled trial. Diabetes Care 2008;31:631–636

96. Argenta LC, Morykwas MJ, Marks MW, DeFranzo AJ, Molnar JA, David LR. Vacuum-assisted closure: state of clinic art. Plast Reconstr Surg 2006;117(Suppl.):127S–142S

97. Löndahl M, Katzman P, Nilsson A, Hammarlund C. Hyperbaric oxygen therapy facilitates healing of chronic foot ulcers in patients with diabetes. Diabetes Care 2010;33:998–1003

98. Santema KTB, Stoekenbroek RM, Koelemay MJW, et al.; DAMO2CLES Study Group. Hyperbaric oxygen therapy in the treatment of ischemic lower-extremity ulcers in patients with diabetes: results of the DAMO2CLES multicenter randomized clinical trial. Diabetes Care 2018;41:112–119

99. Fedorko L, Bowen JM, Jones W, et al. Hyperbaric oxygen therapy does not reduce indications for amputation in patients with diabetes with nonhealing ulcers of the lower limb: a prospective, double-blind, randomized controlled clinical trial. Diabetes Care 2016;39: 392–399

100. Lalieu RC, Brouwer RJ, Ubbink DT, Hoencamp R, Bol Raap R, van Hulst RA. Hyperbaric oxygen therapy for nonischemic diabetic ulcers: a systematic review. Wound Repair Regen 2020;28: 266–275

101. Niederauer MQ, Michalek JE, Liu Q, Papas KK, Lavery LA, Armstrong DG. Continuous diffusion of oxygen improves diabetic foot ulcer healing when compared with a placebo control: a randomised, double-blind, multicentre study. J Wound Care 2018;27(Suppl. 9):S30–S45

102. Serena TE, Bullock NM, Cole W, Lantis J, Li L, Moore S, et al. Topical oxygen therapy in the treatment of diabetic foot ulcers: a multicentre, open,

randomised controlled clinical trial. J Wound Care 2021;30(Suppl. 5):S7–S14

103. Sun XK, Li R, Yang XL, Yuan L. Efficacy and safety of topical oxygen therapy for diabetic foot ulcers: an updated systematic review and metaanalysis. Int Wound J. 5 May 2022 [Epub ahead of print]. DOI: 10.1111/iwj.13830

104. Frykberg RG. Topical wound oxygen therapy in the treatment of chronic diabetic foot ulcers. Medicina (Kaunas) 2021;57:917

105. Sethi A, Khambhayta Y, Vas P. Topical oxygen therapy for healing diabetic foot ulcers: a systematic review and meta-analysis of randomised control trials. Health Sci Rep 2022;3:100028

106. van Netten JJ, Price PE, Lavery LA, et al.; International Working Group on the Diabetic Foot. Prevention of foot ulcers in the at-risk patient with diabetes: a systematic review. Diabetes Metab Res Rev 2016;32(Suppl. 1):84–98

107. Frykberg RG, Vileikyte L, Boulton AJM, Armstrong DG. The at-risk diabetic foot: time to focus on prevention. Diabetes Care 2022;45: e144–e145

Chapter 20
Hypertension

CHEYENNE FRAZIER, PHARMD, BCACP

H ypertension is defined as a sustained systolic blood pressure >130 mmHg or a diastolic blood pressure > 80 mmHg and is common among patients with diabetes.[1] It is estimated that over half of U.S. patients with diabetes also have hypertension; of these patients with hypertension, less than half are achieving blood pressure goals. Hypertension is a well-established risk factor for CVD, HF, and microvascular complications. The prevalence of hypertension increases with aging as do other CVD risk factors.[2] CVD is the most prevalent cause of mortality and morbidity for patients with diabetes, and thus it is imperative to address these risk factors.[3]

Antihypertensive therapy reduces cardiovascular events, HF, and microvascular complications in patients with diabetes.[4-8] In addition to pharmacologic therapy, lifestyle modifications are an important consideration for hypertension. Effective lifestyle modifications to lower blood pressure include reducing excess body weight through caloric restriction, restricting sodium intake to less than 2,300 mg/day, increasing consumption of fruits and vegetables and low-fat dairy products, avoiding excessive alcohol consumption, smoking cessation, reducing sedentary time, and increasing physical activity levels to 150 min per week.[9-11]

Because of the high prevalence of hypertension and the availability of effective treatments to positively impact patient outcomes, it is recommended that patients' blood pressure be measured at every routine clinical visit.[12] This helps provide early diagnoses for patients and identifies patients who are not achieving blood pressure goals and who would benefit from therapy intensification. Blood pressure should be measured by a trained individual and should follow the guidelines established for the general population: measurement in the seated position, with feet on the floor and arm supported at heart level, after 5 min of rest. Cuff size should be appropriate for the upper-arm circumference. Orthostatic blood pressure measurements should be checked on initial visit and as indicated. Patients with "white coat hypertension" experience feelings of anxiety in medical environments, which causes a higher reading than the patient's normal reading when blood pressure is measured in a medical setting. Patients with "masked hypertension" have normal blood pressure when they are in medical settings but elevated blood pressure readings outside of medical settings. Home blood pressure self-monitoring and 24 h ambulatory blood pressure monitoring may provide evidence of white coat hypertension, masked hypertension, or other discrepancies between office and "true" blood pressure.[12] In addition to confirming or refuting a diagnosis of hypertension, home blood pressure assessment may be useful to monitor antihypertensive treatment. Moreover, home blood pressures may improve patient medication adherence and thus help reduce cardiovascular risk.[13]

GOALS OF TREATMENT

There is robust evidence that treatment of hypertension reduces macrovascular and microvascular complications.[4-8,14,15] In recent years, there has been debate on the optimal blood pressure goals for patients, with different clinical guidelines recommending slightly different goals. Currently the American Diabetes Association, the American College of Cardiology, and the International Society of Hypertension have reached consensus of recommending a blood pressure goal of less than 130/80 mmHg for people with diabetes, if it can be attained safely.[1,12,16] While there is no randomized controlled trial specifically demonstrating decreased incidence of cardiovascular events in people with diabetes by targeting a goal <130/80mm Hg, this goal has been derived from collective evidence of several randomized controlled trials.[17-20] Absolute benefit from blood pressure reduction correlates with baseline cardiovascular risk, indicating patients with high cardiovascular risk would most greatly benefit from intensive blood pressure control.[12,17] Hypertension treatment should be individualized and should not be targeted to <120/80 mmHg due to association of adverse effects.[1]

OVERVIEW OF MEDICATIONS AND RATIONALE FOR USE

Antihypertensive medications do not cure high blood pressure; they reduce blood pressure only when taken and must be taken indefinitely to keep blood pressure at goal if no significant lifestyle modifications to reduce blood pressure are adopted. Many antihypertensive classes and medications are available; however, only a few have been shown to have clinical benefits, and some have significant adverse effects. It is recommended that the initial antihypertensive medication be from a drug class that has demonstrated reduction in cardiovascular events in patients with diabetes. These classes are *1)* ACE inhibitors,[21,22] *2)* ARBs,[21,22] *3)* thiazide-like diuretics,[23] or *4)* dihydropyridine calcium channel blockers.[24] The general recommendations for initial therapy should be re-evaluated in patients with medical conditions in whom specific agents might offer benefits independent of blood pressure control.

There are certain patient characteristics that make ACE inhibitors or ARBs optimal therapy, and other factors that make ACE inhibitors and ARBs a less favorable prospect. For patients with albuminuria (urine albumin-to-creatinine ratio >30 mg/g), initial treatment should include an ACE inhibitor or ARB in order to reduce the risk of progressive kidney disease.[12] However, in the absence of albuminuria, risk of progressive kidney disease is low, and ACE inhibitors and ARBs have not been found to provide superior cardioprotection when compared to thiazide-like diuretics or dihydropyridine calcium channel blockers.[25] ACE inhibitors or ARBs are also first line in patients who have HF or have had an ST-segment elevation myocardial infarction (STEMI).[11] ACE inhibitors and ARBs are teratogenic and should be avoided in pregnancy. ACE inhibitors and ARBs are not recommended as initial monotherapy in black patients because they have shown inferior efficacy in major cardiovascular outcomes compared to calcium channel blockers.[26–29] If patients experience a cough with an ACE inhibitor, they can be switched to an ARB, as ARBs have much lower incidence of cough than ACE inhibitors.[30] ACE inhibitors and ARBs should be avoided in combination except in rare circumstances.

Previously, β-blockers were also considered appropriate initial antihypertensive therapy, but they are no longer preferred unless there are specific comorbidities.[11,12,31] Compared to other antihypertensive medications in the primary treatment of hypertension, β-blockers may be associated with inferior protection against stroke risk.[31–33] β-Blockers may be used for the rate-control treatment in atrial fibrillation, prior MI, active angina, or HF, but have not been shown to reduce mortality as blood pressure-lowering agents in the absence of these conditions.[5] Therefore, β-blockers should not be recommended for antihypertensive therapy unless there is a compelling indication.

There is some evidence that there may be a benefit of evening versus morning dosing of antihypertensive medications with regard to blood pressure control and reduction of cardiovascular outcomes.[34,35] The mechanism underlying this benefit is not well understood. Switching to bedtime dosing can also be a beneficial way to reduce symptoms of hypotension, but should be recommended cautiously in patients who routinely have to get up at night to urinate because of risk of syncope and falls.[12]

Resistant hypertension is defined as blood pressure >130/80 mmHg despite a therapeutic strategy that includes appropriate lifestyle management plus a diuretic and two other antihypertensive drugs belonging to different classes at adequate doses.[1] Prior to diagnosing resistant hypertension, a number of other conditions should be excluded, including medication nonadherence, white coat hypertension, and secondary hypertension. Mineralocorticoid receptor antagonists are effective for management of resistant hypertension in patients with T2D when added to existing treatment with an ACE inhibitor or ARB, thiazide-like diuretic, and dihydropyridine calcium channel blocker.[36] Mineralocorticoid receptor antagonists also reduce albuminuria and reduce the risk of morbidity and mortality in some patients who have HF with reduced ejection fraction.[1,37,38]

An important side effect to monitor for antihypertensive medications is orthostatic hypotension. The definition of orthostatic hypotension is a decrease in systolic blood pressure of 20 mmHg or a decrease in diastolic blood pressure of 10 mmHg within 3 min of standing when compared with blood pressure from the sitting or supine position.[39] Orthostatic hypotension can be caused by volume depletion or diabetic autonomic neuropathy, and can be further exacerbated by antihypertensive medications.[40] Orthostatic hypotension is common in people with T2D and hypertension and is associated with an increased risk of mortality and HF.[37] It is important to re-evaluate blood pressure goals when new information about patients' risks for events or side effects arises.

Table 20.1—Medication Overview by Class

Medication class	Medication	Mechanism of action	Adverse effects	Considerations
Thiazide and Thiazide-type Diuretic	▪ Chlorthalidone ▪ Hydrochlorothiazide	▪ Increases excretion of sodium and chloride in equal amounts at the distal renal tubule of the kidney nephron	▪ Phototoxicity ▪ Hyponatremia ▪ Hypercalcemia ▪ Hypokalemia ▪ Hypophosphatemia ▪ Hypomagnesemia ▪ Hyperuricemia ▪ Male sexual dysfunction	▪ Chlorthalidone may be preferred over hydrochlorothiazide as it has shown a superior reduction in cardiovascular events[38] ▪ Monitor serum electrolytes and creatinine within the first 1–2 weeks of therapy ▪ Can exacerbate gout by increasing serum uric acid
Calcium Channel Blockers, Dihydropyridine	▪ Amlodipine ▪ Felodipine	▪ Lowers blood pressure by causing a direct vasodilation in the peripheral arteries of the vascular smooth muscle; also blocks the influx of calcium ions into cardiac and vascular smooth muscles	▪ Peripheral edema ▪ Dizziness ▪ Flushing ▪ Headache ▪ Nausea ▪ Fatigue ▪ Palpitations	▪ Peripheral edema is dose dependent, and dose reduction may resolve edema ▪ Also indicated for angina and Raynaud's phenomenon ▪ Significant drug-drug interactions with clopidogrel, simvastatin, cyclosporine and tacrolimus
Calcium Channel Blockers, Non-dihydropyridine	▪ Diltiazem SR ▪ Verapamil SR	▪ Blocks calcium ion influx during depolarization of cardiac and vascular smooth muscle; decreases peripheral vascular resistance and causes relaxation of the vascular smooth muscle, resulting in a decrease of both systolic and diastolic blood pressure	▪ Bradyarrhythmia ▪ Peripheral edema ▪ Dizziness ▪ Headache ▪ Fatigue ▪ Constipation ▪ Heart failure	▪ Avoid with β-blockers due to risk of bradycardia or heart block ▪ Both are CYP3A4 liver enzyme substrates and also a moderate CYP3A4 inhibitor; therefore they have many drug-drug interactions

(continued)

Table 20.1 (continued)

Medication class	Medication	Mechanism of action	Adverse effects	Considerations
ACE Inhibitor	■ Enalapril ■ Lisinopril ■ Ramipril	■ ACE inhibition prevents the conversion of angiotensin I to angiotensin II, which is a potent vasoconstrictor; decreased angiotensin II leads to decreased vasopressor activity and decreased aldosterone secretion	■ Angioedema ■ Cough ■ Syncope ■ Dizziness ■ Headache ■ Hyperkalemia ■ Renal impairment	■ Because of constriction of the efferent renal arteriole, increase in serum creatinine within a week of initiation is frequently observed; if serum creatinine stabilizes, it is appropriate to continue the ACE inhibitor ■ Monitor serum potassium and creatinine within the first 1–2 weeks of therapy ■ Dose titration can occur every 1–2 weeks ■ Teratogenic
ARB	■ Candesartan ■ Olmesartan ■ Losartan	■ Blocks the vasoconstrictor effects of angiotensin II by selectively blocking the binding of angiotensin II to the angiotensin II receptor type 1 in vascular smooth muscle, which decreases vasoconstriction, synthesis and release of aldosterone, and renal absorption of sodium	■ Angioedema ■ Dizziness ■ Renal impairment ■ Upper respiratory tract infections	■ Because of constriction of the efferent renal arteriole, increase in serum creatinine within a week of initiation is frequently observed; if serum creatinine stabilizes, it is appropriate to continue the ARB ■ Monitor serum potassium and creatinine within the first 1–2 weeks of therapy ■ Losartan increases urine excretion of uric acid and can be beneficial for patients with gout ■ Dose titration can occur every 1–2 weeks ■ Teratogenic
Aldosterone Antagonist	■ Spironolactone ■ Eplerenone	■ Inhibits the effect of aldosterone by competing for the aldosterone–dependent sodium–potassium exchange site in the distal tubule cells; this increases the secretion of water and sodium, while decreasing the excretion of potassium	■ Hyperkalemia ■ ED* ■ Irregular menses* ■ Gynecomastia* *Eplerenone does not cause gynecomastia or menses disruption, and causes less ED	■ Drug of choice for resistant hypertension ■ Monitor serum potassium and creatinine within the first 1–2 weeks of therapy ■ 4 weeks to full effect and between dose titrations

(continued)

Table 20.1 (continued)

Medication class	Medication	Mechanism of action	Adverse effects	Considerations
β-adrenergic Blockers— β-1-selective/ Cardioselective	■ Atenolol ■ Bisoprolol ■ Metoprolol ■ Nebivolol	■ Blocks the binding of epinephrine and norepinephrine, decreases contractility of cardiac muscles, reduces cardiac output, suppresses renin production	■ Bradyarrhythmia ■ Pruritus ■ Dyspnea ■ Dizziness ■ Fatigue ■ Depression ■ Diarrhea ■ ED ■ Hyperglycemia	■ β-2 adrenergic receptors are responsible for respiratory dilation ■ Avoid nonselective β-adrenergic blockers in patients with reactive airway disease β-1-selective adrenergic blockers preferred for reactive airway disease ■ α-1 and nonselective β-blockers may be more effective at blood pressure control because they reduce cardiac contractility and cause peripheral vasodilation ■ Mask symptoms of hypoglycemia—patient may only experience sweating ■ Taper off to avoid rebound tachycardia
β-adrenergic Blockers— β-Nonselective	■ Nadolol ■ Propranolol	■ Blocks the binding of epinephrine and norepinephrine, decreases contractility of cardiac muscles, reduces cardiac output, suppresses renin production		
β-Blockers—α-1 and Nonselective β-Blockers	■ Carvedilol ■ Labetalol	■ Blocks the binding of epinephrine and norepinephrine, decreases contractility of cardiac muscles, reduces cardiac output, suppresses renin production ■ The α-1 adrenergic blocking activity blunts the pressor effect of phenylephrine, causes vasodilation, and reduces peripheral vascular resistance		
Loop Diuretics	■ Bumetanide ■ Furosemide ■ Torsemide	■ Inhibits the reabsorption of sodium and chloride in the ascending limb of the loop of Henle causing an increase in urine output, reducing plasma and extracellular fluid volume; cardiac output also decreases. Eventually, cardiac output returns to normal with an accompanying decrease in peripheral resistance.	■ Hyperuricemia ■ Hypomagnesemia ■ Hypochloremia ■ Hypokalemia	■ Beneficial in patients with edema or symptomatic congestive heart failure ■ More potent diuretic effect than thiazide in patients with eGFR <30 mL/min

(continued)

Table 20.1 (continued)

Medication class	Medication	Mechanism of action	Adverse effects	Considerations
Direct Vasodilators	■ Hydralazine	■ Decreases blood pressure by exhibiting a peripheral-vaso-dilating effect through a direct relaxation of vascular smooth muscle; also indirectly increases renin secretion, ultimately leading to sodium reabsorption, as a response to reflex sympathetic discharge	■ Palpitations ■ Tachycardia ■ Edema ■ Angina ■ Headache	■ Short half-life, dosed four times a day, difficult for patients to adhere to regimen
Centrally Acting α-2 Adrenergic Agonist	■ Clonidine	■ Stimulates α-2 adrenergic receptors in the brain, resulting in reduced sympathetic outflow from the CNS and decreased peripheral resistance, renal vascular resistance, heart rate, and blood pressure	■ Somnolence ■ Xerostomia ■ Fatigue ■ Orthostatic hypotension	■ When discontinuing therapy, gradually decrease the dose over 2–4 days to reduce the risk of withdrawal symptoms and rebound hypertension ■ Avoid alcohol and other CNS depressants ■ Available as an oral tablet and a transdermal patch applied once weekly
Diuretics—Potassium Sparing	■ Triamterene ■ Amiloride	■ Inhibits the reabsorption of sodium in exchange for potassium and hydrogen ions by exerting a direct effect on the distal renal tubule	■ Hypercalcemia ■ Hyperuricemia ■ Orthostatic hypotension	■ Minimally effective as monotherapy; can be used in combination with thiazide-type diuretic to overcome hypokalemia
■ α-1 Adrenergic Antagonists	■ Doxazosin ■ Terazosin	■ Directly relaxes vascular smooth muscle and causes vasodilation by inhibiting α-1 adrenergic receptors	■ Orthostatic hypotension ■ Palpitations ■ Asthenia ■ Dizziness ■ Headache ■ Lethargy ■ Somnolence ■ First dose effect of somnolence or hypotension	■ Not recommended for monotherapy because increased risk of heart failure[39] ■ Initiate at low doses at bedtime to reduce orthostatic hypotension ■ Taper off medication slowly to avoid rebound hypertension ■ Also indicated for benign prostatic hypertrophy

A BRIEF OVERVIEW OF EACH CLASS OF MEDICATION

See Table 20.1.

A BRIEF OVERVIEW OF COMBINATION THERAPY

Most patients will require multiple antihypertensive medications to achieve goal blood pressure.[40] When initiating therapy, how far patients are above their goal blood pressure should be considered. If patients have blood pressure between 130/80 mmHg and 159/99 mmHg, pharmacologic therapy can be initiated with a single medication. For patients with blood pressure ≥160/100 mmHg, it is recommended to start with two antihypertensive medications.[1] Other patients may achieve goal blood pressure with monotherapy initially, but with aging, the elasticity of vessels reduces as does the body's ability to process sodium, which leads to increasing blood pressure. Therefore, patients may need to add on additional antihypertensive therapy as they age. There is consensus that the amount of blood pressure reduction is the major determinant in reduction of cardiovascular risk in patients with hypertension, not the choice of antihypertensive drug (assuming that the patient does not have an indication for a particular drug).[45-48] When selecting how to optimize hypertensive medications, it may be advantageous to add an agent rather than titrating to the maximum dose of an agent. Using maximum doses of blood pressure medications generally produces a lesser blood pressure response and more toxicity than adding an additional blood pressure medication at a low dose.[49-51] Although many patients will require multiple blood pressure medications, fixed-dose combination preparations may improve patient adherence and blood pressure control.[52,53]

There are many blood pressure medications with different mechanisms of action that can be taken together; however, there are some combinations to avoid or to be cautious of using. Multiple diuretics are efficacious for hypertension, but combinations have the additive risk of combined dehydration, hypovolemia, hypoperfusion, and renal injury. Patients should maintain adequate hydration, and their renal function should be monitored if combination diuretics are used. Mineralocorticoid receptor antagonists are recommended for patients with resistant hypertension who are already taking three or more medications, but may increase the risk of hyperkalemia when combined with an ACE inhibitor or ARB, emphasizing the importance of regular monitoring of serum creatinine and potassium in these patients.[1] ACE inhibitors and ARBs should not routinely be combined. The dual blockade of the renin-angiotensin-aldosterone system, which may increase the risk of adverse events such as hyperkalemia, hypotension, and renal failure, argues against the use of this combination.[54] With the exception of combining ACE inhibitors and ARBs, all other combinations of first-line medication classes (i.e., thiazide-like diuretics, calcium channel blockers, ACE inhibitors, and ARBs) are considered safe.

Table 20.2—Doses and Dose Adjustments for the Most Prominent Antihypertensives

Class	Medication	Dose	Dose adjustment
ACE Inhibitors	Benazepril	10–40 mg once daily or in 2 divided doses	■ eGFR <30 mL/min/1.73 m²: initial dose is 5 mg daily
	Enalapril	5–40 mg once daily or in 2 divided doses	■ CrCl <30 mL/min: initial dose is 2.5 mg daily
	Fosinopril	10–80 mg once daily or in 2 divided doses	
	Lisinopril	10–40 mg once daily or in 2 divided doses	■ CrCl 10–30 mL/min: initial dose is 5 mg daily ■ CrCl <10 mL/min or hemodialysis: initial dose is 2.5 mg daily ■ Combination with diuretic: initial dose is 5 mg daily
	Quinapril	10–80 mg once daily or in 2 divided doses	■ Combination with diuretic: initial dose is 5 mg daily ■ Renal impairment: – CrCl 30–60 mL/min: initial dose is 5 mg daily – CrCl 10–30 mL/min: initial dose is 2.5 mg daily
	Ramipril	2.5–20 mg once daily or in 2 divided doses	■ CrCl <60 mL/min: initial dose is 1.25 mg once daily, max dose is 5 mg daily
ARBs	Irbesartan	150–300 mg once daily	■ Volume- or salt-depleted (e.g., vigorous diuretic therapy, hemodialysis): initial dose is 75 mg orally once daily
	Losartan	50–100 mg once daily	■ Renal impairment in volume-depleted patients: initiate at 25 mg daily; depending on blood pressure response, a 25-mg dose given twice daily may be needed ■ Hepatic impairment (mild to moderate): initial dose 25 mg orally once daily ■ Intravascular depletion: initiate at 25 mg orally once daily
	Olmesartan	20–40 mg once daily	
	Telmisartan	20–80 mg once daily	
	Valsartan	40–320 mg once daily	
Thiazide and Thiazide-Type Diuretics	Chlorthalidone	12.5–100 mg once daily	■ Anuria: use is contraindicated
	Hydrochlorothiazide	12.5–50 mg once daily or in 2 divided doses	■ Anuria: use is contraindicated ■ Geriatric: initial doses, 12.5–25 mg, with slower titration than with younger patients

(continued)

Table 20.2 (continued)

Class	Medication	Dose	Dose adjustment
Calcium Channel Blockers—Nondihydropyridine	Diltiazem	120–540 mg once daily	■ Geriatric: initiate at low end of dosing range
	Verapamil	Immediate release: 80–120 mg three times daily Sustained release: 180–480 mg once daily	■ Hepatic impairment (severe): Use 30% of dose given to patients with normal hepatic function ■ Low-weight patients: 40 mg orally three times daily for immediate-release tablets, 120 mg once daily for sustained release
Calcium Channel Blockers—Dihydropyridine	Amlodipine	2.5–10 mg once daily	
	Felodipine	2.5–10 mg once daily	

Aldosterone Antagonist	Spironolactone	50–200 mg once daily or in divided doses	■ Renal impairment:
			  – eGFR ≥50 mL/min/1.73 m²: initial dose is 12.5–25 mg once a day; maintenance dose, may increase to 25 mg once or twice a day after 4 weeks
			  – eGFR 30–49 mL/min 1.73 m²: initial dose is 12.5 mg orally once daily or every other day; maintenance dose, may increase to 12.5–25 mg once a day after 4 weeks

	Eplerenone	50 mg once daily	■ CrCl ≤50 mL/min: contraindicated ■ Concomitant moderate CYP3A inhibitor (e.g., erythromycin, saquinavir, verapamil, fluconazole): initial dose is 25 mg orally once daily; may increase to a maximum of 25 mg twice daily if blood pressure response is inadequate
β-Blockers	Bisoprolol	2.5–20 mg once daily	■ Liver disease: initial dose is 2.5 mg once daily, maximum dose is 10 mg once daily ■ Renal impairment: initial dose is 2.5 mg once daily, maximum dose is 10 mg once daily
	Nebivolol	5–40 mg once daily	■ Liver disease (moderate): initial dose is 2.5 mg daily, titrate dose cautiously ■ Renal impairment (CrCl <30 mL/min): initial dose is 2.5 mg per day, titrate dose cautiously
	Carvedilol	6.25–25 mg twice daily	■ Hepatic impairment (severe): use is contraindicated ■ Hepatic impairment (liver cirrhosis): initial dosage, consider reduction of approximately 20%
	Labetalol	100–800 mg twice daily	■ Hepatic impairment: average required dose is 50% of usual dosing ■ Geriatric: maximum dose is 200 mg b.i.d.
Loop Diuretics	Furosemide	40 mg twice daily	■ Concomitant medication: reduce dosage of other antihypertensive agents by at least 50% when furosemide is added to a regimen, further reduction in dosage or discontinuation of other agents may be necessary

DIURETIC COMBINATIONS

- HCTZ/Spironolactone: 25 mg/25 mg
- HCTZ/Triamterene: 25 mg/37.5 mg, 25 mg/50 mg, 50 mg/75 mg

ACE INHIBITORS AND DIURETICS

- Benazepril/HCTZ: 5 mg/6.25 mg, 10 mg/12.5 mg, 20 mg/12.5 mg, 20 mg/25 mg
- Enalapril/HCTZ: 5 mg/12.5 mg, 10 mg/25 mg
- Lisinopril/HCTZ: 10 mg/12.5 mg, 20 mg/12.5 mg, 20 mg/25 mg

ARBs AND DIURETICS

- Losartan/HCTZ: 50 mg/12.5 mg, 100 mg/12.5 mg, 100 mg/25 mg
- Valsartan/HCTZ: 80 mg/12.5 mg, 160 mg/12.5 mg, 320 mg/12.5 mg, 160 mg/25 mg, 320 mg/25 mg

CALCIUM CHANNEL BLOCKERS AND ACE INHIBITORS

- Amlodipine/Benazepril: 2.5 mg/10 mg, 5 mg/10 mg, 5 mg/20 mg, 5 mg/40 mg, 10 mg/20 mg, 10 mg/40 mg

MONOGRAPHS (COMBINATION PRODUCTS EXCLUDED)

ACE INHIBITORS

Benazepril (Lotensin): https://dailymed.nlm.nih.gov/dailymed/drugInfo.cfm?setid=60f0fb82-d870-4f07-82af-e4aeb79ed023

Enalapril (Vasotec): https://dailymed.nlm.nih.gov/dailymed/drugInfo.cfm?setid=ac0289a6-9533-4f8c-b46c-506dce1b90b5

Lisinopril (Prinivil, Zestril): https://dailymed.nlm.nih.gov/dailymed/drugInfo.cfm?setid=27ccb2f4-abf8-4825-9b05-0bb367b4ac07

Ramipril (Altace): https://dailymed.nlm.nih.gov/dailymed/drugInfo.cfm?setid=8b59207a-ea5c-4697-a8b6-94c3015a00de

ARBs

Losartan (Cozaar): https://dailymed.nlm.nih.gov/dailymed/drugInfo.
cfm?setid=5ac32c20-169d-475a-fc8a-934f758d6ab0

Olmesartan (Benicar): https://dailymed.nlm.nih.gov/dailymed/drugInfo.
cfm?setid=d5658d8a-f8e9-454d-89a9-34884e753001

DIURETICS

Chlorthalidone (Thalitone): https://dailymed.nlm.nih.gov/dailymed/drugInfo.
cfm?setid=193c85ba-43c2-4be2-82cf-7b394a83390e

Furosemide (Lasix): https://dailymed.nlm.nih.gov/dailymed/drugInfo.
cfm?setid=a15d7845-5827-481d-ba3f-e4883489a5ef

Hydrochlorothiazide (Microzide): https://dailymed.nlm.nih.gov/dailymed/drugInfo.cfm?setid=7b38ac8a-4540-4eb2-aedd-9aa966d22190

Spironolactone (Aldactone): https://dailymed.nlm.nih.gov/dailymed/drugInfo.
cfm?setid=8a96e2c9-049a-43ab-abf3-21baedeb736f

CALCIUM CHANNEL BLOCKERS

Amlodipine (Norvasc): https://dailymed.nlm.nih.gov/dailymed/drugInfo.
cfm?setid=b52e2905-f906-4c46-bb24-2c7754c5d75b

Diltiazem (Cardizem): https://dailymed.nlm.nih.gov/dailymed/drugInfo.
cfm?setid=5e39be50-ea17-4077-a2dc-668267049f6a

Verapamil (Calan, Isoptin): https://dailymed.nlm.nih.gov/dailymed/drugInfo.
cfm?setid=0742cf97-601b-4c13-a6c3-1a6a616ed292

β-BLOCKERS

Carvedilol (Coreg): https://dailymed.nlm.nih.gov/dailymed/drugInfo.
cfm?setid=7d485d38-5d43-4a54-bc63-82734035c66a

REFERENCES

1. ElSayed NA, Aleppo G, Aroda VR, et al., American Diabetes Association. Standards of Care in Diabetes—2023. *Diabetes Care* 2023;46(Suppl. 1): S158–S190

2. Keenan NL, Rosendorf KA; Centers for Disease Control and Prevention. Prevalence of hypertension and controlled hypertension—United States 2005–2008. *Morbidity and Mortality Weekly Report (MMWR)* Suppl.

2011;60(1):94–97. Available from www.cdc.gov/mmwr/preview/mmwrhtml/su6001a21.htm

3. Matheus AS, Tannus LR, Cobas RA, et al. Impact of diabetes on cardiovascular disease: an update. *Int J Hypertens* 2013:653789

4. Emdin CA, Rahimi K, Neal B, et al. Blood pressure lowering in type 2 diabetes: a systematic review and meta-analysis. *JAMA* 2015;313(6):603–615

5. Ettehad D, Emdin CA, Kiran A, et al. Blood pressure lowering for prevention of cardiovascular disease and death: a systematic review and meta-analysis. *Lancet* 2016;387:957–967

6. Brunström M, Carlberg B. Effect of antihypertensive treatment at different blood pressure levels in patients with diabetes mellitus: systematic review and meta-analyses. *BMJ* 2016;352:i717

7. Bangalore S, Kumar S, Lobach I, Messerli FH. Blood pressure targets in subjects with type 2 diabetes mellitus/impaired fasting glucose: observations from traditional and Bayesian random-effects meta-analyses of randomized trials. *Circulation* 2011;123:2799–2810

8. Thomopoulos C, Parati G, Zanchetti A. Effects of blood-pressure-lowering treatment on outcome incidence in hypertension: 10—Should blood pressure management differ in hypertensive patients with and without diabetes mellitus? Overview and meta-analyses of randomized trials. *J Hypertens* 2017;35:922–944

9. Sacks FM, Svetkey LP, Vollmer WM, et al.; DASH-Sodium Collaborative Research Group. Effects on blood pressure of reduced dietary sodium and the Dietary Approaches to Stop Hypertension (DASH) diet. *N Engl J Med* 2001;344:3–10

10. Young DR, Hivert MF, Alhassan S, et al.; Endorsed by the Obesity Society; Physical Activity Committee of the Council on Lifestyle and Cardiometabolic Health; Council on Clinical Cardiology; Council on Epidemiology and Prevention; Council on Functional Genomics and Translational Biology; and Stroke Council. Sedentary behavior and cardiovascular morbidity and mortality: a science advisory from the American Heart Association. *Circulation* 2016;134:e262–e279

11. James PA, Oparil S, Carter BL, et al. 2014 evidence-based guideline for the management of high blood pressure in adults: report from the panel members appointed to the Eighth Joint National Committee (JNC 8). *JAMA* 2014;311:507–520

12. de Boer IH, Bangalore S, Benetos A, et al. Diabetes and hypertension: a position statement by the American Diabetes Association. *Diabetes Care* 2017;40:1273–1284

13. Omboni S, Gazzola T, Carabelli G, Parati G. Clinical usefulness and cost effectiveness of home blood pressure telemonitoring: meta-analysis of ran-

domized controlled studies. *J Hypertens* 2013;31:455–467; discussion 467–468

14. Arguedas JA, Leiva V, Wright JM. Blood pressure targets for hypertension in people with diabetes mellitus. *Cochrane Database Syst Rev* 2013;10:CD008277

15. Xie X, Atkins E, Lv J, et al. Effects of intensive blood pressure lowering on cardiovascular and renal outcomes: updated systematic review and meta-analysis. *Lancet* 2016;387:435–443

16. Unger T, Borghi C, Charchar F, et al. 2020 International Society of Hyperten-sion Global Hypertension Practice Guidelines. *Hypertension* 2020; 75:1334–1357

17. Wright JT Jr, Williamson JD, Whelton PK, et al.; SPRINT Research Group. A ran-domized trial of intensive versus standard blood-pressure control. *N Engl J Med* 2015;373:2103–2116

18. Zhang W, Zhang S, Deng Y, et al.; STEP Study Group. Trial of intensive blood-pressure control in older patients with hypertension. *N Engl J Med* 2021;385:1268–1279

19. Cushman WC, Evans GW, Byington RP, et al.; ACCORD Study Group. Effects of intensive bloodpressure control in type 2 diabetes mellitus. *N Engl J Med* 2010;362:1575–1585

20. Patel A, MacMahon S, Chalmers J, et al.; ADVANCE Collaborative Group. Effects of a fixed combination of perindopril and indapamide on macrovascular and microvascular outcomes in patients with type 2 diabetes mellitus (the ADVANCE trial): a randomised controlled trial. *Lancet* 2007;370:829–840STEP

21. Catalá-López F, Macías Saint-Gerons D, González-Bermejo D, et al. Cardiovascular and renal outcomes of renin-angiotensin system blockade in adult patients with diabetes mellitus: a systematic review with network meta-analyses. *PLoS Med* 2016;13:e1001971

22. Palmer SC, Mavridis D, Navarese E, et al. Comparative efficacy and safety of blood pressure-lowering agents in adults with diabetes and kidney disease: a network meta-analysis. *Lancet* 2015;385:2047–2056

23. Barzilay JI, Davis BR, Bettencourt J, et al.; ALLHAT Collaborative Research Group. Cardiovascular outcomes using doxazosin vs. chlorthalidone for the treatment of hypertension in older adults with and without glucose disorders: a report from the ALLHAT study. *J Clin Hypertens* (Greenwich) 2004;6:116–125

24. Weber MA, Bakris GL, Jamerson K, et al.; ACCOMPLISH Investigators. Cardiovascular events during differing hypertension therapies in patients with diabetes. *J Am Coll Cardiol* 2010;56:77–85

25. Bangalore S, Fakheri R, Toklu B, Messerli FH. Diabetes mellitus as a compelling indication for use of renin angiotensin system blockers: systematic review and meta-analysis of randomized trials. *BMJ* 2016;352:i438

26. Flack JM, Sica DA, Bakris G, et al.; International Society on Hypertension in Blacks. Management of high blood pressure in Blacks: an update of the International Society on Hypertension in Blacks consensus statement. *Hypertension* 2010;56(5):780–800

27. Julius S, Alderman MH, Beevers G, et al. Cardiovascular risk reduction in hypertensive black patients with left ventricular hypertrophy: the LIFE study. *J Am Coll Cardiol* 2004;43(6):1047–1055

28. ALLHAT Officers and Coordinators for the ALLHAT Collaborative Research Group. Major outcomes in high-risk hypertensive patients randomized to angiotensin-converting enzyme inhibitor or calcium channel blocker vs diuretic: the Antihypertensive and Lipid-Lowering Treatment to Prevent Heart Attack Trial (ALLHAT). *JAMA* 2002;288:2981–2997

29. Wright JT Jr., Dunn JK, Cutler JA, et al. Outcomes in hypertensive black and nonblack patients treated with chlorthalidone, amlodipine, and lisinopril. *JAMA* 2005;293:1595–1608

30. ONTARGET Investigators, Yusuf S, Teo KK, Pogue J, et al. Telmisartan, ramipril, or both in patients at high risk for vascular events. *N Engl J Med* 2008;358(15):1547–1559

31. Medical Research Council trial of treatment of hypertension in older adults: principal results. MRC Working Party. *BMJ* 1992;304(6824):405–412

32. Lindholm LH, Carlberg B, Samuelsson O. Should beta blockers remain first choice in the treatment of primary hypertension? A meta-analysis. *Lancet* 2005;366(9496):1545–1553

33. Wiysonge CS, Bradley HA, Volmink J, et al. Beta-blockers for hypertension. *Cochrane Database Syst Rev* 2012;11:CD002003

34. Zhao P, Xu P, Wan C, Wang Z. Evening versus morning dosing regimen drug therapy for hypertension. *Cochrane Database Syst Rev* 2011;(10):CD004184

35. Hermida RC, Ayala DE, Mojón A, Fernández JR. Influence of time of day of blood pressure-lowering treatment on cardiovascular risk in hypertensive patients with type 2 diabetes. *Diabetes Care* 2011;34:1270–1276

36. Zoungas S, de Galan BE, Ninomiya T, et al.; ADVANCE Collaborative Group. Combined effects of routine blood pressure lowering and intensive glucose control on macrovascular and microvascular outcomes in patients with type 2 diabetes: new results from the ADVANCE trial. *Diabetes Care* 2009;32:2068–2074

37. Margolis KL, O'Connor PJ, Morgan TM, et al. Outcomes of combined cardiovascular risk factor management strategies in type 2 diabetes: the ACCORD randomized trial. *Diabetes Care* 2014;37:1721–1728

38. Patel A, MacMahon S, Chalmers J, et al.; ADVANCE Collaborative Group. Effects of a fixed combination of perindopril and indapamide on macrovascular and microvascular outcomes in patients with type 2 diabetes mellitus (the ADVANCE trial): a randomised controlled trial. *Lancet* 2007;370: 829–840

39. Freeman R, Wieling W, Axelrod FB, et al. Consensus statement on the definition of orthostatic hypotension, neurally mediated syncope and the postural tachycardia syndrome. *Auton Neurosci* 2011;161:46–48

40. Pop-Busui R, Boulton AJM, Feldman EL, et al. Diabetic neuropathy: a position statement by the American Diabetes Association. *Diabetes Care* 2017;40:136–154

41. Fleg JL, Evans GW, Margolis KL, et al. Orthostatic hypotension in the ACCORD (Action to Control Cardiovascular Risk in Diabetes) blood pressure trial: prevalence, incidence, and prognostic significance. *Hypertension* 2016;68:888–895

42. Dorsch MP, Gillespie BW, Erickson SR, et al. Chlorthalidone reduces cardiovascular events compared with hydrochlorothiazide: a retrospective cohort analysis. *Hypertension* 2011;57(4):689–694

43. ALLHAT Collaborative Research Group. Major cardiovascular events in hypertensive patients randomized to doxazosin vs chlorthalidone: the antihypertensive and lipid-lowering treatment to prevent heart attack trial (ALLHAT) [erratum, *JAMA* 2000;283(23):2976]. *JAMA* 2000;283(15):1967–1975

44. Mancia G. Effects of intensive blood pressure control in the management of patients with type 2 diabetes mellitus in the Action to Control Cardiovascular Risk in Diabetes (ACCORD) trial. *Circulation* 2010;122(8):847–849

45. Bakris GL, Weir MR; Study of Hypertension and the Efficacy of Lotrel in Diabetes (SHIELD) Investigators. Achieving goal blood pressure in patients with type 2 diabetes: conventional versus fixed-dose combination approaches. *J Clin Hypertens* (Greenwich) 2003;5:202–209

46. Law MR, Morris JK, Wald NJ. Use of blood pressure lowering drugs in the prevention of cardiovascular disease: meta-analysis of 147 randomised trials in the context of expectations from prospective epidemiological studies. *BMJ* 2009;338:b1665

47. Rosendorff C, Black HR, Cannon CP, et al. Treatment of hypertension in the prevention and management of ischemic heart disease: a scientific statement from the American Heart Association Council for High Blood Pres-

sure Research and the Councils on Clinical Cardiology and Epidemiology and Prevention. *Circulation* 2007;115:2761–2788

48. Mancia G, Fagard R, Narkiewicz K, et al. 2013 ESH/ESC guidelines for the management of arterial hypertension: the task force for the management of arterial hypertension of the European Society of Hypertension (ESH) and of the European Society of Cardiology (ESC). *J Hypertens* 2013;31:1281–1357

49. Materson BJ, Reda DJ, Cushman WC, et al. Single-drug therapy for hypertension in men. A comparison of six antihypertensive agents with placebo. The Department of Veterans Affairs Cooperative Study Group on Antihypertensive Agents [erratum, *N Engl J Med* 1994;330(23):1689]. *N Engl J Med* 1993;328(13):914–921

50. Epstein M, Bakris G. Newer approaches to antihypertensive therapy. Use of fixed-dose combination therapy. *Arch Intern Med* 1996;156(17):1969–1978

51. Bakris GL. Maximizing cardiorenal benefit in the management of hypertension: achieve blood pressure goals. *J Clin Hypertens* (Greenwich) 1999;1(2):141–147

52. Brixner DI, Jackson KC 2nd, Sheng X, et al. Assessment of adherence, persistence, and costs among valsartan and hydrochlorothiazide retrospective cohorts in free- and fixed-dose combinations. *Curr Med Res Opin* 2008;24(9):2597–2607

53. Bangalore S, Kamalakkannan G, Parkar S, Messerli FH. FixeΔ350

54. d-dose combinations improve medication compliance: a meta-analysis. *Am J Med* 2007;120(8):713–719

55. Lotensin (oral tablets) [product information], 2014; Micardis (oral tablets) [product information], 2014

Chapter 21
Lipids

Cheyenne Frazier, PharmD, BCACP

rteriosclerosis is a thickening, hardening, and loss of elasticity of the walls of the arteries. Atherosclerosis is a specific type of arteriosclerosis, but the terms are sometimes used interchangeably. Atherosclerosis refers to when the buildup of fats, cholesterol, and other substances in and on the artery walls leads to narrowing of the vessel lumen and restricts blood flow. Abnormalities of plasma lipoproteins result in a predisposition to ASCVD.[1] ASCVD is defined as ACS, MI, angina, coronary or other arterial revascularization, stroke, transient ischemic attack, or PAD. Premature coronary arteriosclerosis is the most common and significant consequence of dyslipidemia. Patients with T2D have an increased prevalence of lipid abnormalities, contributing to their high risk of ASCVD.[2] Treatments for patients who are at risk but who have not yet experienced their first cardiovascular or cerebrovascular event are termed primary prevention, whereas those for patients who already have manifestations of vascular disease are termed secondary prevention.

Lipids are essential substrates for cell membrane formation and hormone synthesis, and provide a source of free fatty acids for cellular functions. Cholesterol, triglycerides, and phospholipids are the major lipids in the body and are known as lipoproteins. The three major classes of lipoproteins are low-density lipoproteins (LDL), high-density lipoproteins (HDL), and very-low-density lipoproteins (VLDL). HDL transports excess cholesterol from peripheral tissue (called reverse cholesterol transport) to the liver and has been shown to be cardioprotective for the occurrence of ASCVD.[3] Although HDL is beneficial, LDL is a major contributor to ASCVD. Atherosclerotic lesions are thought to arise from transport and retention of plasma LDL cholesterol in the epithelial cell wall. Once in the artery, LDL undergoes oxidation, which leads to decreased LDL-receptor expression and increased levels of coagulation promoters and vasoactive substances, with a reduction in vasodilator and antiplatelets. This results in massive accumulation of cholesterol on the arterial walls. An imbalance between plaque synthesis and degradation can lead to a weakened plaque prone to rupture. LDL is catabolized through interaction with cell surface receptors on liver, adrenal, and smooth muscle cells. Increased intracellular cholesterol resulting from LDL catabolism inhibits the activity of 3-hydroxy-3-methylglutaryl coenzyme A reductase (HMG-CoA reductase), the rate-limiting enzyme for intracellular cholesterol biosynthesis. Increased intracellular cholesterol also causes reduced synthesis of LDL receptors, which limits subsequent cholesterol uptake from the plasma.[1] Triglycerides are also an important component of lipids, as hypertriglyceridemia has been associated with increased ASCVD independent of other lipid abnormalities, and high levels of triglycerides also increase the risk of developing acute pancreatitis.[4] Obesity and insulin resistance are common causes of a high triglycerides, thus hypertriglyceridemia is common in patients with T2D.[2]

Lifestyle modification focusing on weight loss (if indicated); reducing intake of saturated fat, trans fat, and cholesterol; increasing intake of dietary n-3 fatty acids, viscous fiber, and plant sterols; and increasing physical activity should be recommended to improve the lipid profile, specifically HDL, in patients with diabetes. Glycemic control may also beneficially modify plasma lipid levels, particularly in patients with very high triglycerides and poor glycemic control. Abstinence from alcohol may also reduce triglycerides.[2]

GOALS OF TREATMENT

The goal of treatment for most patients with diabetes is to maintain adherence to statin therapy long term to reduce the risk of ASCVD. The intensity of statin therapy, as well as the addition of other medications, is based on a patient's ASCVD risk. For patients without a history of ASCVD, it is recommended to target an LDL of <70mg/dL. For patients with established ASCVD, the recommended LDL target is <55mg/dL.[2] Patients with elevated triglycerides may also benefit from medication therapy, not to reduce ASCVD, but instead to reduce the risk of pancreatitis. It is preferred for fasting triglycerides to be lower than 175 mg/dL, and pharmacotherapy should be considered if triglycerides are above 500 mg/dL.[2]

OVERVIEW OF MEDICATIONS AND RATIONALE FOR USE

Statins are the cornerstone for ASCVD reduction for patients with diabetes. Multiple clinical trials have demonstrated the beneficial effects of statin therapy on ASCVD outcomes in patients with and without preexisting heart disease.[7,8] Specific trials in patients with diabetes showed significant primary and secondary prevention of ASCVD events and death from cardiovascular causes in patients with diabetes.[9,10] Meta-analyses, including data from over 18,000 patients with diabetes from trials of statin therapy, demonstrate clinically significant reduction in all-cause mortality and vascular mortality.[11] Accordingly, statins are the drugs of choice for LDL cholesterol lowering and cardioprotection, and the only class recommended as initial therapy for ASCVD reduction.

For primary prevention, moderate-dose statin therapy is recommended for people with diabetes aged 40–75 years. For people 45–75 years of age with one or more ASCVD risk factors, it is recommended to use high-intensity statin therapy to reduce LDL by >50% of baseline and to target an LDL goal of <70 mg/dL. If patients aged 45–75 years with multiple ASCVD risk factors and LDL is >70 mg/dL on maximally tolerated statin therapy, adding ezetimibe or a PCSK9 inhibitor may be reasonable.[2] The evidence of benefit is strong for patients with diabetes aged 40–75 years, an age group well represented in statin trials. There is less evidence of statins for primary prevention in patients over 75 years; relatively few older patients with diabetes have been enrolled in primary prevention trials. However, heterogeneity by age has not been seen in the relative benefit of lipid-lowering therapy in trials that included older participants; because older age confers higher risk, the absolute benefits are actually greater.[8,12] Moderate-intensity statin therapy may be appropriate in patients with diabetes who are 75 years of age or older, and it is reasonable to continue statin therapy if patients were on it before age 75. However, the risk-benefit profile should be routinely evaluated in this population, with downward titration of dose performed as needed for tolerability.[2] In adults with diabetes mellitus who are <40 or >75 years of age, it is reasonable to evaluate the potential effects of statins on ASCVD reduction, adverse effects, and drug-drug interactions, and to consider patient preferences when deciding to initiate, continue, or intensify statin therapy.

For secondary prevention, high-intensity statin therapy is recommended for all patients with diabetes and ASCVD. This recommendation is based on the Cholesterol Treatment Trialists' Collaboration involving 26 statin trials, of which 5 compared high-intensity to moderate-intensity statins. Together, they found reductions in nonfatal cardiovascular events with more intensive therapy in patients with and without diabetes.[8,12,13] For patients with clinical ASCVD who do not achieve a 50% reduction in LDL or an LDL of less than 55 mg/dL on maximally tolerated statin therapy, the addition of ezetimibe or a PCSK9 inhibitor is recommended.[2]

Table 21.1 shows the recommended lipid-lowering strategies, and Table 21.2 shows the two statin-dosing intensities that are recommended for use in clinical practice. High-intensity statin therapy will achieve approximately 50% reduction in LDL cholesterol, and moderate-intensity statin regimens achieve 30–50% reductions in LDL cholesterol. Low-dose statin therapy is generally not recommended in patients with diabetes but is sometimes the only dose of statin that a patient can tolerate. For patients who do not tolerate the intended intensity of statin, the maximally tolerated statin dose should be used; even a less-than-daily statin dosing (i.e., once or twice a week) may be beneficial.[14] Mild myalgia and arthralgia are common side effects of statins. However, rhabdomyolysis may occur. Rhabdomyolysis is a rare but serious adverse reaction that causes muscle cells to break down as well as complications of kidney failure. If patients receiving statin therapy express they are experiencing muscle pain, tenderness, stiffness, cramping, weakness, or fatigue, a thorough history should be conducted to identify alternative causes to avoid unnecessary discontinuation of statins. If rhabdomyolysis is suspected, a serum creatinine kinase level can be drawn for diagnosis.

OVERVIEW OF COMBINATION THERAPY

Over the past few years, there have been multiple large randomized trials investigating the benefits of adding nonstatin agents to statin therapy, including two that evaluated further lowering of LDL cholesterol with ezetimibe[12] or PCSK9 inhibitors.[13] Both trials found a significant benefit in the reduction of ASCVD events that was directly related to the degree of further LDL cholesterol lowering. Approximately one-third of participants in these trials had diabetes. For patients

Table 21.1—Recommendations for Statin and Combination Treatment in Adults with Diabetes

Age	ASCVD	Recommended statin intensity^ and combination treatment*
<40 years	No	None†
	Yes	High
		■ If LDL cholesterol ≥70 mg/dL despite maximally tolerated statin dose, consider adding additional LDL-lowering therapy (such as ezetimibe or PCSK9 inhibitor)#
≥40 years	No	Moderate‡
	Yes	High
		■ If LDL cholesterol ≥70 mg/dL despite maximally tolerated statin dose, consider adding additional LDL-lowering therapy (such as ezetimibe or PCSK9 inhibitor)

*In addition to lifestyle therapy. ^For patients who do not tolerate the intended intensity of statin, the maximally tolerated statin dose should be used. †Moderate-intensity statin may be considered based on risk-benefit profile and presence of ASCVD risk factors. ASCVD risk factors include LDL cholesterol ≥100 mg/dL (2.6 mmol/L), high blood pressure, smoking, CKD, albuminuria, and family history of premature ASCVD. ‡High-intensity statin may be considered based on risk-benefit profile and presence of ASCVD risk factors. #Adults aged <40 years with prevalent ASCVD were not well represented in clinical trials of nonstatin-based LDL reduction. Before initiating combination lipid-lowering therapy, consider the potential for further ASCVD risk reduction, drug-specific adverse effects, and patient preferences.

with ASCVD who are on high-intensity (and maximally tolerated) statin therapy and have an LDL cholesterol >70 mg/dL, the addition of nonstatin LDL-lowering therapy is recommended after considering the potential for further ASCVD risk reduction, drug-specific adverse effects, and patient preference.

STATINS AND EZETIMIBE

IMPROVE-IT was a randomized controlled trial with 18,144 patients, comparing the addition of ezetimibe to simvastatin therapy versus simvastatin alone. Individuals were ≥50 years of age, had been hospitalized for ACS (not marking going forward) within 10 days of therapy initiation, and were treated for an average of 6 years. Overall, the addition of ezetimibe led to a 6.4% relative benefit and a 2% absolute reduction in major adverse cardiovascular events. The degree of benefit was directly proportional to the change in LDL cholesterol, which was 70 mg/dL in the statin group on average and 54 mg/dL in the combination group. In those with diabetes (27% of participants), the combination of moderate-intensity simvastatin (40 mg) and ezetimibe (10 mg) showed a significant reduction of major adverse cardiovascular events, with an absolute risk reduction of 5%

Table 21.2 — High-Intensity and Moderate-Intensity Statin Therapy*

High-intensity statin therapy (lowers LDL cholesterol by ≥50%)	Moderate-intensity statin therapy (lowers LDL cholesterol by 30–50%)
Atorvastatin 40–80 mg	Atorvastatin 10–20 mg
Rosuvastatin 20–40 mg	Rosuvastatin 5–10 mg
	Simvastatin 20–40 mg
	Pravastatin 40–80 mg
	Lovastatin 40 mg
	Fluvastatin XL 80 mg
	Pitavastatin 2–4 mg

*Once-daily dosing. XL, extended release.

(40% vs. 45%) and relative risk reduction of 14% (RR 0.86 [95% CI 0.78–0.94]) over moderate-intensity simvastatin (40 mg) alone.[12]

STATINS AND PCSK9 INHIBITORS

Placebo-controlled trials evaluating the addition of the PCSK9 inhibitors evolocumab and alirocumab to maximally tolerated doses of statin therapy in participants who were at high risk for ASCVD demonstrated an average reduction in LDL cholesterol ranging from 36–59%. These agents have been approved as adjunctive therapy for patients with ASCVD or familial hypercholesterolemia who are receiving maximally tolerated statin therapy but require additional lowering of LDL cholesterol.[15,16]

The effects of PCSK9 inhibition on ASCVD outcomes were investigated in the FOURIER trial, which enrolled 27,564 patients with prior ASCVD and an additional high-risk feature who were receiving their maximally tolerated statin therapy (two-thirds were on high-intensity statin) but who still had an LDL cholesterol >70 mg/dL or a non-HDL cholesterol >100 mg/dL.[17] Patients were randomized to receive subcutaneous injections of evolocumab (either 140 mg every 2 weeks or 420 mg every month based on patient preference) versus placebo. Evolocumab reduced LDL cholesterol by 59% from a median of 92–30 mg/dL in the treatment arm.

During the median follow-up of 2.2 years, the composite outcome of cardiovascular death, MI, stroke, hospitalization for angina, or revascularization occurred in 11.3% vs. 9.8% of the placebo and evolocumab groups, respectively, representing a 15% relative risk reduction (*P* = 0.001). The combined endpoint of cardiovascular death, MI, or stroke was reduced by 20%, from 7.4% to 5.9% (*P* = 0.001). Importantly, similar benefits were seen in a prespecified subgroup of patients with diabetes, comprising 11,031 patients (40% of the enrolled participants).[18]

STATINS AND SMALL INTERFERING RIBONUCLEIC ACID AGENT

Inclisiran is a first-in-class medication of antilipemic small interfering ribonucleic acid (siRNA) agents. It was approved by the FDA in December 2021 for patients with clinical ASCVD or heterozygous familial hypercholesterolemia who do not meet cholesterol goals with other lipid-lowering therapies (that is, maximally tolerated statin plus ezetimibe and/or PCSK9 inhibitors). Inclisiran is administered by subcutaneous injection 3 months after an initial dose and then every 6 months thereafter. Inclisiran should be reserved for patients who cannot use a PCSK9 inhibitor and should not be combined with a PCSK9 inhibitor since there is no evidence for additive LDL lowering.[19] Trials assessing inclisiran found it reduced LDL by around 50% from baseline to 17 months.[20] A cardiovascular outcome trial using inclisiran in people with established cardiovascular disease is currently ongoing.[21]

STATINS AND BEMPEDOIC ACID

Bempedoic acid is a novel LDL cholesterol–lowering agent approved by the FDA in February 2020 as an adjunct to diet and maximally tolerated statin therapy for the treatment of adults with heterozygous familial hypercholesterolemia or established ASCVD who require additional lowering of LDL cholesterol.

A pooled analysis suggests that bempedoic acid therapy lowers LDL cholesterol levels by about 23% compared with placebo.[22] Currently, studies are limited to showing a reduction in LDL and there are no completed trials demonstrating a cardiovascular outcomes benefit of bempedoic acid. Bempedoic acid may be considered for patients who cannot use or tolerate other evidence-based LDL cholesterol–lowering approaches, or for whom those other therapies are inadequately effective.[23]

STATINS AND OMEGA-3 FATTY ACIDS

The main lipid parameter benefit of omega-3 fatty acids is reduction in triglycerides. The Combination of Prescription Omega-3 With Simvastatin (COMBOS) study evaluated the change in lipid parameters of prescription omega-3 fatty acids when added to stable moderate-intensity statin therapy in patients with persistent hypertriglyceridemia. The addition of prescription omega-3 fatty acids reduced triglyceride levels by 29.5% ($P < 0.001$).[24] LDL was relatively unchanged in this study, while other studies of omega-3 fatty acids have shown increases in LDL of 5–10%.[25] Omega-3 fatty acids eicosapentaenoic acid (EPA) and docosahexaenoic acid (DHA) are responsible for the decrease in triglycerides. DHA-containing omega-3 fatty acids are more associated with LDL increase than EPA-only prescription omega-3 fatty acids.[26,27] Icosapent ethyl, a prescription fatty acid containing EPA only became available in the U.S. in 2012.

The Reduction of Cardiovascular Events with Icosapent Ethyl-Intervention Trial (REDUCE-IT) enrolled patients receiving statin therapy with triglycerides between 135 and 499 mg/dL, and either cardiovascular disease or diabetes plus one additional cardiovascular risk factor. Patients were randomized to either placebo or icosapent ethyl 4 g/day. There was a 25% relative risk reduction ($P < 0.001$)

for the composite end point of cardiovascular death, nonfatal MI, nonfatal stroke, coronary revascularization, or unstable angina.[28] Because of this trial, the addition of icosapent ethyl for patients with ASCVD or diabetes and another ASCVD risk factor on a statin with controlled LDL cholesterol, but elevated triglycerides (between 135 and 499 mg/dL) can be considered to reduce ASCVD risk. It is important to note that data are lacking with other n-3 fatty acid formulations and the reults of the REDUCE-IT trial should not be extrapolated to other n-3 fatty acid products.

STATINS AND FIBRATES

Fibrate-statin combinations produce significant additional decreases in triglycerides (30–50%) and increases in HDL cholesterol (10–20%) in comparison with statin monotherapy. The combination of a statin and fibrate is associated with an increased risk for abnormal transaminase levels, myositis, and rhabdomyolysis. The risk of rhabdomyolysis is more common with higher doses of statins and renal insufficiency and appears to be higher when statins are combined with gemfibrozil (compared with fenofibrate).[29] For this reason, statins are contraindicated with gemfibrozil, and statins should be dose reduced if combined with fenofibrate. In the ACCORD study, in patients with T2D who were at high risk for ASCVD, the combination of fenofibrate and simvastatin did not reduce the rate of fatal cardiovascular events, nonfatal MI, or nonfatal stroke compared with simvastatin alone. Prespecified subgroup analyses suggested heterogeneity in treatment effects, with possible benefit for men with both a triglyceride level of ≥204 mg/dL and an HDL cholesterol level of ≤34 mg/dL.[30] The combination of statin plus fibrate is generally not recommended because it has not been shown to improve ASCVD outcomes and there is increased risk of adverse effects.

STATINS AND NIACIN

In combination with statins, niacin further reduces LDL cholesterol (10–20%), non-HDL cholesterol, and triglycerides (10–30%), and increases HDL cholesterol (20–40%). The AIM-HIGH trial randomized over 3,000 patients (about one-third with diabetes) with established ASCVD, LDL cholesterol levels <180 mg/dL, low HDL cholesterol levels (men <40 mg/dL and women <50 mg/dL), and triglyceride levels of 150–400 mg/dL to statin therapy plus extended-release niacin or placebo. The trial was halted early due to lack of efficacy on the primary ASCVD outcome (first event of the composite of death from CHD, nonfatal MI, ischemic stroke, hospitalization for ACS, or symptom-driven coronary or cerebral revascularization) and a possible increase in ischemic stroke in those on combination therapy.[31]

The much larger HPS2-THRIVE trial also failed to show a benefit of adding niacin to background statin therapy.[32] A total of 25,673 patients with prior vascular disease were randomized to receive 2 g of extended-release niacin and 40 mg of laropiprant (an antagonist of the prostaglandin D2 receptor DP1 that has been shown to improve adherence to niacin therapy) versus a matching placebo daily and followed for a median follow-up period of 3.9 years. There was no significant difference in the rate of coronary death, MI, stroke, or coronary revascularization

Table 21.3—Overview of Each Class of Medication

Medication class	Medication	Mechanism of action	Adverse effects	Considerations
HMG-CoA Reductase Inhibitors (Statins)	Rosuvastatin Atorvastatin Lovastatin Pitavastatin Fluvastatin Pravastatin Simvastatin	Selectively and competitively inhibits HMG-CoA reductase, a rate-limiting enzyme in cholesterol synthesis	Myalgia Arthralgia Constipation, nausea, diarrhea Stomach pain/cramps	■ Monitor liver function and lipid panel at baseline and as clinically warranted ■ Creatinine kinase should be measured in individuals with muscle symptoms ■ Hepatic function should be measured if symptoms suggesting hepatotoxicity arise (abdominal pain, dark-colored urine, or yellowing of the skin or sclera) ■ Patients on simvastatin and lovastatin should not eat large amounts of grapefruit or drink more than 1 L/day of grapefruit juice
PCSK9 Inhibitors	Alirocumab Evolocumab	Inhibits the binding of PCSK9 to LDL receptors on hepatocytes, thus reducing degradation of the LDL receptors. Increased LDL receptors are then available to clear LDL from circulation and lower LDL levels	Neurocognitive Swelling, pain, or bruising at injection site Back pain Influenza Nasopharyngitis	■ Monitoring: LDL at baseline and within 4–8 weeks of treatment initiation or dosage increase ■ If dose is missed, take as soon as possible if there are at least 7 days before the next scheduled dose. If less than 7 days remain, skip the missed dose ■ Requires injection ■ Very high cost relative to other agents
Cholesterol Absorption Inhibitors	Ezetimibe	Reduces blood cholesterol by acting at the brush border of the small intestine to inhibit the absorption of cholesterol, leading to a decrease in the delivery of intestinal cholesterol to the liver. This reduces hepatic cholesterol stores and increases the clearance of cholesterol from the blood	Stomach pain Fatigue Myalgia Arthralgia Diarrhea	
Omega-3 Fatty Acids	Omega-3 Acid Ethyl Esters Omega-3 Carboxylic Acids Icosapent ethyl	Not fully known; may increase hepatic mitochondrial and peroxisomal β-oxidation to reduce hepatic synthesis of triglycerides or increase plasma lipoprotein lipase activity	Belching Fishy taste Indigestion	■ Can cause significant increase in LDL due to DHA component (up to 50%) ■ Icosapent ethyl is an EPA-only formulation

(continued)

Table 21.3 (continued)

Medication class	Medication	Mechanism of action	Adverse effects	Considerations
Bile Acid Sequestrants	Colesevelam Cholestyramine Colestipol	Binds to bile acids to prevent reabsorption in the intestine. Serum bile acids are depleted, which activates conversion of cholesterol into bile acids. Demand for cholesterol in liver is increased, and there is an increase in LDL receptors, which increases clearance of LDL from the blood	Constipation Bloating Indigestion Nausea Flatulence	▪ Must be taken with a meal ▪ Bile acid sequestrants can reduce absorption of medications and vitamins. Administer medications with a narrow therapeutic window (warfarin, levothyroxine) 4 h before or after administration of a bile acid sequestrant ▪ Contraindicated in patients with triglycerides >500 mg/dL
Niacin	Niacin	Not fully known; may reduce esterification of hepatic triglycerides, decrease release of free fatty acids from adipose tissue, and enhance the removal of triglycerides from plasma	Facial and neck flushing Nausea, vomiting, diarrhea Increased uric acid Increased glucose Peptic ulcers	▪ To reduce flushing, patients can take aspirin or eat a low-fat snack 30–60 min prior to administration of niacin ▪ Monitor liver function, A1C, uric acid
Fibric Acid Derivatives	Fenofibrate Gemfibrozil	Stimulates peroxisome proliferator activated receptor α (PPAR-α), which leads to 1) VLDL catabolism, 2) fatty acid oxidation, and 3) elimination of triglyceride-rich particles	Abdominal pain Gallstones Increased liver function tests Increased serum creatinine Indigestion Nausea Stomach pain	▪ Monitoring: liver function, renal function ▪ Significant reduction in triglycerides
Adenosine Triphosphate-Citrate Lyase (ACL) Inhibitor	Bempedoic Acid	Inhibition of ACL results in decreased cholesterol synthesis in the liver and lowers LDL-C in blood via upregulation of LDL receptors.	Hyperuricemia Tendon rupture Nasopharyngitis Myalgia Upper respiratory tract infection	▪ Caution in patients with gout ▪ Monitoring: serum uric acid, symptoms of hyperuricemia, symptoms of tendon rupture

(continued)

Table 21.3 (continued)

Medication class	Medication	Mechanism of action	Adverse effects	Considerations
Antilipemic Small Interfering Ribonucleic Acid (siRNA)	Inclisiran	Utilizes RNA interference mechanism and directs catalytic breakdown of mRNA for PCSK9 in hepatocytes. This increases LDL receptor recycling and expression on the hepatocyte cell surface, which increases LDL uptake and lowers LDL levels in the circulation.	Injection site reactions Arthralgia Bronchitis Antibody development	■ If a dose is missed by <3 months from the usual day of administration, administer the dose as soon as possible and then resume the original schedule. If a dose is missed by >3 months, skip the missed dose and restart with a new dosing schedule as initial dose, then again at 3 months, and then every 6 months.

HMG-CoA, 3-hydroxy-3-methylglutaryl coenzyme A reductase; VLDL, very-low-density lipoproteins.

with the addition of niacin–laropiprant versus placebo (13.2% vs. 13.7%; rate ratio 0.96; $P = 0.29$). Niacin–laropiprant was associated with an increased incidence of new onset diabetes (absolute excess, 1.3 percentage points; $P < 0.001$) and disturbances in diabetes control among those with diabetes. In addition, there was an increase in serious adverse events associated with the gastrointestinal system, musculoskeletal system, skin, and, unexpectedly, infection and bleeding. Therefore, combination therapy with a statin and niacin is not recommended, given the lack of efficacy on major ASCVD outcomes and the side effects, including worsening of diabetes.

STATINS AND BILE ACID SEQUESTRANTS

In combination with moderate-intensity statins, bile acid sequestrants can reduce LDL cholesterol by an additional 10–25% and may slightly increase triglycerides and HDL.[33-35] In addition to LDL lowering, colesevelam, a second-generation bile acid sequestrant, is approved as an adjunct to antidiabetes therapy for improving glycemic control in adults with T2D. A reduction in A1C of 0.32–0.41% was observed when colesevelam was added to monotherapy or combination therapy with metformin, sulfonylureas, or insulin.[36-38] However, there are not any clinical outcomes data for bile acid sequestrants in combination with statins, which limits the support of combining them with statins for the goal of ASCVD reduction.

IMPORTANT COMBINATION PRODUCTS

- Simcor: simvastatin and niacin
- Advicor: niacin and lovastatin
- Vytorin: simvastatin and ezetimibe

MONOGRAPHS (COMBINATION PRODUCTS EXCLUDED)

HMG-CoA REDUCTASE INHIBITORS

Atorvastatin (Lipitor): https://dailymed.nlm.nih.gov/dailymed/drugInfo.cfm?setid=c6e131fe-e7df-4876-83f7-9156fc4e8228

Rosuvastatin (Crestor): https://dailymed.nlm.nih.gov/dailymed/drugInfo.cfm?setid=bb0f3b5e-4bc6-41c9-66b9-6257e2513512

Simvastatin (Zocor): https://dailymed.nlm.nih.gov/dailymed/drugInfo.cfm?setid=fdbfe194-b845-42c5-bb87-a48118bc72e7

Pitavastatin (Livalo): https://dailymed.nlm.nih.gov/dailymed/drugInfo.cfm?setid=44dcbf97-99ec-427c-ba50-207e0069d6d2

Table 21.4—Doses and Dose Adjustments for Prominent Medications in the Chapter

Medication	Dose	Dose adjustment
HMG-CoA Reductase Inhibitors		
Rosuvastatin	5–40 mg once daily	■ CrCl less than 30 mL/min: 5 mg orally once daily; maximum 10 mg orally once daily ■ Contraindicated in patients with active liver disease ■ Concomitant gemfibrozil: avoid if possible; if concomitant use is required, initiate at 5 mg orally once daily, maximum 10 mg/day ■ Rosuvastatin is a CYP3A4 substrate, and CYP3A4 inhibitors will increase the concentrations: reduce to 5–10 mg once daily ■ Asian descent: initial, consider 5 mg orally once daily
Atorvastatin	10–80 mg once daily	■ Avoid or reduce dose with CYP3A4 enzyme inhibitors ■ No adjustment needed for renal impairment or dialysis ■ Contraindicated in patients with active liver disease ■ Avoid use with gemfibrozil
Lovastatin, Immediate Release	10–80 mg once daily or in divided doses	■ Lovastatin is a CYP3A4 substrate, and CYP3A4 inhibitors will increase the concentrations: reduce dose or do not use ■ Avoid use with gemfibrozil
Lovastatin, Extended Release	20–60 mg once daily	■ Renal insufficiency: initial, 20 mg orally once daily ■ Geriatric: initial, 20 mg orally once daily in the evening at bedtime ■ Avoid use with gemfibrozil ■ Lovastatin is a CYP3A4 substrate, and CYP3A4 inhibitors will increase the concentrations: reduce dose or do not use
Pitavastatin	1–4 mg once daily	■ Renal impairment (moderate, eGFR 30–59 mL/min/1.73 m²): initial, 1 mg orally once daily; maximum 2 mg/day ■ Renal impairment (severe, eGFR 15–29 mL/min/1.73 m², not receiving hemodialysis): initial, 1 mg orally once daily; maximum 2 mg/day ■ Active liver disease (including unexplained persistent elevations of hepatic transaminases): use is contraindicated ■ Hemodialysis: initial, 1 mg orally once daily; maximum 2 mg/day ■ Avoid use with gemfibrozil
Fluvastatin, Immediate Release	20–40 mg once or twice daily	■ Fluvastatin is a CYP3A4, CYP2C8, and CYP2C9 substrate. CYP3A4, CYP2C8, and CYP2C9 inhibitors will increase the concentrations: reduce dose or do not use ■ Avoid use with gemfibrozil
Fluvastatin, Extended Release	80 mg daily	

(continued)

Table 21.4 (continued)

Medication	Dose	Dose adjustment
Pravastatin	40–80 mg daily	■ Renal impairment (severe): initial, 10 mg orally once daily ■ Hepatic impairment (active liver disease or unexplained, persistent elevations of serum transaminases): use is contraindicated ■ Pravastatin is a CYP3A4 substrate, and CYP3A4 inhibitors will increase the concentrations: dose reduction may be needed ■ Avoid use with gemfibrozil
Simvastatin	5–40 mg daily	■ Renal impairment (mild or moderate): no adjustment necessary ■ Renal impairment (severe): initial, 5 mg orally once daily ■ Simvastatin is a CYP3A4 substrate, and CYP3A4 inhibitors will increase the concentrations: reduce dose or do not use ■ Avoid use with gemfibrozil
PCSK9 Inhibitors		
Alirocumab	75–150 mg subcutaneously once every 2 weeks or 300 mg subcutaneously once every 4 weeks	■ Renal impairment (mild or moderate): no adjustment necessary ■ Hepatic impairment (mild or moderate): no adjustment necessary
Evolocumab	140 mg subcutaneously every 2 weeks or 420 mg subcutaneously monthly	■ Renal impairment (mild or moderate): no adjustment necessary ■ Hepatic impairment (mild or moderate): no adjustment necessary
Cholesterol Absorption Inhibitors		
Ezetimibe	10 mg once daily	■ Hepatic impairment (moderate to severe, Child-Pugh score 7–15): use not recommended
Fibric Acid Derivatives		
Fenofibrate	120–160 mg daily	■ Renal impairment (mild to moderate): 40–54 mg daily ■ Renal impairment (severe) or hemodialysis: contraindicated ■ Active liver disease, primary biliary cirrhosis, or unexplained persistent liver function abnormalities: contraindicated
Gemfibrozil	600 mg orally twice daily 30 min before the morning and evening meal	■ Severe renal impairment: avoid use
Colesevelam	3,750 mg orally once daily or in two divided doses	
Cholestyramine	4–24 g per day, in divided doses if over 8 g	

(continued)

Table 21.4 (continued)

Medication	Dose	Dose adjustment
Colestipol	2–16 g per day	
Niacin, Extended Release	500–2,000 mg once daily at bedtime	Hepatic impairment, active liver disease, unexplained transaminase elevations, and significant or unexplained hepatic dysfunction: contraindicated
Niacin, Immediate Release	250–6,000 mg, in divided doses if >1,500 mg per day	
Omega-3 Acid Ethyl Esters	4 g daily, may be given once daily or divided into two doses	
Bempedoic Acid	180 mg daily	

Pravastatin (Pravachol): https://dailymed.nlm.nih.gov/dailymed/drugInfo.cfm?setid=897ad8b7-921d-eb02-a61c-3419e662a2da

Fluvastatin (Lescol): https://dailymed.nlm.nih.gov/dailymed/drugInfo.cfm?setid=e38126a5-9d6a-422f-812c-a01610108162

Lovastatin (Mevacor): https://dailymed.nlm.nih.gov/dailymed/drugInfo.cfm?setid=10a557fe-6620-4b15-862a-d3ff5dece612

OMEGA-3 FATTY ACIDS

Omega-3 Acid Ethyl Esters (Lovaza): https://dailymed.nlm.nih.gov/dailymed/drugInfo.cfm?setid=5ada82f0-a5fd-46c9-aecc-f106f614c9f0

Icosapent Ethyl Capsule (Vascepa): https://dailymed.nlm.nih.gov/dailymed/drugInfo.cfm?setid=9c1a2828-1583-4414-ab22-a60480e8e508

CHOLESTEROL ABSORPTION INHIBITORS

Ezetimibe (Zetia): https://dailymed.nlm.nih.gov/dailymed/drugInfo.cfm?setid=a773b0b2-d31c-4ff4-b9e8-1eb2d3a4d62a

NIACIN

Niacin (Niaspan): https://dailymed.nlm.nih.gov/dailymed/drugInfo.cfm?setid=35433c7b-556c-49a0-bfb5-0d498359925b

FIBRIC ACID DERIVATIVES

Fenofibrate (Tricor): https://dailymed.nlm.nih.gov/dailymed/drugInfo.cfm?setid=b693e68d-f812-4993-54b6-852e3517c344

Gemfibrozil (Lopid): https://dailymed.nlm.nih.gov/dailymed/drugInfo.
cfm?setid=c48855b7-215e-453b-b3b1-a0f9dee7221f

PCSK9 INHIBITORS

Alirocumab (Praluent): https://dailymed.nlm.nih.gov/dailymed/drugInfo.
cfm?setid=446f6b5c-0dd4-44ff-9bc2-c2b41f2806b4

Evolocumab (Repatha): https://dailymed.nlm.nih.gov/dailymed/drugInfo.
cfm?setid=709338ae-ab8f-44a9-b7d5-abaabec3493a

BILE ACID SEQUESTRANTS

Cholestyramine (Questran): https://dailymed.nlm.nih.gov/dailymed/search.cfm?l
abeltype=all&query=questran&pagesize=20&page=1

Colesevelam (Welchol): https://dailymed.nlm.nih.gov/dailymed/drugInfo.
cfm?setid=4a06d3b2-7229-4398-baba-5d0a72f63821

REFERENCES

1. Talbert RL. Hyperlipidemia. In *Pharmacotherapy: A Pathophysiologic Approach*, 9th ed. DiPiro JT, Talbert RL, Yee GC, et al., Eds. New York, McGraw-Hill, 2014, p. 291–317

2. American Diabetes Association. *Standards of Care in Diabetes—2023*. *Diabetes Care* 2023;46(Suppl. 1):S158–S190

3. Rader DL. Mechanisms of disease: HDL metabolism as a target for novel therapies. *Nat Clin Pract Cardiovasc Med* 2007;4:102–109

4. McBride P. Triglycerides and risk for coronary artery disease. *Curr Atheroscler Rep* 2008;10(5):386–390

5. Jellinger PS, Handelsman Y, Rosenblit PD, et al. American Association of Clinical Endocrinologists and American College of Endocrinology guidelines for the management of dyslipidemia and prevention of cardiovascular disease. *Endocr Pract* 2017;23:1–87

6. Stone NJ, Robinson J, Lichtenstein AH, et al. 2013 ACC/AHA guideline on the treatment of blood cholesterol to reduce atherosclerotic cardiovascular risk in adults: a report of the American College of Cardiology/American Heart Association Task Force on Practice Guidelines. *Circulation* 2014; (25 Suppl. 2):S1–S45

7. Mihaylova B, Emberson J, Blackwell L, et al.; Cholesterol Treatment Trialists' (CTT) Collaborators. The effects of lowering LDL cholesterol with statin therapy in people at low risk of vascular disease: meta-analysis of individual data from 27 randomised trials. *Lancet* 2012;380:581–590

8. Baigent C, Keech A, Kearney PM, et al.; Cholesterol Treatment Trialists' (CTT) Collaborators. Efficacy and safety of cholesterol-lowering treatment: prospective meta-analysis of data from 90,056 participants in 14 randomised trials of statins. *Lancet* 2005;366:1267–1278

9. Knopp RH, d'Emden M, Smilde JG, Pocock SJ. Efficacy and safety of atorvastatin in the prevention of cardiovascular end points in subjects with type 2 diabetes: the Atorvastatin Study for Prevention of Coronary Heart Disease Endpoints in Non-Insulin-Dependent Diabetes Mellitus (ASPEN). *Diabetes Care* 2006;29:1478–1485

10. Colhoun HM, Betteridge DJ, Durrington PN, et al.; CARDS investigators. Primary prevention of cardiovascular disease with atorvastatin in type 2 diabetes in the Collaborative Atorvastatin Diabetes Study (CARDS): multicentre randomised placebo-controlled trial. *Lancet* 2004;364:685–696

11. Kearney PM, Blackwell L, Collins R, et al.; Cholesterol Treatment Trialists' (CTT) Collaborators. Efficacy of cholesterol-lowering therapy in 18,686 people with diabetes in 14 randomised trials of statins: a meta-analysis. *Lancet* 2008;371:117–125

12. Cannon CP, Blazing MA, Giugliano RP, et al.; IMPROVE-IT Investigators. Ezetimibe added to statin therapy after acute coronary syndromes. *N Engl J Med* 2015;372:2387–2397

13. Shepherd J, Barter P, Carmena R, et al. Effect of lowering LDL cholesterol substantially below currently recommended levels in patients with coronary heart disease and diabetes: the Treating to New Targets (TNT) study. *Diabetes Care* 2006;29:1220–1226

14. Meek C, Wierzbicki AS, Jewkes C, et al. Daily and intermittent rosuvastatin 5 mg therapy in statin intolerant patients: an observational study. *Curr Med Res Opin* 2012;28:371–378

15. Moriarty PM, Jacobson TA, Bruckert E, et al. Efficacy and safety of alirocumab, a monoclonal antibody to PCSK9, in statin-intolerant patients: design and rationale of ODYSSEY ALTERNATIVE, a randomized phase 3 trial. *J Clin Lipidol* 2014;8:554–561

16. Zhang X-L, Zhu Q-Q, Zhu L, et al. Safety and efficacy of anti-PCSK9 antibodies: a meta-analysis of 25 randomized, controlled trials. *BMC Med* 2015;13:123

17. Sabatine MS, Giugliano RP, Keech AC, et al.; FOURIER Steering Committee and Investigators. Evolocumab and clinical outcomes in patients with cardiovascular disease. *N Engl J Med* 2017;376:1713–1722

18. Sabatine MS, Leiter LA, Wiviott SD, et al. Cardiovascular safety and efficacy of the PCSK9 inhibitor evolocumab in patients with and without diabetes and the effect of evolocumab on glycaemia and risk of new-onset diabetes: a prespecified analysis of the FOURIER randomised controlled trial. *Lancet Diabetes Endocrinol* 2017;5(12):941–950

19. Lloyd-Jones DM, Morris PB, Ballantyne CM, et al. 2022 ACC expert consensus decision path-way on the role of nonstatin therapies for LDL-cholesterol lowering in the management of atherosclerotic cardiovascular disease risk: a report of the American College of Cardiology Solution Set Oversight Committee. *J Am Coll Cardiol* 2022;80(14):1366–1418

20. Ray KK, Wright RS, Kallend D, et al.; ORION-10 and ORION-11 Investigators. Two phase 3 tri-als of inclisiran in patients with elevated LDL cholesterol. *N Engl J Med* 2020;382:1507–1519

21. University of Oxford. A Randomized Trial Assessing the Effects of Inclisiran on Clinical Out-comes Among People With Cardiovascular Disease (ORION-4). In: ClinicalTrials.gov. Bethes-da, MD, National Library of Medicine. NLM Identifier: NCT03705234. Accessed 8 March 2023. Available from https://clinicaltrials.gov/ct2/show/ NCT03705234

22. Dai L, Zuo Y, You Q, Zeng H, Cao S. Efficacy and safety of bempedoic acid in patients with hypercholesterolemia: a systematic review and meta-analysis of randomized controlled trials. *Eur J Prev Cardiol* 2021;28:825–833

23. Di Minno A, Lupoli R, Calcaterra I, et al. Efficacy and safety of bempedoic acid in patients with hypercholesterolemia: systematic review and meta-analysis of randomized controlled trials. *J Am Heart Assoc* 2020;9:e016262

24. Davidson MH, Stein EA, Bays HE, et al.; COMBination of prescription Omega-3 with Simvastatin (COMBOS) Investigators. Efficacy and tolerability of adding prescription omega-3 fatty acids 4 g/d to simvastatin 40 mg/d in hypertriglyceridemic patients: an 8-week, randomized, double-blind, placebo-controlled study. *Clin Ther* 2007;29(7):1354–1367

25. Harris WS. N-3 fatty acids and serum lipoproteins: human studies. *Am J Clin Nutr* 1997;65:1645S–1654S

26. Mori TA, Burke V, Puddey IB, et al. Purified eicosapentaenoic and docosahexaenoic acids have differential effects on serum lipids and lipoproteins, LDL particle size, glucose, and insulin in mildly hyperlipidemic men. *Am J Clin Nutr* 2000;71:1085–1094

27. Wei MY, Jacobson TA. Effects of eicosapentaenoic acid versus docosahexaenoic acid on serum lipids: a systematic review and meta-analysis. *Curr Atheroscler Rep* 2011;13:474–483

28. Cannon CP, Blazing MA, Giugliano RP, et al.; IMPROVE-IT Investigators. Ezetimibe added to statin therapy after acute coronary syndromes. *N Engl J Med* 2015;372:2387–2397

29. Jones PH, Davidson MH. Reporting rate of rhabdomyolysis with fenofibrate + statin versus gemfibrozil + any statin. *Am J Cardiol* 2005;95:120–122

30. Ginsberg HN, Elam MB, Lovato LC, et al.; ACCORD Study Group. Effects of combination lipid therapy in type 2 diabetes mellitus. *N Engl J Med* 2010;362:1563–1574

31. Boden WE, Probstfield JL, Anderson T, et al.; AIM-HIGH Investigators. Niacin in patients with low HDL cholesterol levels receiving intensive statin therapy. *N Engl J Med* 2011;365:2255–2267

32. Landray MJ, Haynes R, Hopewell JC, et al.; HPS2-THRIVE Collaborative Group. Effects of extended-release niacin with laropiprant in high-risk patients. *N Engl J Med* 2014;371:203–212

33. Davidson MH, Toth P, Weiss S, et al. Low-dose combination therapy with colesevelam hydrochloride and lovastatin effectively decreases low-density lipoprotein cholesterol in patients with primary hypercholesterolemia. *Clin Cardiol* 2001;24(6):467–474

34. Hunninghake D, Insull W Jr., Toth P, et al. Coadministration of colesevelam hydrochloride with atorvastatin lowers LDL cholesterol additively. *Atherosclerosis* 2001;158(2):407–416

35. Knapp HH, Schrott H, Ma P, et al. Efficacy and safety of combination simvastatin and colesevelam in patients with primary hypercholesterolemia. *Am J Med* 2001;110(5):352–360

36. Bays HE, Goldberg RB, Truitt KE, Jones MR. Colesevelam hydrochloride therapy in patients with type 2 diabetes mellitus treated with metformin: glucose and lipid effects. *Arch Intern Med* 2008;168:1975–1983

37. Fonseca VA, Rosenstock J, Wang AC, et al. Colesevelam HCl improves glycemic control and reduces LDL cholesterol in patients with inadequately controlled type 2 diabetes on sulfonylurea-based therapy. *Diabetes Care* 2008;31:1479–1484

38. Goldberg RB, Fonseca VA, Truitt KE, Jones MR. Efficacy and safety of colesevelam in patients with type 2 diabetes mellitus and inadequate glycemic control receiving insulin-based therapy. *Arch Intern Med* 2008;168: 1531–1540

Chapter 22
Antiplatelets

Megan Willson, PharmD, BCPS
Kimberly C. McKeirnan, PharmD, BCACP

INTRODUCTION

Platelets play an integral role in homeostasis and coagulation. Thrombosis occurs through the process of platelet activation, adhesion, and aggregation because of tissue injury.[1] Although platelets are critical in homeostasis with injury to prevent hemorrhage, the platelet cascade and formation of clots in CVD lead to significant morbidity and mortality. CVD comprises CHD, including acute MI; cerebrovascular disease, including stroke; PAD; and atherosclerosis. Therapy that modulates platelet activity is an important component of the treatment and prevention of these diseases.

The staggering statistics reported in the Heart Disease and Stroke Statistics 2021 Update illustrate the importance of treating heart disease. Heart disease is the second-leading cause of death in 2021 following COVID-19, with stroke the fifth-leading cause of death.[2] It is estimated that 1 in 3 deaths in the U.S. are due to CVD claimed over 928,000 lives in the U.S. during 2020. Stroke statistics are similarly frightening, with 1 in 20 deaths due to stroke; stroke remains the leading cause of long-term disability. Prevention and treatment of heart disease and stroke are important targets for improving health in the U.S. and are reflected in the American Heart Association (AHA) goals. Although rates of CVD and stroke are decreasing with lifestyle modifications and medical advancement, the prevalence remains high.[3]

CVD significantly impacts morbidity and mortality and can also cause significant economic burden. Costs include the direct costs of caring for individuals with heart disease, as well as the indirect costs of the loss of affected individuals' productivity. It is estimated that both direct and indirect costs for heart disease (including stroke) are approximately $407.3 billion annually.[3]

Risk factors for CVD include hypertension, dyslipidemia, smoking, diabetes mellitus, family history of premature CHD, obesity, CKD, and albuminuria.[4] Risk-enhancing factors specific to diabetes are a long duration of diabetes, albuminuria, eGFR <60 mL/min/1.73m^2, retinopathy, neuropathy, and ankle-bracial index <0.95. Diabetes mellitus alone is an independent risk factor for CVD.[4] Control of risk factors is extremely important to modifying long-term outcomes and risk for patients. The American Diabetes Association recommends that patients are assessed for risk yearly to guide therapy and risk-reduction strategies for CVD.[4] CVD is the leading cause of death for patients with diabetes.[4] Not only do diabetes and elevated blood glucose increase risk of events, but patients who experience cardiovascular events have worse outcomes, with more complicated hospital stays and more cardiovascular event reoccurrences.[4-6]

Atherosclerosis and thrombosis both contribute to CVD in patients with diabetes. Atherosclerosis leads to a blockage of a vessel, which then leads to platelet aggregation, activation, and adhesion. Platelet function is altered in diabetes with increased propensity toward thrombosis. Diabetes enhances platelet aggregation, adhesion, and thrombin generation. Specific changes in lipid membrane fluidity have led to hyperreactivity of platelets. Increasing production of thromboxane A2 may increase the sensitivity of platelets to stimuli. Alterations in nitric oxide production and increased expression of activation adhesion molecules glycoprotein IIb-IIIa and P-selection may also be contributing to platelet dysfunction. Other changes affecting platelet activity are alterations of intracellular calcium and magnesium levels, increased arachidonic acid metabolism, decreased prostacyclin production, and decreased antioxidant levels.[5]

This chapter will discuss the following antiplatelet therapies commonly used today: aspirin, prasugrel, clopidogrel, ticagrelor, dipyridamole/aspirin, cilostazol, and vorapaxar. Many trials have been conducted for primary and secondary prevention of cardiovascular events. The data from some of the trials will be summarized here. Many of the trials had high subsets of patients with diabetes mellitus.

GOALS OF THERAPY

Table 22.1—Goals of Therapy

- Reduce morbidity and mortality from CVD
- Prevent primary and secondary occurrence of CVD events including stroke, MI, and heart failure
- Control risk factors to decrease risk of diabetes-related complications
    - Glycemic control
    - Blood pressure management
    - Lipid management
    - Utilization of agents with cardiovascular and kidney benefit
    - Lifestyle modification and diabetes education
- Reduce risk of bleeding and other adverse effects of antiplatelet therapy
- Reduce symptoms of atherosclerotic disease
    - Chest pain or angina
    - Leg pain
    - Numbness

Source: American Diabetes Association.[4]

ASPIRIN

Aspirin reduces platelet aggregation by irreversibly inhibiting prostaglandin cyclooxygenase-1 (COX-1).[8] Aspirin has greater potency for inhibiting platelet aggregation than any other salicylic acid derivative.[8] Aspirin is indicated to reduce the risk of death and nonfatal stroke for patients who have had an ischemic stroke or transient ischemia of the brain; to reduce the risk of vascular mortality in patients with a suspected acute MI; to reduce the risk of death or nonfatal MI in patients with a previous MI or unstable angina pectoris; to reduce the risk of MI and death in patients with chronic stable angina pectoris; and specifically in patients who have undergone revascularization procedures or for patients who had a preexisting indication for aspirin.[8]

The recommend aspirin dosing as shown in Table 22.2.

Table 22.2—Aspirin Dosing

Indication	Dose
Acute Coronary Syndrome	75–100 mg once daily[26]
Initial	162–325 once at time of diagnosis[18]
Maintenance	75–100 mg once daily[26]
Diabetes—Primary prevention with increased cardiovascular risk. Secondary prevention of ASCVD.	75–162 mg daily[4]
Ischemic Stroke and Transient Ischemic Attack	
Initial	160–325 mg at time of diagnosis and then daily for 21–90 days[32,36]
Maintenance	81–325 mg daily[32]
Peripheral atherosclerotic disease	75–100 mg once daily[38]
Post-CABG—Secondary prevention	75–81 mg once daily beginning preoperatively; continue indefinitely following surgery[26]
Stable ischemic heart disease	75–100 mg once daily[9]

Aspirin is available in a multitude of doses and combination products. Doses should be administered with a full glass of water to minimize gastrointestinal distress. Aspirin is not recommended for patients under the age of 12 years due to the risk for Reye's syndrome.[9] The manufacturer also warns against stomach bleeding as an important side effect.[9] The risk of stomach bleeding is increased in patients who are over 60 years of age, take aspirin at a higher dose or for longer than recommended, take additional blood-thinning medications or corticosteroids, drink three or more alcoholic beverages per day, have a history of stomach ulcers or bleeding problems, or take prescription or nonprescription NSAIDs.[9]

PRASUGREL

Prasugrel, a thienopyridine, inhibits platelet activation and aggregation by irreversibly binding to the $P2Y_{12}$ class of adenosine diphosphate (ADP) receptors on platelets. This medication is indicated for use in patients with unstable angina or non-ST-elevated myocardial infarction (NSTEMI) and patients with STEMI when managing with percutaneous coronary intervention (PCI).[10]

Doses are available as a 5-mg tablet and a 10-mg tablet.[10] Initial dosing should begin with a single 60-mg oral loading dose on day 1, followed by a 10-mg dose thereafter administered orally once a day, with or without food. Patients taking prasugrel should also take 75–325 mg of aspirin daily. After receiving a 60-mg loading dose, 90% of patients achieved 50% inhibition of platelet aggregation within 1 h.[10] Average steady-state platelet aggregation inhibition was approximately 70% and occurred after 3–5 days of receiving a 10-mg daily dose following the single 60-mg loading dose. The elimination half-life is approximately 7 h. Patients weighing less than 60 kg have increased levels following a 10-mg dose. A maintenance dose of 5 mg for patients weighing less than 60 kg can be considered; however, prospective studies have not been done with this dose.[10] Also consider 5-mg daily dose for patients of East Asian descent after 30 days of maintenance therapy.[11]

Prasugrel carries a boxed warning of increased bleeding risk and is contraindicated for patients who have an active pathological bleed (i.e. peptic ulcer, intracranial hemorrhage), those who have had a prior transient ischemic attack or stroke, and those allergic to any component of the product. Because of the increased risk of bleeding, caution should be used in patients over the age of 75, those with an increased likelihood of bleeding such as from recent trauma or surgery, and those taking medications that may cause bleeding, such as NSAIDs or other oral anticoagulants. Although not generally recommended in patients over 75 years of age, patients with diabetes or a history of MI may still benefit from therapy.[10]

Prasugrel is converted into an active metabolite primarily by CYP3A4 and CYP2B6, although CYP2C9 and CYP2C19 are involved to a lesser extent. However, medications that potentially inhibit or induce these enzymes, such as ketoconazole and rifampin, do not appear to have a clinically significant impact on pharmacokinetics or platelet aggregation when used in combination with prasugrel. This can be beneficial for patients with a complex medication regimen.[10]

Prasugrel has no data in pregnant women to inform a drug risk assessment. Reproductive studies in rats and rabbits receiving doses up to 30 times the recommended human dose showed no evidence of fetal harm. However, prasugrel should be recommended for pregnant women only if the benefits outweigh the potential fetal risk related to risk of bleeding.

Dose adjustments are not necessary for patients with mild to moderate hepatic impairment, although severe hepatic disease has been associated with an increased bleeding risk. Prasugrel has not been studied in these patients. Renal impairment does not require dose adjustment either, but there are limited data for patients with ESRD.[10]

CLOPIDOGREL

Clopidogrel, another medication in the thienopyridine class, is indicated for patients with unstable angina (UA), NSTEMI, STEMI, and those who have suffered from a recent stroke, recent MI, or with established PAD. Contraindications for use of clopidogrel include active bleeding and hypersensitivity to components of the medication.[12]

Clopidogrel is supplied as a 75-mg tablet. An additional 300-mg tablet is also available for the loading dose. Dosing for patients with UA/NSTEMI/STEMI includes a loading dose of 300–600 mg followed by a 75-mg once-daily dose.[12] Initiate aspirin (75–325 mg once daily) and continue in combination with clopidogrel.[12] For patients with a recent MI, recent stroke, or established PAD, the dose is also 75 mg daily with or without food, but the loading dose is not recommended.[12]

Clopidogrel must be activated to an active metabolite by CYP2C19. Clopidogrel carries a boxed warning due to diminished antiplatelet effect in patients who are poor metabolizers of CYP2C19. Although a higher dosage regimen could be considered, there are not currently recommended dosing guidelines for this patient population. In cases where the patient is suspected to be a poor metabolizer, genetic testing or choosing an alternative product is recommended.[12] Because some proton pump inhibitors (PPIs), such as omeprazole, are moderate inhibitors of CYP2C19, coadministration is not recommended. An alternate PPI or different class of acid-reducing medication may be preferred.

Although clopidogrel does not have the boxed warning for bleeding that prasugrel carries, bleeding is still a concern due to the nature of this medication. Although clopidogrel has a relatively short half-life, only 6 h, the inhibitory effect on platelet aggregation exists for the lifetime of the platelet, approximately 7–10 days after exposure. For patients who are undergoing surgery, clopidogrel should be discontinued for at least 5 days prior to surgery. In an emergency, hemostasis may be restored by administering exogenous platelets, although even this may not be effective within 4 h of the 300-mg loading dose or 2 h of the 75-mg maintenance dose. Taking NSAIDs, warfarin, and aspirin with clopidogrel increases the risk of bleeding and should be given only when benefits outweigh the risk.

Clopidogrel has not demonstrated any risks for birth defects from case reports or postmarketing surveillance. Dose adjustment is not necessary for geriatric patients or those with hepatic impairment. In patients with severe (CrCl 5–15 mL/min) or moderate renal impairment (CrCl 30–60 mL/min), taking clopidogrel resulted in low inhibition of aggregation of 25%.[12] Dosing guidelines for patients with renal impairment are not provided by the manufacturer, but choosing an alternative medication in this class may be preferred. Cross-reactivity is seen with the thienopyridine class regarding hypersensitivity reactions like angioedema, rash, and hematologic reactions.[12]

TICAGRELOR

Like the other thienopyridines, ticagrelor is a $P2Y_{12}$ platelet inhibitor used to reduce the risk of cardiovascular death, MI, and stroke in patients with ACS. For the first 12 months following ACS, ticagrelor has been shown to be superior to clopidogrel.[13] Additional indications include primary prevention of MI and stroke for high-risk individuals with coronary artery disease and for secondary stroke prevention.[13] Unlike clopidogrel, ticagrelor doses exhibit low inhibition of aggregation in patients with impaired renal function. Ticagrelor dosing changes per indication: For secondary prevention after ACS, administer a 180-mg loading dose followed by a 90-mg dose twice daily for the first year after an ACS event. After the first year, the dose may be decreased to 60 mg twice daily. Dosing for primary prevention in high-risk patients is 60 mg twice daily. For secondary stroke prevention, ticagrelor is administered as a 180-mg load followed with 90 mg twice daily for 30 days. The dose of 60 mg twice daily is recommended for pateints with CAD and no prior stroke or MI. Patients taking ticagrelor should also be taking a daily aspirin dose of 75–100 mg. Aspirin loading is also suggested at a dose of 300–325 mg once, followed by standard maintenance dosing for patient with acute stroke. Ticagrelor is available in a round, 90-mg tablet and a round, 60-mg tablet. [13]

Ticagrelor is contraindicated in patients who have a history of intracranial hemorrhage, hypersensitivity to any of the medication components, or any active bleeding. Ticagrelor has two boxed warnings: one because of the risk of fatal bleeding associated with the mechanism of action of this medication, and the other to warn about the concomitant use with aspirin doses >100 mg daily. Higher aspirin doses do not have an established benefit in the ACS setting, and there is a strong suggestion from the Platelet Inhibition and Patient Outcomes (PLATO) trial that use of such doses reduces the effectiveness of ticagrelor.[13] During clinical trials, 14–21% of patients taking ticagrelor reported experiencing dyspnea, although pulmonary function tests did not detect any abnormalities. For patients who have a preexisting pulmonary condition or develop dyspnea that is problematic, an alternative thienopyridine may be preferred.[13]

CYP3A4 is the primary enzyme responsible for metabolizing ticagrelor and forming the major active metabolite. Strong inhibitors of CYP3A4, such as ketoconazole and clarithromycin, substantially increase the effects of ticagrelor and increase patient risk of experiencing an adverse bleeding event. Strong inducers of CYP3A4 have the opposite effect and reduce the potency of ticagrelor. Use with strong inducers or inhibitors is recommended to avoid. Ticagrelor may also increase serum concentrations of medications metabolized by CYP3A4, such as simvastatin and lovastatin.

Ticagrelor does not have an identified drug-associated risk of birth defects, miscarriage, or adverse outcomes during human pregnancy; however, animal studies showed structural abnormalities at maternal doses five to seven times the maximum recommended human dose. If a patient is of childbearing age, an alternative thienopyridine may be a better option. Additionally, ticagrelor does not require dose adjustment in patients with renal impairment, making it a better choice for these patients than clopidogrel. Since ticagrelor is metabolized by the liver, use should be avoided for patients with severe hepatic impairment and caution should be used in patients with moderate hepatic impairment.

DIPYRIDAMOLE/ASPIRIN

Another antiplatelet option is the combination of dipyridamole and aspirin. This combination product is used to reduce the risk of stroke for patients who have had an ischemic stroke or transient ischemia of the brain. Dipyridamole inhibits platelet aggregation by reducing the uptake of adenosine into platelets, which results in an increased concentration of local adenosine, stimulating platelet adenylate cyclase and increasing cAMP levels. Aspirin inhibits platelet aggregation by irreversibly inhibiting cyclooxygenase, inhibiting generation of thromboxane A2, and reducing induction of aggregation.[14]

This combination product is supplied as a capsule with 25 mg of aspirin and 200 mg of extended-release dipyridamole. The recommended dosing is one capsule given with or without food twice daily. Some patients report experiencing intolerable headaches when first taking this medication. If this is the case, the manufacturer recommends starting with one capsule at bedtime and a low-dose aspirin in the morning. When the headache is reduced, patients can return to the usual dose.[14]

Dipyridamole/aspirin is contraindicated for patients with an allergy to aspirin or any other component of the product. Use should be avoided in children and teenagers due to the risk of Reye's syndrome. Aspirin/dipyridamole is not recommended in pregnancy due to the teratogenic effects. Adverse serious events associated with this combination include increased bleeding risk, elevated hepatic enzymes, and hepatic failure. Hypotension and chest pain may also occur due to the vasodilatory effect. Because it contains aspirin, this medication should also be avoided in patients with renal failure (eGFR <10 mL/min/1.73 m²).[14]

There are many drug interactions to be aware of that could be concerning for patients with diabetes. The most concerning is the risk for increased potency of oral hypoglycemics. Moderate doses of aspirin may increase the effectiveness of oral medications used to lower blood glucose and may lead to hypoglycemia. Other notable drug interactions include ACE inhibitors, other anticoagulants, anticonvulsants, β-blockers, diuretics, methotrexate, and NSAIDs.[14]

CILOSTAZOL

Cilostazol has yet another mechanism of action for inhibiting platelet aggregation. Cilostazol inhibits platelet aggregation by suppressing cAMP degradation, leading to an increase in cAMP in platelets and blood vessels. This medication is indicated for reducing symptoms of intermittent claudication. The recommended dose is 100 mg twice daily. Cilostazol should be taken at least half an hour before or 2 h after breakfast and dinner. Patients should be counseled that medication may work within 2–4 weeks, but may take up to 12 weeks before the full effect is seen. Cilostazol is available as 50-mg and 100-mg tablets.[15]

Cilostazol is contraindicated for patients with HF due to the inhibition of phosphodiesterase III, a mechanism that has been shown to decrease survival in patients will class III and IV HF. Tachycardia may occur with cilostazol, so it should be used with caution for patients who have a history of heart disease. White blood cell counts and platelets should also be monitored because of the risk of agranulocytosis. Other common side effects include headache (27%), infection (14%), diarrhea (12%), abnormal stool (12%), and rhinitis (12%) at the 50 mg dose and higher rates with the 100 mg dose.[15]

Cilostazol has shown teratogenicity in rats at high doses and is pregnancy category C. No significant differences have been observed for geriatric populations, so dose adjustment with age is not necessary. Dose adjustments are also not required for patients with renal impairment or mild hepatic impairment.[15]

The effect of cilostazol is seen as early as 3 h after dosing and lasts for 12 h following a single dose. Cilostazol and the active metabolite have half-lives of 11 h and 13 h, respectively. Metabolism occurs predominantly through CYP3A4 and CYP2C19, leading to the need for a dose reduction to 50 mg twice daily when administered in combination with strong or moderate inhibitors of either CYP3A4 or CYP2C19.[15]

VORAPAXAR

Vorapaxar is another antiplatelet agent with a unique mechanism of action. It works by acting as a protease-activated receptor-1 (PAR-1) antagonist, which inhibits thrombin-induced and thrombin receptor agonist peptide–induced platelet aggregation. It is currently indicated for the reduction of thrombotic cardiovascular events in patients with a history of MI or with PAD. The dose of vorapaxar is 2.08 mg by mouth daily. It can be taken with or without food. This medication has only been studied either in combination with either aspirin or clopidogrel. Study outcomes demonstrated a reduction in composite endpoint of cardiovascular death, MI, stroke, and urgent revascularization.[16]

Vorapaxar is contraindicated in patients with a history of stroke, transient ischemic attack, or intracranial hemorrhage due to the increased risk of intracranial hemorrhage and active pathological bleeding. A major side effect is bleeding, which was significantly increased. It is recommended to avoid the use of vorapaxar with anticoagulants, such as warfarin. Currently, there is no reversal agent for vorapaxar. Other side effects that occurred included anemia, depression, rash, and diplopia or ocular motor disturbances.[16]

Vorapaxar is not considered safe during pregnancy due to increased risk of maternal bleeding. It is known to cross into the breast milk of rats and should be used with caution when breast-feeding. It is currently unknown if vorapaxar is excreted into human breast milk. There is no contraindication or dosing adjustment in the geriatric population, but bleeding risk should be evaluated prior to initiating therapy. No dosage adjustments are needed for renal dysfunction or for mild to moderate hepatic dysfunction. It is not recommended to be used in patients who have severe hepatic dysfunction due to increased risk of bleeding.[16]

Eighty percent or more of the antiplatelet effect is achieved at approximately 1 week and steady state is achieved at 21 days. The terminal half-life is 8 days, which can yield a continued antiplatelet effect of approximately 50% at 4 weeks after discontinuation of the medication. Metabolism occurs through CYP3A4 and CYP2J2. Vorapaxar should be avoided in patients who are receiving strong inducers or inhibitors of CYP3A.[16]

COMBINATION THERAPY

CORONARY HEART DISEASE AND MYOCARDIAL INFARCTION

Combination use of antiplatelet therapy has long been established for secondary prevention of MI. Currently, dual antiplatelet therapy is recommended for management of patients who received either medical management, PCI, or CABG.[17,18] The Clopidogrel in Unstable Angina to Prevent Recurrent Events (CURE) trial and Clopidogrel for the Reduction of Events During Observation (CREDO) trial established that dual antiplatelet therapy with clopidogrel and aspirin is better than aspirin for patients experiencing ACS with regard to death from cardiovascular causes, nonfatal MI, and refractory ischemia.[19] The CREDO trial demonstrated that the combination of clopidogrel and aspirin prior to elective PCI reduced death, MI, and need for urgent revascularization.[20] The TRial to assess Improvement in Therapeutic Outcomes by optimizing platelet InhibitioN with prasugrel Thrombolysis In Myocardial Infarction 38 (TRITON-TIMI 38) trial demonstrates that prasugrel for treatment of ACS with scheduled PCI is superior to clopidogrel in the reduction of the combined cardiovascular outcome of death from cardiovascular causes, nonfatal MI, and nonfatal stroke. However, patients in the prasugrel group had increased rates of bleeding. Based on post hoc analysis, prasugrel should not be used in patients aged 75 years or older, patients who weigh ≤ 60 kg, and patients who have had prior TIA or stroke, due to increased rates of bleeding.[21] Subgroup analysis was conducted to further elucidate the benefits of prasugrel versus clopidogrel. The major benefit appears to be from the reduction of MIs. Specifically, looking at the subpopulation of patients with diabetes mellitus demonstrated a significant net clinical benefit with prasugrel compared to clopidogrel (14.6% vs 19.2%, $P = 0.001$). Subgroup analysis data suggest benefits in patients with diabetes outweigh safety risks.[22] Ticagrelor was also compared to clopidogrel in patients experiencing ACS. Ticagrelor demonstrated improved rates of the composite outcome of death from vascular causes, MI, or stroke, while showing no difference in rates of major bleeding.[23]

The recommended duration of dual antiplatelet therapy is continuing to evolve with new evidence. Dual antiplatelet therapy has been studied up to 18–36 months. Prasugrel and clopidogrel combined with aspirin have demonstrated improved efficacy compared to aspirin alone but had increased rates of moderate and severe bleeding.[23] In another study, ticagrelor taken with aspirin was associated with an improved composite efficacy endpoint at 3 years compared to aspirin alone, but the combination had increased risk of major bleeding.[24] Recognition of individual patient-risk characteristics may have increased benefit with prolonged dual antiplatelet (DAPT). Patients with diabetes mellitus are recognized as a group who may benefit from extend duration of DAPT.[25] Results from a DAPT trial demonstrated reduced rates of stent thrombosis, major cardiovascular and cerebrovascular events, and myocardial infarctions; however, rates of moderate and serious bleeding were increased.[25] Current guideline recommendations are outlined in Table 22.3.[26]

Table 22.3—Duration of Dual Antiplatelet Therapy[26]

Indication	Intervention	Duration (medication)	Additional notes
Stable Ischemic Heart Disease	BMS	1 month (clopidogrel)	May be reasonable for >1 month in those with low risk of bleeding
	DES	6 months (clopidogrel)	May be reasonable for >1 month in those with low risk of bleeding
	CABG	May be reasonable for 12 months of therapy (clopidogrel)	
Recent ACS	Medical Therapy	At least 12 months (clopidogrel, ticagrelor)	Not high risk of bleeding or no significant bleeding on DAPT >12 months may be reasonable
	Lytic (STEMI)	Minimum 14 days and ideally 12 months (clopidogrel)	Not high risk of bleeding or no significant bleeding on DAPT >12 months may be reasonable
	PCI (BMS or DES)	At least 12 months (clopidogrel, prasugrel, ticagrelor)	Not high risk of bleeding or no significant bleeding on DAPT >12 months may be reasonable
	CABG	Resume DAPT to complete 1 year	

BMS, bare metal stent; CABG, coronary artery bypass graft; DAPT, dual antiplatelet therapy; DES, drug eluting stent.

Bleeding with DAPT continues to be a concern. Finding the ideal regimen to balance the risk of thrombosis and bleeding for post stent continues to evolve. The TWILIGHT trial examined the use of ticagrelor monotherapy to ticagrelor-aspirin combination therapy after 3 months of therapy with ticagrelor and aspirin. Results at 1 year showed a reduced rate of bleeding with monotherapy (4.0% vs 7.1% $P < 0.001$), with no increased risk of a composite of death from any cause, nonfatal myocardial infarction, or nonfatal stroke (at 3.9% in both groups).[27] Results from the SMART-CHOICE trial demonstrated similar outcomes after 1 month DAPT then a transition to any P2Y12 inhibitor; however, the trial was conducted in Korea, potentially decreasing its external validity.[28] STOPDAPT-2 trial demonstrated that monotherapy with clopidogrel following 1 month of DAPT was superior to DAPT for 12 months in the composite endpoint of both cardiovascular and bleeding (2.36% vs 3.70% $P = 0.04$). Again, the trial population decreases the generalizability to the U.S. population.[29] Contradictory results were found in the GLOBAL LEADERS trial. Ticagrelor monotherapy for 23 months was compared to DAPT (clopidogrel/aspirin or ticagrelor/aspirin) for 12 months, then aspirin. Both arms followed 1 month DAPT. Results showed no improve-

Table 22.4—Dose and Dose Adjustments for Commonly Used Medications

Drug	Usual dose	Dose adjustments
Aspirin	■ Prevention of MI: 81 mg p.o. daily[30] ■ Stroke prevention: 160–300 mg daily[32] ■ Acute treatment of MI: 162–325 mg chewed as soon as possible[17,18] ■ PAD: 75–325 mg p.o. daily[38]	■ Must use doses <100 mg daily in combination with ticagrelor[20]
Prasugrel[10]	■ ACS: 60-mg loading dose followed by 10 mg once daily	■ Consider reducing dose to 5 mg daily in patients who weigh less than 60 kg ■ Use in combination with aspirin
Clopidogrel[12]	■ ACS: 300-mg load followed by 75 mg daily ■ Recent MI, stroke, or PAD: 75 mg daily	■ Avoid use with CYP2C19 inhibitors
Ticagrelor[13]	■ ACS: 180-mg loading dose followed by 90 mg twice daily for the first year. After 1 year of therapy, lower dose to 60 mg twice daily	■ Use in combination with aspirin at doses <100 mg daily
Aspirin/Dipyridamole[14]	■ Stroke and TIA: 1 (25-mg/200-mg) capsule twice daily with or without food	■ For intolerable headaches, consider reducing dose to bedtime and aspirin 81 mg daily in the morning
Cilostazol[15]	■ Intermittent claudication: 100 mg twice daily	■ Reduce dose to 50 mg twice daily when used in combination with CYP2C19 inhibitors and strong or moderate CYP3A4 inhibitors
Vorapaxar[16]	■ Prevention of cardiovascular events in patients with history of MI or PAD: 2.08 mg once daily	■ Avoid with inducers or inhibitors of CYP3A

ment in bleeding events or difference in all-cause mortality or myocardial infarction.[30]

The THEMIS further increases evidence for DAPT. The trial included patients with stable coronary artery disease and T2D at high risk of CV events for primary prevention. The results demonstrated ticagrelor given in combination with aspirin had a reduced incidence of ischemic CV events (7.7% vs 8.5%; $P = 0.04$), but had a higher rate of bleeding (2.2% vs 1.0%; $P < 0.001$) compared to aspirin alone.[31]

STROKE

Dual antiplatelet therapy is not as well defined in stroke prevention as it is in prevention of MI. Current stroke guidelines recommend use of dual antiplatelet therapy (clopidogrel and aspirin) for 21 days for minor strokes or TIAs.[32] This recommendation is based on the Clopidogrel in High-risk patients with Acute Nondisabling Cerebrovascular Events (CHANCE) trial, which demonstrated a reduction in ischemic stroke with no increase in hemorrhagic strokes at 90 days.[33] The trial was conducted in China, potentially limiting the external validity of the trial.[34] The Platelet-Oriented Inhibition in New TIA and minor ischemic stroke (POINT) trial demonstrated similar results in an expanded population. Ischemic stroke was significantly reduced when clopidogrel was added to aspirin for a total of 90 days in patients with minor stroke or TIA when initiated within 12 h of stroke symptom onset. However, major hemorrhage was increased in the dual antiplatelet therapy arm. Approximately 25% of patients in both trial arms had diabetes.[35] The THALES trial compared ticagrelor (180 mg load followed by 90 mg twice daily) plus aspirin (300–325 mg load followed by 75–100 mg daily) to aspirin for minor stroke or TIA for 30 days. Results demonstrated a reduction in the primary composite outcome (stroke or death) and ischemic stroke in the ticagrelor/aspirin group.[36] Currently, dual antiplatelet therapy is limited to minor stroke and TIA for a short duration (21 days) after the event. Data are unavailable to support dual antiplatelet therapy for moderate and severe stroke. For intercranial large artery atherosclerosis, dual aspirin and clopidogrel are recommended for 90 days.[32] Triple antiplatelet therapy (aspirin, clopidogrel, and dipyridamole) for stroke prevention is not recommended.[37]

PERIPHERAL ARTERIAL DISEASE

Aspirin, clopidogrel, ticagrelor, and cilostazol alone are all effective in treating PAD. Limited data are available looking at dual antiplatelet therapy for treatment of PAD comparing mono to dual antiplatelet therapy.[38] A recent meta-analysis reviewed dual antiplatelet therapy compared to mono antiplatelet therapy after lower limb revascularization procedures in symptomatic PAD. Ten trials were included in the analysis. Conclusions of the meta-analysis found lower rates of all-cause mortality, major adverse limb effects and amputation in dual antiplatelet therapy group. While no difference was seen in the major bleeding, dual antiplatelet therapy group had a significantly increase rate of minor bleeding. The authors stated more data is still needed.[39]

MONOGRAPHS

Aspirin: https://dailymed.nlm.nih.gov/dailymed/drugInfo.cfm?setid=baf5a1ba-14a7-4e0d-ba0c-a34c4befd8ae

Aspirin/extended-release dipyridamole (Aggrenox): https://dailymed.nlm.nih.gov/dailymed/drugInfo.cfm?setid=92222dd3-7802-2a03-7d30-58cf-192cc33e

Cilostazol: https://dailymed.nlm.nih.gov/dailymed/drugInfo.cfm?setid=db0278e9 -4ece-4aaf-9216-6bcbec58206a#ID_5c96e74b-a47c-453b-80bb-9ff624 fa9e16

Clopidogrel (Plavix): https://dailymed.nlm.nih.gov/dailymed/drugInfo.cfm?setid =de8b0b67-eb25-4684-83b5-7ad785314227

Prasugrel (Effient): https://dailymed.nlm.nih.gov/dailymed/drugInfo.cfm?setid =69ea2d58-5353-4222-b61f-cab976fa7e5e

Ticagrelor (Brilinta): https://dailymed.nlm.nih.gov/dailymed/drugInfo. cfm?setid=f7b3f443-e83d-4bf2-0e96-023448fed9a8

Vorapaxar (Zontivity): https://dailymed.nlm.nih.gov/dailymed/drugInfo. cfm?setid=f001f406-8cf1-40a4-bbf5-1775fe020122

REFERENCES

1. Periayah MH, Halim AS, Saad AZM. Mechanism action of platelets and crucial blood coagulation pathways in hemostasis. *Int J Hematol Oncol Stem Cell Res* 2017;11(4):319–327

2. Xu JQ, Murphy SL, Kochanek KD, Arias E. Mortality in the United States, 2021. *NCHS Data Brief*, no 456. Hyattsville, MD: National Center for Health Statistics, 2022. DOI: https://dx.doi.org/10.15620/cdc:122516

3. Taso CW, Aday AW, Almarzooq ZI, et al. Heart disease and stroke statistics—2023 update: a report from the American Heart Association. *Circulation* 2023;147:e93-e621

4. American Diabetes Association. 10. Cardiovascular disease and risk management: *Standards of Care in Diabetes—2023*. *Diabetes Care* 2023;46(Suppl.1):S159–S190

5. Arnett DK, Blumenthal RS, Albert MA, et al. 2019 ACC/AHA guideline on the primary prevention of cardiovascular disease: a report of the American College of Cardiology/American Heart Association Task Force on Clinical Practice Guidelines. *J Am Coll Cardiol* 2019;74:e177–232

6. Colwell JA, Nesto RW. The platelet in diabetes: focus on prevention of ischemic events. *Diabetes Care* 2003;26:2181–2188

7. Sharma A, Garg A, Elmariah S, et al. Duration of dual antiplatelet therapy following drug-eluting stent implantation in diabetic and non-diabetic patients: a systematic review and meta-analysis of randomized controlled trials. *Progress Cardiovasc Dis* 2018;60:500–507

8. Bayer Aspirin: The Wonder Drug. Available from https://www.bayeraspirinhcp.com/static/documents/Bayer_Aspirin_Wonder_Drug.pdf. Accessed 11 February 2021

9. Adult Aspirin Regimen Low Dose [package information]. Available from https://dailymed.nlm.nih.gov/dailymed/drugInfo.cfm?setid=7f5d9ebe-8119-49a2-9380-eca18a5e5e85. Accessed 11 February 2021

10. Effient (prasugrel) [prescribing information]. Bridgewater, NJ, Cosette Pharmaceuticals, 2022. Available from https://dailymed.nlm.nih.gov/dailymed/drugInfo.cfm?setid=69ea2d58-5353-4222-b61f-cab976fa7e5e

11. Kim HS, Kang J, Hwang D, et al; HOST-REDUCE-POLYTECH-ACS investigators. Prasugrel-based de-escalation of dual antiplatelet therapy after percutaneous coronary intervention in patients with acute coronary syndrome (HOST-REDUCE-POLYTECH-ACS): an open-label, multi-centre, non-inferiority randomised trial. *Lancet* 2020;396(10257):1079–1089. DOI:10.1016/S0140-6736(20)31791-8

12. Plavix (clopidogrel) [prescribing information]. Bridgewater, NJ, Sanofi-Aventis U.S. LLC, 2022. Available from https://dailymed.nlm.nih.gov/dailymed/drugInfo.cfm?setid=de8b0b67-eb25-4684-83b5-7ad785314227

13. Brilinta (ticagrelor) [prescribing information]. Wilmington, DE, AstraZeneca Pharmaceuticals LP, 2020. Available from https://dailymed.nlm.nih.gov/dailymed/drugInfo.cfm?setid=f7b3f443-e83d-4bf2-0e96-023448fed9a8

14. Aggrenox (aspirin/extended-release dipyridamole) [prescribing information]. Ridgefield, CT, Boehringer Ingelheim Pharmaceuticals, Inc., 2015. Available from https://dailymed.nlm.nih.gov/dailymed/drugInfo.cfm?setid=938ab0b5-8377-404a-8f61-5c630bda5932

15. Pletal (cilostazol) [prescribing information]. Rockville, MD, Otsuka America Pharmaceuticals Inc., 2017. Available from https://www.accessdata.fda.gov/drugsatfda_docs/label/2017/020863s024lbl.pdf

16. Zontivity (vorapaxar) [prescribing information]. Princeton, NJ, Aralez Pharmaceuticals US Inc., 2019. Available from https://dailymed.nlm.nih.gov/dailymed/drugInfo.cfm?setid=f001f406-8cf1-40a4-bbf5-1775fe020122#S12.3

17. O'Gara PT, Kushner FG, Ascheim DD, et al. 2013 ACCF/AHA guideline for the management of ST-elevation myocardial infarction: a report of the American College of Cardiology Foundation/American Heart Association Task Force on Practice Guidelines. *J Am Coll Cardiol* 2013;61:e78–e140

18. Amsterdam EA, Wenger NK, Brindis RG, et al. 2014 ACC/AHA guideline for the management of patients with non-ST elevation acute coronary syndromes: a report of the American College of Cardiology/American Heart Association Task Force on Practice Guidelines. *Circulation* 2014;130:e344–e426

19. Yusuf S, Zhao F, Mehta SR, et al. the Clopidogrel in Unstable Angina to Prevent Recurrent Events (CURE) Trial Investigators. Effects of clopidogrel in addition to aspirin in patients with acute coronary syndromes without ST-segment elevation. *N Engl J Med* 2001;345:494–502

20. Steinhubl SR, Berger PB, Mann JT 3rd, et al. Early and sustained dual oral antiplatelet therapy following percutaneous coronary intervention: a randomized controlled trial. *JAMA* 2002;288(19):2411–2420

21. Wiviott SD, Braunwald E, McCabe CH, et al. Prasugrel versus clopidogrel in patients with acute coronary syndromes. *N Engl J Med* 2007;357(20): 2001–2015

22. Montalescot G. Benefits for specific subpopulations in TRITON-TIMI 38. *Eur Heart J Supplements* 2009;11(Suppl. G):G18–G24

23. Wallentin L, Becker RC, Budaj A, et al.; PLATO Investigators. Ticagrelor versus clopidogrel in patients with acute coronary syndromes. *N Engl J Med* 2009;361(11):1045–1057

24. Bonaca MP, Bhatt DL, Cohen M, et al. Long-term use of ticagrelor in patients with prior myocardial infarction. *N Engl J Med* 2015;372(19): 1791–1800

25. Howard CE, Nambi V, Jneid H, and Khalid U. Extended duration of dual-antiplatelet therapy after percutaneous coronary intervention: How long is too long? *JAMA* 2019;8(20). DOI:10.1161/JAHA.119.012639

26. Levine GN, Bates ER, Bittl JA, et al.; 2016 ACC/AHA guideline focused update on duration of dual antiplatelet therapy in patients with coronary artery disease: a report of the American College of Cardiology/American Heart Association Task Force on Clinical Practice Guidelines: an update of the 2011 ACCF/AHA/SCAI guideline for percutaneous coronary intervention, 2011 ACCF/AHA guideline for coronary artery bypass graft surgery, 2012 ACC/AHA/ACP/AATS/PCNA/SCAI/STS guideline for the diagnosis and management of patients with stable ischemic heart disease, 2013 ACCF/AHA guideline for the management of ST-elevation myocardial infarction, 2014 ACC/AHA guideline for the management of patients with non–ST-elevation acute coronary syndromes, and 2014 ACC/AHA guideline on perioperative cardiovascular evaluation and management of patients undergoing noncardiac surgery. *Circulation* 2016;134:e123–e155. DOI: 10.1161/CIR.0000000000000404

27. Mehran R, Usman B, Sharma SK, et al. Ticagrelor with or without aspirin in high-risk patients after PCI. *N Engl J Med* 2019;381:2032–2042

28. Hahn JY, Song YB and Oh JH. Effect of P2Y12 inhibitor monotherapy vs dual antiplatelet therapy on cardiovascular events in patients undergoing percutaneous coronary intervention. *JAMA* 2019;321(24):2428–2437

29. Watanabe H, Domei T, Morimoto T. Effect of 1-month dual antiplatelet therapy followed by clopidogrel 12-month dual antiplatelet therapy on cardiovascular and bleeding events in patients receiving PCI. *JAMA* 2019;321(24):2414–2427

30. Vranckx P, Valgimigli M, Jüni P, et al. Ticagrelor plus aspirin for 1 month followed by ticagrelor monotherapy for 23 months vs aspirin plus clopidogrel or ticagrelor for 12 months, followed by aspirin monotherapy for 12

months after implantation of a drug-eluting stent: A multicenter, open-label, randomized superiority trial. *Lancet* 2018;392(10151):940–949

31. Steg PG, Bhatt DL, Simon T, et al. Ticagrelor in patients with stable coronary disease and diabetes. *N Engl J Med* 2019;381(14):1309–1320

32. Kleindorfer DO, Chaturvedi S, Cockroft KM, et al. 2021 Guideline for the Prevention of Stroke in Patients with Stroke and Transient Ischemic Attack: A guideline from the American Heart Association/American Stroke Association. *Stroke* 2021;52(7):e364–e467

33. Wang Y, Wang Y, Zhao X, et al.; CHANCE Investigators. Clopidogrel with aspirin in acute minor stroke or transient ischemic attack. *N Engl J Med* 2013;369(1):11–19

34. Johnston SC, Easton JD, Farrant M, et al. Clopidogrel and aspirin in acute ischemic stroke and high-risk TIA. *N Engl J Med* 2018;379:215–225

35. Peeters Weem SM, van Haelst ST, den Ruijter HM, et al. Lack of evidence for dual antiplatelet therapy after endovascular arterial procedures: A meta-analysis. *Eur J Vasc Endovasc Surg* 2016;52:253–262

36. Johnston SC, Amarenco P, Denison H, et al. Ticagrelor and Aspirin or Aspirin Alone in Acute Ischemic Stroke or TIA. *NEJM* 2020;383:207–217

37. Bath PM Woodhouse LJ, Appleton JP, et al. Antiplatelet therapy with aspirin, clopidgrel, and dipyridamole versus clopidogrel alone or aspiring and dipyridamole in patients with acute cerebral ischaemia (TARDIS): A randomized, open-label, phase 3 superiority trial. *Lancet* 2018;391(10123):850–859

38. Gerhard-Herman MD, Gornik HL, Barrett C, et al. 2016 AHA/ACC guideline on the management of patients with lower extremity peripheral artery disease: executive summary: a report of the American College of Cardiology/American Heart Association Task Force on Clinical Practice Guidelines. *Circulation* 2017;135:e686–e725

39. Tsai SY, Li YS, Lee CH, et al. Mono or dual antiplatelet therapy for treating patients with peripheral artery disease after lower extremity revascularization: A systematic review and meta-analysis. *Pharmaceuticals* (Basel) 2022;15(5):596

Chapter 23
Medications for Smoking Cessation

Anne P. Kim, PharmD, MPH, MIT

INTRODUCTION

Nicotine is an addictive compound that can be delivered in a number of ways—cigarettes, smokeless tobacco (e.g., oral snuff, chewing tobacco), electronic cigarettes (e-cigarettes), and heat-not-burn (HNB) products.[1] For adults, the most commonly used tobacco product is cigarettes; for youth, the most commonly used is e-cigarettes.[2,3] Although the prevalence of cigarette smoking in adults has declined over the years, it is estimated that 19% or 47.1 million U.S. adults used any tobacco product in 2020.[2] There is also a high prevalence of youths who reported ever using tobacco products in 2022 (24.8% or 6.77 million) with 11.3% reporting current use (high school students: 16.5% or 2.51 million; middle school students: 4.5% or 530,000).[3] There is concern that a marked increase in e-cigarette use by youth will lead to quicker, early initiation of cigarette smoking by acting as a gateway device.[4,5] A recent study showed that adolescents who use e-cigarettes, particularly modifiable devices, are more likely to report future cigarette smoking.[6]

Cigarette smoking continues to be the leading cause of preventable disease (e.g., cancer, COPD, CVD, and diabetes) and premature death. Cigarettes are the most commonly used tobacco product, leading to an estimated 480,000 smoking-related deaths per year, in 2014.[2,7] Recent data from the Centers for Disease Control and Prevention indicate that e-cigarettes are contributing to the high rate of smoking-related hospitalizations and deaths due to e-cigarette or vaping use-associated lung injury (EVALI).[8] Although the number of EVALI cases has decreased since its peak in 2019, EVALI cases and deaths continue to be reported and monitored. Use of e-cigarettes to encourage smoking cessation as a form of "step-down therapy" is not recommended.[9]

The 2014 U.S. Surgeon General's report indicates that new research data have expanded the list of diseases caused by smoking cigarettes, including diabetes mellitus.[7,10] Active smokers have a 30–40% increased risk of developing T2D, in a dose-dependent manner, compared to nonsmokers.[7]

It is well established that cigarette smoking is associated with increased risk of cardiovascular morbidity and mortality and that diabetes also is associated with increased risk of cardiovascular morbidity and mortality. The Multiple Risk Factor Intervention Trial (MRFIT), the prospective study of women in Finland, and the Paris Prospective Study showed that cigarette smoking is a significant risk factor for increased risk of cardiovascular events.[11-13] A meta-analysis that included 89 prospective cohort studies demonstrated active cigarette smoking significantly increases the risk of cardiovascular mortality, total CVD, CHD, and stroke in patients with diabetes.[14]

The American Diabetes Association states that smoking cessation is one intervention of few that is safe and cost-effective for all patients who smoke.[15] Smoking cessation has been shown to decrease cardiovascular events. A meta-analysis of 46 prospective cohort or nested case-controlled studies on patients with diabetes reported lower risks of cardiovascular outcomes (e.g., stroke, MI) in those who quit smoking cigarettes compared to those who actively smoke cigarettes.[16] Another meta-analysis of 68 cohort and randomized controlled trials determined smoking cessation compared to continued smoking decreases risk of cardiovascular mortality and major adverse cardiovascular events (MACE; e.g., myocardial infarction).[17] Unfortunately, as few as 20% of patients are counseled on smoking cessation, with a common barrier being time limitations of healthcare providers.[18]

Goals of smoking cessation counseling and pharmacotherapy include:

- Prevention/mitigation of symptoms of nicotine withdrawal.
- Cessation of tobacco use (or decreased use) and maintained abstinence.
- Decreased risk of morbidity and mortality from smoking-related diseases (including diabetes).

The American Diabetes Association recommendations for smoking cessation and prevention are provided in Table 23.1.

Table 23.1 — Recommendations Regarding Diabetes and Smoking

Assessment of smoking status and history
■ Systematic documentation of a history of tobacco use must be obtained from all adolescent and adult individuals with diabetes.
Counseling on smoking prevention and cessation
■ All healthcare providers should advise individuals with diabetes not to initiate smoking. This advice should be consistently repeated to prevent smoking and other tobacco use among children and adolescents with diabetes under age 21 years.
■ Among smokers, cessation counseling must be completed as a routine component of diabetes care.
■ Every smoker should be urged to quit in a clear, strong, and personalized manner that describes the added risks of smoking and diabetes.
■ Every diabetic smoker should be asked if he or she is willing to quit at this time.
– If no, initiate brief and motivational discussion regarding need to stop using tobacco, risks of continued use, and encouragement to quit as well as support when ready.
– If yes, assess preference for and initiate either minimal, brief, or intensive cessation counseling and offer pharmacological supplements as appropriate.
Effective systems for delivery of smoking cessation
■ Training of all diabetes healthcare providers in the Public Health Service guidelines regarding smoking should be implemented.
■ Follow-up procedures designed to assess and promote quitting status must be arranged for all diabetic smokers.

Source: American Diabetes Association.[15]

Table 23.2—The "5 A's" Model for Treating Tobacco Use and Dependence

Ask about tobacco use.	Identify and document tobacco use status for every patient at every visit.
Advise to quit.	In a clear, strong, and personalized manner, urge every tobacco user to quit.
Assess willingness to make a quit attempt.	Is the tobacco user willing to make a quit attempt at this time?
Assess in quit attempt.	For patients willing to make a quit attempt, offer medication and provide or refer for counseling or additional treatment to help quit. For patients unwilling to quit at the time, provide interventions designed to increase future quit attempts.
Arrange for follow-up.	For patients willing to make a quit attempt, arrange for follow-up contacts, beginning within the first week after the quit date. For patients unwilling to make a quit attempt at the time, address tobacco dependence and willingness to quit at next clinic visit.

Source: Fiore.[19]

The U.S. Department of Health and Human Services created the "5 A's" model for healthcare providers to use as a tool to promote smoking cessation.[18] Table 23.2 lists the steps of the "5 A's" model.

The American College of Cardiology recently published the "Pathway for Tobacco Cessation Treatment" that builds on the "5 A's" model (Figure 23.1).[1]

Studies have shown the individual efficacy of counseling and pharmacotherapy, but the combination of counseling and pharmacotherapy is better than either alone in smoking cessation rates.[19–21] Thus, it is recommended that both are provided to all patients, if feasible and appropriate.[19]

The intent of pharmacotherapy interventions is to prevent or reduce any symptoms of nicotine withdrawal and thus assist the patient in achieving smoking cessation. Common symptoms of nicotine withdrawal include irritability, anxiety, depression, difficulty concentrating, headaches, difficulty sleeping, increased appetite, and restlessness.[22,23] First-line pharmacotherapies that are FDA approved for smoking cessation include nicotine replacement therapy (NRT), varenicline, and bupropion sustained release (SR). Second-line, non-FDA-approved medications include nortriptyline and clonidine. Other options have been assessed to have little to no proven clinical benefit in increasing smoking cessation rates (e.g., selective serotonin reuptake inhibitors, e-cigarettes).[19,21] The medications detailed below are those that have sufficient evidence to support their use in clinical practice.

FIRST-LINE MEDICATIONS FOR SMOKING CESSATION

- Nicotine Replacement Therapy
- Long-acting Nicotine Replacement Therapy
- Short-acting Nicotine Replacement Therapy
- Varenicline
- Bupropion SR

NICOTINE REPLACEMENT THERAPY

NRT is an FDA-approved, first-line intervention for smoking cessation.[19] NRT is available in a variety of formulations: transdermal patch, gum, lozenge, inhaler, and nasal spray. The transdermal patch formulation is long-acting, and the others are short-acting formulations of NRT. NRT patches, lozenges, and gum are available over the counter (OTC). A meta-analysis of 150 randomized trials concluded that all NRT formulations are efficacious in achieving smoking cessation.[24] Any of the NRT products may be administered, depending on a number of factors such as patient preference, cost, and side effects.[25]

Mechanism of Action

NRT partially replaces the nicotine that was previously supplied from cigarettes or other forms of tobacco at the site of nicotine receptors. Stimulated nicotine receptors in the peripheral and central nervous systems diminish the severity of nicotine withdrawal symptoms, including nicotine craving, associated with smoking cessation.[25]

Because of the different NRT formulations, specific drug administration instructions, pharmacokinetic parameters, efficacy data, and adverse events will be discussed under each product below, after the following sections on common adverse events/warnings and precautions and drug interactions. Dosages are outlined in Table 23.3 (see page 388).

Adverse Events/Warnings and Precautions

Adverse events associated with NRT include gastrointestinal effects (e.g., nausea, vomiting), insomnia, and increased heart rate.[21,26]

NRT should be used with caution in those who have acute CVD (e.g., recent MI, unstable angina pectoris) because of nicotine's sympathomimetic effect, which can increase heart rate and contractility and constrict blood vessels. Benefits may outweigh risk in patients with CVD who continue to smoke, as clinical studies have not shown increased risk of adverse cardiovascular events with use of NRT.[25,27]

NRT has not been intentionally studied in pregnant smokers, and the insufficient evidence available is limited and conflicting.[21] Nicotine is suspected to cause reproductive toxicity, including fetal neuro-teratogenicity.[26] It is recommended that pregnant smokers be encouraged to quit smoking without the aid of medications.[19]

Adolescents who smoke may be prone to poisoning (in some cases, fatal poisoning) from NRT. Symptoms of NRT overdose in adolescents include nausea, vomiting, diarrhea, increased salivation, pallor, sweating, headache, dizziness, mental confusion, marked weakness, tremor, respiratory failure, and auditory or visual disturbance. These symptoms may be followed by hypotension, breathing difficulties, circulatory collapse, and convulsions with higher levels of unwanted NRT exposure.[26]

Drug Interactions

The sympathomimetic nature of NRT products may cause the following effects:[19]

- Decrease in the sedative effects of benzodiazepines.
- Decrease in subcutaneous absorption of insulin.

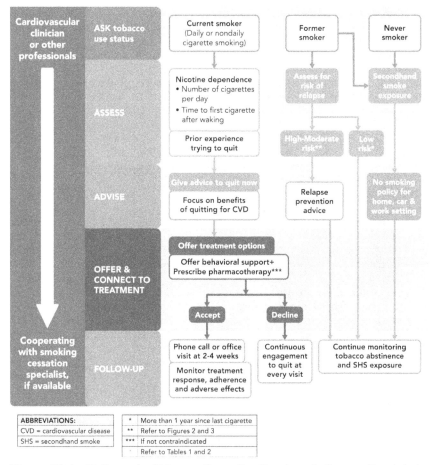

Figure 23.1—Pathway for Tobacco Cessation Treatment. *Source*: Reprinted with permission from Barua.[1]

- Decrease in the capacity of β-blockers to decrease blood pressure and heart rate.
- Decrease in the analgesic effect of opioids.

It may be necessary to adjust these medications when NRT therapy is discontinued.[19]

LONG-ACTING NRT

Nicotine transdermal patches provide nicotine at a continuous rate over a long duration and can be worn for up to 24 h. Patients may wear the 16-h patch if they are having trouble sleeping.[19,25] The pharmacokinetics of nicotine vary, depending on the NRT formulation administered. Nicotine transdermal patches are manufactured in a variety of delivery designs, which results in differing pharmacokinetic parameters. In general, the maximum rate of nicotine absorption is reached after 6–12 h of patch administration. Peak blood levels are reached after 16–24 h. Absolute bioavailability is about 82%.[28] Compared to placebo, use of the transdermal patch increased the likelihood of long-term smoking cessation by nearly twofold (OR 1.9 [95% CI 1.7–2.2]) in a meta-analysis of 25 clinical trials. A longer duration of therapy (>14 weeks) with the patch was similarly effective (OR 1.9 [95% CI 1.7–2.3]) and did not increase the rate of smoking cessation.[19] Despite rotating administration sites, NRT transdermal patches may produce local skin reactions that tend to be mild and self-limiting. Skin reactions may be treated with topical hydrocortisone cream or triamcinolone cream. If skin reactions are intolerable, patient should discontinue nicotine patch therapy.[19]

SHORT-ACTING NRT

Nicotine gum is available in several flavors and in the original flavor. There is a specific chewing technique ("chew and park") that optimizes nicotine release from the gum. Gum should be chewed until a taste emerges, then park the gum between the cheek and upper or lower gums until the taste disappears. This should be repeated for 30 min or until there is no more taste released upon chewing, which indicates all the nicotine has been released.[19] Buccal absorption of nicotine may be disrupted by acidic beverages (e.g., coffee). Patients should be advised to only consume water 15 min before and during chewing.[19] Nicotine gum is formulated so that one piece of gum provides NRT for 1–2 h each. Because the rate of nicotine release depends on the patient's chewing speed, another piece of gum may be needed within the hour to appease strong cravings.[28] Compared to placebo, use of nicotine gum increased the likelihood of long-term smoking cessation by about 50% (OR 1.5 [95% CI 1.2–1.7]) in a meta-analysis of nine clinical trials. However, many patients do not administer the gum as frequently as needed. They should be advised to chew the gum on a fixed schedule to achieve optimal benefit.[19] Nicotine gum is associated with mild, transient side effects such as mouth soreness, hiccups, dyspepsia, headache, and jaw pain, especially if not using proper chewing technique.[19,28]

Nicotine lozenges release nicotine as they slowly dissolve in the mouth. They are not to be chewed or swallowed. Similar to nicotine gum, lozenges are affected by acidic beverages, which should be avoided 15 min before and during administration.[19] Compared to placebo, the lower, 2-mg dose doubled and the higher, 4-mg dose nearly tripled the odds of achieving smoking cessation. Many patients do not use enough as-needed nicotine lozenges to achieve maximal benefit. They should be advised to administer lozenges per the schedule detailed in Table 23.3.[19] Lozenge-specific side effects include mouth/throat irritation, nausea, hiccups, and heartburn. The higher-dose lozenge is also associated with headache and coughing.[19,25]

Nicotine inhalers consist of a cartridge and mouthpiece that resemble a cigarette.[28] They deposit nicotine in the oropharynx, allowing nicotine to be absorbed through the buccal mucosa rather than the pulmonary route.[19,28] An advantage of the inhaler formulation is potentially addressing the hand-to-mouth behaviors and sensory cues reminiscent of cigarette smoking.[26] Cold temperatures (below around 40°F) decrease the amount of nicotine delivered from the inhaler (poor absorption and bioavailability). It is recommended that the inhaler/cartridge be kept in a warm area (e.g., inside pocket).[19,28] Compared to placebo, use of the nicotine inhaler increased the likelihood of long-term smoking cessation by about twofold (OR 2.1 [95% CI 1.5–2.9]) in a meta-analysis of six clinical trials.[18] As another as-needed NRT product, many patients do not use inhalers as often as needed for optimal benefit. Patients should be advised on appropriate frequency and duration of inhaler administration.[19] Nicotine inhalers are associated with mild, transient mouth/throat irritation, coughing, and rhinitis.[19]

Nicotine nasal spray (Nicotrol) delivers nicotine at higher levels than the other NRT formulations, which has raised concerns for dependence potential. Patients have reported using nicotine nasal sprays longer than the recommended 6–12 months of therapy, and some have reported using the product at a dose higher than recommended.[19] Blood nicotine levels peak after 5–10 min of administration. Nicotine is delivered faster with the nasal spray than with gum or the inhaler, but it is still slower than the delivery of nicotine from smoking cigarettes.[28] The nasal spray should be administered with the head slightly tilted back, without sniffing, swallowing, or inhaling through the nose at time of administration to avoid increased side effects.[19] Compared to placebo, nasal spray administration more than doubled (OR 2.3 [95% CI 1.7–3.0]) the likelihood of achieving smoking cessation in a meta-analysis of four clinical trials.[19] Nicotine nasal spray is associated with persistent nasal/throat irritation, rhinitis/nasal congestion, coughing, and transient changes in taste and smell.[19,25] Patients with severe reactive airway disease should use another NRT formulation besides the nasal spray.[19,25]

VARENICLINE (CHANTIX)

Varenicline is a nicotine receptor partial agonist—a non-nicotine medication—that is approved by the FDA as a first-line intervention for smoking cessation.[19]

Mechanism of Action

Varenicline is an analog of cytisine, which comes from a plant called *Cytisus laburnum* (false tobacco).[28] Varenicline is a selective partial agonist at the α4β2 neuronal nicotinic acetylcholine receptor (nAchR), which is central to the development of nicotine addiction. Because it is selective, varenicline does not bind to other nicotine or non-nicotine receptors/transporters.[28] As a partial agonist, varenicline promotes the release of a lower amount of dopamine than triggered by nicotine from tobacco products, but enough to minimize nicotine withdrawal symptoms and cravings. In addition to exerting agonistic effects, varenicline competitively inhibits the binding of nicotine and thus prevents full stimulation and release of dopamine to activate the mesolimbic region of the CNS (associated with reinforcement and reward).[25,29] Studies show that patients who concomitantly take varenicline and smoke cigarettes experience a lower level of satisfaction.[29,30] Figure 23.2 illustrates the effects of varenicline.

Dosage and Administration

Varenicline should be initiated 1 week prior to the quit date with the following recommended titration schedule:[19,29]

- 0.5 mg once daily for 3 days, then
- 0.5 mg twice daily for 4 days, and then
- 1 mg twice daily for 3 months (may be extended to 6 months).

On day 8 (quit date), when the dosage is first increased to 1 mg twice daily, patients should be instructed to quit smoking.[19,29] If they are unwilling or unable to quit on day 8, patients may gradually approach cessation with varenicline therapy by decreasing smoking by 50% every 4 weeks with the goal of quitting smok-

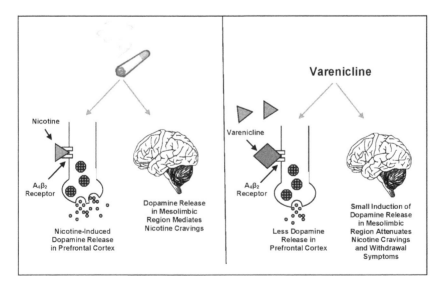

Figure 23.2—Pharmacological effects of varenicline in smoking cessation. Courtesy of JJ Neumiller.

ing by the end of 12 weeks.[29] After successfully achieving smoking cessation at 12 weeks of therapy, an additional 12 weeks of therapy is recommended, for all patients, to maintain smoking abstinence.[29]

There is no need to adjust the dose for patients with mild to moderate renal impairment. For those with severe renal impairment (CrCl <30 mL/min), the starting dose is the same (0.5 mg once daily) but it can only be titrated, as needed, to a maximum dose of 0.5 mg twice daily.[29]

Varenicline should be taken with food to reduce nausea, and the second dose of the day may be taken with dinner rather than at bedtime to reduce insomnia.[19,29]

Pharmacokinetics

Within 3–4 h of oral administration, maximum plasma concentration of varenicline is reached, and steady-state concentrations are reached after approximately 4 days of therapy. Varenicline follows linear pharmacokinetics. The oral bioavailability of about 90% is not affected by food or time of dosing. Varenicline is ≤20% bound to plasma proteins.[29]

Varenicline is primarily excreted unchanged in the urine (92%), with a half-life of about 24 h.[29]

Clinical Efficacy

Compared to placebo, use of varenicline increased the likelihood of long-term smoking cessation by about twofold (OR 2.1 [95% CI 1.5–3.0]) with the lower 1 mg dose and by about threefold (OR 3.1 [95% CI 2.5–3.8]) with the higher 2-mg dose in meta-analyses of two clinical trials and of four clinical trials, respectively. These findings suggest that 1 mg per day could be used in patients who experience intolerable side effects from the 2-mg dosage regimen.[18] Head-to-head trials against bupropion SR (and placebo) showed varenicline had higher rates of smoking cessation than bupropion SR. (Varenicline and bupropion SR were each better than placebo.)[29–31] The American Thoracic Society Clinical Practice Guideline recommends use of varenicline over the nicotine patch and bupropion, based on a moderate level of certainty in the estimated effects.[32] The likelihood of long-term smoking cessation was greater with 24 weeks of varenicline therapy than with the standard 12 weeks.[29] Varenicline therapy for extended periods of time (up to 1 year) has been shown to reduce relapse rates.[13]

Choosing a quit date beyond day 8 but within 5 weeks of initiating varenicline was successful in achieving smoking cessation compared to placebo.[29] Another study showed that varenicline therapy and a gradual reduction in smoking for 12 weeks before quitting resulted in improved smoking cessation rates compared to concomitant placebo therapy. Upon quitting smoking at week 12, patients continued varenicline or placebo therapy for an additional 12 weeks.[29]

Compared to placebo, varenicline increased the rate of smoking cessation in patients who had failed previous attempts to quit smoking with varenicline therapy.[29]

Varenicline has been studied as a smoking cessation aid in patients with CVD, COPD, or major depressive disorder (MDD). Varenicline was found to be superior to placebo in achieving smoking cessation in all three patient populations. In addition, a postmarketing trial on neuropsychiatric safety outcomes demonstrated that varenicline is better than placebo at attaining smoking cessation and that exposure to varenicline does not increase the risk of neuropsychiatric adverse events in either patients with a history of psychiatric disorder or patients without. There were, however, neuropsychiatric adverse events that occurred during varenicline therapy, so it remains in the warning and precautions section of the prescribing information document.[29,33]

Adverse Events/Warnings and Precautions

Common adverse events associated with exposure to varenicline include nausea, vomiting, constipation, difficulty sleeping, and abnormal vivid dreams.[19,29]

The FDA issued a black box warning in July 2009 regarding observed serious neuropsychiatric events (e.g., depression, agitation, suicidal ideation and behavior) in adult patients who received varenicline therapy, but it was removed in December 2016 after new study data presented lower-than-suspected rates of serious neuropsychiatric events.[29,34] It is important to note, however, that the risk still remains, particularly for those with a history of mental illnesses such as depression, anxiety disorders, or schizophrenia.[35] Healthcare providers should gather a complete psychiatric history prior to initiating varenicline and monitor patients for any evidence of neuropsychiatric adverse events. Patients who are already taking varenicline should stop therapy and contact their healthcare providers if they experience any changes in mood, thoughts, or behavior so that the healthcare provider may weigh the benefits against the risks and consider the following options: dose reduction, continued treatment with close monitoring, or discontinuing therapy.[19,29]

Varenicline may increase the risk for nonfatal cardiovascular events (e.g., nonfatal MI, nonfatal stroke, hospitalization for angina pectoris). Even though these events were not statistically significant, they were consistent in occurrence; thus, healthcare providers should weigh the benefits and risks of prescribing varenicline therapy to smokers with CVD.[29]

Varenicline has been associated with seizures. The benefits and risks should be assessed before initiating varenicline in patients with a history of seizures or lowered seizure threshold. Patients should immediately stop therapy and contact their healthcare providers if they experience a seizure.[29]

There are insufficient data on varenicline in pregnant smokers. It is not known whether the benefits of using varenicline to quit smoking outweigh the unknown maternal and fetal risks of harm from varenicline exposure.[29] It is recommended that pregnant smokers be encouraged to quit smoking without the aid of medications.[19]

Exposure to varenicline therapy has been associated with postmarketing reports of hypersensitivity reactions (e.g., angioedema) and serious skin reactions (e.g., Stevens-Johnson syndrome). Varenicline should be discontinued immediately upon any signs of hypersensitivity or skin rash.[29]

Increased intoxicating effects of alcohol with concomitant administration of varenicline have been reported postmarketing. It is recommended that patients decrease alcohol consumption until they assess how varenicline affects their ability to tolerate alcohol.[29]

Somnambulism or sleepwalking has been associated with exposure to varenicline therapy. Some cases report harmful behavior to self, other people, or property. Patients should discontinue varenicline and contact their healthcare providers if somnambulism occurs.[29]

Varenicline has also been reported to cause somnolence, dizziness, or difficulty concentrating while driving, which have led to traffic accidents. It is recommended that patients use caution when driving until they assess how varenicline affects them.[29]

Drug Interactions

Because varenicline is mainly eliminated via the kidneys, there are no metabolic interactions.[19] Medications that inhibit varenicline renal excretion, such as cimetidine, may increase the levels of varenicline, but this potential interaction is considered to be not clinically significant. Thus, there are no significant drug interactions with varenicline.[19]

BUPROPION SUSTAINED RELEASE (ZYBAN)

Bupropion SR is an atypical antidepressant that is an FDA-approved medication for smoking cessation. The U.S. Department of Health and Human Services recommends bupropion SR as another first-line intervention available for aiding in smoking cessation, and it may be used in combination with NRT products.[19]

Mechanism of Action

The mechanism of action for facilitating smoking cessation is not fully understood, but bupropion SR's efficacy in smoking cessation is thought to be related to its noradrenergic and/or dopaminergic activity (i.e., its weak inhibition of the synaptic reuptake of norepinephrine and dopamine in the CNS). Bupropion SR has also been shown to act as a nicotine receptor antagonist, which would contribute to its utility in smoking cessation.[28,29]

Dosage and Administration

Bupropion SR should be initiated 1–2 weeks prior to the quit date with the following recommended titration schedule to minimize seizure risk:[19,36]

- 150 mg once daily for 3 days and then
- 150 mg twice daily (at least 8 h apart) for 7–12 weeks (may be extended to 6 months)

Dosages for smoking cessation should not exceed the maximum dose of 300 mg per day. Bupropion SR may be taken with or without food, but it is not to be split, crushed, or chewed. Bupropion SR must be swallowed as a whole tablet to be delivered at the rate intended.[36]

Based on limited data, it is recommended that bupropion SR is used with caution in patients with renal impairment (CrCl <90 mL/min). Healthcare providers may consider a reduction in dose and/or frequency of administration in this population.[36] The same considerations (lower dose and/or frequency) should be applied to patients with mild hepatic impairment (Child-Pugh score of 5 or 6). Patients with moderate to severe hepatic impairment (Child-Pugh score of 7–15) should not exceed a maximum dose of 150 mg every other day.[36]

The second bupropion SR dose of the day may be taken earlier in the afternoon, but at least 8 h after the first dose, instead of in the evening to reduce major changes in sleep pattern (i.e., insomnia).[19]

Pharmacokinetics

Within 3 h of oral administration, maximum plasma concentration of bupropion SR is reached, and steady-state concentrations are reached after approximately 8 days of therapy. Bupropion SR follows linear pharmacokinetics. Based on preclinical animal study data, the bioavailability of orally administered bupropion SR ranges from 5 to 20%, and it is not significantly increased with food intake. Bupropion SR is 84% bound to plasma proteins.[36]

Bupropion SR is mainly metabolized in the liver to many metabolites (three of which are active). Only 0.5% of bupropion SR is excreted as unchanged parent drug. Bupropion SR and the metabolites have long half-lives. Bupropion SR has a half-life of about 21 h, and metabolites have half-lives that range from about 20–37 h.[36]

Clinical Efficacy

Compared to placebo, bupropion SR increased the likelihood of long-term smoking cessation by approximately twofold (OR 2.0 [95% CI 1.8–2.2]) in a meta-analysis of 24 clinical trials.[19] Similar to varenicline, bupropion SR was investigated in patients with COPD, and postmarketing data on neuropsychiatric safety outcomes were analyzed. Bupropion SR demonstrated superiority over placebo in achieving smoking cessation in smoking patients with COPD and in patients with or without a history of a psychiatric disorder. The postmarketing trial also concluded that bupropion SR does not have an increased risk of neuropsychiatric adverse events compared to placebo. Due to the small but consistent occurrence of neuropsychiatric adverse events in adults, however, it remains in the prescribing document under the warnings and precautions section.[36]

Contraindications

Bupropion SR is contraindicated in patients with a history of seizures or eating disorders (bulimia or anorexia nervosa) because of a dose-dependent risk of seizures with bupropion SR exposure. There is increased risk of seizures at dosages higher than 300 mg per day, so doses should not exceed the maximum of 300 mg per day. If patients experience a seizure, bupropion SR should be discontinued and not reinitiated.[36]

Bupropion SR is contraindicated in patients who are taking monoamine oxidase inhibitors (MAOIs) (e.g., linezolid, methylene blue) or have been treated with an MAOI within 14 days, due to increased risk of hypertensive reactions. Bupropion SR alone is associated with increased blood pressure. The risk of hypertension is increased with concomitant administration of MAOIs.[36]

Bupropion SR is also contraindicated in patients who are abruptly discontinuing the use of alcohol, benzodiazepines, barbiturates, and antiepileptic medications.[36]

Adverse Events/Warnings and Precautions

Adverse events associated with bupropion SR therapy include insomnia and dry mouth. Decreasing the dose may help provide relief.[36]

Despite Zyban being used as a smoking-cessation agent, it contains the same active ingredient as the antidepressant Wellbutrin. Thus, bupropion SR has a black box warning regarding suicidal thoughts and behaviors because of short-term trial data that showed increased risk of suicidal thinking and behavior in children, adolescents, and young adults.[36] It is recommended that all patients taking antidepressant therapy be closely monitored for any occurrence or worsening of suicidal thoughts and behaviors. Those who are close in relation to the patient (e.g., family members, caregivers) should be advised about the daily need to observe and communicate any concerns with the healthcare provider.[36]

Antidepressant therapy is known to trigger manic, mixed, or hypomanic episodes in patients with bipolar disorder. Bupropion SR should not be used to treat bipolar depression.[36]

Similar to varenicline, the FDA issued a black box warning in July 2009 regarding observed serious neuropsychiatric events (e.g., depression, agitation, suicidal ideation and behavior) in adult patients who received bupropion SR therapy, but it was removed in May 2017 after new study data presented lower than suspected rates of serious neuropsychiatric events.[34,36] It is important to note, however, that the risk still remains, particularly for those with a history of mental illnesses such as depression, anxiety disorders, or schizophrenia.[35] Healthcare providers should gather a complete psychiatric history prior to initiating bupropion SR and monitor patients for any evidence of neuropsychiatric adverse events. Patients who are already taking bupropion SR should stop therapy and contact their healthcare providers if they experience any changes in mood, thoughts, or behavior so that the healthcare provider may weigh the benefits against the risks and consider the following options: dose reduction, continued treatment with close monitoring, or discontinuing therapy.[36]

Bupropion SR therapy may precipitate angle-closure glaucoma in patients with anatomically narrow angles without a patent iridectomy by dilating pupils.[36]

There are epidemiological study data available that show that bupropion SR is not associated with increased risk of congenital malformations in the first trimester of pregnancy, but there are no data regarding its effectiveness in this population.[19,36] It is recommended that pregnant smokers be encouraged to quit smoking without the aid of medications, and only use bupropion SR when potential benefits clearly justify potential risks of fetal harm.[19,36]

Drug Interactions

As mentioned earlier, bupropion SR should not be administered with MAOIs. Bupropion SR may be initiated after waiting a minimum of 14 days from discontinuing MAOI therapy.[36]

Because bupropion SR can lower seizure threshold, caution should be used when coadministering with other medications that lower seizure threshold.[19]

Bupropion SR is primarily metabolized by CYP2B6, so drugs that inhibit CYP2B6 activity (e.g., ticlopidine, clopidogrel) will increase bupropion SR concentrations. Conversely, drugs that induce the CYP2B6 enzyme (e.g., ritonavir, lopinavir, efavirenz) will decrease bupropion SR levels. Additionally, drugs that are known to be strong inducers (e.g., carbamazepine, phenobarbital, phenytoin) will decrease bupropion SR concentrations, while strong inhibitors (e.g., valproate, cimetidine) will increase bupropion SR concentrations because bupropion SR is extensively metabolized by the liver.[19,36]

Bupropion SR and its metabolites inhibit CYP2D6. Coadministration of bupropion SR may lead to increased concentrations of drugs that are metabolized by CYP2D6 (e.g., tricyclic antidepressants, antipsychotics, β-blockers). Bupropion SR may also lower the efficacy of drugs that are activated by CYP2D6, such as tamoxifen. Higher doses may be needed to reach normal therapeutic benefit of these drugs when administered with bupropion SR.[36]

Digoxin levels may decrease when coadministered with bupropion SR. It is recommended that digoxin levels are monitored with this combination.[36]

SECOND-LINE MEDICATIONS FOR SMOKING CESSATION

- Clonidine
- Nortriptyline

CLONIDINE

Clonidine is a centrally acting α_2 adrenergic receptor agonist that is FDA approved to treat hypertension and is not approved for smoking cessation, but it may be used off-label as a second-line intervention for smoking cessation.[18] It is also used off-label for a variety of other conditions (e.g., chronic pain syndromes, Tourette syndrome, menopausal flushing).[28] Clonidine may be used when first-line therapies are contraindicated or when their use is unsuccessful in achieving smoking cessation.[19]

Mechanism of Action

Clonidine's efficacy in smoking cessation is thought to be related to its effects on the CNS, which likely mitigate symptoms of nicotine withdrawal, including craving.[25] As an α_2 adrenergic receptor agonist, clonidine decreases sympathetic outflow from the CNS.[37]

Dosage and Administration

Clonidine is available as an oral tablet and as a transdermal patch. It should be initiated up to 3 days prior to the quit date.[19] Although there is no specific dosing regimen established for using clonidine as a smoking cessation aid, the recommended/common initial dose is 0.1 mg twice daily for the oral tablet and 0.1 mg once daily for the transdermal patch.[19,38] The dose may be increased by 0.1 mg/day in weekly intervals to a maximum of approximately 0.4 mg per day, if necessary.[19,38] The duration of clonidine therapy ranged from 3–10 weeks in clinical trials, but some recommend that clonidine treatment be given for a maximum of 3–4 weeks for smoking cessation.[19,28] Due to the risk of rebound hypertension (i.e., rapid increase in blood pressure, agitation, headache, confusion, and/or tremor) upon abrupt discontinuation, clonidine should be slowly tapered down over 2–4 days (or longer).[19,37,38]

For the transdermal patch, patients should be counseled to place a new patch on skin that is relatively hairless between the neck and waist, once a week.[19]

Pharmacokinetics

Within 1–3 h of oral administration, maximum plasma concentration of clonidine is reached.[36] Oral bioavailability ranges from 70–80% and transdermal bioavailability is about 60%.[36,38] Clonidine is metabolized by the liver (~50%) and renally excreted as unchanged drug (40–60%), with a half-life of 12–16 h (up to 41 h with severe renal impairment).[36] The transdermal patch formulation releases clonidine at a constant rate over 7 days and, once the patch is removed, clonidine plasma levels slowly decline with a half-life of 20 h.[38]

Clinical Efficacy

Compared to placebo, clonidine increased the likelihood of long-term smoking cessation by approximately twofold (OR 2.1 [95% CI 1.2–3.7]) in a meta-analysis of three clinical trials.[19] Another meta-analysis showed that clonidine was better than placebo in successfully quitting smoking but that many experienced side effects from clonidine therapy. Thus, the therapeutic benefits of clonidine must be weighed against the side-effect profile of this drug, which may limit its usefulness as an intervention for smoking cessation.[38]

Adverse Events/Warnings and Precautions

Adverse events associated with clonidine therapy are mainly due to the anticholinergic properties of clonidine, commonly presenting with dry mouth, dizziness, sedation, and constipation.[37] The transdermal patch may cause some local skin irritation, but in terms of the anticholinergic adverse events listed above, patients may experience them to a lesser degree because of the more constant release of clonidine with the patch.[39]

As clonidine is used to treat hypertension, it may lower blood pressure and cause orthostatic hypotension.[38] Blood pressure should be monitored while on clonidine for smoking cessation, particularly for those who are older (>65 years) as fall risk is a concern in older adults.

The efficacy and safety of clonidine have not been adequately studied in pregnant smokers.[37] It is recommended that pregnant smokers be encouraged to quit smoking without the aid of medications.[19]

Clonidine can cause sedation, so patients should be careful when driving or operating large machinery.[19,37]

Drug Interactions

Clonidine in combination with alcohol, barbiturates, or other sedating medications may enhance CNS depression.[37] Patients should avoid this combination.

Risk of hypotension is increased when clonidine is coadministered with other antihypertensive agents or an antipsychotic agent.[37] Older adults in particular should be monitored for orthostatic hypotension and fall risk.

Caution should be used when administering clonidine with drugs that slow heart rate (e.g., β-blockers, calcium-channel blockers). There have been cases of sinus bradycardia due to this interaction.[37]

NORTRIPTYLINE

Nortriptyline is a tricyclic antidepressant that is FDA approved to treat depression and may be used off-label as a second-line intervention for smoking cessation.[19,40] Second-line therapies, such as nortriptyline, may be used when first-line therapies are contraindicated or when their use is unsuccessful in achieving smoking cessation.[19]

Mechanism of Action

The mechanism of action for assisting in smoking cessation is unknown, as nortriptyline has not been formally studied for this indication in preclinical or clinical trials. It is known that nortriptyline inhibits the reuptake of norepinephrine and serotonin, which may contribute to its efficacy in smoking cessation. Some proposed rationales are briefly described below:[41]

- Smoking cessation causes depression, and depression increases need for smoking or relapse. Nortriptyline is an antidepressant that can prevent depression while quitting smoking.
- The noradrenergic effects of nicotine are replaced with the noradrenergic effects of nortriptyline. This modulation of the noradrenergic receptor systems decreases withdrawal symptoms, including craving.
- Nortriptyline is a weak nicotine receptor antagonist (i.e., having anticholinergic properties), which causes dry mouth and altered taste perception and thus decreases craving.

Dosage and Administration

Nortriptyline should be initiated at 25 mg per day and gradually increased over a period of 10 days to 5 weeks until reaching the target dose of 75–100 mg per day. Therapy should begin 10–28 days prior to the quit date to reach steady-state concentrations by the time target dose is reached. The duration of nortriptyline therapy is 12 weeks, but it may be extended up to 6 months.[19,41] Nortriptyline should be slowly tapered off when discontinuing therapy to avoid withdrawal symptoms (e.g., nausea, headache, malaise).[40]

Therapeutic drug monitoring levels have not been established for the efficacy of nortriptyline in smoking cessation; however, nortriptyline plasma levels may be monitored for patients with depression and/or monitored as needed to prevent toxicity.[19,41]

Pharmacokinetics

Nortriptyline is rapidly absorbed following oral administration, with maximum plasma concentrations achieved within 4–9 h.[41] Oral bioavailability ranges from 46–70%.[43] There is high interindividual variability in time to steady-state concentrations; it may take 6–15 days to reach steady state. Nortriptyline is highly bound to plasma proteins.[42]

Nortriptyline is metabolized in the liver by CYP2D6 to produce primarily the major active metabolite 10-hydroxynortriptyline, which has the potential to accumulate in older adults.[43,44] Additionally, the half-life of nortriptyline is longer in older adults than in younger patients. Nortriptyline half-life ranges from 14–79 h: 14–51 h, with an average of 26 h, for younger patients; 23.5–79 h, with an average of 45 h, for older adults.[45] Thus, lower doses may be warranted for older adults than younger patients. Nortriptyline is mainly excreted as metabolites in the urine (>80%).[42]

Clinical Efficacy

Although nortriptyline has not been evaluated in as many smokers as NRT and bupropion SR have been, nortriptyline appears to be efficacious in quitting smoking.[25] Compared to placebo, nortriptyline about doubled (OR 1.8 [95% CI 1.3–2.6]) the likelihood of achieving smoking cessation in a meta-analysis of four clinical trials.[19] Nortriptyline is recommended as second-line therapy because it is associated with serious side effects that the healthcare provider and patient must weigh against the benefits of using a non-FDA-approved medication for smoking cessation.[19]

Contraindications

Coadministration with MAOIs is contraindicated due to increased risk of developing serotonin syndrome. A minimum of 14 days must pass from time of discontinuing nortriptyline and initiating an MAOI, and vice versa.[40]

Nortriptyline is contraindicated in patients who are recovering from an acute MI episode because nortriptyline is associated with increased risk of arrhythmias and impaired myocardial contractility.[19,40]

Adverse Events/Warnings and Precautions

Common adverse events associated with exposure to nortriptyline include dry mouth, sedation, constipation, urinary retention, blurred vision, dizziness, and tremors.[19,40] Patients should be advised to use caution while driving or operating large machinery since nortriptyline can cause sedation and impair mental/physical abilities.[19,40] Nortriptyline has been associated with risk of both hyperglycemia and hypoglycemia.[40] Patients with diabetes should be able to recognize signs and symptoms of having low and high blood glucose levels and monitor their glucose levels more closely while on nortriptyline.

Similar to bupropion SR, because nortriptyline is an antidepressant, it has a black box warning regarding suicidal thoughts and behaviors in children, adolescents, and young adults. Patients should be closely monitored for suicidality or changes in behavior, and families/caregivers should be advised to keep close observation and to communicate concerns with the healthcare providers.[40]

Consider the risk of overdose prior to initiating nortriptyline in patients because ingestion of an excessive amount of nortriptyline can result in seizures, coma, and/or severe, life-threatening cardiovascular toxicity (death included).[19,40]

Nortriptyline may trigger mania in patients with bipolar disorder and thus should not be used to treat bipolar depression.[40]

Nortriptyline, which dilates pupils, may precipitate angle-closure glaucoma in patients with anatomically narrow angles without a patent iridectomy.[40]

The efficacy and safety of nortriptyline have not been adequately studied in pregnant smokers.[40] It is recommended that pregnant smokers be encouraged to quit smoking without the aid of medications.[19]

Drug Interactions

As mentioned above, nortriptyline should not be coadministered with MAOIs. Serotonin syndrome may also be precipitated by the concomitant use of serotonergic drugs such as triptans, buspirone, and St. John's Wort. Patients should be monitored for symptoms of serotonin syndrome (e.g., agitation, coma, tachycardia, hyperthermia, rigidity, seizures, vomiting, diarrhea).[40]

There are a number of drugs that may interact with nortriptyline. In general, the following should be used with caution when administered with nortriptyline: other tricyclic antidepressants, other anticholinergic drugs, other sympathomimetic drugs, and alcohol. Patients should be monitored for amplified side-effect profiles of either interacting drug.[40]

Nortriptyline is metabolized by CYP2D6. Drugs that inhibit this enzyme (e.g., quinidine, cimetidine, antidepressants, flecainide) will increase nortriptyline levels. Changes in nortriptyline doses may be necessary during times of drug initiation or discontinuation.[40]

COMBINATION THERAPY FOR SMOKING CESSATION

Studies have demonstrated that combination therapy prevents nicotine withdrawal symptoms better than a single intervention alone, but selection of treatments will heavily depend on patient preference (e.g., tolerability of side effects, cost of product).[19]

The U.S. Department of Health and Human Services recognizes combination therapies comprising first-line medications as first-line combination therapies and those combinations mixed with a second-line medication as second-line combination therapies.[19]

A few studies have shown promising results with varenicline plus nicotine transdermal patch and varenicline plus bupropion SR;[19] however, other studies have shown no significant difference when comparing varenicline plus nicotine transdermal patch to varenicline monotherapy.[46,47,48] Additional studies will be needed to support use of combination therapy with varenicline.[49,50]

- First-line combination therapy
  - Nicotine transdermal patch + bupropion SR
  - Nicotine transdermal patch + nicotine inhaler
  - Nicotine transdermal patch + nicotine gum/nasal spray
- Second-line combination therapy
  - Nicotine transdermal patch + nortriptyline
  - Nicotine transdermal patch + second-generation antidepressants

Table 23.3—Medications for Smoking Cessation

Medication	Dosage
First-Line Medications	
Nicotine Transdermal Patch[19,51]	■ >10 cigarettes per day: Initially 21 mg/24 h for 6–8 weeks; then 14 mg/24 h for 2–4 weeks; then 7 mg/24 h for 2–4 weeks ■ ≤10 cigarettes per day: Initially 14 mg/24 h for 6 weeks; then 7 mg/24 h for 2–4 weeks ■ There are single-dose patches for lighter smokers: 22 mg/24 h and 11 mg/24 h
Nicotine Gum[19]	■ ≥25 cigarettes per day: 4 mg ■ <25 cigarettes per day: 2 mg ■ Initially 1 piece every 1–2 h for 6 weeks; then 1 piece every 2–4 h for 3 weeks; then 1 piece every 4–8 h for 3 weeks ■ Maximum of 24 pieces per day
Nicotine Lozenge[19]	■ First cigarette within 30 min of waking: 4 mg ■ First cigarette more than 30 min after waking: 2 mg ■ Initially at least 9 lozenges per day for 6 weeks; continue use for up to 12 weeks ■ Maximum of 20 lozenges per day
Nicotine Inhalers[19]	■ One dose is equal to 1 inhalation; each cartridge delivers >80 inhalations or 4 mg total ■ Initially 6–16 cartridges per day for up to 6 months ■ Gradually reduce dose for last 3 months of therapy
Nicotine Nasal Spray[19]	■ 1 dose is equal to 1 spray; each spray delivers 0.5 mg (1 spray in each nostril equals 1 mg total); each bottle delivers ~100 doses ■ Initially 1–2 doses per hour, increase as needed for symptom relief; continue use for 3–6 months ■ Recommended minimum of 8 doses per day ■ Maximum of 40 doses per day (i.e., 5 doses per hour)
Varenicline[6,29]	■ Begin 1 week before quit date ■ Initially 0.5 mg once daily for 3 days; then 0.5 mg twice daily for 4 days; then on day 8 (quit day) 1 mg twice daily for 3 months or up to 6 months ■ Dose adjustment for severe renal impairment: maximum of 0.5 mg twice daily
Bupropion SR[19,36]	■ Begin 1–2 weeks before quit date ■ Initially 150 mg once daily for 3 days; then 150 mg twice daily (at least 8 h apart) for 7–12 weeks or up to 6 months (post-quit day) ■ Maximum of 300 mg per day ■ Dose adjustment for moderate to severe hepatic impairment: maximum of 150 mg every other day
Second-Line Medications	
Clonidine[19]	■ Begin up to 3 days before quit date ■ Oral tablet: initially 0.1 mg twice daily ■ Transdermal patch: initially 0.1 mg once daily ■ Increase by 0.1 mg/day every week, as needed; continue use for 3–10 weeks ■ Maximum ~0.4 mg per day ■ Gradually reduce dose over 2–4 days at end of therapy
Nortriptyline[19]	■ Begin 10–28 days before quit date ■ Initially 25 mg per day; gradually increase over 10 days to 5 weeks until at target dose of 75–100 mg per day; continue use for 12 weeks or up to 6 months ■ Gradually reduce dose at end of therapy

NICOTINE TRANSDERMAL PATCH + BUPROPION SR

A meta-analysis of three clinical trials showed that the combination of nicotine transdermal patch and bupropion SR at recommended doses and treatment duration was superior to placebo in maintaining long-term smoking cessation (OR 2.5 [95% CI 1.9–3.4]).[19]

NICOTINE TRANSDERMAL PATCH + NICOTINE INHALER

A meta-analysis of two clinical trials that studied the efficacy of nicotine patch (15 mg) plus nicotine inhaler compared to placebo determined that the NRT combination was better at achieving long-term smoking cessation (OR 2.2 [95% CI 1.3–3.6]).[19]

NICOTINE TRANSDERMAL PATCH + NICOTINE GUM/NASAL SPRAY

A meta-analysis of three clinical trials concluded that chronic nicotine transdermal patch therapy (>14 weeks; ranging from 18–24 weeks) plus ad libitum short-acting NRT (gum or nasal spray) was better than placebo for long-term smoking cessation (OR 3.6 [95% CI 2.5–5.2]).[19]

NICOTINE TRANSDERMAL PATCH + NORTRIPTYLINE

A meta-analysis of two clinical trials that compared the efficacy of nicotine transdermal patch plus nortriptyline to that of placebo showed that combination therapy was superior for achieving long-term smoking cessation (OR 2.3 [95% CI 1.3–4.2]).[19]

NICOTINE TRANSDERMAL PATCH + SECOND-GENERATION ANTIDEPRESSANTS

A meta-analysis of three clinical trials determined that the combination of nicotine transdermal patch (highest dose being 21 or 22 mg) and second-generation antidepressants (paroxetine 20 mg or venlafaxine 22 mg) was better than placebo in maintaining long-term smoking cessation (OR 2.0 [95% CI 1.2–3.4]).[18]

Table 23.4—Combination Therapy for Smoking Cessation

- First-line combination therapy options
  - Nicotine transdermal patch + bupropion SR
  - Nicotine transdermal patch + nicotine inhaler
  - Nicotine transdermal patch + nicotine gum
  - Nicotine transdermal patch + nicotine nasal spray
- Second-line combination therapy options
  - Nicotine transdermal patch + nortriptyline
  - Nicotine transdermal patch + second-generation antidepressants

MONOGRAPHS

Bupropion SR (Zyban): https://dailymed.nlm.nih.gov/dailymed/drugInfo. cfm?setid=a3327c31-d987-40ec-b3b5-097bbf2f4f8c

Clonidine (Catapres-TTS): https://dailymed.nlm.nih.gov/dailymed/drugInfo. cfm?setid=a842ab83-3531-44dd-a8a8-64dd89e87026 and https://dailymed. nlm.nih.gov/dailymed/drugInfo.cfm?setid=fe0f5dcb-65dd-4d31-80d6-8b97eb040063

Nicotine gum: https://dailymed.nlm.nih.gov/dailymed/drugInfo.cfm?setid=3872c622-1a30-459c-b878-61648bb30627

Nicotine inhaler (Nicotrol): https://dailymed.nlm.nih.gov/dailymed/drugInfo. cfm?setid=62245d7d-b50d-48d9-9f03-071c61620ccf

Nicotine lozenge (Nicorette): https://dailymed.nlm.nih.gov/dailymed/drugInfo. cfm?setid=fdee1637-8049-4bc5-b196-b6d854c9f9f3

Nicotine nasal spray (Nicotrol): https://dailymed.nlm.nih.gov/dailymed/drugInfo.cfm?setid=acb7d02d-249b-4645-ac1b-8ff9a56dd244

Nicotine transdermal patch: https://dailymed.nlm.nih.gov/dailymed/drugInfo. cfm?setid=8a5c7835-3ab1-b3f8-e9db-e5d0cb42b59e

Nortriptyline: https://dailymed.nlm.nih.gov/dailymed/drugInfo.cfm?setid=b58d473a-b19f-4d2a-b1ae-dd398d7a29e1

Varenicline (Chantix): https://dailymed.nlm.nih.gov/dailymed/drugInfo. cfm?setid=f0ff4f27-5185-4881-a749-c6b7a0ca5696

REFERENCES

1. Barua RS, Rigotti NA, Benowitz NL, et al. 2018 ACC expert consensus decision pathway on tobacco cessation treatment. *J Am Coll Cardiol* 2018;72(25):3332–3365. DOI:10.1016/j.jacc.2018.10.027

2. Cornelius ME, Loretan CG, Wang TW, Jamal A, Homa DM. Tobacco product use among adults – United States, 2020. *MMWR Morb Mortal Wkly Rep* 2022;71(11):397-405 DOI:http://dx.doi.org/10.15585/mmwr. mm7111a1

3. Park-Lee E, Ren C, Cooper M, Cornelius M, Jamal A, Cullen KA. Tobacco product use among middle and high school students—United States, 2022. *MMWR Morb Mortal Wkly Rep* 2022;71(45):1429-1435 DOI:http://dx.doi. org/10.15585/mmwr.mm7145a1

4. Glantz SA, Bareham DW. E-cigarettes: use, effects on smoking, risks, and policy implications. *Annu Rev Public Health* 2018;39:215–235

5. Miech R, Patrick ME, O'Malley PM, Johnston LD. E-cigarette use as a predictor of cigarette smoking: results from a 1-year follow-up of a national sample of 12th grade students. *Tob Control* 2017;26(e2):e106–e111

6. Barrington-Trimis JL, Yang Z, Schiff S, et al. E-cigarette product characteristics and subsequent frequency of cigarette smoking. Pediatrics. 2020; 145(5):e20191652

7. U.S. Department of Health and Human Services. *The health consequences of smoking—50 years of progress: a report of the surgeon general.* Atlanta, Centers for Disease Control and Prevention, Coordinating Center for Health Promotion, National Center for Chronic Disease Prevention and Health Promotion, Office on Smoking and Health, 2014. Available from http://www.surgeongeneral.gov/library/reports/50-years-of-progress/full-report.pdf

8. Centers for Disease Control and Prevention. Outbreak of lung injury associated with e-cigarette use, or Vaping, Products, 2020 [Internet]. Accessed 8 February 2023. Available from https://www.cdc.gov/tobacco/basic_information/e-cigarettes/severe-lung-disease.html

9. American Diabetes Association. 5. Facilitating behavior change and well-being to improve health outcomes: *Standards of Care in Diabetes—2023. Diabetes Care* 2023;46(Suppl. 1):S68–S96

10. Foy CG, Bell RA, Farmer DF, et al. Smoking and incidence of diabetes among U.S. adults: findings from the Insulin Resistance Atherosclerosis Study. *Diabetes Care* 2005;28(10):2501–2507

11. Multiple Risk Factor Intervention Trial Research Group. Multiple risk factor intervention trial: risk factor changes and mortality results. *JAMA* 1982;248(12):1465–1477

12. Jousilahti P, Vartiainen E, Tuomilehto J, Puska P. Sex, age, cardiovascular risk factors, and coronary heart disease: a prospective follow-up study of 14,786 middle-aged men and women in Finland. *Circulation* 1999;99(9): 1165–1172

13. Richard JL, Ducimetiere P, Cambien F. [Tobacco, mortality and morbidity of atherosclerotic cardiovascular diseases: a prospective study in Paris]. In French. *Bull Schwiez Akad Med Wiss* 1979;35(1–3):51–69

14. Pan A, Wang Y, Talaei M, Hu FB. Relation of smoking with total mortality and cardiovascular events among patients with diabetes: a meta-analysis and systematic review. *Circulation* 2015;132(19):1795–1804

15. American Diabetes Association. Smoking and diabetes. *Diabetes Care* 2004;27(Suppl. 1):S74–S75

16. Qin R, Chen T, Lou Q, Yu D. Excess risk of mortality and cardiovascular events associated with smoking among patients with diabetes: meta-analysis of observational prospective studies. *Int J Cardiol* 2013;167(2):342–350

17. Wu AD, Lindson N, Hartmann-Boyce J, et al. Smoking cessation for secondary prevention of cardiovascular disease. *Cochrane Database Syst Rev* 2022;8(8):CD014936

18. Thorndike AN, Regan S, Rigotti NA. The treatment of smoking by US physicians during ambulatory visits: 1994–2003. *Am J Public Health* 2007; 97(10):1878–1883

19. Fiore MC, Jaen CR, Baker TB, et al. *Treating tobacco use and dependence: 2008 update. Clinical Practice Guideline.* Rockville, MD, Agency for Healthcare Research and Quality, May 2008. Available from https://www.ahrq.gov/ professionals/clinicians-providers/guidelines-recommendations/tobacco/ clinicians/update/index.html. Accessed 8 February 2023

20. Stead LF, Loilpillai P, Fanshawe T, Lancaster T. Combined pharmacotherapy and behavioural interventions for smoking cessation. *Cochrane Database Syst Rev* 2016;3:CD008286. DOI:10.1002/14651858.CD008286.pub3

21. Krist AH; U.S. Preventive Services Task Force. Interventions for tobacco smoking cessation in adults, including pregnant persons: U.S. Preventive Services Task Force recommendation statement. *JAMA* 2021;325(3):265–279

22. Hughes JR, Hatsukami D. Signs and symptoms of tobacco withdrawal. *Arch Gen Psychiatry* 1986;43(3):289–294

23. Hughes JR. Tobacco withdrawal in self-quitters. *J Consult Clin Psychol* 1992;60(5):689–697

24. Stead LF, Perera R, Bullen C, et al. Nicotine replacement therapy for smoking cessation. *Cochrane Database Syst Rev* 2012;11:CD000146. DOI:10.1002/14651858.CD000146.pub4

25. Nides M. Update on pharmacologic options for smoking cessation treatment. *Am J Med* 2008;121(4A):S20–S31

26. Drug and Therapeutics Bulletin. Republished: nicotine and health. *BMJ* 2014;349:2014.7.0264rep. DOI:10.1136/bmj.2014.7.0264rep

27. Woolf KJ, Zabad MN, Post JM, et al. Effect of nicotine replacement therapy on cardiovascular outcomes after acute coronary syndromes. *Am J Cardiol* 2012;110(7):968–970

28. Frishman WH. Smoking cessation pharmacotherapy: nicotine and non-nicotine preparations. *Prev Cardio* 2007;10(2 Suppl. 1):10–22

29. Chantix (varenicline) [prescribing information]. New York, Pfizer Labs— Division of Pfizer, Inc., December 2016. Available from https://dailymed. nlm.nih.gov/dailymed/drugInfo.cfm?setid=f0ff4f27-5185-4881-a749-c6b7a0ca5696

30. Gonzales D, Rennard SI, Nides M, et al. Varenicline, an alpha4beta2 nicotinic acetylcholine receptor partial agonist, vs sustained-release bupropion and placebo for smoking cessation: a randomized controlled trial. *JAMA* 2006;296(1):47–55

31. Jorenby DE, Hays JT, Rigotti NA, et al. Efficacy of varenicline, an alpha-4beta2 nicotinic acetylcholine receptor partial agonist, vs placebo or sus-

tained-release bupropion for smoking cessation: a randomized controlled trial. *JAMA* 2006;296(1):56–63

32. Leone FT, Zhang Y, Evers-Casey S, et al. Initiating pharmacologic treatment in tobacco-dependent adults. An official American Thoracic Society Clinical Practice Guideline. *Am J Respir Crit Care Med* 2020;202(2):e5-e31

33. Anthenelli RM, Benowitz NL, West R, et al. Neuropsychiatric safety and efficacy of varenicline, bupropion, and nicotine patch in smokers with and without psychiatric disorders (EAGLES): a double-blind, randomised, placebo-controlled clinical trial. *Lancet* 2016;387(10037):2507–2520

34. U.S. Food and Drug Administration. Information for healthcare professionals: varenicline (marketed as Chantix) and bupropion (marketed as Zyban, Wellbutrin, and generics). Published 1 July 2009. Available from http://wayback.archive-it.org/7993/20170112032419/http://www.fda.gov/Drugs/DrugSafety/PostmarketDrugSafetyInformationforPatientsandProviders/DrugSafetyInformationforHeathcareProfessionals/ucm169986.htm. Accessed 8 February 2023

35. FDA Drug Safety Communication. FDA revises description of mental health side effects of the stop-smoking medicines Chantix (varenicline) and Zyban (bupropion) to reflect clinical trial findings. Published 16 December 2016. Available from https://www.fda.gov/Drugs/DrugSafety/ucm532221.htm. Accessed 8 February 2023

36. Zyban (bupropion hydrochloride) [prescribing information]. Research Triangle Park, NC, GlaxoSmithKline, May 2017. Available from https://dailymed.nlm.nih.gov/dailymed/drugInfo.cfm?setid=a3327c31-d987-40ec-b3b5-097bbf2f4f8c

37. Catapres (clonidine hydrochloride) [prescribing information]. Ridgefield, CT, Boehringer Ingelheim Pharmaceuticals, Inc., September 2016. Available from https://dailymed.nlm.nih.gov/dailymed/drugInfo.cfm?setid=d7f569dc-6bed-42dc-9bec-940a9e6b090d

38. Gourlay SG, Stead LF, Benowitz N. Clonidine for smoking cessation. *Cochrane Database Syst Rev* 2004;3:CD000058. DOI:10.1002/14651858.CD000058.pub2

39. Catapres-TTS (clonidine) [prescribing information]. Ridgefield, CT, Boehringer Ingelheim Pharmaceuticals, Inc., August 2016. Available from https://dailymed.nlm.nih.gov/dailymed/drugInfo.cfm?setid=fe0f5dcb-65dd-4d31-80d6-8b97eb040063

40. Pamelor (nortriptyline hydrochloride) [prescribing information]. North Wales, PA, TEVA Pharmaceuticals USA, Inc., June 2016. Available from https://dailymed.nlm.nih.gov/dailymed/drugInfo.cfm?setid=b58d473a-b19f-4d2a-b1ae-dd398d7a29e1

41. Hughes JR, Stead LF, Lancaster T. Nortriptyline for smoking cessation: a review. *Nicotine Tob Res* 2005;7(4):491–499

42. Alexanderson B. Pharmacokinetics of nortriptyline in man after single and multiple oral doses: the predictability of steady-state plasma concentrations from single-dose plasma-level data. *Eur J Clin Pharmacol* 1972;4(2):82–91

43. Rubin EH, Biggs JT, Preskorn SH. Nortriptyline pharmacokinetics and plasma levels: implications for clinical practice. *J Clin Psychiatry* 1985;46(10):418–424

44. Venkatakrishnan K, von Moltke LL, Greenblatt DJ. Nortriptyline E-10-hydroxylation in vitro is mediated by human CYP2D6 (high affinity) and CYP3A4 (low affinity): implications for interactions with enzyme-inducing drugs. *J Clin Pharmacol* 1999;39(6):567–577

45. Dawling S, Crome P, Braithwaite R. Pharmacokinetics of single oral doses of nortriptyline in depressed elderly hospital patients and young healthy volunteers. *Clin Pharmacokinet* 1980;5(4):394–401

46. Hajek P, Smith KM, Dhanji AR, McRobbie H. Is a combination of varenicline and nicotine patch more effective in helping smokers quit than varenicline alone? A randomized controlled trial. *BMC Med* 2013;11:140

47. Ramon JM, Morchon S, Baena A, Masuet-Aumatell C. Combining varenicline and nicotine patches: a randomized controlled trial study in smoking cessation. *BMC Med* 2014;12:172

48. Baker TB, Piper ME, Smith SS, Bolt DM, Stein JH, Fiore MC. Effects of combined varenicline with nicotine patch and of extended treatment duration on smoking cessation: A randomized clinical trial. *JAMA* 2021;326(15):1485-1493

49. Chang PH, Chiang CH, Ho WC, et al. Combination therapy of varenicline with nicotine replacement therapy is better than varenicline alone: a systematic review and meta-analysis of randomized controlled trials. *BMC Public Health* 2015;15:689

50. Vogeler T, McClain C, Evoy KE. Combination bupropion SR and varenicline for smoking cessation: a systematic review. *Am J Drug Alcohol Abuse* 2016;42(2):129–139

51. NicoDerm CQ (nicotine patch, extended release) [prescribing information]. Moon Township, PA, GlaxoSmithKline, May 2016. Available from https://dailymed.nlm.nih.gov/dailymed/drugInfo.cfm?setid=93b2d1b9-83c1-40b5-b6af-90c38c8d6cef

Chapter 24

Medications for the Management of Neuropathy

DAMIANNE BRAND-EUBANKS, PHARMD

Neuropathy, a disease or dysfunction of one or more nerves, is most commonly linked to metabolic, vascular, and/or immune origins, and is one of the leading complications associated with T1D and T2D. There are three primary types of neuropathy found in patients with diabetes: diabetic polyneuropathy, autonomic neuropathy, and focal neuropathy (see Table 24.1). The two most common types of diabetic-induced neuropathy are diabetic polyneuropathy, also known as distal symmetric sensorimotor polyneuropathy (DSPN), and diabetic autonomic neuropathy (DAN).

DSPN is a chronic, nerve-length-dependent, sensorimotor neuropathy that affects at least one-third of those with T1D or T2D and up to one-quarter of those with impaired glucose tolerance.[1] Progression of DSPN differs between T1D and T2D. With T2D, there is a milder functional defect early on that can progress to structural degenerative changes, eventually resulting in nerve fiber loss. In comparison, the late structural phase of DSPN affects people with T1D more severely.[2] People with DSPN often have length-dependent symptoms—which usually affect the feet first, as they are the longest nerves in the body—with these symptoms progressing proximally.[3,4] The symptoms begin as sensory and are categorized as either "positive," due to excess or inappropriate nerve activity, or "negative," due to reduced nerve activity (see Table 24.2).[1] Although positive symptoms can lead to the need for pharmacological modulation of varied levels of pain, negative symptoms, such as decreased sensation, can increase risk of painless foot ulcers or both proprioceptive impairment and loss of balance, leading to falls. Negative symptoms are usually not treated; rather, there is an attempt to avoid further damage through better glycemic control.

Chronic hyperglycemia, resulting in microvascular and neuronal damage, is one of the main mechanisms by which DSPN is theorized to develop; however, more needs to be known to understand why glucose control as a treatment works better for T1D. Nerve biopsies of patients diagnosed with DSPN have shown a thickening of the basement membranes of vessels feeding damaged neurons and a greater variation overall of vessel lumen thickness. Damaged blood vessels display a poor vasodilatory response to nitric oxide, and ischemia is prominent in the microvasculature. Following this cascade, hypoxia will eventually result, leading to neuronal starvation and death. Increased influx of glucose and other sugar molecules may increase basement membrane thickening through the polyol flux pathway.[5] This pathway may also be responsible for the destruction of neuronal

Table 24.1—Primary Types of Diabetes-Induced Neuropathy

Origin	Common presentations
Peripheral Polyneuropathy	
Distal Symmetrical	■ Most common in T2D ■ Glove/stocking loss of sensation (pain, vibration, temperature, proprioception) ■ Loss of motor nerve function with clawed toes and small muscle wasting in hands and flexor muscles ■ Charcot joints (loss of sensation results in joint and ligament degeneration, particularly in the foot, causing deterioration of weight-bearing joints in foot and ankle) ■ Acute painful neuropathy with burning pain in legs and feet
Autonomic Neuropathy	
Gastrointestinal	■ Constipation ■ Gastroparesis ■ Diarrhea (hallmark nocturnal)
Cardiac	■ Resting tachycardia ■ Exercise intolerance ■ Orthostatic hypotension (sleep in sitting or semirecumbent position due to risk of silent MI or cardiac death)
Urogenital	■ Loss of bladder tone ■ Urinary retention ■ Risk for bladder infection ■ Decreased sensation of bladder fullness/urge ■ Overflow incontinence ■ ED ■ Female sexual dysfunction
Sweat Glands	■ Anhidrosis: sudomotor dysfunction ■ Gustatory sweating (usually after eating)
Focal Neuropathy	
Amyotrophic	■ Uncommon (occur more often in elderly with poor glycemic control) ■ Proximal thigh muscle pain and weakness ■ Wrist or foot drop

Source: Triplitt.[8]

supporting cells, more specifically the Schwann cells, perpetuating eventual axonal changes. This is thought to be more damaging to those neurons less protected by the blood-nerve barrier, such as the dorsal root ganglia. These changes may include an increase of intra-neuronal sodium, which slows nerve conduction in both sensory and motor neurons. Oxidative stress, in tandem with the resultant mitochondrial dysfunction through the polyol pathway is another mechanism by which neuronal damage and ultimately DSPN is theorized to occur, with free radicals damaging neuronal tissue.[6] Antioxidant levels in patients with diabetes are depleted, allowing formation of free radicals through the oxidation of glucose and

Table 24.2—Positive and Negative Symptoms of Polyneuropathy

Common symptoms of peripheral neuropathy		
	Sensory Symptoms	Motor Symptoms
Positive	■ Paresthesia ■ Pain: burning, squeezing or tightness, electric shock-like, hypersensitivity	■ Fasciculation ■ Cramps
Negative	■ Numbness ■ Reduced or absent sensation ■ Postural instability	■ Weakness ■ Atrophy

Source: Triplitt.[8]

other cellular mechanisms. Free radicals form, and the damage produced can ultimately lead to neuronal cell death.[7]

DAN is the most diverse form of neuropathy affecting patients with diabetes, as this can involve the cardiovascular, gastrointestinal, and genitourinary systems (see Table 24.1). Autonomic neuropathy does not primarily involve large nerve fibers, as previously described for DSPN. Cardiovascular complications associated with DAN can lead to hypotensive episodes, irregular heartbeat, instability related to anesthetic administration, and an increased risk for both MI and sudden death. Gastrointestinal neuropathy can involve the gastrointestinal tract as a whole and is commonly identified by gastroparesis and esophageal difficulties. Genitourinary neuropathy occurs through loss of coordination of smooth muscle and often results in urinary incontinence issues and sexual dysfunction in both men and women with diabetes. Therapies are available to treat all forms of DAN, although most include intensive glucose and metabolic control coupled with medications addressing the symptoms associated with the affected organ system.

Previously investigated pharmacological interventions for pain associated with diabetic neuropathy include pregabalin, gabapentin, certain tricyclic antidepressants (TCAs), opioids, antidepressants, and other anticonvulsants.

ANTICONVULSANTS

GABA ANALOGS

The GABA analogs, gabapentin and pregabalin, are structurally related to the neurotransmitter γ-aminobutyric acid (GABA), but do not influence GABA receptors or use this pathway as a mechanism of action. These agents bind to the α_2-δ subunit of neural presynaptic voltage-gated calcium channels, which decrease calcium flux.[9] Subsequently, decreased neurotransmitter release from these neurons occurs, thus limiting neuronal excitation. This mechanism is theorized to account for the analgesic effect and decrease in neuropathic pain.[10]

Gabapentin was initially introduced for treatment of seizures and was later found to have use in diabetic-induced neuropathic pain, though it still does not have FDA approval for this indication. Oral gabapentin has a nonlinear kinetic profile. For instance, the bioavailability of oral gabapentin is reduced from 60 to 33% as the dose increases from 900 to 3,200 mg/day. In addition, administering gabapentin with food increases bioavailability by 10%, without a change in time to maximum concentration (T_{max}). This is considered to be a slight change, so gabapentin may be administered with or without food. Although gabapentin does have a manufacturer-approved maximum dose of 3,600 mg/day, it has been studied at higher doses with similarly successful response.[10]

Pregabalin was approved for use by the FDA for DSPN in 2004. Pregabalin displays linear kinetics, with peak concentrations achieved 1.5 h after administration and steady-state concentrations achieved after 1–2 days of continuous dosing. Pregabalin dosing is recommended to not exceed 300 mg/day in order to mitigate side effects that are observed at higher doses, even though greater response has been observed at doses of up to 600 mg/day.[11,12,13]

Tolerance may develop with continued gabapentin use, while tolerance to pregabalin has not been reported to develop. Continued monitoring to assure successful therapy is still recommended for pregabalin therapy.[11] Common side effects of the GABA analogs include sedation, dizziness, CNS depression, blurred vision, balance issues, tremors, and confusion.

Both gabapentin and pregabalin are primarily cleared by the renal system. Dosing adjustments based on renal impairment may be required. It is important to note that both agents are dialyzable. The half-lives for these agents are 5–7 h, which may be increased in patients with impaired renal function. Current investigation in this area suggests caution with both gabapentin and pregabalin, as they have been associated with an increased risk of cardiac events linked to alteration of myogenic tone and the resultant fluid retention. GABA analogs have not been adequately studied in patients who are pregnant or breast-feeding. They should only be used when the benefit of therapy outweighs the potential risk of maternal/fetal harm.[14] Administration of GABA analogs with other CNS depressants may increase risk of sedation and other similar side effects. Also, caution should be exercised if administering pregabalin with TZDs (e.g., pioglitazone and rosiglitazone), as this combination may increase the risk of weight gain and edema. Discontinuation of either gabapentin or pregabalin should be performed in a downward titration, as withdrawal-like symptoms including sweating, dizziness, sleep disturbances, and muscle pain may occur with abrupt discontinuation of therapy.[11]

OTHER ANTICONVULSANTS

Carbamazepine and valproic acid and its sodium salt (sodium valproate) are other anticonvulsants used off-label to treat DSPN, though more studies are needed to prove both effectiveness in pain treatment and safety for this indication. The mechanism of action for carbamazepine is related to its ability to block voltage-dependent sodium channels, thus reducing ectopic nerve discharge and stabilizing neural membranes while minimizing the effect of normal nerve conductance. Although chemically related to the TCAs, carbamazepine is not considered to have a mechanistic effect on neural transmitters. Carbamazepine has shown to be effective in the treatment of trigeminal neuralgia, but may be used for treating DSPN if patients are refractory to other treatments, due to its difficult-to-manage dosage and side-effect profile.[15]

Valproic acid, in addition to its inhibition of glutamate/N-methyl-D-aspartate (NMDA) receptor-mediated neuronal excitation, has been shown to be a potent inhibitor of histone deacetylase (HDAC) enzymes. HDAC regulation is a possible new approach in the treatment of T2D to modify the metabolism of glucose and fatty acid and the secondarily associated neuronal damage. HDAC is thought to promote the development, proliferation, differentiation, and function of pancreatic β-cells and ameliorate microvascular complications in later stages of the disease.[16] Valproic acid (potentially teratogenic) and carbamazepine should be avoided in women of childbearing age with diabetes.[16]

ANTIDEPRESSANTS

DULOXETINE

Duloxetine is FDA approved for the treatment of DSPN as a dose-dependent, dual-acting selective serotonin-norepinephrine reuptake inhibitor (SNRI). Its effects on serotonin (5-HT) and norepinephrine are considered to be responsible for the analgesic effect of duloxetine.[17] Serotonin and norepinephrine elicit neurogenic transmission in the brainstem and spinal column, and are theorized to minimize pain transmission from the periphery to the CNS via these transmission pathways. Duloxetine is extensively metabolized in the liver and is a substrate of the enzymes CYP2D6 and CYP1A2. It is also a moderate inhibitor of both enzymes, so care should be taken to avoid drug-drug interactions when given concurrently. Common side effects with duloxetine may include nausea/vomiting, dizziness, fatigue, and somnolence. These side effects can occur within the first 8 weeks of treatment or at times of dosage increase, but they typically dissipate with time. Duloxetine has been shown in multiple studies to be well tolerated with slow titration in elderly patients. Dose adjustments for hepatic and renally impaired patients are not necessary.[12,18]

OTHER ANTIDEPRESSANTS: SELECTIVE SEROTONIN-NOREPINEPHRINE REUPTAKE INHIBITORS

Venlafaxine and desvenlafaxine have similar mechanisms of action to those of duloxetine, but little evidence is available to support their effectiveness in DSPN. They are usually considered second-line DSPN treatment medications. These SNRIs are often better tolerated and have fewer drug interactions when compared to TCAs (e.g., amitriptyline), but have shown comparatively less effectiveness in treatment outcomes.[18] Dosing adjustments may be necessary for both renal and hepatic impairment. Though there are no controlled studies in pregnant women, there are reported concerns associated with other SNRIs used in the third trimes-

Table 24.3—Recommended Dose and Dose Adjustment of First-, Second-, and Third-Line Medications for Diabetic-Induced Neuropathy

Class	Agent	Initial dose	Maximum dose	Dose adjustment
Anticonvulsants	Pregabalin	25–75 mg 1–3 times/day	600 mg/day	Renal: ■ CrCl 30–60 mL/min: 300 mg maximum ■ CrCl 15–29 mL/min: 150 mg maximum ■ CrCl <15 mL/min: 75 mg maximum
	Gabapentin	100–300 mg/day	3,600 mg/day	Renal: ■ CrCl 30–60 mL/min: 1,500 mg maximum ■ CrCl 16–29 mL/min: 700 mg maximum ■ CrCl 15 mL/min: 300 mg maximum
Antidepressants (Serotonin-Norepinephrine Reuptake Inhibitors)	Duloxetine	20–30 mg/day	120 mg/day	Renal and Hepatic: ■ CrCl <30 mL/min or hepatic cirrhosis: avoid use
	Venlafaxine	37.5 mg/day	225 mg/day	Renal and Hepatic: ■ CrCl 10–50 mL/min ■ Child-Pugh Class B: decrease dose by 50%
Tricyclic Antidepressants	Amitriptyline	10–25 mg/day	100 mg/day	■ N/A
Opioids	Tramadol ER	50 mg 1–2 times/day	300 mg/day	Renal and Hepatic: ■ CrCl <30 mL/min ■ Child-Pugh Class C: avoid use
	Tapentadol ER	50 mg 2 times/day	500 mg/day	Hepatic: ■ Child-Pugh Class B: start 50 mg/24 hr with 100 mg maximum ■ Child-Pugh Class C: not recommended
Topical Medications (Adjunct)	Lidocaine 5% patch	1 patch/day	3 patches/day	■ Small treatment areas advised
	Capsaicin 0.075%	4 times daily		■ N/A
	Capsaicin 8% patch	Apply up to 4 patches to feet for 30 min (can repeat every 3 months)		■ Must be administered by physician supervised provider
	Isosorbide dinitrate spray	30 mg daily at bedtime to bottom of feet		■ N/A
	Glyceryl trinitrate spray	400 mcg daily at bedtime to top of feet		■ N/A

First-line therapies   Second-line therapies   Adjunct therapies

Source: Adapted from Vinik,[3] Schwartz,[19] Griebeler,[22] and American Diabetes Association.[37]

ter, resulting in a pregnancy category C designation. Avoidance in breast-feeding is suggested, due to excretion into breast milk.[19]

TRICYCLIC ANTIDEPRESSANTS

TCAs were the first medication class used in placebo-controlled trials for neuropathic pain, yet there is still not an FDA-approved TCA for treatment of such pain. The primary mechanism of action of TCAs occurs through inhibition of serotonin and norepinephrine reuptake. The analgesic effect is considered to be independent of the primary antidepressant effect and is theorized to be related to a secondary mechanism, such as α-adrenergic, H_1-histaminergic, and muscarinic receptor blockade; sodium-channel blockade; or possibly NMDA blockade. Dopamine is not directly affected by this class of medications, although dopamine reuptake may fluctuate through indirect effects on adrenergic receptors. Similar to other antidepressants, peak plasma levels may occur within 24 h, but the peak effect may not be seen until 2–4 weeks. TCAs are also highly protein bound, particularly to albumin, and interactions with other protein-bound medications (e.g., warfarin) need to be monitored. Hypothetically, TCAs can displace other protein-bound medications from their binding sites. This displacement could lead to increased serum levels, and in the case of warfarin, increased anticoagulation. Close monitoring of labs, including the INR and especially of narrow therapeutic medications like warfarin, should be done if given concurrently.[17] TCAs can be separated into two categories: secondary amines (e.g., amitriptyline, imipramine) and tertiary amines (e.g., nortriptyline, desipramine). Secondary amines are relatively norepinephrine-selective and have been shown to produce a markedly lower incidence of adverse effects. As such, they are considered more favorable for the treatment of neuropathic disorders than are tertiary amines.[19] The dose of TCAs for neuropathic pain is usually only half that required for depression. An example of this dosing variance would be amitriptyline, which has been proven effective in neuropathic pain at doses of 25–75 mg daily, while the recommended dose for use in depression is 150–300 mg daily.[18] Caution is advised for using any TCA during pregnancy, especially in the third trimester, due to the concern of possible unknown risks of neonatal withdrawal symptoms. There is currently no known risk of infant harm in breast-feeding, based on limited human data and drug properties. Patients already taking antidepressant therapy must be monitored for the possibility of serotonin syndrome when started on a TCA, as this can potentiate serotonin levels on their current medications.

OPIOID AND ATYPICAL OPIOID ANALGESIA

Opioid agonists have been studied for use in many forms of noncancer chronic neuropathies. Two such opioids showing 50% greater efficacy than placebo in the treatment of pain specifically associated with diabetic neuropathy are tramadol and tapentadol. Both medications are centrally acting synthetic opioids with affinity for the μ-opioid receptor. Tramadol is a partial agonist and has a secondary mechanism of transporter inhibition for both serotonin (5HT) and norepinephrine (NE) reuptake from the synaptic cleft. It is theorized that this blockade potentiates the additional analgesic properties when compared to other opioid agonists. Tramadol is extensively metabolized through CYP enzymes 3A4 and

2D6. CYP2D6 metabolism results in a more potent metabolite, though this does not equate to higher analgesic properties, but can contribute to toxicity in patients who exhibit rapid metabolism. In contrast, tapentadol, approved for DSPN in 2012, is a full opioid agonist and secondarily participates in neurotransmitter modulation, like tramadol, but with a greater affinity for the NE transporters and very little inhibition to the 5HT transporters. This lessor inhibition of the 5HT transporters, and only mild reliance on CYP enzymes for metabolism, allow this medication to be given without worry of the severity of adverse drug reactions associated with tramadol, including serotonin syndrome, drug-drug interactions, and labile blood pressure. Tapentadol is primarily excreted through the kidneys with a half-life of approximately 4.25 h.[19] Though both medications have shown some effect, there is little evidence to support use long term, as most studies did not exceed 12 weeks of use with relatively small sample sizes and were subject to bias.[20,21] With the increasing concern associated with opioid dependency and the additional data needed to define efficacy and safety for use of these opioids long term, current evidence does not support use opioid analgesics for first or even second line in chronic diabetic neuropathic pain treatment.

TOPICAL MEDICATIONS

LIDOCAINE

Topical 5% lidocaine patches have been clinically studied for use in the treatment of localized DSPN. The mechanism of action for lidocaine functions through inhibition of voltage-gated sodium channels, which are theorized to activate spontaneously in damaged neurons. Lidocaine has been shown to decrease perceived pain levels, as well as increase patient quality of life through reduction of the negative impact neuropathy may have on activities of daily living. Topical lidocaine reaches systemic levels equal to one-tenth the level necessary to treat cardiac arrhythmias and is not considered to have a significant effect on the cardiovascular system. Distribution of topical lidocaine is negligible. Metabolism of lidocaine occurs primarily in the liver, with excretion occurring primarily through the kidneys. Lidocaine patches can be used as an adjunct to oral therapy and are not considered a primary agent for pain control in widespread neuropathic damage. When comparing lidocaine and pregabalin for use with localized pain, comparable pain relief (30–50% response) to that of pregabalin has been shown, with fewer adverse effects (primarily dermatological) and higher quality-of-life scores for localized pain.[13]

CAPSAICIN

Capsaicin, an active component of chili peppers, is thought to produce analgesia by selectively stimulating unmyelinated C-fiber afferent neurons causing release and depletion of substance P. Capsaicin binds to the sensory vanilloid transient receptor potential cation channel (TRPV1), which is part of the communication pathway for painful stimuli. Currently, 2 dosage forms with this substance have been studied and shown efficacy. The first treatment, a 0.075% capsaicin cream was studied at a dosing interval of every 6 h, not to exceed 4 times per day. It showed significant pain relief of 50% from the patient's baseline level, but adverse effects, such as burning at the site of application, led to early subject withdrawal from the study. Pain relief with capsaicin cream has been observed as soon as 2 weeks after initiation with continual administration, but can take up to 6–8 weeks to reach maximal desired effect.[22,23]

The second treatment contains capsaicin at a higher concentration delivered in an 8% transdermal patch (Qutenza, Acorda therapeutics). A large multicenter study showed reduction of pain scores by upward of 28% when compared to placebo. This patch requires application by a healthcare provider supervised by a physician due to the potential for substantial procedural pain upon application and the transient increases in blood pressure, averaging <10mm/Hg due to pain response following patch application. Most subjects in primary studies found the erythema and pain following application to be transient and self-limited. To mediate this pain on application, it is suggested a topical anesthetic be applied before the patch, followed by a cleansing gel after its removal. Pain relief using the patch formulation was seen to improve symptoms over a range of 2 days to 2 weeks with resulting analgesia lasting up to 3 months.

Capsaicin, in both the cream and patch delivery systems, was found to be only negligibly absorbed systemically through topical administration and so is not expected to result in fetal exposure in utero or through breast feeding. Animal models have supported this.[24]

ISOSORBIDE DINITRATE AND GLYCERYL TRINITRATE SPRAYS

Impaired nitric oxide synthesis or release is thought to contribute to the pathogenesis of diabetic neuropathy and hyperalgesia. Isosorbide dinitrate and glyceryl trinitrate are nitric oxide donors, vasodilators, and smooth muscle relaxants that theoretically modulate impaired nitric oxide synthesis or release.[25] Both sprays reported decrease in pain scores when applied on affected areas, but more studies are needed to show consistency in treatment and side-effect profile over a longer duration of treatment.[26,27]

COMBINATION THERAPY

There was some evidence to support superiority to placebo for the combination of gabapentin and nortriptyline, and no significant difference when the combination of duloxetine and pregabalin at moderate doses were compared against monotherapy at high doses.[13]

DIABETIC GASTROPARESIS

Gastroparesis is a delay in gastric emptying without an obstruction of the stomach. It occurs in 30–50% of patients with T1D or T2D. Chronically elevated blood glucose and A1C levels are associated with an increased risk of gastroparesis, but the severity of clinical symptoms does not always correspond with the rate of gastric emptying. The mechanism by which diabetic gastroparesis occurs is mainly associated with central autonomic neuropathy affecting the vagus nerve and a decrease in the number of inhibitory neurons associated with gastrointestinal motor control. High blood glucose causes chemical changes in the nerves and damages the blood vessels feeding those nerves. Increased levels of glucagon are also considered a factor in gastroparesis. It slows the rate at which food is delivered for digestion in the small intestine. All of these processes together lead to a decrease in fundic and antral motor activity, a reduction of interdigestive migration control, and an increase in digestive and gastric spasmodic problems. To further complicate the issue, there is a bidirectional relationship between gastric emptying and glycemic control. Hyperglycemia can delay gastric emptying and this delay can affect glycemic control. This relationship should be taken into account when determining the treatment definition of "glycemic control."

The common symptoms associated with diabetic gastroparesis are early satiety, nausea, erratic glycemic control, weight loss, abdominal pain, and bloating.[26] In addition to gastrointestinal symptoms, diabetic gastroparesis can have a negative impact on the patient's quality of life and psychological health. When attempting treatment, it is important to exclude other known causes of altered gastric emptying, including, but not limited to, infection, gastric obstruction, or even some medications. Several therapies are available for the symptomatic treatment of diabetic gastroparesis including prokinetics and antiemetics, although a combination of strict glycemic control and dietary changes may result in the best outcome for the patient.[29,30]

Investigational medications include ghrelin receptor agonist, motilin receptor agonists and 5HT4 receptor agonists.

METOCLOPRAMIDE

Metoclopramide is FDA approved for short-term use in the treatment of gastroparesis, but it should be reserved for severe refractory cases of the disease.[28] This medication acts on a diverse number of neurotransmitters: it is a serotonin-4 receptor ($5HT_4$) agonist, a weak serotonin-3 receptor ($5HT_3$) antagonist, a central and peripheral dopamine D_2 antagonist, and a cholinesterase inhibitor. Metoclopramide is prokinetic through $5HT_4$ receptor agonism and antagonism at the peripheral dopamine D_2 receptors, which decreases fundal relaxation and increases antral contractions, thereby improving gastric emptying. It also acts as an antiemetic through antagonism of $5HT_3$ receptors and the central dopamine D_2 receptors in the area postrema.

Metoclopramide is available in oral, parenteral, and nasal spray dosage forms. Onset of action varies, taking 30–60 min for oral and nasal (Gimoti, Evoke Pharma), 10–15 min for intramuscular, and 1–3 min for intravenous administration. Metoclopramide is only 30% protein-bound and crosses the blood-brain barrier. The half-life for metoclopramide is 2.5–6 h, requiring multiple doses a day with meals.[28]

Despite its efficacy, use of metoclopramide is limited by the presence of unfavorable side effects, including neuroendocrine effects such as inappropriate lactation either in men or women, gynecomastia, impotence, and serious extrapyramidal symptoms such as tardive dyskinesia. Though increased gastric emptying is the goal, if achieved, it can also alter the absorption of coadministered medications. Plasma levels should be monitored initially for drugs with a narrow therapeutic index (e.g., lithium, digoxin) to ensure safety and efficacy. Metoclopramide is cleared renally, and the adjustment of metoclopramide dosing may be necessary in the renally impaired patient, as accumulation and toxicity may occur.[29] Metoclopramide has been shown to cross into breast milk, so caution is warranted when using metoclopramide in a breast-feeding patient.[28] Finally, Gimoti nasal spray (15 mg/70 µL) is not recommended in geriatric patients as initial therapy, but can be switched if used as an alternative to the other dosage forms if currently taking. Use not to exceed 8 weeks for all patient populations.

MACROLIDE ANTIBIOTICS: ERYTHROMYCIN

Erythromycin, a motilin agonist, induces high-amplitude gastric propulsive contractions and stimulates fundic contractility, mimicking the effect of the polypeptide motilin, which increases motility and improves gastric emptying of both liquids and solids.[29] In a systematic review of five clinical trials involving oral erythromycin for gastroparesis, 26 of 60 patients (43%) had an improvement in symptoms of gastroparesis, though the studies had a small sample size and a short duration.[30] Clinical responsiveness tends to wane after a few weeks, associated with tachyphylaxis, due to down regulation of the motilin receptor.[31] Common adverse effects of erythromycin include nausea/vomiting, diarrhea, abdominal pain, headache, rash, and possible cardiac QT interval prolongation. It is also a potent inhibitor and a substrate of the CYP3A4 enzyme, so care should be taken to avoid interactions with concurrent medications and food. Patients with a diagnosed heart rhythm disorder or a prolonged QT interval should receive erythromycin with caution, as this medication has been shown to cause ventricular arrhythmias of the torsade de pointes type. Erythromycin may be used with caution in pregnant patients and is considered safe for use in breast-feeding patients.[30]

Erythromycin is available in oral and intravenous form. It was found to be a more potent agent for treatment of diabetic gastroparesis when given intravenously; among oral formulations, suspension was found to be more effective than tablets. Finally, erythromycin efficacy is negatively affected by hyperglycemia, so adequate control of blood glucose must be established to maximize its effect. Newer motilin and synthetic ghrelin agonists are being researched to expand the options available for the treatment of gastroparesis.[32,33]

ERECTILE DYSFUNCTION

ED is the inability to achieve or maintain an erection sufficient for sexual intercourse. Causes for ED are multifactorial, and may relate to psychological, neurological, hormonal, vascular, mediation, or age factors, or a combination of these. Autonomic neurotransmission controls the corpora cavernosa and detrusor smooth muscle tone and function. Endothelial dysfunction is also a common cause of ED, as well as the common link between ED, diabetes, and subsequent vascular disease. Endothelial dysfunction in the pudendal penile arteries/arterioles leads to a loss of vascular patency and increased risk of atherosclerosis, thrombosis, plaque formation, and occlusive artery disease. The endothelium is responsible for the release of nitric oxide into the smooth vascular cells, which ultimately increases release of cyclic guanosine monophosphate (cGMP), leading to increased relaxation of smooth vascular muscle cells. Endothelial dysfunction lowers nitric

Table 24.4 — Phosphodiesterase Inhibitors[31]

Pde5-i	Dose/day	Onset of action	Duration	Comments
Sildenafil Available in tablets, suspension, and injectable	Initial p.r.n. dose: 50 mg Dose range: 25–100 mg >65 years: 25 mg	60 min	4 h	▪ Possible color visual disturbances ▪ Renal dosing: p.r.n. = CrCl 30–50 mL/min: max 5 mg OR 10 mg every 48 h. CrCl <30 mL/min: max 5 mg ▪ Hepatic dosing: Child-Pugh Class A or B: max of 10 mg daily
Tadalafil Available in tablets	Initial p.r.n. dose: 10 mg Dose range (p.r.n.): 5–20 mg Initial daily dose: 2.5 mg Dose range (daily): 2.5–5 mg >65 years: 5 mg	30–45 min	Up to 36 h	▪ Renal dosing: – p.r.n. = CrCl 30–50 mL/min: max 5 mg/day. CrCl <30 mL/min: max 5 mg/72 h – Daily = CrCl <30 mL/min: avoid use ▪ Hepatic dosing: avoid use in Child-Pugh Class C
Vardenafil Available in tablets and ODT	Initial p.r.n. dose: 10 mg Dose range: 5–20 mg >65 years: 5 mg	60 min	5 h	▪ Hepatic dosing: Child-Pugh Class B: start 5 mg x 1, max 10 mg per dose ▪ Child-Pugh Class C: avoid use
Avanafil Available in tablets	Initial p.r.n. dosing: 100 mg Dose range: 50–200 mg	15–30 min	6 h	▪ Renal dosing: CrCl <30 mL/min: avoid use ▪ Hepatic dosing: avoid use in Child-Pugh Class C

ODT, orally dissolving tablet. *Source*: Huang.[35]

oxide formation and release, which was identified as a key contributor to ED.[3,28] Although therapy may be initiated to modify or treat ED, it is also recommended to educate the patient regarding other underlying conditions (e.g., diabetes mellitus, CVD), and make sure that control of these conditions is established to reduce any risk of further damage and worsening ED.[1] Outside of pharmacology, weight loss has shown benefit through reducing conversion of testosterone to β-estradiol in the adipose tissue as well as improving other concurrent metabolic disease states (e.g., hypertension and dyslipidemia).

PHOSPHODIESTERASE TYPE 5 INHIBITORS (PDE5-Is): SILDENAFIL, TADALAFIL, VARDENAFIL, AND AVANAFIL

Sildenafil was the first phosphodiesterase inhibitor studied for the treatment of ED, and has since been followed by vardenafil, tadalafil, and avanafil, which are more selective for phosphodiesterase type 5 (PDE5) (see Table 24.4). PDE5-Is, such as sildenafil, exert their action through blockade of cGMP-specific phosphodiesterase-5 degradation. Normally, the endothelium of the corpus cavernosum releases nitric oxide during sexual stimulation. The nitric oxide stimulates release of cGMP, which relaxes the smooth muscle of the corpus cavernosum and allows blood flow to occur. In ED, cGMP levels are decreased and smooth muscle relaxation may not occur, leading to the failure of erection. By inhibiting PDE5, sildenafil raises levels of cGMP and improves smooth muscle relaxation in the corpus cavernosum, improving erectile function. Repeated dosing is recommended, with continued exposure showing improved responses. Common adverse effects associated with PDE5-I use include headache, flushing, dizziness, and rash. Combined use of PDE5-Is with known CYP3A4 inhibitors (e.g., erythromycin, ketoconazole) may increase plasma concentrations of sildenafil through inhibition of metabolism, leading to a greater risk of side effects. Caution should also be exercised when using sildenafil in a patient with a previous history of cardiovascular events (e.g., MI, stroke). PDE5-Is should not be used concurrently with nitrate therapy, due to the additive effect of vasodilation and acute hypotension that could potentially lead to death.[28,35,36]

ALPROSTADIL

Alprostadil is a naturally occurring prostaglandin E found in the seminal vesicles and cavernous tissues of the penis. Alprostadil acts on the smooth muscles of the corpus cavernosum, thereby stimulating the activity of adenylate cyclase. As a result, an increase of intracellular cAMP and a decrease in intracellular calcium occur. A decrease in norepinephrine also occurs through this mechanism, leading to smooth muscle relaxation and increased blood flow. Additionally, alprostadil directly dilates cavernosal arteries, increasing arterial blood flow, and thereby enhancing erectile function.

Alprostadil is available as an intracavernosal injection and an intraurethrally applied tablet, allowing for administration of an ED medication in patients unable to take PDE5-Is (e.g., patients taking concurrent antianginal nitrates). Systemic absorption of alprostadil is minimal, with little to no adverse effects associated with this medication. No dosing adjustments are necessary for known disease states, such as hepatic or renal impairment. Side effects noted during use include hypotension and syncope. Alprostadil should be used cautiously in patients who have experienced priapism (erection ≥4 h). Although no dosing guidelines have been outlined for this medication, the manufacturer recommendations state initial dosing is to begin at 1.25 μg for injection and 125 μg per intraurethral tablet, with titration based on physiological response. Injections should be given no more than three times per week, with at least a 24 h period between doses following initial titration.[2,35]

MONOGRAPHS

Alprostadil injection: https://dailymed.nlm.nih.gov/dailymed/drugInfo. cfm?setid=4dec1dbd-c63b-4a1b-81cb-c8d29696cc40

Alprostadil suppository: https://dailymed.nlm.nih.gov/dailymed/drugInfo.cfm?setid=4c55f3f9-c4cf-11df-851a-0800200c9a66

Amitriptyline: https://dailymed.nlm.nih.gov/dailymed/drugInfo.cfm?setid=1e6d2c80-fbc8-444e-bdd3-6a91fe1b95bd

Avanafil: https://dailymed.nlm.nih.gov/dailymed/drugInfo.cfm?setid=a8726f90-9329-46ca-9379-2b50c78fe0e2

Capsaicin cream 0.075%: https://dailymed.nlm.nih.gov/dailymed/drugInfo.cfm?setid=5a9e970c-7e67-469d-b9ad-010c031ed35b

Carbamazepine: https://dailymed.nlm.nih.gov/dailymed/drugInfo.cfm?setid=8d409411-aa9f-4f3a-a52c-fbcb0c3ec053

Desipramine: https://dailymed.nlm.nih.gov/dailymed/drugInfo.cfm?setid=a3b4b25d-0ddb-4531-badb-f1ba3168ac07

Desvenlafaxine ER: https://dailymed.nlm.nih.gov/dailymed/drugInfo.cfm?setid=0f43610c-f290-46ea-d186-4f998ed99fce

Duloxetine: https://dailymed.nlm.nih.gov/dailymed/drugInfo.cfm?setid=2f7d4d67-10c1-4bf4-a7f2-c185fbad64ba

Erythromycin: https://dailymed.nlm.nih.gov/dailymed/drugInfo.cfm?setid=86d6353c-2b58-4219-b31d-fb5b97789094

Gabapentin: https://dailymed.nlm.nih.gov/dailymed/drugInfo.cfm?setid=ee9ad9ed-6d9f-4ee1-9d7f-cfad438df388

Gimoti: https://dailymed.nlm.nih.gov/dailymed/drugInfo.cfm?setid=95269b1f-779c-4ca0-9f86-e74e677f9900

Glyceryl trinitrate: https://dailymed.nlm.nih.gov/dailymed/drugInfo.cfm?setid=1b7cb5e7-e1f7-093d-e054-00144ff8d46c

Imipramine: https://dailymed.nlm.nih.gov/dailymed/drugInfo.cfm?setid=2f7d5e7f-79aa-4f3a-b9a6-758d9f3ce74d

Lidocaine patch 5%: https://dailymed.nlm.nih.gov/dailymed/drugInfo.cfm?setid=f1c40164-4626-4290-9012-c00e33420a33

Metoclopramide: https://dailymed.nlm.nih.gov/dailymed/drugInfo.cfm?setid=de55c133-eb08-4a35-91a2-5dc093027397

Nortriptyline: https://dailymed.nlm.nih.gov/dailymed/drugInfo.cfm?setid=e17dc299-f52d-414d-ab6e-e809bd6f8acb

Pregabalin: https://dailymed.nlm.nih.gov/dailymed/drugInfo.cfm?setid=60185c88-ecfd-46f9-adb9-b97c6b00a553

Qutenza 8% patch: https://dailymed.nlm.nih.gov/dailymed/drugInfo.cfm?setid=3ffbbcb0-ad93-4f15-bb38-5da76a71c735

Sildenafil: https://dailymed.nlm.nih.gov/dailymed/drugInfo.cfm?setid=0b0be196-0c62-461c-94f4-9a35339b4501

Tadalafil: https://dailymed.nlm.nih.gov/dailymed/drugInfo.cfm?setid=bcd8f8ab-81a2-4891-83db-24a0b0e25895

Tapentedol: https://dailymed.nlm.nih.gov/dailymed/drugInfo.cfm?setid=f4c911f3-484b-44fa-833e-2d970d39be8

Tramadol: https://dailymed.nlm.nih.gov/dailymed/drugInfo.cfm?setid=0f799e5c-f782-4f3d-bdb6-52bd413a19cf

Valproate: https://dailymed.nlm.nih.gov/dailymed/drugInfo.cfm?setid=6b4331f5-4475-417a-6a9d-09c2f8334235

Vardenafil: https://dailymed.nlm.nih.gov/dailymed/drugInfo.cfm?setid=a01def95-c0ef-43b9-bd9e-5565b2385ad3

Venlafaxine ER: https://dailymed.nlm.nih.gov/dailymed/drugInfo.cfm?setid=53c3e7ac-1852-4d70-d2b6-4fca819acf26

REFERENCES

1. Vinik A. Diabetic sensory and motor neuropathy. *N Engl J Med* 2016;374:1455–1464

2. Sima AA, Kamiya H. Diabetic neuropathy differs in type 1 and type 2 diabetes. *Ann N Y Acad Sci* 2006;1084:235–249

3. Vinik A, Nevoret M-L, Casellini C, Parson H. Diabetic neuropathy. In *Acute and Chronic Complications of Diabetes*. Poretsky L, Liao EP, Eds. Amsterdam, Elsevier, 2013, p. 747–787

4. Ziegler D, Papanas N, Vinik AI, Shaw JE. Epidemiology of polyneuropathy in diabetes and prediabetes. In *Diabetes and the Nervous System*. Zochodne DW, Malik RA, Eds. Vol. 126 of *Handbook of Clinical Neurology*. 3rd series. Amsterdam, Elsevier, 2014, p. 3–22

5. Rahman H, Jha MK, Suk K. Evolving insights into the pathophysiology of diabetic neuropathy: implications of malfunctioning glia and discovery of novel therapeutic targets. *Curr Pharm Des* 2016,22:738–757

6. Tomlinson DR, Gardiner NJ. Glucose neurotoxicity. *Nat Rev Neurosci* 2008;9:36–45

7. Hinder LM, Vivekanandan-Giri A, McLean LL, et al. Decreased glycolytic and tricarboxylic acid cycle intermediates coincide with peripheral nervous system oxidative stress in a murine model of type 2 diabetes. *J Endocrinol* 2013;216:1–11

8. Triplitt CL, Repas T, Alvarez C. Diabetes mellitus. In *Pharmacotherapy: A Physiological Approach*. 10th ed. Dipiro DT, Talbert RL, et al., Eds. New York, McGraw-Hill, 2017, p. 1174

9. Neurontin (gabapentin) Clinical Pharmacology. Pfizer Medical Information. Available from https://www.pfizermedicalinformation.com/en-us/neurontin/clinical-pharmacology. Accessed 25 January 2022

10. Bockbrader HN, Wesche D, Miller R, et al. A comparison of the pharmacokinetics and pharmacodynamics of pregabalin and gabapentin. *Clin Pharmacokinet* 2010;49(10):661–669

11. Wiffen PJ, Derry S, Bell RF, et al. Gabapentin for chronic neuropathic pain in adults. *Cochrane Database Syst Rev* 2017;6:CD007938

12. Arnold L, McCarberg B, Clair AG, et al. Dose-response of pregabalin for diabetic peripheral neuropathy, postherpetic neuralgia, and fibromyalgia. *Postgrad Med* 2017;129(8):921–933

13. Finnerup NB, Attal N, Haroutounian S, et al. Pharmacotherapy for neuropathic pain in adults: a systematic review and meta-analysis. *Lancet Neurol* 2015;14(2):162–173

14. Kristensen JH, Ilett KF, Hackett PL, Kohan R. Gabapentin and breastfeeding: a case report. *J Human Lactation* 2006;22(4):426–428

15. Saeed T, Nasrullah M, Ghafoor A, et al. Efficacy and tolerability of carbamazepine for the treatment of painful diabetic neuropathy in adults: a 12-week, open-label, multicenter study. *Int J Gen Med* 2014;7:339–343

16. Rakitin A. Does Valproic acid have potential in the treatment of diabetes mellitus? *Front Endocrinol* (Lausanne) 2017;8:147

17. Bril V, England J, Franklin GM, et al. Evidence-based guideline: treatment of painful diabetic neuropathy: report of the American Academy of Neurology, the American Association of Neuromuscular and Electrodiagnostic Medicine, and the American Academy of Physical Medicine and Rehabilitation. *Neurology* 2011;76(20):1758–1765

18. Sansone RA, Sansone LA. Pain, pain, go away: antidepressants and pain management. *Psychiatry* (Edgmont) 2008;5:16–19

19. Schwartz S, Etropolski M, Shapiro DY, et al. A randomized withdrawl, placebo-controlled study evaluating the efficacy and tolerability of tapentadol extended release in patients with chronic painful diabetic peripheral neuropathy. *Diabetes Care* 2014;2302–2309

20. McNicol ED, Midbari A, Eisenberg E. Opioids for neuropathic pain. The Cochrane database of systemic reviews. 2013. CD006146

21. Sommer C, Kolse P, Welsch P, Petzke F, and Häuser W. Opioids for chronic non-cancer neuropathic pain. An updated systematic review and meta-analysis of efficacy, tolerability and safety in randomized placebo-controlled studies of at least 4 weeks duration. *Eur J Pain*. Epub 2019

22. Griebeler ML, Morey-Vargas OL, Brito JP, et al. Pharmacological interventions for painful diabetic neuropathy: an umbrella systematic review and

comparative effectiveness network meta-analysis. *Ann Intern Med* 2014;161:639–649

23. Snyder MJ, Gibbs LM, Lindsay TJ. Treating painful diabetic peripheral neuropathy: an update. *Am Fam Physician* 2016;94(3):227–234

24. Simpson DM, Robinson-Papp J, Van J, et al. Capsaicin 8% patch in painful diabetic peripheral neuropathy: a randomized, double-blind, placebo-controlled study. *J Pain* 2017;18(1):42–53. DOI:10.1016/j.jpain.2016.09.008

25. Lindsay TJ, Rodgers BC, Savath V, Hettinger K. Treating diabetic peripheral neuropathic pain. *Am Fam Physician* 2010;82(2):151–158

26. Agrawal RP, Choudhary R, Sharma P, et al. Glyceryl trinitrate spray in the management of painful diabetic neuropathy: a randomized double blind placebo controlled cross-over study. *Diabetes Res Clin Pract* 2007 Aug;77(2):161–167

27. Yuen K, Baker N, Rayman G. Treatment of chronic painful diabetic neuropathy with isosorbide dinitrate spray. *Diabetes Care* 2002;25(10): 1699–1703

28. Pop-Busui R, Boulton AJ, Feldman EL, et al. Diabetic neuropathy: a position statement by the American Diabetes Association. *Diabetes Care* 2017;40(1):136–154

29. Kumar M, Chapman A, Javed S, et al. The investigation and treatment of diabetic gastroparesis. *Clin Ther* 2018;40(6):850–861

30. Youssef AS, Parkman HP, Nagar S. Drug-drug interactions in pharmacologic management of gastroparesis. *Neurogastroenterol Motil* 2015;27 (11):1528–1541

31. Ali T, Hasan M, Hamadani M, Harty RF. Gastroparesis. *South Med J* 2007;100:281–286

32. Keshavarzian A, Isaac RM. Erythromycin accelerates gastric emptying of indigestible solids and transpyloric migration of the tip of an enteral feeding tube in fasting and fed states. *Am J Gastroenterol* 1993;88:193

33. Maganti K, Onyemere K, Jones MP. Oral erythromycin and symptomatic relief of gastroparesis: a systematic review. *Am J Gastroenterol* 2003;98:259

34. Camilleri M, Parkman HP, Shafi MA, et al.; American College of Gastroenterology. Clinical guideline: management of gastroparesis. *Am J Gastroenterol* 2013;108:18–37

35. Huang SA, Lie JD. Phosphodiesterase-5 (PDE5) inhibitors in the management of erectile dysfunction. *P T* 2013;38(7):407–419

36. Kamenov ZA. A comprehensive review of erectile dysfunction in men with diabetes. *Exp Clin Endocrinol Diabetes* 2015;123(3):141–158

Chapter 25
Medications for the Management of Nephropathy

Emmeline Tran, PharmD

CKD resulting from diabetes is known as diabetic kidney disease (DKD) or diabetic nephropathy. DKD is typically characterized by the presence of albuminuria and/or reduced eGFR not attributable to other causes of renal injury.[1] This broad definition of DKD has made it difficult to compare and contrast relevant results from trials since renal endpoints in these trials have not always been consistent.

Approximately 20–40% of patients with diabetes have DKD.[1] Risk factors for DKD are both modifiable and nonmodifiable. Modifiable risk factors include poor glycemic control, hypertension, dyslipidemia, and obesity. Nonmodifiable risk factors include older age; male sex; early age of onset of diabetes; family history; African American, Native American, Hispanic, Asian, or Pacific Islander race or ethnicity; and genetics.[2,3] Progression of DKD to ESRD can occur. In fact, the major cause of ESRD in the U.S. is diabetes.[4] Moreover, patients with DKD have a substantial cost burden. This is principally driven by the strong association with CVD among this patient population and by the development of ESRD.[4-6]

The pathophysiology of DKD involves a multifactorial process driven by histological changes in the glomeruli. Mesangial expansion occurs initially followed by thickening of the glomerular basement membrane and, lastly, glomerular sclerosis.[7] Collectively, these changes result in glomerular hyperfiltration, glomerular hypertension, and renal hypertrophy, which are clinically manifested as albuminuria and hypertension.[7] The natural history of DKD aligns with the histological changes, moving from progressive albuminuria to declining GFR, and ultimately ESRD.[3] However, it must be noted that not all patients with DKD present in the conventional manner described. Some patients may present with GFR loss independent from albuminuria.[8]

Considerable morbidity, mortality, and costs are associated with DKD.[4] Once DKD is established, it is only possible to slow progression. Additionally, DKD is strongly associated with CVD, and most patients with DKD die from CVD prior to needing dialysis.[3,9] Consequently, the goals of DKD treatment are to prevent DKD development and progression, to improve quality of life, and to reduce morbidity and mortality.

Despite limitations in these surrogate markers, it is generally accepted that GFR (estimating kidney function) and albuminuria (assessing kidney injury) are used to help identify and monitor DKD. In general, an eGFR of <60 mL/min/1.73 m^2, and a urinary albumin excretion (UAE) ≥30 mg/g creatinine are considered to be abnormal.[1] However, variations may be seen in the literature, especially in regard to studies examining the efficacy of treatment options in DKD. Of note, the terms "microalbuminuria" (30–300 mg/g creatinine) and "macroalbuminuria" (>300 mg/g creatinine) are no longer favored. Instead, reporting of urine albumin level as a continuous variable is preferred.[10] Although there is guidance correlating these laboratory parameters with initiation of pharmacological treatment, guidance on use of these parameters to monitor efficacy of the treatment implemented is less clear.[1,10] Furthermore, correlation of specific targets with improved patient-centered outcomes is inconclusive. A meta-analysis of two large clinical trials suggests that a 30% reduction in albuminuria may translate into a 30% reduction in risk of ESRD.[11]

MEDICATIONS

Development and progression of DKD is believed to be driven by glomerular hyperfiltration, and in turn, glomerular hypertension. Under diabetic conditions, afferent arterioles are dilated, and blood flow into the glomeruli is increased, causing elevated intraglomerular pressure. These changes induce inflammation and oxidative stress in the glomeruli, leading to the excessive production of extracellular matrix, which plays a key role in the development of glomerulosclerosis. Studies have shown that reducing intraglomerular pressure is associated with renal protection.[12,13] Medications targeting this pathogenesis mechanism are a central focus and therapeutic option in patients with DKD. Although inflammation, oxidative stress, and fibrosis also contribute to the pathogenesis of DKD, attempts to target these mechanisms have been less successful.

Although a targeted mechanistic approach on the kidneys is described, prevention and treatment of DKD lies heavily with glycemic control, hypertension, and cardiovascular risk reduction. Several landmark trials have proven the benefits of glycemic control on reducing progression of DKD in both patients with T1D[14,15] and patients with T2D.[16–20] The effect of antihypertensive therapy on DKD will be discussed below. Although statin therapy has not been found to inhibit the progression of kidney disease,[21] it has been shown to be beneficial in reducing CVD events and mortality in patients with non-dialysis-dependent CKD, with or without diabetes.[22] Conversely, benefits of statin therapy on CVD events or mortality have not been found in patients on dialysis.[23] Therefore, initiating statin therapy in patients on dialysis is not recommended. However, continuation of statin therapy in those who progress to dialysis may be considered.

RENIN-ANGIOTENSIN SYSTEM INHIBITORS

Renin-angiotensin system (RAS) inhibition, through the use of ACE inhibitors, ARBs, or direct renin inhibitors, slows the progression of DKD. Benefits, specifically those related to mortality and cardiovascular events, extend even to patients with an eGFR <30 mL/min/1.73m^2.[24] ACE inhibitors, ARBs, and renin inhibitors favorably affect intraglomerular pressure by lowering systemic blood pressure and reducing efferent arteriolar vasoconstriction.[25]

Furthermore, the beneficial effects of ACE inhibitors and ARBs are found to be independent of their effects on systemic blood pressure.[26–30] Specifically, long-term renoprotective effects are believed to be related to an initial rise in serum creatinine of up to 30% and decreased intraglomerular pressure.[12,13] The level of evidence supporting the efficacy of these classes of medications on renal outcomes is driven by the studied patient population, specifically type of diabetes mellitus, presence of hypertension, and presence of albuminuria.

T1D with Hypertension and Albuminuria

The Captopril Study established the role of ACE inhibitors in the treatment of DKD in patients with T1D, mild to moderate hypertension (mean blood pressure of 139/86 mmHg), and established nephropathy (mean urinary protein excretion of 2,750 mg per 24 h).[26] Specifically, captopril statistically significantly reduced the risk of doubling of serum creatinine and the decline in creatinine clearance rate, and decreased the risk of the composite endpoint of death, dialysis, and transplantation compared with placebo over a median follow-up of 3 years. Moreover, remission of nephrotic syndrome in a subset of these patients with nephrotic-range proteinuria was established and sustained at approximately 8 years. Remission was defined as a decrease in proteinuria from >3,500 mg per 24 h to <1,000 mg per 24 h and sustained for at least 6 months at <1,500 mg per 24 h.[31,32]

T1D with Normotension and Albuminuria

Use of ACE inhibitors to prevent worsening renal function in patients with T1D who have albuminuria but no hypertension has been studied and was found to be efficacious. The combined results of two large clinical trials in patients with T1D, normotension (mean blood pressure of 122/77 mmHg), and albuminuria (geometric mean albumin excretion rate of 59 μg/min) showed that captopril statistically significantly decreased the risk of progression to overt clinical albuminuria, UAE rate, and decline in CrCl compared with placebo at 24 months.[33–35] Follow-up to one of the studies at 8 years found statistically significant benefits related to UAE rate, but not in rate of decline in GFR.[36]

A Cochrane review found that ACE inhibitors reduced the risk of new onset kidney disease by 29% and the risk of death by 16% in individuals with diabetes.[37] Clear renal benefits were observed among individuals without hypertension at baseline and in comparison to calcium channel blockers (CCBs). These effects were consistent regardless of type of diabetes, presence of hypertension, or comparator group (placebo-controlled studies or studies comparing ACE inhibitors to other blood pressure agents). In contrast, use of ARBs did not find the same benefits. Most ARB studies in this meta-analysis recruited mainly normotensive patients at lower renal and vascular risk. Consequently, study power was limited.[37]

T1D with Hypertension and Normoalbuminuria

Studies specifically examining DKD outcomes in patients with T1D, hypertension, and normoalbuminuria are lacking. This may be explained by the more common presence of microalbuminuria prior to the onset of hypertension in patients with T1D. The onset of hypertension appears to be an effect of DKD rather than a cause.[38]

T1D with Normotension and Normoalbuminuria

Literature supporting the use of RAS inhibitors in patients with normotension and normoalbuminuria is equivocal. Patients with T1D, normotension (median blood pressure of 122/80 mmHg), and mainly normoalbuminuria (84%) were studied to investigate the effects of lisinopril on prevention of diabetic nephropathy in the EUCLID study.[39] Although lisinopril was found to have a statistically significant effect on decreasing the progression of microalbuminuria in those with albuminuria at baseline, no difference was found in those with normoalbuminuria.

On the other hand, another study found benefits with the use of an ACE inhibitor on primary prevention of diabetic nephropathy. The Renal and Retinal Effects of Enalapril and Losartan in Type 1 Diabetes (RASS) study examined the renal preventative effects of enalapril and losartan in patients with T1D, normotension (mean blood pressure of 120/70 mmHg), and normoalbuminuria (median UAE rate of 5.1 µg/min).[40] When compared to placebo, enalapril statistically significantly prevented the increase of UAE rate and decreased the incidence of albuminuria at 5 years, but losartan did not. No effects on GFR were found with either medication.

The Diabetic Retinopathy Candesartan Trials Renal (DIRECT-Renal) study pooled three clinical trials to determine whether candesartan prevents the onset of albuminuria in patients with T1D or T2D.[41] Of the patients with diabetes, about 64% had T1D. All patients were normotensive and normoalbuminuric. Similarly, no difference was found on development of albuminuria (defined as a UAE rate of ≥20 µg/min) or on change in UAE rate compared with placebo.

T2D with Hypertension and Albuminuria

Although there has been much less information, similar findings with ACE inhibitors have been observed in patients with T2D. The MICRO-Heart Outcomes Prevention Evaluation (MICRO-HOPE) substudy of the HOPE trial assessed whether or not similar renal protective effects with ACE inhibitors seen in patients with T1D could be obtained in patients with T2D.[42] Approximately one-third of the patients were defined as having a urinary ACR of 17.7 mg/g creatinine or higher. Additionally, about 56% of patients had a history of hypertension, and the mean blood pressure at baseline was 142/80 mmHg. When compared with placebo, ramipril statistically significantly decreased the progression to overt nephropathy. In patients with normoalbuminuria, the risk of development of albuminuria was reduced, but not significantly. Of note, although the term is no longer in use, microalbuminuria, as defined by the study, is slightly different than what has been previously considered the cutoff (30–300 mg/g creatinine). Moreover, the benefit on mortality found in the trial can be attributable only to patients with T2D at an increased risk for CVD but without established diabetic nephropathy.

More data are available on the efficacy of ARBs in T2D than in T1D. As with the ACE inhibitors, efficacy findings correlate with level of albuminuria. The Irbesartan in Patients with Type 2 Diabetes and Microalbuminuria (IRMA-2) trial examined the effect of irbesartan on the development of diabetic nephropathy in patients with T2D, hypertension (mean blood pressure of 153/90 mmHg), and albuminuria between 20–200 µg/min (geometric mean UAE rate of 57 µg/min).[27] Irbesartan achieved statistical significance in decreasing the progression to overt nephropathy, reducing UAE rate, and restoring normoalbuminuria compared with placebo. No statistically significant difference was found in the rate of decline in CrCl. The MicroAlbuminuria Reduction With VALsartan (MARVAL) study examined a similar patient population (T2D, hypertension with mean blood pressure of 148/86 mmHg, and albuminuria between 20–200 µg/min with a mean of UAE rate of 57 µg/min), but compared an ARB (valsartan) to amlodipine instead of placebo.[28] Valsartan statistically significantly reduced the UAE rate compared with amlodipine regardless of baseline blood pressure.

Benefits of ARBs on patients with higher levels of albuminuria at baseline have also been established. The Irbesartan Diabetic Nephropathy Trial (IDNT)[29] and Reduction of Endpoints in NIDDM with the Angiotensin II Antagonist Losartan (RENAAL)[43] trials examined the effects of ARBs in patients with T2D, hypertension (mean blood pressures of 159/87 mmHg and 153/82 mmHg, respectively), and nephropathy (median UAE rate of 1,900 mg per 24 h and median urinary ACR of 1,249 mg/g creatinine, respectively). In the IDNT trial, irbesartan was associated with a statistically significant decrease in the risk of the composite endpoint (doubling of serum creatinine, onset of ESRD, or death) compared with amlodipine and placebo.[29] The composite outcome was driven mainly by statistically significant benefits achieved by irbesartan in decreasing the risk of doubling serum creatinine and ESRD. Losartan achieved similar results compared with placebo using the same composite endpoint in the RENAAL trial.[43]

Although most trials examining aliskiren were in combination with ACE inhibitors or ARBs, there are a few studies examining aliskiren monotherapy on progression of diabetic nephropathy. In a small exploratory study examining the effect of aliskiren in patients with T2D, hypertension (mean blood pressure of 146/76 mmHg), and albuminuria (median urinary ACR of 158 mg/g creatinine), aliskiren was found to reduce urinary ACR significantly, but not eGFR, at 28 days compared with baseline.[44] Another larger study compared the antiproteinuric effect of aliskiren to that of ramipril.[45] Patients had T2D, hypertension (mean blood pressure of 159/94 mmHg), and albuminuria defined as a UAE rate of >200 and <300 mg per day (mean UAE rate of 258 mg per day). Aliskiren was found to have a statistically significantly greater and more prolonged effect on decreasing UAE rate compared with ramipril. The authors attribute this finding to a higher degree of intrarenal renin-angiotensin-aldosterone system (RAAS) blockade.

T2D with Normotension and Albuminuria

A small trial compared the effects of enalapril to placebo on patients with T2D, normotension, and microalbuminuria defined as a UAE rate of 30–300 mg per 24 h.[46] Enalapril statistically significantly slowed progression to nephropathy compared with placebo. Benefits persisted through 7 years.

T2D with Hypertension and Normoalbuminuria

Use of an RAS inhibitor for primary prevention in patients with T2D is supported by a few trials. The Bergamo Nephrologic Diabetes Complication Trial

(BENEDICT) trial examined the effects of trandolapril with verapamil, trandolapril monotherapy, verapamil monotherapy, or placebo on the development of albuminuria defined as an overnight UAE rate of ≥20 μg/min.[47] Patients had T2D, hypertension (mean blood pressure of 151/88 mmHg), and normoalbuminuria (median UAE rate of 5.3 μg/min). Development of albuminuria was significantly delayed in patients receiving trandolapril with verapamil or trandolapril monotherapy, but not verapamil monotherapy, compared with placebo.

Instead of an ACE inhibitor, the Randomized Olmesartan And Diabetes MicroAlbuminuria Prevention (ROADMAP) trial investigated the effects of an ARB (olmesartan) for primary prevention of albuminuria in patients with T2D and hypertension (mean blood pressure of 136/81 mmHg).[48] Albuminuria was defined as a urinary ACR of >35 mg/g creatinine in females and >25 mg/g creatinine in males. The geometric mean baseline urinary ACR was 6.1 mg/g creatinine. Olmesartan was associated with a statistically significantly longer time to the development of albuminuria compared with placebo.

T2D with Normotension and Normoalbuminuria

Again, in patients with normotension and normoalbuminuria, the literature is less clear. The Appropriate Blood Pressure Control in Diabetes (ABCD) study examining the effects of enalapril or nisoldipine on primary prevention of diabetic nephropathy found that a lower percentage of patients progressed from normoalbuminuria to microalbuminuria regardless of antihypertensive agent used, but observed no difference in CrCl.[49] Patients in this study had T2D and normotension (mean blood pressure of 136/84 mmHg). Approximately 66% of patients had normoalbuminuria. Similarly, another study in patients with T2D, normotension (mean systolic blood pressure of 97 mmHg), and normoalbuminuria (mean UAE rate of 11.2 mg per 24 h) found benefits of enalapril on decreasing the risk of new onset microalbuminuria and UAE, and preventing CrCl in declining substantially.[50]

Patients with T2D in the DIRECT-Renal study (36%) were generally normotensive or well controlled on antihypertensive medications.[41] All patients were normoalbuminuric. As previously mentioned, candesartan was not found to have a benefit in preventing the development of albuminuria or decreasing UAE rate when compared with placebo.

Of note, two randomized controlled trials examining the renoprotective effects of olmesartan in patients with T2D observed an increase in the number of cardiovascular-related deaths in the olmesartan group compared with the placebo group.[48,51] The FDA conducted a safety review and found no clear evidence of increased cardiovascular risk associated with the use of olmesartan in patients with diabetes. A meta-analysis also confirmed no difference in cardiovascular risk.[52]

ACE Inhibitors versus ARBs

Comparisons of ACE inhibitors to ARBs on their effects in diabetic nephropathy are relatively limited.[53] The majority of evidence from controlled clinical trials supports the use of ACE inhibitors in patients with T1D and ARBs in patients with T2D. A noninferiority study (Diabetics Exposed to Telmisartan And enaprIL [DETAIL]) comparing the effect of telmisartan and enalapril on the change in GFR in patients with T2D, mild to moderate hypertension (mean blood pressure of 152/86 mmHg), and albuminuria with a UAE rate between 11–999 μg/min (median UAE rate 53 μg/min) found telmisartan to be not inferior to enalapril in change in GFR over 5 years.[54]

Limitations in comparative studies of ACE inhibitors and ARBs make it difficult to clearly define superiority of one class over another in the prevention and treatment of diabetic nephropathy. Mixed findings showing benefits of one class over another have been observed in reviews and meta-analyses.[53,55-58] Clinical determination of using one class over another may be driven by side-effect profile. ACE inhibitors have traditionally been associated with a dry cough whereas ARBs have not.[53]

In summary, studies investigating the use of RAS inhibitors on improving renal outcomes in patients with normotension and albuminuria are lacking. Furthermore, the data supporting use of RAS inhibitors in the setting of normoalbuminuria are inconsistent and suggest no clear benefit over other antihypertensive agents. In those patients with hypertension and albuminuria, it is generally accepted that the renal protective benefit is a class effect. However, studies examining specific dosing of each medication within each class are not available. Consequently, equivalent doses that may confer renoprotective effects are unknown when converting from one medication to another within a class.

SGLT2 INHIBITORS

SGLT2 inhibitors are believed to exert renoprotection through direct and indirect effects. The direct renal effects of SGLT2 inhibitors are thought to be related to activation of tubuloglomerular feedback through reduction in sodium reabsorption in the proximal tubules and consequently increased distal sodium delivery to the macula densa.[59] The increased sodium delivery is perceived as an increase in circulating volume causing constriction of the afferent renal arterioles and reduction in intraglomerular pressure. Indirect effects occur through suppression of renal glucose reabsorption for improved glycemic control.[59]

In cardiovascular trials of SGLT2 inhibitors, exploratory results suggest that these medications positively affect renal outcomes in patients with T2D. The potential efficacy of canagliflozin on progression of diabetic nephropathy was examined in the CANVAS-R[60] and CANTATA-SU[61] trials as secondary outcomes or analyses. All patients in the CANVAS-R trial had T2D (mean A1C of 8.2%) and high cardiovascular risk, 30% of patients had albuminuria, and 80% of patients were on a RAAS inhibitor at baseline.[60] Outcomes of *1*) progression to albuminuria and *2*) the composite endpoint of 40% reduction in GFR, need for renal replacement therapy, or death from renal causes occurred less frequently in patients receiving canagliflozin compared with placebo. Additionally, regression of albuminuria occurred more frequently among patients on canagliflozin compared with placebo. A subgroup analysis of the CANVAS-R trial found that benefits of canagliflozin on renal outcomes were not impacted by baseline renal function down to an eGFR of 30 mL/min/1.73 m^2.[62] As with the CANVAS-R trial, all patients in the CANTATA-SU trials had T2D (mean A1C of 7.8%).[61] The median urinary ACR at baseline in the CANTATA-SU was 8.5 mg/g creatinine; approximately 16% of patients had a baseline urinary ACR ≥30 mg/g creatinine; and approximately 61% of patients received background RAAS inhibition. Canagliflozin at both the 100-mg and 300-mg dose was associated with a decreased rate of decline in GFR compared with glimepiride, and canagliflozin 300 mg was associated with a decreased urinary ACR compared with glimepiride. Changes in A1C were similar in both groups. Therefore, the renal benefits found are thought to be independent of the glycemic effects of canagliflozin.

A secondary analysis of prespecified renal outcomes was also conducted in the EMPA-REG OUTCOME trial to assess the renal effects of empagliflozin in patients with T2D (mean A1C of 8.1%) at high risk for cardiovascular events.[63] Approximately 30% of patients had a urinary ACR of 30–300 mg/g creatinine and ~13% had a urinary ACR of >300 mg/g creatinine. Most patients (82%) were on a RAAS inhibitor at baseline. Significant benefits were found in those receiving empagliflozin compared with placebo in incident or worsening nephropathy, progression to albuminuria of >300 mg/g creatinine, doubling of serum creatinine, and initiation of renal replacement therapy. However, no difference was found in regard to rate of incident albuminuria in patients with a normal albumin level at baseline.

Dapagliflozin was assessed for renal effects as secondary outcomes in patients with T2D (mean A1C of 8.3%) and mildly reduced renal function (mean eGFR of 85.3 mL/min/1.73 m²) in the DECLARE-TIMI 58.[64,65] Of those patients with available data for urinary ACR, a majority had normoalbuminuria or microalbuminuria. It is important to note that study patients were required to have a CrCl ≥60 mL/min, but no minimum eGFR was specified. RAAS inhibitor use occurred in most patients (81.3%). The percentage of patients with the renal composite outcome of ≥40% decrease in eGFR to <60 mL/min/1.73 m², ESRD, or death from renal cause was lower in patients receiving dapagliflozin compared to placebo (1.5% vs 2.8%).

Lastly, the effects of ertugliflozin on renal outcomes in patients with T2D (mean A1C of 8.2%) were assessed as a secondary outcome of the VERTIS-CV trial.[66] Of note, patients with an eGFR below 30 mL/min/1.73 m² were excluded (mean eGFR of approximately 76 mL/min/1.73 m²) and about 80% of individuals in each group were on an RAAS inhibitor. Renal outcomes were defined as a composite of doubling of serum creatinine level, renal replacement therapy, or death due to renal causes. A nonsignificant trend toward improved renal outcomes was observed. This was primarily driven by a lower percentage of patients with a doubling of serum creatinine level in the ertugliflozin group (3.1%) compared with those in the placebo group (3.8%).

Unlike the aforementioned trials, the CREDENCE trial,[67] DAPA-CKD trial,[68] and EMPA-KIDNEY trial[69] were conducted to specifically examine the effects of canagliflozin, dapagliflozin, and empagliflozin respectively on renal outcomes. Included patients in the CREDENCE trial had T2D (mean A1C of 8.3%), were at high risk of kidney disease (mean eGFR of 56.2 mL/min/1.73 m², median urinary ACR of 927 mg/g creatinine), and were on a stable dose of an ACE inhibitor or ARB.[67] The trial was stopped early for positive efficacy findings. The primary composite outcome of ESRD, doubling of serum creatinine, and renal or cardiovascular death occurred less frequently in patients receiving canagliflozin compared with placebo. Moreover, the renal-specific composite of ESRD, a doubling of serum creatinine, or renal death was lower in the canagliflozin group than in the placebo group. Benefits were consistently seen throughout various stages of renal disease.

However, due to the exclusion of patients with normoalbuminuria, microalbuminuria, and eGFR <30 mL/min/1.73 m², findings from the study may not be generalizable to these populations.

Although patients with and without T2D were included in the DAPA-CKD trial, a majority of patients had T2D (67.5%).[68] Compared with the CREDENCE trial, patients with a slightly more severe degree of CKD were included (eGFR of 25 to 75 mL/min/1.73 m², mean of 43.1 mL/min/1.73 m²; urinary ACR of 200 to 5,000 mg/g creatinine, median of 950 mg/g creatinine). Study participants were required to be on a stable dose of an ACE inhibitor or ARB unless documented as being unable to take these medications. Greater efficacy, as measured by the primary composite outcome of sustained decline in eGFR of at least 50%, ESRD, or renal or cardiovascular mortality, was observed in patients in the dapagliflozin group compared with patients in the placebo group. The beneficial findings remained regardless of the presence of T2D.

The EMPA-KIDNEY trial was designed specifically to address the efficacy and safety of empagliflozin in patients with a wider range of eGFRs and degrees of albuminuria (eGFR of 20 to <45 mL/min/1.73 m² with any degree of albuminuria or eGFR of 45 to <90 mL/min/1.73 m² with urinary ACR of at least 200 mg/g creatinine; mean eGFR 37.4 mL/min/1.73 m², median urinary ACR 329 mg/g creatinine).[69] Unlike previous trials, a little over half of all patients did not have diabetes. Notably, 85.2% of patients were on an RAAS inhibitor at baseline. The trial was stopped early due to efficacy benefits found. Specifically, a significantly lower percentage of the primary composite outcome of progression of kidney disease or death from cardiovascular causes was observed in patients receiving empagliflozin compared with placebo. This appeared to be primarily driven by a decrease in progression of kidney disease. Findings were consistent across various eGFR ranges. Subgroup analyses examining patients not on RAAS inhibitors or patients with normoalbuminuria found similar outcomes between groups. Consequently, it is unclear whether or not the addition of SGLT2 inhibitors would benefit these patient populations.

Although they do not have such an FDA-approved indication, SGLT2 inhibitors have been studied in patients with T1D. In particular, a post-hoc analysis of the DEPICT trials found greater improvements in urinary ACR from baseline in those on dapagliflozin compared with those on placebo in patients with T1D.[70] No significant difference was found in eGFR between groups. Further research is needed in this patient population to fully determine the effects of this class of medication on renal outcomes.

No head-to-head trials are available. Differences in renal outcomes found between trials are likely attributed to differing baseline renal function, definitions of the renal composite outcome, glomerular filtration estimating equations, and duration of T2D and follow-up. Although canagliflozin and dapagliflozin are the only SGLT2 inhibitors to currently have an FDA-labeled indication for diabetic nephropathy with albuminuria, it is generally accepted that albuminuria reduction and preservation of eGFR are class effects.

Overall, there is growing evidence to show that SGLT2 inhibitors offer beneficial effects on renal outcomes in patients with T2D. Extrapolating from the patient populations studied in the aforementioned trials and landmark SGLT2 inhibitor trials focused on other disease states, recommendations focus on supporting use of SGLT2 inhibitors in patients with eGFR ≥20 mL/min/1.73 m² and urinary ACR ≥200 mg/g creatinine.[1,67–74] More trials are being conducted to evaluate the effect of SGLT2 inhibitors in patients with DKD. The benefits are not just limited to urinary ACR, but extend to hard renal endpoints such as ESRD. Moreover, these benefits were seen across different degrees of albuminuria and stages of kidney disease. That said, due to the attenuated effects on blood glucose control at eGFR of <45 mL/min/1.73 m²,[75] and limited data in patients with eGFR <30 mL/min/1.73 m², evidence for use of SGLT2 inhibitors must be carefully considered in patients with increasing severity of renal impairment. Most patients, regardless of baseline renal function, will experience a drop in eGFR by 4 to 6 mL/min/1.73 m² a few weeks after starting therapy due to afferent vasoconstriction caused by these agents.[76,77]

Common side effects related to this class include an increased risk of genital infections.[78] The FDA released a warning on the increased risk of a serious rare genital infection, Fournier's gangrene, with the use of SGLT2 inhibitors. Of note, renal function was not found to be a clinical risk factor in predicting genital fungal infections in patients taking SGLT2 inhibitors.[79] However, safety outcomes are still being explored. The increased risk of lower limb amputation observed in the CANVAS trial in patients taking canagliflozin was not confirmed in the CREDENCE trial; other observational studies report conflicting results.[80] Consequently, use of an SGLT2 inhibitor, especially canagliflozin, should be avoided in patients with prior amputations or existing foot ulcerations. It is also important to take into account the FDA alerts regarding the risk of AKI in patients taking canagliflozin and dapagliflozin. Subsequent studies have found no increased risk to a reduction in risk of AKI with the use of SGLT2 inhibitors.[81]

The impact of SGLT2 inhibitors on volume depletion is important to take into consideration, especially in the context of a patient population that may be on diuretics. This class of medications exerts a loop-diuretic sparing effect. Management of diuretic therapy was not required in the landmark randomized controlled trials above. Consequently, it is difficult to ascertain the impact these medications may have had on outcomes. However, it is prudent to assess volume status and blood pressure when initiating and during therapy.[82]

GLP-1 RAs AND DPP-4 INHIBITORS

In addition to their effects on glycemic control, GLP-1 RAs and DPP-4 inhibitors potentially have direct beneficial effects on renal function independent of their glucose-lowering effects. Most studies investigating the mechanisms of action of these medications on diabetic nephropathy have been in animal studies or models. Elucidated mechanisms of actions include inhibition of inflammatory markers, attenuation of angiotensin II–mediated effects, and modulation of sodium-water homeostasis.[83] Extrapolation of these findings to humans should be done cautiously, and data are insufficient to discriminate whether the effect of these medications on nephropathy is due to improvement of glycemic control or direct action on the kidneys.

In general, like the SGLT2 inhibitors, the renal effects of these medications are mainly derived from secondary analyses of trials with primary outcomes related to cardiovascular effects of these agents in patients with T2D.

The LEADER trial examined the effects of liraglutide on prespecified secondary renal outcomes in patients with T2D (mean A1C of 8.7%).[84] Microalbuminuria was present in 26.3% of patients and macroalbuminuria was present in 10.5% of patients at randomization. Approximately 84% of patients received RAAS inhibitors at baseline. The composite renal outcome of new-onset persistent macroalbuminuria, persistent doubling of serum creatinine and eGFR of 45 mL/min/1.73 m^2 or less, the need for renal replacement therapy, or death from renal disease occurred in fewer patients receiving liraglutide than in those receiving placebo. The statistical significance achieved in the composite outcome was driven primarily by differences found in new-onset persistent macroalbuminuria in those on liraglutide compared with placebo. Additionally, the urinary ACR increased less in patients receiving liraglutide compared with placebo. Although the decrease in eGFR was lower in the liraglutide group, this is likely not clinically significant (difference of 0.38 mL/min/1.73 m^2). A prespecified subgroup analysis of the composite outcome found the renal benefit of liraglutide to be independent of baseline renal function.

Semaglutide and its effects on renal function were investigated as a prespecified secondary outcome in the SUSTAIN-6 trial.[85] Patients had T2D (mean A1C of 8.7%), and a majority were on an ACE inhibitor or ARB (~84%). Albuminuria status at baseline was not reported. The same composite outcome used in the LEADER trial was examined and found to have similar results: patients in the semaglutide group experienced the composite outcome less frequently than those in the placebo group. Again, this was driven by benefits seen with semaglutide on the development of new-onset persistent macroalbuminuria. Renal outcomes have not been assessed or reported for the oral formulation of semaglutide.

An exploratory analysis of the REWIND trial examined the effects of dulaglutide or placebo on the renal component of composite microvascular outcome, defined as the first occurrence of new macroalbuminuria (urinary ACR >300 mg/g creatinine), a sustained decline in eGFR of 30% or more from baseline, or chronic renal replacement therapy.[86] The mean A1C was 7.4%. Patients had a mean eGFR of 76.9 mL/min/1.73 m^2 and urinary ACR of 16.3 mg/g creatinine. Approximately 84% of individuals were on an ACE inhibitor or ARB at baseline. The significant difference found in the renal component of the composite microvascular outcome favoring dulaglutide was driven mainly by progression to macroalbuminuria.

Dulaglutide efficacy and safety was assessed in patients with T2D (mean A1C 8.6%) and moderate-to-severe chronic kidney disease (eGFR 38.3 mL/min/1.73 m^2) in the AWARD-7 trial.[87] Patients were also required to be treated with a maximum tolerated dose of ACE inhibitor or ARB (93%). A majority of patients had microalbuminuria or macroalbuminuria (78%). The decline in eGFR was smaller for dulaglutide compared to insulin glargine. Overall, decreases from baseline in urinary ACR were achieved with dulaglutide and insulin glargine with no statistical differences between groups. However, in patients with macroalbuminuria, urinary ACR decreases were significantly larger in patients taking dulaglutide 1.5 mg

Table 25.1—Medications and Dosing*

Class	Medication	Typical dose(s)	Renal dose adjustment(s)	Hepatic dose adjustment(s)
ACE Inhibitors	Captopril (Capoten)	Initial: 25 mg t.i.d.	Reduce initial dose and titrate slowly	None
	Enalapril (Vasotec)	Initial: 2.5 mg b.i.d. Max: 40 mg/day	CrCl ≤30 mL/min: initial 2.5 mg daily; titrate upward as needed HD: initial 2.5 mg after dialysis on dialysis days; adjust dose on non-dialysis days depending on blood pressure response	None or not specified
	Lisinopril (Prinivil, Zestril)	Initial: 2.5–5 mg daily Max: 80 mg/day	HD: initial 2.5 mg daily after dialysis	None or not specified
	Ramipril (Altace)	Initial: 1.25–2.5 mg daily Max: 20 mg/day	CrCl <40 mL/min: administer 25% of normal dose	None or not specified
ARBs	Candesartan (Atacand)	Initial: 4–8 mg daily Max: 32 mg/day	None or not specified	None or not specified
	Irbesartan (Avapro)	Initial: 150 mg daily Max: 300 mg/day	None or not specified	None or not specified
	Losartan (Cozaar)	Initial: 25–50 mg daily Max: 100 mg/day	None or not specified	Mild to moderate hepatic impairment: initial 25 mg once daily Severe hepatic impairment: not studied
	Olmesartan (Benicar)	Initial: 20 mg daily Max: 40 mg/day	None or not specified	None or not specified
	Telmisartan (Micardis)	Initial: 20–40 mg daily Max: 80 mg/day	None or not specified	Initiate therapy with low dose; titrate slowly and monitor closely
	Valsartan (Diovan)	Initial: 80 mg daily Max: 320 mg/day	None or not specified	None or not specified
Direct Renin Inhibitor	Aliskiren (Tekturna)	Initial: 150 mg daily Max: 300 mg/day	None or not specified	None or not specified

(continued)

Table 25.1 (continued)

Class	Medication	Typical dose(s)	Renal dose adjustment(s)	Hepatic dose adjustment(s)
SGLT2 Inhibitors	Canagliflozin (Invokana)	Initial: 100 mg daily Max: 300 mg/day	eGFR 30 to <60 mL/min/1.73 m²: 100 mg daily eGFR <30 mL/min/1.73 m² with UAE ≤300 mg/day: not recommended for initiation of therapy eGFR <30 mL/min/1.73 m² with UAE >300 mg/day: not recommended for initiation of therapy; in patients previously on canagliflozin, may continue 100 mg daily HD: contraindicated	None or not specified
	Dapagliflozin (Farxiga)	Initial: 5 mg daily Max: 10 mg/day	eGFR <25 mL/min/1.73 m²: not recommended for initiation of therapy; in patients previously on dapagliflozin, may continue 10 mg daily HD: contraindicated	None or not specified
	Empagliflozin (Jardiance)	Initial: 10 mg daily Max: 25 mg/day	eGFR <20 mL/min/1.73 m²: not recommended; in patients previously on empagliflozin may continue 10 mg daily HD: contraindicated	None or not specified
	Ertugliflozin (Steglatro)	Initial: 5 mg daily Max: 15 mg/day	eGFR <45 mL/min/1.73 m²; not recommended HD: contraindicated	None or not specified

(continued)

Table 25.1 (continued)

Class	Medication	Typical dose(s)	Renal dose adjustment(s)	Hepatic dose adjustment(s)
GLP-1 RAs	Dulaglutide (Trulicity)	Initial: 0.75 mg SQ once weekly Max: 1.5 mg SQ weekly	None or not specified	None or not specified
	Exenatide (Bydureon)	2 mg SQ once weekly	eGFR <45 mL/min/1.73 m², ESRD: not recommended	None or not specified
	Liraglutide (Victoza)	Initial: 0.6 mg SQ daily for 1 week; then increase to 1.2 mg daily Max: 1.8 mg SQ daily	None or not specified	None or not specified
	Lixisenatide (Adlyxin)	Initial: 10 µg SQ daily for 14 days; on day 15 increase to 20 µg daily Maintenance dose: 20 µg SQ daily	eGFR <15 mL/min/1.73 m²: not recommended	None or not specified
	Semaglutide (Ozempic)	Initial: 0.25 mg SQ once weekly for 4 weeks then increase to 0.5 mg once weekly for at least 4 weeks Max: 1 mg SQ once weekly	None or not specified	None or not specified
DPP-4 Inhibitors	Alogliptin (Nesina)	25 mg daily	CrCl ≥30 to <60 mL/min: 12.5 mg daily CrCl ≥15 to <30 mL/min: 6.25 mg daily CrCl <15 mL/min or HD: 6.25 mg daily	None or not specified
	Linagliptin (Tradjenta)	5 mg daily	None or not specified	None or not specified
	Saxagliptin (Onglyza)	2.5–5 mg daily	eGFR <45 mL/min/1.73 m²: 2.5 mg daily HD: 2.5 mg daily; administer post dialysis	None or not specified
	Sitagliptin (Januvia)	100 mg daily	eGFR ≥30 to <45 mL/min/1.73 m²: 50 mg daily eGFR <30 mL/min/1.73 m²: 25 mg daily HD: 25 mg daily	None or not specified

(continued)

Table 25.1 (continued)

Class	Medication	Typical dose(s)	Renal dose adjustment(s)	Hepatic dose adjustment(s)
NDCAs	Diltiazem (Cardizem, Tiazac)	Initial: 120–180 mg daily Max: 480–540 mg/day	None or not specified	None or not specified
	Verapamil (Calan, Verelan)	Initial: 40–80 mg t.i.d. Max: 480 mg/day	None or not specified	Severe hepatic impairment: 30% of the normal dose
MRAs	Spironolactone (Aldactone)	Initial: 12.5–25 mg daily Max: 100–200 mg	Use with caution due to risk of hyperkalemia	None or not specified
	Eplerenone (Inspra)	Initial: 25 mg daily Max: 100 mg/day	Use with caution due to risk of hyperkalemia	None or not specified
	Finerenone (Kerendia)	Typical dose(s): 10 mg daily Max: 20 mg daily	Initial: eGFR ≥25 to <60 mL/min/1.73m²: 10 mg daily; eGFR < 25 mL/min/1.73m²: not recommended Maintenance: determined by serum potassium measured 4 weeks after initiation or a dose adjustment and periodically	Severe hepatic impairment: avoid use

ACE, angiotensin-converting enzyme; ARB, angiotensin receptor blocker; CrCl, creatinine clearance; DPP-4, dipeptidyl peptidase 4; eGFR, estimated glomerular filtration rate; ESRD, end-stage renal disease; GLP-1 RA, glucagon-like peptide-1 receptor agonist; HD, hemodialysis; MRA, mineralocorticoid receptor antagonist; NDCA, nondihydropyridine calcium antagonist; SGLT2, sodium–glucose cotransporter 2; SQ, subcutaneously; UAE, urinary albumin excretion. * Not inclusive of all medications within each class (focused on medications discussed in the chapter); § Oral route unless otherwise indicated; ^ General doses, not necessarily specific to indication of diabetic nephropathy.

compared with insulin glargine. No significant difference was found in urinary ACR decrease with dulaglutide 0.75 mg compared to insulin glargine.

Lixisenatide was found to decrease the percentage change in urinary ACR from baseline favorably compared with placebo in the ELIXA trial.[88] As with the previous trials, renal outcomes were considered to be an additional efficacy variable examined. Patients had T2D (mean A1C of 7.7%) and normoalbuminuria (median urinary ACR of 10.3 mg/g creatinine). About 85% of patients were taking an ACE inhibitor or ARB at baseline. The change in urinary ACR was found to be statistically significant in favor of lixisenatide. However, this may not be clinically significant (difference of 1.5 mg/g creatinine between groups). An exploratory analysis of the ELIXA trial confirmed the above finding in regard to change in urinary ACR, and associated the significant difference to those with macroalbuminuria.[89] Patients with normoalbuminuria or microalbuminuria did not achieve statistical significance.

In the safety analysis of the EXSCEL trial, once-weekly exenatide was found to have a similar incidence of microalbuminuira (exenatide 7.2% vs. placebo 7.5%), macroalbuminuria (exenatide 2.2% vs. placebo 2.8%), and ESRD needing chronic peritoneal dialysis, hemodialysis, or renal transplantation (exenatide 0.7% vs. placebo 0.9%) between groups.[90] Patients in this trial had a median A1C of 8.0% and median eGFR of 76.3 mL/min/1.73m². Approximately 80% of individuals were on an ACE inhibitor or ARB.

Meta-analyses examining the effects of GLP-1 RAs on diabetic nephropathy have shown conflicting results.[91–93]

In regard to DPP-4 inhibitors, similar benefits on diabetic nephropathy have been seen, but, again, the data are limited and mainly derived from secondary analyses of controlled clinical trials.

A pooled analysis of all randomized, double-blind, and placebo-controlled trials of linagliptin was conducted to assess the renal effects of the medication.[94] Patients had T2D (mean A1C of 8.2%); 66% of patients had a urinary ACR of 30 mg/g creatinine or less. Approximately 45% of patients were on ACE inhibitors or ARBs at enrollment. The primary outcome examined was a composite of first occurrence of six individual and clinically relevant kidney disease endpoints. The six endpoints were new onset of moderate elevation of albuminuria, new onset of severe elevation of albuminuria, reduction in kidney function, halving of eGFR, incidence of acute renal failure, and death from any cause. This composite outcome occurred less frequently in patients receiving linagliptin compared with placebo, and was driven by differences seen with new onset of moderate elevation of albuminuria in favor of linagliptin. Changes in urinary ACR also favored linagliptin.

The CARMELINA trial specifically examined patients with T2D (mean A1C of 8.0%) at high risk of kidney events (median urinary ACR 162 mg/g creatinine, mean eGFR 54.6 mL/min/1.73 m²).[95] A majority of patients were on an ACE inhibitor or ARB (81.1%). Although it was assessed as a secondary outcome, the study did not find a difference in the renal composite outcome of sustained ESRD, death due to kidney failure, or sustained decrease of ≥40% in eGFR from baseline between those receiving linagliptin and those receiving placebo. However, in an exploratory analysis of renal outcomes, progression of albuminuria occurred less frequently in patients on linagliptin compared with placebo (35.3% vs. 38.5%). It is unclear whether or not this positive outcome can be attributed to the effect of glucose control.

The SAVOR-TIMI 53[96,97] (saxagliptin vs. placebo), EXAMINE[98] (alogliptin vs. placebo), and TECOS[99,100] (sitagliptin vs. placebo) trials reported renal outcomes as other efficacy or safety endpoints. Benefits in change in urinary ACR were seen with saxagliptin and sitagliptin compared with placebo in patients in which urinary ACR data were available. The difference in mean change in urinary ACR in patients receiving saxagliptin compared with placebo was mainly driven by differences in change in urinary ACR among patients with urinary ACRs >300 mg/g creatinine at baseline, but was statistically significant at any level of albuminuria.[97]

An observational cohort study was conducted to determine the renoprotective effects of DPP-4 inhibitors and found benefit with use of these agents, especially in patients with macroalbuminuria.[101] Patients with macroalbuminuria experienced significant reductions in albumin levels, but patients with normoalbuminuria or microalbuminuria did not. Similarly, reductions in eGFR were reversed in patients with macroalbuminuria or normoalbuminuria and slowed in patients with microalbuminuria.

In general, evidence supporting the use of GLP-1 RAs or DPP-4 inhibitors for diabetic nephropathy points toward a strong effect on macroalbuminuria. Limited evidence is available for effects on hard renal endpoints.

Mineralocorticoid Receptor Antagonists

Contribution of aldosterone to the development of renal fibrosis and sclerosis has been shown in experimental models or animals.[102] Consequently, medications that reduce the concentration of aldosterone, and hence oxidative stress and inflammation leading to fibrosis and sclerosis, may play a renoprotective role in patients with DKD.

Due to concerns of adverse effects of traditional mineralocorticoid receptor antagonists (MRAs), newer MRAs with different properties have been developed and studied to overcome these limitations.[103] Specifically, finerenone has been found to have less incidence of hyperkalemia, and higher potency and mineralocorticoid receptor selectivity than spironolactone or eplerenone.[103]

The FIDELIO-DKD trial showed promising results on renal outcomes in patients with T2D (mean A1C of 7.7%) and CKD (mean eGFR of 44.3 mL/min/1.73 m², median urinary ACR of 852 mg/g creatinine) on finerenone compared with placebo.[104] Patients were on maximally tolerated doses of ACE inhibitors or ARBs. A significantly lower percentage of patients experiencing the primary composite outcome of a sustained decrease of at least 40% in eGFR, renal failure, or death due to renal causes was seen in patients on finerenone (17.8%) compared with patients on placebo (21.1%). As expected, the incidence of investigator-reported hyperkalemia was higher in the finerenone group (11.8% vs. 4.8%) and led to more permanent discontinuation of the medication due to hyperkalemia (2.3% vs. 0.9%).

Patients with T2D (mean A1C of 7.7%) and a wider range of CKD (mean eGFR of 67.8 mL/min/1.73 m², median urinary ACR of 308 mg/g creatinine) were examined in the FIGARO-DKD trial.[105] Essentially 100% of patients were on baseline ACE inhibitors or ARBs. Renal outcomes were assessed as a secondary composite outcome of a sustained decrease of at least 40% in eGFR, renal failure, or death due to renal causes. Unlike the FIDELIO-DKD trial, no statistically significant difference was found between patients on finerenone (9.5%) and patients on placebo (10.8%) in regard to the composite renal outcome. However, benefits favoring finerenone were seen with incidence of ESRD and reduction in urinary ACR from baseline to month 4. Consistent findings regarding hyperkalemia were noted with a higher incidence and permanent discontinuation in the finerenone group compared with the placebo group.

Results from a prespecified pooled analysis of the FIDELIO-DKD and FIGARO-DKD trials, FIDELITY, confirmed the renal benefits of finerenone.[106] Patients receiving finerenone had a significantly lower incidence of the composite kidney outcome (sustained ≥57% eGFR decline, kidney failure, or renal death) compared with placebo (5.5% vs. 7.1%). Significance in the composite kidney outcome was primarily driven by reductions observed in sustained ≥57% decline in eGFR from baseline over ≥4 weeks and kidney failure, but not renal death.

CCBs

The renoprotective role of CCBs is more equivocal than that of the RAS inhibitors. In part, this may be due to the fact that effects on nephropathy may be highly dependent on the individual CCB. In addition to blood pressure–lowering effects that impact the development and progression of diabetic nephropathy, certain CCBs have intrarenal effects. In general, nondihydropyridine calcium antagonists (NDCAs) reduce glomerular membrane permeability, especially to large molecules such as proteins.[107] On the other hand, dihydropyridine calcium antagonists (DCAs) preferentially vasodilate the afferent arteriole, increasing glomerular pressure and perhaps negating the beneficial effects of blood-pressure reduction.[108] However, there potentially are some exceptions.[109]

NDCAs versus DCAs

The difficulty in establishing the benefits of CCBs for renoprotection in patients with diabetes potentially stems from inconsistent findings in the literature when examining the medication class as a whole. However, when breaking down the class into subclasses, benefits are found beyond blood pressure–lowering effects with the NDCAs compared with the DCAs. A systematic review examining the differences in these subclasses and their effects on proteinuria in individuals with hypertension (mean blood pressure of 162/97 mmHg) found that although these two subclasses of calcium antagonists lower blood pressure to a similar degree, NDCAs provide greater reductions in proteinuria regardless of diabetes status or background ACE inhibitor or ARB therapy.[108] Of note, the number of studies examining patients with diabetes on concomitant calcium antagonists and RAAS inhibitor therapy was limited, and of these, a majority examined ACE inhibitor and NDCA combinations.

CCBs versus RAAS Inhibitors

In studies comparing calcium antagonists to ACE inhibitors or ARBs in patients with diabetes and albuminuria, renoprotection by calcium antagonists was often inferior. However, most of the head-to-head comparison trials included a DCA rather than an NDCA.

A small trial compared the effects of diltiazem to lisinopril on diabetic nephropathy.[110] Patients had T2D, hypertension (mean arterial blood pressure of 118 mmHg), and nephrotic-range proteinuria (mean urinary protein excretion of 4,100 mg per 24 h). Both medications reduced urinary protein excretion by relatively the same amount over 6 weeks.

The MARVAL trial was a larger study that also compared the renal effects of a CCB to an RAAS inhibitor, but in patients with lower albuminuria levels.[28] Specifically, valsartan was compared with amlodipine to determine their effects on UAE rate in patients with T2D and albuminuria of 20–200 μg/min. Valsartan was more effective in lowering UAE rates compared with amlodipine. Similar findings were seen in the IDNT trial, but with irbesartan compared with amlodipine.[29]

COMBINATION THERAPY

DUAL RAAS INHIBITORS

Several studies have investigated the combination of RAAS inhibitors on further improving outcomes in patients with DKD. Combination ACE inhibitor and ARB treatment was studied in three large randomized controlled trials, two of which included only patients with T2D.

Benefits on albuminuria were seen with combination candesartan and lisinopril compared with either agent alone in patients with T2D, hypertension (mean blood pressure of 163/96 mmHg), and albuminuria defined as urinary ACR between 22 and 221 mg/g creatinine (geometric mean urinary ACR of 55 mg/g creatinine).[111] Specifically, combination therapy reduced urinary ACR to a greater extent than candesartan monotherapy, but not lisinopril monotherapy. No clinically significant difference was found in regard to potassium concentrations. On the other hand, the Veterans Affairs Nephropathy in Diabetes (VA-NEPHRON D) trial examining the effects of combination therapy with losartan and lisinopril was stopped early due to safety concerns related to hyperkalemia and AKI in the combination group compared with the monotherapy groups.[112]

The Ongoing Telmisartan Alone and in Combination with Ramipril Global Endpoint Trial (ONTARGET) study examined the effects of telmisartan, ramipril, or a combination of the two drugs on nephropathy as a secondary outcome.[113,114] Approximately 38% of patients had diabetes. In regard to the frequency of the composite renal outcome of dialysis, doubling of serum creatinine, and death, telmisartan and ramipril had similar effects. However, combination therapy resulted in an increased frequency of the composite endpoint. The composite endpoint was primarily driven by differences seen with acute dialysis. eGFR concentrations decreased at a greater rate in those in the telmisartan and combination groups compared with ramipril. Urinary ACRs increased to a lesser extent in those receiving telmisartan or combination therapy than in those receiving ramipril. Overall, although combination therapy reduced albuminuria to a greater extent, major renal outcomes were worse.

Combination therapy with aliskiren and an ACE inhibitor or ARB has also been examined and, like the above trials, found to have inconsistent results. The Aliskiren in the Evaluation of Proteinuria in Diabetes (AVOID) trial investigated aliskiren compared with placebo on top of losartan background therapy in patients with T2D, hypertension (mean blood pressure of 135/78 mmHg), and nephropathy defined as a urinary ACR of >300 mg/g creatinine (geometric mean urinary ACR of 533 mg/g creatinine).[115] Significantly greater reductions in urinary ACR were seen in the aliskiren group compared with the placebo group. Although there was a trend in increased serum potassium levels in those receiving aliskiren compared with those receiving placebo, it was not significant (percentage of patients with at least one value of serum potassium ≥6.0 mmol/L, 4.7% vs. 1.7%). Conversely, the Aliskiren Trial in Type 2 Diabetes Using Cardiovascular and Renal Disease Endpoints (ALTITUDE) trial examining the combination of aliskiren with an ACE inhibitor or ARB was stopped prematurely secondary to an increase in adverse effects.[116]

CCBs + RAAS INHIBITORS

A greater reduction in intraglomerular pressure may be provided with the combined use of a calcium antagonist and RAAS inhibitor due to effects of the calcium antagonist in reducing afferent arteriolar pressure and the RAAS inhibitor in reducing efferent arteriolar pressure.

Direct comparison of the subclasses in an RAAS inhibitor-calcium antagonist combination was examined in a study of patients with T2D, hypertension (mean blood pressure of 142/81 mmHg), and diabetic nephropathy (mean urinary ACR of 830 mg/g creatinine).[117] No difference was found on percentage change in urinary ACR from baseline to week 36 or final visit with trandolapril-verapamil SR compared with benazepril-amlodipine. This trial suggests that a dihydropyridine-RAAS inhibitor combination may negate any negative effects DCAs may have on the kidneys. In fact, in the RENAAL trial examining the effects of losartan compared with placebo on the progression of nephropathy, a majority of patients were on a dihydropyridine at baseline and during study treatment.[43] Again, this suggests that DCAs, when used with an RAAS inhibitor, do not counteract the benefits of the RAAS inhibitor on nephropathy progression.

Another study observed significant reductions of proteinuria from baseline with a combination NDCA-ACE inhibitor (verapamil-trandolapril) over either agent alone.[118] This study examined patients with T2D, hypertension (mean blood pressure of 172/105 mmHg), and urinary protein excretion of >300 mg per day (mean UAE rate of 631 mg per day). However, the trial was relatively small, with 37 participants.

MRAs + RAAS INHIBITORS

The concept of aldosterone breakthrough lends to the mechanistic understanding of combining an MRA and RAAS inhibitor. Aldosterone breakthrough is typically defined as an elevated plasma aldosterone concentration after treatment compared with pretreatment concentrations.[119] In regard to diabetic nephropathy, aldosterone breakthrough can be thought of as sustained aldosterone synthesis during long-term RAAS inhibitor therapy.

Combination therapy with an RAAS inhibitor has been examined with both traditional[120,121] and non-traditional[104–106] MRAs. Studies of concomitant spironolactone or eplerenone with RAAS inhibitors have generally been limited by small sample size. As mentioned above, randomized controlled trials assessing finerenone required patients to be on background ACE inhibitor or ARB therapy (see previous "Mineralocorticoid Receptor Antagonists" section). Benefits in renal outcomes found in these studies need to be balanced with the increased risk of hyperkalemia.

SGLT2 INHIBITORS + RAAS INHIBITORS

The different roles that SGLT2 inhibitors and RAAS inhibitors play in the kidney may theoretically promote synergistic activity when used as combination therapy in DKD. Although this has mechanistically been seen in animal models, extrapolation to humans must be done with caution.[122] In general, in the trials assessing SGLT2 inhibitors, patients received background ACE inhibitor or ARB therapy (see previous "SGLT2 Inhibitors" section).

SGLT2 INHIBITORS + GLP-1 RAS

The differing mechanisms of action of SGLT2 inhibitors and GLP-1 RAs likely explain the differing effects found with each class on renal outcomes. Moreover, due to the largely distinct mechanisms, combining medications from these classes may have an additive beneficial effect. No clinical trial examining renal outcomes with combination SGLT2 inhibitors and GLP-1 RAs has been reported to date. However, a post hoc analysis of the EXSCEL trial examined patients who took SGLT2 inhibitors and GLP-1 RAs in parallel or sequentially over the course of the trial.[123] Outcomes were compared between patients on combination therapy and patients on placebo or exenatide alone. The number of renal events (persistent 40% reduction in eGFR, renal dialysis, renal transplant, new macroalbuminuria) were fairly similar between groups. Moreover, although benefits were seen in regard to eGFR slope in those on combination therapy compared with placebo or exenatide alone, the observed eGFR slope improvement appeared to be primarily due to the SGLT2 inhibitor.

SGLT2 INHIBITORS + DPP-4 INHIBITORS

Analyses of secondary outcomes in trials of patients on combined SGLT2 inhibitors and DPP-4 inhibitors suggest potential benefit of this combination on renal outcomes. Specifically, one study found that combination empagliflozin-linagliptin had more patients regress in proteinuria compared with each medication at 52 weeks.[124]

SGLT2 INHIBITORS + MRAS

Differences in mechanism of action between SGLT2 inhibitors and MRAs may provide additional benefits beyond those seen with each individual therapy. A subset of patients in the FIDELIO-DKD[104] (4.6%) and FIGARO-DKD[105] (8.4%) trials received concomitant SGLT2 inhibitor treatment during the trial. In the pooled analysis of both trials (FIDELITY), reduction in the composite kidney outcome was found irrespective of SGLT2 inhibitor use at baseline, but tended to be greater among patients on SGLT2 inhibitors at baseline. Furthermore, the rate of treatment-emergent hyperkalemia-related adverse events were lower in patients who received an SGLT2 inhibitor at baseline compared to those who did not.[125]

COMBINATION PRODUCTS

Ccbs + RAAS INHIBITORS

- Amlodipine-benazepril (Lotrel)
- Verapamil-trandolapril (Tarka)

MONOGRAPHS

ACE INHIBITORS

Captopril (Capoten): https://dailymed.nlm.nih.gov/dailymed/drugInfo.cfm?setid=01cca91e-0374-4b89-a25a-be05e8b64346

Enalapril (Vasotec): https://dailymed.nlm.nih.gov/dailymed/drugInfo.cfm?setid=39631f1f-5d19-43c1-b504-bf56d991ed97

Lisinopril (Prinivil, Zestril): https://dailymed.nlm.nih.gov/dailymed/drugInfo.cfm?setid=27ccb2f4-abf8-4825-9b05-0bb367b4ac07

Ramipril (Altace): https://dailymed.nlm.nih.gov/dailymed/drugInfo.cfm?setid=0fc34cd8-86e6-4034-73bd-4263a68ba046

ARBs

Candesartan (Atacand): https://dailymed.nlm.nih.gov/dailymed/drugInfo.cfm?setid=0f2b2fa3-249b-4756-a3f1-3223a004d9cb

Irbesartan (Avapro): https://dailymed.nlm.nih.gov/dailymed/drugInfo.cfm?setid=7885b2a8-be4e-48ab-8113-4e6ab791eb98

Losartan (Cozaar): https://dailymed.nlm.nih.gov/dailymed/drugInfo.cfm?setid=5ac32c20-169d-475a-fc8a-934f758d6ab0

Olmesartan (Benicar): https://dailymed.nlm.nih.gov/dailymed/drugInfo.cfm?setid=33770d80-754f-11de-8dba-0002a5d5c51b

Telmisartan (Micardis): https://dailymed.nlm.nih.gov/dailymed/drugInfo.cfm?setid=cfb9309f-e0df-4a55-9542-0e869fce05fb

Valsartan (Diovan): https://dailymed.nlm.nih.gov/dailymed/drugInfo.cfm?setid=9402b022-5809-4251-dfef-54f6ef5723fe

DIRECT RENIN INHIBITORS

Aliskiren (Tekturna): https://dailymed.nlm.nih.gov/dailymed/drugInfo. cfm?setid=3dd61fa5-1620-4ebf-bbdb-ede29b92fce2

SGLT2 INHIBITORS

Canagliflozin (Invokana): https://dailymed.nlm.nih.gov/dailymed/drugInfo. cfm?setid=b9057d3b-b104-4f09-8a61-c61ef9d4a3f3

Dapagliflozin (Farxiga): https://dailymed.nlm.nih.gov/dailymed/drugInfo. cfm?setid=72ad22ae-efe6-4cd6-a302-98aaee423d69

Empagliflozin (Jardiance): https://dailymed.nlm.nih.gov/dailymed/drugInfo. cfm?setid=faf3dd6a-9cd0-39c2-0d2e-232cb3f67565

Ertugliflozin (Steglatro): https://dailymed.nlm.nih.gov/dailymed/drugInfo. cfm?setid=e6f3e718-bb99-48f1-ab94-b9f0af05fed6

GLP-1 RAs

Dulaglutide (Trulicity): https://dailymed.nlm.nih.gov/dailymed/drugInfo. cfm?setid=463050bd-2b1c-40f5-b3c3-0a04bb433309

Exenatide (Bydureon): https://dailymed.nlm.nih.gov/dailymed/drugInfo. cfm?setid=71fe88be-b4e6-4c2d-9cc3-8b1864467776

Liraglutide (Victoza): https://dailymed.nlm.nih.gov/dailymed/drugInfo. cfm?setid=5a9ef4ea-c76a-4d34-a604-27c5b505f5a4

Lixisenatide (Adlyxin): https://dailymed.nlm.nih.gov/dailymed/drugInfo. cfm?setid=1727cc16-4f86-4f13-b8b5-804d4984fa8c

Semaglutide (Ozempic): https://dailymed.nlm.nih.gov/dailymed/drugInfo. cfm?setid=adec4fd2-6858-4c99-91d4-531f5f2a2d79

DPP-4 INHIBITORS

Alogliptin (Nesina): https://dailymed.nlm.nih.gov/dailymed/drugInfo. cfm?setid=a3768c7e-aa4c-44d3-bc53-43bb7346c0b0

Linagliptin (Tradjenta): https://dailymed.nlm.nih.gov/dailymed/drugInfo. cfm?setid=c797ea5c-cab7-494b-9044-27eba0cfe40f

Saxagliptin (Onglyza): https://dailymed.nlm.nih.gov/dailymed/drugInfo. cfm?setid=c5116390-e0fe-4969-94cb-e9de5165fbab

Sitagliptin (Januvia): https://dailymed.nlm.nih.gov/dailymed/drugInfo. cfm?setid=f85a48d0-0407-4c50-b0fa-7673a160bf01

NDCAs

Diltiazem (Cardizem, Tiazac): https://dailymed.nlm.nih.gov/dailymed/drugInfo.
cfm?setid=73b3607a-99d0-44d8-92ef-0074684c9d7d

Verapamil (Calan, Verelan): https://dailymed.nlm.nih.gov/dailymed/drugInfo.
cfm?setid=ed1e0c14-3571-43f9-88fc-5a4d2b598263

MRAs

Spironolactone (Aldactone): https://dailymed.nlm.nih.gov/dailymed/drugInfo.
cfm?setid=0fed2822-3a03-4b64-9857-c682fcd462bc

Eplerenone (Inspra): https://dailymed.nlm.nih.gov/dailymed/drugInfo.
cfm?setid=a55a39ff-1bd5-428b-a64f-c44262e2f3ed

Finerenone (Kerendia): https://dailymed.nlm.nih.gov/dailymed/lookup.
cfm?setid=fc726765-5d5a-4d6e-b037-b847bda9fb7c

REFERENCES

1. American Diabetes Association; 11. Chronic Kidney Disease and Risk Management: *Standards of Care in Diabetes—2023. Diabetes Care* 2023; 46(Suppl. 1):S191–S202

2. Harjutsalo V, Groop PH. Epidemiology and risk factors for diabetic kidney disease. *Adv Chronic Kidney Dis* 2014;21(3):260–266

3. Alicic RZ, Rooney MT, Tuttle KR. Diabetic kidney disease: challenges, progress, and possibilities. *Clin J Am Soc Nephrol* 2017;12(12):2032–2045

4. Johansen KL, Chertow GM, Gilbertson DT, et al. US renal data system 2020 annual data report: Epidemiology of kidney disease in the United States. *Am J Kidney Dis* 2022;79(4 Suppl 1):A8–A12

5. Ozieh MN, Dismuke CE, Lynch CP, Egede LE. Medical care expenditures associated with chronic kidney disease in adults with diabetes: United States 2011. *Diabetes Res Clin Pract* 2015;109(1):185–190

6. United States Renal Data System. Chapter 6: healthcare expenditures for persons with CKD. Available from https://www.usrds.org/2017/view/v1_06.aspx. Accessed 25 January 2022

7. Toth-Manikowski S, Atta MG. Diabetic kidney disease: pathophysiology and therapeutic targets. *J Diabetes Res* 2015;2015:697010

8. Kramer HJ, Nguyen QD, Curhan G, Hsu CY. Renal insufficiency in the absence of albuminuria and retinopathy among adults with type 2 diabetes mellitus. *JAMA* 2003;289(24):3273–3277

9. Afkarian M, Sachs MC, Kestenbaum B, et al. Kidney disease and increased mortality risk in type 2 diabetes. *J Am Soc Nephrol* 2013;24(2):302–308

10. Tuttle KR, Bakris GL, Bilous RW, et al. Diabetic kidney disease: a report from an ADA Consensus Conference. *Diabetes Care* 2014;37(10):2864–2883

11. Heerspink HJ, Kropelin TF, Hoekman J, de Zeeuw D. Drug-induced reduction in albuminuria is associated with subsequent renoprotection: a meta-analysis. *J Am Soc Nephrol* 2015;26(8):2055–2064

12. Apperloo AJ, de Zeeuw D, de Jong PE. A short-term antihypertensive treatment-induced fall in glomerular filtration rate predicts long-term stability of renal function. *Kidney Int* 1997;51(3):793–797

13. Holtkamp FA, de Zeeuw D, Thomas MC, et al. An acute fall in estimated glomerular filtration rate during treatment with losartan predicts a slower decrease in long-term renal function. *Kidney Int* 2011;80(3):282–287

14. DCCT/EDIC Research Group. Effect of intensive diabetes treatment on albuminuria in type 1 diabetes: long-term follow-up of the Diabetes Control and Complications Trial and Epidemiology of Diabetes Interventions and Complications study. *Lancet Diabetes Endocrinol* 2014;2(10):793–800

15. de Boer IH, Sun W, Cleary PA, et al.; DCCT/EDIC Research Group. Intensive diabetes therapy and glomerular filtration rate in type 1 diabetes. *N Engl J Med* 2011;365(25):2366–2376

16. UK Prospective Diabetes Study (UKPDS) Group. Effect of intensive blood-glucose control with metformin on complications in overweight patients with type 2 diabetes (UKPDS 34). *Lancet* 1998;352(9131):854–865

17. Ismail-Beigi F, Craven T, Banerji MA, et al. Effect of intensive treatment of hyperglycaemia on microvascular outcomes in type 2 diabetes: an analysis of the ACCORD randomised trial. *Lancet* 2010;376(9739):419–430

18. Zoungas S, Arima H, Gerstein HC, et al. Effects of intensive glucose control on microvascular outcomes in patients with type 2 diabetes: a meta-analysis of individual participant data from randomised controlled trials. *Lancet Diabetes Endocrinol* 2017;5(6):431–437

19. Patel A, MacMahon S, Chalmers J, et al.; ADVANCE Collaborative Group. Intensive blood glucose control and vascular outcomes in patients with type 2 diabetes. *N Engl J Med* 2008;358(24):2560–2572

20. Zoungas S, Chalmers J, Neal B, et al. Follow-up of blood-pressure lowering and glucose control in type 2 diabetes. *N Engl J Med* 2014;371(15):1392–1406

21. Haynes R, Lewis D, Emberson J, et al. Effects of lowering LDL cholesterol on progression of kidney disease. *J Am Soc Nephrol* 2014;25(8):1825–1833

22. Palmer SC, Craig JC, Navaneethan SD, et al. Benefits and harms of statin therapy for persons with chronic kidney disease: a systematic review and meta-analysis. *Ann Intern Med* 2012;157(4):263–275

23. Palmer SC, Navaneethan SD, Craig JC, et al. HMG CoA reductase inhibitors (statins) for dialysis patients. *Cochrane Database Syst Rev* 2013(9):CD004289

24. Qiao Y, Shin JI, Chen TK, et al. Association between renin-angiotensin system blockade discontinuation and all-cause mortality among persons with low estimated glomerular filtration rate. *JAMA Intern Med* 2020;180(5):718–726

25. Brown NJ, Vaughan DE. Angiotensin-converting enzyme inhibitors. *Circulation* 1998;97(14):1411–1420

26. Lewis EJ, Hunsicker LG, Bain RP, Rohde RD; for the Collaborative Study Group. The effect of angiotensin-converting-enzyme inhibition on diabetic nephropathy. *N Engl J Med* 1993;329(20):1456–1462

27. Parving HH, Lehnert H, Brochner-Mortensen J, et al. The effect of irbesartan on the development of diabetic nephropathy in patients with type 2 diabetes. *N Engl J Med* 2001;345(12):870–878

28. Viberti G, Wheeldon NM. Microalbuminuria reduction with valsartan in patients with type 2 diabetes mellitus: a blood pressure-independent effect. *Circulation* 2002;106(6):672–678

29. Lewis EJ, Hunsicker LG, Clarke WR, et al. Renoprotective effect of the angiotensin-receptor antagonist irbesartan in patients with nephropathy due to type 2 diabetes. *N Engl J Med* 2001;345(12):851–860

30. Kasiske BL, Kalil RS, Ma JZ, et al. Effect of antihypertensive therapy on the kidney in patients with diabetes: a meta-regression analysis. *Ann Intern Med* 1993;118(2):129–138

31. Hebert LA, Bain RP, Verme D, et al.; for the Collaborative Study Group. Remission of nephrotic range proteinuria in type I diabetes. *Kidney Int* 1994;46(6):1688–1693

32. Wilmer WA, Hebert LA, Lewis EJ, et al. Remission of nephrotic syndrome in type 1 diabetes: long-term follow-up of patients in the Captopril Study. *Am J Kidney Dis* 1999;34(2):308–314

33. Laffel LM, McGill JB, Gans DJ; on behalf of the North American Microalbuminuria Study Group. The beneficial effect of angiotensin-converting enzyme inhibition with captopril on diabetic nephropathy in normotensive IDDM patients with microalbuminuria. *Am J Med* 1995;99(5):497–504

34. Viberti G, Mogensen CE, Groop LC, Pauls JF, et al. Effect of captopril on progression to clinical proteinuria in patients with insulin-dependent diabetes mellitus and microalbuminuria. European Microalbuminuria Captopril Study Group. *JAMA* 1994;271(4):275–279

35. The Microalbuminuria Captopril Study Group. Captopril reduces the risk of nephropathy in IDDM patients with microalbuminuria. *Diabetologia* 1996;39(5):587–593

36. Parving HH, Hommel E, Jensen BR, Hansen HP. Long-term beneficial effect of ACE inhibition on diabetic nephropathy in normotensive type 1 diabetic patients. *Kidney Int* 2001;60(1):228–234

37. Lv J, Perkovic V, Foote CV, et al. Antihypertensive agents for preventing diabetic kidney disease. *Cochrane Database Syst Rev* 2012;12:CD004136

38. Van Buren PN, Toto R. Hypertension in diabetic nephropathy: epidemiology, mechanisms, and management. *Adv Chronic Kidney Dis* 2011;18(1): 28–41

39. The EUCLID Study Group. Randomised placebo-controlled trial of lisinopril in normotensive patients with insulin-dependent diabetes and normoalbuminuria or microalbuminuria. *Lancet* 1997;349(9068):1787–1792

40. Mauer M, Zinman B, Gardiner R, et al. Renal and retinal effects of enalapril and losartan in type 1 diabetes. *N Engl J Med* 2009;361(1):40–51

41. Bilous R, Chaturvedi N, Sjolie AK, et al. Effect of candesartan on microalbuminuria and albumin excretion rate in diabetes: three randomized trials. *Ann Intern Med* 2009;151(1):11–20, W13–14

42. Heart Outcomes Prevention Evaluation Study Investigators. Effects of ramipril on cardiovascular and microvascular outcomes in people with diabetes mellitus: results of the HOPE study and MICRO-HOPE substudy. *Lancet* 2000;355(9200):253–259

43. Brenner BM, Cooper ME, de Zeeuw D, et al. Effects of losartan on renal and cardiovascular outcomes in patients with type 2 diabetes and nephropathy. *N Engl J Med* 2001;345(12):861–869

44. Persson F, Rossing P, Schjoedt KJ, et al. Time course of the antiproteinuric and antihypertensive effects of direct renin inhibition in type 2 diabetes. *Kidney Int* 2008;73(12):1419–1425

45. Fogari R, Mugellini A, Zoppi A, et al. Time course of antiproteinuric effect of aliskiren in arterial hypertension associated with type 2 diabetes and microalbuminuria. *Expert Opin Pharmacother* 2013;14(4):371–384

46. Ravid M, Lang R, Rachmani R, Lishner M. Long-term renoprotective effect of angiotensin-converting enzyme inhibition in non-insulin-dependent diabetes mellitus. A 7-year follow-up study. *Arch Intern Med* 1996;156(3):286–289

47. Ruggenenti P, Fassi A, Ilieva AP, et al. Preventing microalbuminuria in type 2 diabetes. *N Engl J Med* 2004;351(19):1941–1951

48. Haller H, Ito S, Izzo JL Jr., et al. Olmesartan for the delay or prevention of microalbuminuria in type 2 diabetes. *N Engl J Med* 2011;364(10):907–917

49. Schrier RW, Estacio RO, Esler A, Mehler P. Effects of aggressive blood pressure control in normotensive type 2 diabetic patients on albuminuria, retinopathy and strokes. *Kidney Int* 2002;61(3):1086–1097

50. Ravid M, Brosh D, Levi Z, et al. Use of enalapril to attenuate decline in renal function in normotensive, normoalbuminuric patients with type 2 diabetes mellitus. A randomized, controlled trial. *Ann Intern Med* 1998;128(12 Pt 1):982–988

51. Imai E, Chan JC, Ito S, et al. Effects of olmesartan on renal and cardiovascular outcomes in type 2 diabetes with overt nephropathy: a multicentre, randomised, placebo-controlled study. *Diabetologia* 2011;54(12):2978–2986

52. Wang AC, Stellmacher U, Schumi J, et al. Assessment of the cardiovascular risk of olmesartan medoxomil-based treatment: meta-analysis of individual patient data. *Am J Cardiovasc Drugs* 2016;16(6):427–437

53. Strippoli GF, Craig M, Deeks JJ, et al. Effects of angiotensin converting enzyme inhibitors and angiotensin II receptor antagonists on mortality and renal outcomes in diabetic nephropathy: systematic review. *BMJ* 2004;329(7470):828

54. Barnett AH, Bain SC, Bouter P, et al. Angiotensin-receptor blockade versus converting-enzyme inhibition in type 2 diabetes and nephropathy. *N Engl J Med* 2004;351(19):1952–1961

55. Wu HY, Peng CL, Chen PC, et al. Comparative effectiveness of angiotensin-converting enzyme inhibitors versus angiotensin II receptor blockers for major renal outcomes in patients with diabetes: a 15-year cohort study. *PLoS One* 2017;12(5):e0177654

56. Casas JP, Chua W, Loukogeorgakis S, et al. Effect of inhibitors of the renin-angiotensin system and other antihypertensive drugs on renal outcomes: systematic review and meta-analysis. *Lancet* 2005;366(9502):2026–2033

57. Palmer SC, Mavridis D, Navarese E, et al. Comparative efficacy and safety of blood pressure-lowering agents in adults with diabetes and kidney disease: a network meta-analysis. *Lancet* 2015;385(9982):2047–2056

58. Wu HY, Huang JW, Lin HJ, et al. Comparative effectiveness of renin-angiotensin system blockers and other antihypertensive drugs in patients with diabetes: systematic review and bayesian network meta-analysis. *BMJ* 2013;347:f6008

59. Fioretto P, Zambon A, Rossato M, et al. SGLT2 inhibitors and the diabetic kidney. *Diabetes Care* 2016;39(Suppl. 2):S165–S171

60. Neal B, Perkovic V, Matthews DR. Canagliflozin and cardiovascular and renal events in type 2 diabetes. *N Engl J Med* 2017;377(21):2099

61. Heerspink HJ, Desai M, Jardine M, et al. Canagliflozin slows progression of renal function decline independently of glycemic effects. *J Am Soc Nephrol* 2017;28(1):368–375

62. Neuen BL, Ohkuma T, Neal B, et al. Cardiovascular and renal outcomes with canagliflozin according to baseline kidney function. *Circulation* 2018;138(15):1537–1550

63. Wanner C, Inzucchi SE, Lachin JM, et al. Empagliflozin and progression of kidney disease in type 2 diabetes. *N Engl J Med* 2016;375(4):323–334

64. Wiviott SD, Raz I, Bonaca MP, et al. Dapagliflozin and cardiovascular outcomes in type 2 diabetes. *N Engl J Med* 2019;380(4):347–357

65. Mosenzon O, Wiviott SD, Cahn A, et al. Effects of dapagliflozin on development and progression of kidney disease in patients with type 2 diabetes: an analysis from the DECLARE-TIMI 58 randomised trial. *Lancet Diabetes Endocrinol* 2019;7(8):606–617

66. Cannon CP, Pratley R, Dagogo-Jack S, et al. Cardiovascular outcomes with ertugliflozin in type 2 diabetes. *N Engl J Med* 2020;383(15):1425–1435

67. Perkovic V, Jardine MJ, Neal B, et al. Canagliflozin and renal outcomes in type 2 diabetes and nephropathy. *N Engl J Med* 2019;380(24):2295–2306

68. Heerspink HJL, Stefánsson BV, Correa-Rotter R, et al. Dapagliflozin in patients with chronic kidney disease. *N Engl J Med* 2020;383(15):1436-1446

69. The EMPA-KIDNEY Collaborative Group. Empagliflozin in patients with chronic kidney disease. *N Engl J Med* 2023;388(2):117–127

70. Groop PH, Dandona P, Phillip M, et al. Effect of dapagliflozin as an adjunct to insulin over 52 weeks in individuals with type 1 diabetes: post-hoc renal analysis of the DEPICT randomised controlled trials. *Lancet Diabetes Endocrinol* 2020;8(10):845-854

71. Chertow GM, Vart P, Jongs N, et al. Effects of dapagliflozin in stage 4 chronic kidney disease. *J Am Soc Nephrol* 2021;32(9):2352–2361

72. Zannad F, Ferreira JP, Pocock SJ, et al. Cardiac and kidney benefits of empagliflozin in heart failure across the spectrum of kidney function: insights from EMPEROR-Reduced. *Circulation* 2021;143(4):310–321

73. Zannad F, Kraus B, Zeller C, et al. EMPEROR-Preserved: empagliflozin and outcomes in heart failure with a preserved ejection fraction and CKD. Paper presented at: American Society of Nephrology Kidney Week; November 5, 2021 [virtual]

74. Mosenzon O, Wiviott SD, Heerspink HJL, et al. The effect of dapagliflozin on albuminuria in DECLARE-TIMI 58. *Diabetes Care* 2021;44(8):1805–1815

75. Davidson JA. SGLT2 inhibitors in patients with type 2 diabetes and renal disease: Overview of current evidence. Postgrad Med 2019;131(4):251–260

76. Wang C, Zhou Y, Kong Z, et al. The renoprotective effects of sodium-glucose cotransporter 2 inhibitors versus placebo in patients with type 2 diabetes with or without prevalent kidney disease: A systematic review and meta-analysis. *Diabetes Obes Metab* 2018;21(4):1018–1026

77. Heerspink HJL, Kosiborod M, Inzucchi SE, Cherney DZI. Renoprotective effects of sodium-glucose cotransporter-2 inhibitors. *Kidney Int* 2018;94(1):26–39

78. Liu J, Li L, Li S, et al. Effects of SGLT2 inhibitors on UTIs and genital infections in type 2 diabetes mellitus: a systematic review and meta-analysis. *Sci Rep* 2017;7(1):2824

79. Thong KY, Yadagiri M, Barnes DJ, et al. Clinical risk factors predicting genital fungal infections with sodium-glucose cotransporter 2 inhibitor treatment: The ABCD nationwide dapagliflozin audit. *Prim Care Diabetes* 2018;12(1):45–50

80. Papadokostaki E, Rizos E, Tigas S, Liberopoulos EN. Canagliflozin and amputation risk: Evidence so far. *Int J Low Extrem Wounds* 2019:21–26

81. Sridhar VS, Tuttle KR, Cherney DZI. We can finally stop worrying about SGLT2 inhibitors and acute kidney injury. *Am J Kidney Dis* 2020;76(4):454-456

82. Cherney DZ, Udell JA. Use of sodium glucose cotransporter 2 inhibitors in the hands of cardiologists: With great power comes great responsibility. *Circulation* 2016;134(24):1915–1917

83. Filippatos TD, Elisaf MS. Effects of glucagon-like peptide-1 receptor agonists on renal function. *World J Diabetes* 2013;4(5):190–201

84. Mann JFE, Orsted DD, Brown-Frandsen K, et al. Liraglutide and renal outcomes in type 2 diabetes. *N Engl J Med* 2017;377(9):839–848

85. Marso SP, Bain SC, Consoli A, et al. Semaglutide and cardiovascular outcomes in patients with type 2 diabetes. *N Engl J Med* 2016;375(19):1834–1844

86. Gerstein HC, Colhoun HM, Dagenais GR, et al. Dulaglutide and renal outcomes in type 2 diabetes: An exploratory analysis of the REWIND randomised, placebo-controlled trial. *Lancet* 2019;394(10193):131–138

87. Tuttle KR, Lakshmanan MC, Rayner B, et al. Dulaglutide versus insulin glargine in patients with type 2 diabetes and moderate-to-severe chronic kidney disease (AWARD-7): A multicentre, open-label, randomised trial. *Lancet Diabetes Endocrinol* 2018;6(8):605–617

88. Pfeffer MA, Claggett B, Diaz R, et al. Lixisenatide in patients with type 2 diabetes and acute coronary syndrome. *N Engl J Med* 2015;373(23):2247–2257

89. Muskiet MHA, Tonneijck L, Huang Y, et al. Lixisenatide and renal outcomes in patients with type 2 diabetes and acute coronary syndrome: An exploratory analysis of the ELIXA randomised, placebo-controlled trial. *Lancet Diabetes Endocrinol* 2018;6(11):859–869

90. Holman RR, Bethel MA, Mentz RJ, et al. Effects of once-weekly exenatide on cardiovascular outcomes in type 2 diabetes. *N Engl J Med* 2017;377(13):1228–1239

91. Dicembrini I, Nreu B, Scatena A, et al. Microvascular effects of glucagon-like peptide-1 receptor agonists in type 2 diabetes: a meta-analysis of randomized controlled trials. *Acta Diabetol* 2017;54(10):933–941

92. Gargiulo P, Savarese G, D'Amore C, et al. Efficacy and safety of glucagon-like peptide-1 agonists on macrovascular and microvascular events in type 2 diabetes mellitus: a meta-analysis. *Nutr Metab Cardiovasc Dis* 2017;27(12):1081–1088

93. Giugliano D, Maiorino MI, Bellastella G, Longo M, Chiodini P, Esposito K. GLP-1 receptor agonists for prevention of cardiorenal outcomes in type 2 diabetes: An updated meta-analysis including the REWIND and PIONEER 6 trials. *Diabetes Obes Metab* 2019;21(11):2576–2580

94. Cooper ME, Perkovic V, McGill JB, et al. Kidney disease end points in a pooled analysis of individual patient-level data from a large clinical trials program of the dipeptidyl peptidase 4 inhibitor linagliptin in type 2 diabetes. *Am J Kidney Dis* 2015;66(3):441–449

95. Rosenstock J, Perkovic V, Johansen OE, et al. Effect of linagliptin vs placebo on major cardiovascular events in adults with type 2 diabetes and high cardiovascular and renal risk: The CARMELINA randomized clinical trial. *JAMA* 2019;321(1):69–79

96. Scirica BM, Bhatt DL, Braunwald E, et al. Saxagliptin and cardiovascular outcomes in patients with type 2 diabetes mellitus. *N Engl J Med* 2013;369(14):1317–1326

97. Mosenzon O, Leibowitz G, Bhatt DL, et al. Effect of saxagliptin on renal outcomes in the SAVOR-TIMI 53 trial. *Diabetes Care* 2017;40(1):69–76

98. White WB, Cannon CP, Heller SR, et al. Alogliptin after acute coronary syndrome in patients with type 2 diabetes. *N Engl J Med* 2013;369(14):1327–1335

99. Green JB, Bethel MA, Armstrong PW, et al. Effect of sitagliptin on cardiovascular outcomes in type 2 diabetes. *N Engl J Med* 2015;373(3):232–242

100. Cornel JH, Bakris GL, Stevens SR, et al. Effect of sitagliptin on kidney function and respective cardiovascular outcomes in type 2 diabetes: outcomes from TECOS. *Diabetes Care* 2016;39(12):2304–2310

101. Kim YG, Byun J, Yoon D, et al. Renal protective effect of DPP-4 inhibitors in type 2 diabetes mellitus patients: a cohort study. *J Diabetes Res* 2016:1423191

102. Bauersachs J, Jaisser F, Toto R. Mineralocorticoid receptor activation and mineralocorticoid receptor antagonist treatment in cardiac and renal diseases. *Hypertension* 2015;65(2):257–263

103. Dojki FK, Bakris G. Nonsteroidal mineralocorticoid antagonists in diabetic kidney disease. *Curr Opin Nephrol Hypertens* 2017;26(5):368–374

104. Bakris GL, Agarwal R, Anker SD, et al. Effect of finerenone on chronic kidney disease outcomes in type 2 diabetes. *N Engl J Med* 2020;383(23):2219–2229

105. Pitt B, Filippatos G, Agarwal R, et al. Cardiovascular events with finerenone in kidney disease and type 2 diabetes. *N Engl J Med* 2021;385(24):2252–2263

106. Agarwal R, Filippatos G, Pitt B, et al. Cardiovascular and kidney outcomes with finerenone in patients with type 2 diabetes and chronic kidney disease: the FIDELITY pooled analysis. *Eur Heart J* 2022;43(6):474–484

107. Smith AC, Toto R, Bakris GL. Differential effects of calcium channel blockers on size selectivity of proteinuria in diabetic glomerulopathy. *Kidney Int* 1998;54(3):889–896

108. Bakris GL, Weir MR, Secic M, et al. Differential effects of calcium antagonist subclasses on markers of nephropathy progression. *Kidney Int* 2004;65(6):1991–2002

109. Murray KM. Calcium-channel blockers for treatment of diabetic nephropathy. *Clin Pharm* 1991;10(11):862–865

110. Bakris GL. Effects of diltiazem or lisinopril on massive proteinuria associated with diabetes mellitus. *Ann Intern Med* 1990;112(9):707–708

111. Mogensen CE, Neldam S, Tikkanen I, et al. Randomised controlled trial of dual blockade of renin-angiotensin system in patients with hypertension, microalbuminuria, and non-insulin dependent diabetes: the candesartan and lisinopril microalbuminuria (CALM) study. *BMJ* 2000;321(7274):1440–1444

112. Fried LF, Emanuele N, Zhang JH, et al. Combined angiotensin inhibition for the treatment of diabetic nephropathy. *N Engl J Med* 2013;369(20):1892–1903

113. Yusuf S, Teo KK, Pogue J, et al. Telmisartan, ramipril, or both in patients at high risk for vascular events. *N Engl J Med* 2008;358(15):1547–1559

114. Mann JF, Schmieder RE, McQueen M, et al. Renal outcomes with telmisartan, ramipril, or both, in people at high vascular risk (the ONTARGET study): a multicentre, randomised, double-blind, controlled trial. *Lancet* 2008;372(9638):547–553

115. Parving HH, Persson F, Lewis JB, et al. Aliskiren combined with losartan in type 2 diabetes and nephropathy. *N Engl J Med* 2008;358(23):2433–2446

116. Parving HH, Brenner BM, McMurray JJ, et al. Cardiorenal end points in a trial of aliskiren for type 2 diabetes. *N Engl J Med* 2012;367(23):2204–2213

117. Toto RD, Tian M, Fakouhi K, et al. Effects of calcium channel blockers on proteinuria in patients with diabetic nephropathy. *J Clin Hypertens* (Greenwich) 2008;10(10):761–769

118. Bakris GL, Weir MR, DeQuattro V, McMahon FG. Effects of an ACE inhibitor/calcium antagonist combination on proteinuria in diabetic nephropathy. *Kidney Int* 1998;54(4):1283–1289

119. Sato A, Saruta T. Aldosterone breakthrough during angiotensin-converting enzyme inhibitor therapy. *Am J Hypertens* 2003;16(9 Pt 1):781–788

120. Mavrakanas TA, Gariani K, Martin PY. Mineralocorticoid receptor blockade in addition to angiotensin converting enzyme inhibitor or angiotensin II receptor blocker treatment: an emerging paradigm in diabetic nephropathy: a systematic review. *Eur J Intern Med* 2014;25(2):173–176

121. Bolignano D, Palmer SC, Navaneethan SD, Strippoli GF. Aldosterone antagonists for preventing the progression of chronic kidney disease. *Cochrane Database Syst Rev* 2014;(4):CD007004

122. Zou H, Zhou B, Xu G. SGLT2 inhibitors: a novel choice for the combination therapy in diabetic kidney disease. *Cardiovasc Diabetol* 2017;16(1):65

123. Clegg LE, Penland RC, Bachina S, et al. Effects of exenatide and open-label SGLT2 inhibitor treatment, given in parallel or sequentially, on mortality and cardiovascular and renal outcomes in type 2 diabetes: Insights from the EXSCEL trial. *Cardiovasc Diabetol* 2019;18(1):138

124. DeFronzo RA, Lewin A, Patel S, et al. Combination of empagliflozin and linagliptin as second-line therapy in subjects with type 2 diabetes inadequately controlled on metformin. *Diabetes Care* 2015;38(3):384–393

125. Rossing P, Anker SD, Filippatos G, et al. Finerenone in patients with chronic kidney disease and type 2 diabetes by sodium-glucose cotransporter 2 inhibitor treatment: the FIDELITY analysis. *Diabetes Care* 2022;45(12):2991–2998

Chapter 26
Medications for the Management of Retinopathy

Emmeline Tran, PharmD

Diabetic retinopathy is a microvascular complication of diabetes resulting from changes in the blood vessels of the retina.[1] It is the leading cause of vision loss in individuals aged 20–74 years old. Vision loss secondary to diabetic retinopathy occurs as a result of increased vascular permeability and or capillary nonperfusion, distortion of the retina from the development of new blood vessels and fibrous tissue, hemorrhaging of new blood vessels, and damage to retinal neurons.[1]

Global prevalence of diabetic retinopathy is estimated to be about 35%, with a prevalence of 7% for PDR and 7% for diabetic macular edema (DME).[2] Major risk factors for diabetic retinopathy include poor glycemic control, hypertension, dyslipidemia, duration of diabetes, and nephropathy.[3-7] The lifetime risk of diabetic retinopathy is up to approximately 98% in individuals with T1D and up to approximately 80% in individuals with T2D.[8,9]

Diabetic retinopathy occurs in several stages at a slow, nonlinear progression.[1] Initially, patients may present with mild nonproliferative diabetic retinopathy (NPDR) characterized by microaneurysms. Without treatment, patients may progress to moderate or severe NPDR whereby the blood vessels in the retina begin to change shape and become deprived of blood supply. Lack of blood supply causes the body to secrete factors that promote new blood vessel growth leading to the next stage, PDR. The fragile state of the new blood vessels makes them susceptible to leakage and bleeding. Scar tissue can then form and may cause retinal detachment and subsequently permanent vision loss. At any stage, patients can develop macular edema. Macular edema is the swelling of the macula, an area in the center of the retina. Increased vascular permeability due to the breakdown of the blood-retina barrier causes fluid from blood vessels to leak into the retina, resulting in the swelling and thickening of the macula.[1,10] Clinically, patients report blurred vision. In the short term, reductions in visual acuity may be reversible. However, persistent edema may result in irreversible damage and permanent vision loss.[11]

Unfortunately, treatment of diabetic retinopathy usually does not restore lost vision. Additionally, baseline retinopathy greatly shapes the development of this

516

complication. Patients with more severe baseline retinopathy are more likely to progress to vision-threatening retinopathy.[12] Consequently, first and foremost, the goal is to prevent progression of diabetic retinopathy with appropriate management of blood glucose, blood pressure, and lipids. In fact, decreases in the incidence and risk of progression of diabetic retinopathy over the past few decades are a result of improved management in glycemia, blood pressure, and lipid concentration.[13–15]

Tight control of blood glucose in both T1D[16] and T2D[17,18] cannot be overstated in decreasing the risk of development or progression of diabetic retinopathy. The risk of diabetic retinopathy is lowered by approximately 30–50% with each percent reduction in A1C[16,17,19] and effects are long lasting despite loss of glycemic control later on.[20,21] Despite agreement that glycemic control is important in prevention and treatment of diabetic retinopathy, the degree of glucose control is less clear. The ADVANCE trial showed no difference in the development of retinopathy between patients receiving conventional therapy (achieved mean A1C of 7.3%) or intensive therapy (achieved mean A1C of 6.5%) for glucose control.[22] Balancing the risks of hypoglycemia with potential benefit on diabetic retinopathy should be taken into consideration. Additionally, it is important to note that glycemic control may not be the only factor in impacting the incidence and progression of diabetic retinopathy. A1C accounted for only 11% of the risk of retinopathy in the DCCT trial.[23]

Similar to intensive glycemic control, tight blood pressure control has benefits in reducing the risks of diabetic retinopathy progression. The UKPDS study found that the risk for vision loss was decreased by 47%, and need for laser treatment by 34% in patients with T2D.[24] Again, the degree of blood pressure control has been difficult to characterize. The UKPDS study found benefits in lowering systolic blood pressure from a mean of 160 mmHg to a mean of 144 mmHg compared with a mean of 154 mmHg.[24] On the other hand, the ACCORD study did not find a benefit in lowering systolic blood pressure from a median of 137 mmHg to a median of 117 mmHg compared with a median of 133 mmHg.[18] In contrast to glycemic control, benefits seen are only maintained with ongoing blood pressure control.[21]

The impact of lipid control has been more difficult to assess. Although dyslipidemia is a known risk factor for diabetic retinopathy, treatments targeted at lowering lipids have yielded inconsistent results.[25,26] Statin therapy has been evaluated, but studies have mostly been small with conflicting results. Larger studies examining statins were not designed to specifically address diabetic retinopathy outcomes.[25,26] Favorable data regarding lipid-lowering agents have mainly been centered on fenofibrate.

Once diabetic retinopathy develops, the goal is to prevent or arrest progression to avoid vision loss and improve quality of life. The impact of diabetic retinopathy on functions of daily living is significant. Among those with severe NPDR or PDR, approximately half have difficulties with at least one visual function task.[27] Studies examining the effects of certain interventions on diabetic retinopathy have used visual acuity as a marker for improvement in vision. Clinically significant improvement in visual acuity in these studies has generally been defined as a gain of ≥5–15 letters or 1–3 three lines from baseline on the ETDRS chart.[28,29]

Clinically significant macular edema is defined as retinal thickening of the macula or within 500 μm of it, presence of hard exudates at or within 500 μm of the center of the retina with thickening of the adjacent retina, or presence of a zone of retinal thickening one disk area or larger in size, any part of which is within one disk diameter of the center of the retina.[30] This definition generally refers to the threshold at which laser photocoagulation is indicated. Macular edema as defined by central subfield thickness has been described as ≥275 μm on time-domain optical coherence tomography (TD-OCT) with a corresponding Snellen visual acuity decrease of 20/40 to 20/320.[31] This has become a more common measure of clinically significant macular edema in studies examining pharmacologic agents in the treatment of diabetic retinopathy.

MEDICATIONS

In general, outside of medications targeted at metabolic control, pharmacological therapies for diabetic retinopathy are limited, and even then are often costly and require a vitreoretinal ophthalmologist specialist for administration. Pharmacologic treatment options mainly include anti-vascular endothelial growth factor (anti-VEGF) agents and intravitreal corticosteroids. Prior to the advent of anti-VEGF agents, nonpharmacological therapies such as focal laser photocoagulation and panretinal laser photocoagulation (PRP) were standards of care.[30,32,33] Laser photocoagulation improves oxygen availability, thus reducing the secretion of VEGFs and regressing neovascularization.[34] In general, a shift away from these nonpharmacological options has transpired, especially in the setting of DME.

Initiation of treatment is generally guided by the presence of DME and stage of diabetic retinopathy. The threshold for initiation of treatment in DME is the presence of central-involved DME (CIDME). CIDME is defined as edema affecting the diameter of 1 mm in the retinal central subfield.[1] Of note, some trials have found that holding off intiation of anti-VEGF therapy may be considered in patients with CIDME and good visual acuity, defined as ETDRS visual acuity letter score of at least 79 (Snellen equivalent of 20/25 or better).[35,36] In regard to stage of diabetic retinopathy, treatment may be considered with the development of severe NPDR and recommended with PDR. Table 26.1 summarizes treatment recommendations for initiation of intraocular interventions. These treatment options do not reverse vision loss, but instead work to minimize development and progression of vision loss by primarily targeting the angiogenesis and inflammatory pathways.

ANTI-VEGF AGENTS

Angiogenesis is a key component in the pathogenesis of diabetic retinopathy, especially in the later stages. Overexpression of VEGFs induces proliferation of blood vessel development and vascular leakage.[37] There are four FDA-approved anti-VEGF agents, aflibercept, brolucizumab, faricimab, and ranibizumab. Additionally, bevacizumab is used off-label for diabetic retinopathy. Bevacizumab is repackaged in aliquots containing approximately 1/500th of the systemic dose used in cancer therapy.[38] These compounds differ in structure, VEGF-binding

Table 26.1 — Recommended Intraocular Treatment Based on Stage of Diabetic Retinopathy and Presence of DME[1]

Presence of DME	Intraocular treatment
No	None
Yes, non-CIDME	None
Yes, CIDME	Anti-VEGF therapy ± macular laser Alternative: intravitreous steroids
Stage	**Intraocular treatment**
No diabetic retinopathy	None
Mild NPDR	None
Moderate NPDR	None
Severe NPDR	Consider early PRP for patients with T2D
PDR	PRP or anti-VEGF therapy

CIDME, central-involved diabetic macular edema; DME, diabetic macular edema; NPDR, nonproliferative diabetic retinopathy; PDR, proliferative diabetic retinopathy; PRP, panretinal laser photocoagulation; VEGF, vascular endothelial growth factor. *Source*: Solomon.[1]

affinity, and VEGF isoform specificity.[39,40] The effect of these differences in terms of clinical efficacy is not fully known. An advantage of brolucizumab over its counterparts is its small molecular weight, allowing for greater tissue penetration, delivery of higher drug concentrations, and potentially longer durability.[41] In addition to binding to VEGF, faricimab binds to angiopoietin-2, which supports vascular stability and desensitizes blood vessels to the effects of VEGF.[42]

DME

Data supporting the use of anti-VEGF agents are mainly in the treatment of DME. Several randomized controlled trials have established the efficacy of ranibizumab,[43,44] aflibercept,[45] and bevacizumab[46] in visual acuity gain and central retinal thickness reduction when compared with laser therapy. Moreover, a Cochrane review found that use of ranibizumab, aflibercept, and bevacizumab were all more effective than laser photocoagulation for improving vision by three or more lines at 1 year.[47]

Few data are available to guide selection of which VEGF inhibitor should be initiated compared with the others. A large randomized controlled trial compared three agents—aflibercept, bevacizumab, and ranibizumab—and found that all improved vision, but the effect was dependent on baseline visual acuity. In patients who presented with worse baseline levels of visual acuity (20/50 or worse), improvement in vision was greatest with aflibercept.[38] A subsequent post hoc analysis of the trial found a preferential sustained benefit of aflibercept in visual acuity improvement over 2 years compared with bevacizumab, but not ranibizumab among patients with 20/50 or worse vision.[48] Superiority of aflibercept may also be seen in patients with PDR at baseline.[49]

Findings suggesting benefits of aflibercept and ranibizumab over bevacizumab were observed in persistent DME. Persistent DME occurs when, despite anti-VEGF therapy, complete resolution of DME is lacking. A post hoc analysis found that persistent DME at 24 weeks was more common in patients receiving bevacizumab compared with aflibercept or ranibizumab.[50] For patients with persistent DME through 24 weeks, the probability of chronic persistent DME was lower with aflibercept compared with bevacizumab, but not with ranibizumab. However, no difference was found among the anti-VEGF agents in patients with persistent DME with regard to gain of at least 10 letters from baseline through 2 years for patients with chronic persistent DME compared with those without chronic persistent DME. Consequently, these results suggest that meaningful benefits in vision can be gained regardless of anti-VEGF agent given or persistence of DME through 2 years with little risk of vision loss.[50]

Noninferiority of brolucizumab to aflibercept for gain in visual acuity was demonstrated in the KESTREL and KITE studies at 52 weeks.[51] A higher percentage of eyes administered brolucizumab achieved central subfield thickness <280 μm compared with aflibercept. Additionally, the presence of subretinal or intraretinal fluid was seen less in eyes treated with brolucizumab versus aflibercept. Results were sustained at week 100.[52] Similar findings of achievement of noninferiority for gain in visual acuity, and greater reductions in central subfield thickness and number of eyes without intraretinal fluid favoring faricimab over aflibercept, were observed in the YOSEMITE and RHINE trials.[53]

Despite the strong evidence supporting the use of anti-VEGF agents for the treatment of DME, real-world considerations present certain challenges. Administration of these agents is intravitreal and requires multiple injections. Most clinical trials investigating these drugs used at least monthly injections. However, in the real world, patients appear to receive anti-VEGF injections less frequently, resulting in less efficacy than that seen in original trials.[54] Studies have been conducted to determine the potential for tapering the number of injections over a period of time, and suggest no difference in outcomes.[55,56] Although brolucizumab is marketed as a longer-lasting product, the optimal frequency for injections is still unclear. Studies up to 100 weeks suggest durability up to 16 weeks.[52] Longer durability has also been demonstrated with faricimab with more than 70% of patients in the personalized treatment interval group being redosed every 12 weeks or longer at 1 year.[57]

Additional considerations center on cost. Anti-VEGF agents have established cost-effectiveness compared with other interventions in the treatment of DME.[58] The substantial difference in cost with bevacizumab compared with ranibizumab or aflibercept (approximately 20- to 40-fold less) make it an attractive option.[59] A cost-effectiveness study of the three agents emphasized this cost discrepancy, finding that aflibercept and ranibizumab are not cost-effective compared with bevacizumab for the treatment of DME.[60] Conversely, bevacizumab must be compounded to use intravitreally. Issues surrounding compounding such as sterility or requirements for patient-specific prescriptions may limit access to compounded bevacizumab.[59,61] Higher production yields and easier handling attributed to the unique structure of brolucizumab may result in lower manufacturing costs.[41] Moreover, increased durability of brolucizumab[52] and faricimab[57] may also reduce costs long term. However, cost-effectiveness studies of brolucizumab or faricimab for the treatment of DME in the U.S. are lacking.

NPDR

Anti-VEGF therapy for patients with NPDR is not generally recommended.[1] The Protocol W trial examined the role of anti-VEGF therapy in patients with moderate to severe NPDR. The study found that although there was a statistically significant difference favoring those who received aflibercept compared to sham in the 2-year cumulative probability of developing center-involved DME with vision loss or PDR (16.3% vs. 43.5%), there was no difference in mean change in visual acuity from baseline to 2 years.[62] Longer-term results are needed to better elucidate the role of anti-VEGF treatment in patients with NPDR.

PDR

Limited data are available on the use of anti-VEGF agents in the treatment of PDR. Standard of care has traditionally been PRP. A noninferiority study (Protocol S) compared PRP with ranibizumab.[63] The mean treatment group difference in visual acuity letter score improvement between groups was greater than the prespecified noninferiority limit of –5.0 letters. As such, ranibizumab was found to be noninferior to PRP. Visual acuity continued to be good in both groups at 5 years.[64] However, less than 65% of each group was followed up. Another noninferiority study (CLARITY) examined the use of aflibercept compared with PRP and found aflibercept to be noninferior and superior in visual acuity improvement.[65] In patients with vitreous hemorrhage from PDR, the efficacy of aflibercept compared with vitrectomy with PRP is unclear. One study found that at 24 weeks there was no difference in mean visual acuity letter score between the two interventions, and at 2 years, no clear benefits were found regardless of initial intervention.[66] However, the study may have been underpowered.

Reviews of the literature also emphasize the lack of efficacy and safety outcomes available with the use of anti-VEGF agents in the treatment of PDR over standard therapy options. In particular, a Cochrane review, including studies primarily investigating bevacizumab, found potential benefits with the use of anti-VEGF agents, but results were heterogeneous and supported by very low-quality evidence. Limitations of the studies included indirect assessment of visual acuity, lacking of blinding, attrition bias, selective reporting, and lack of prespecified sample size. The review also suggested that a reduction in risk of intraocular bleeding in individuals with PDR is associated with anti-VEGFs.[67] Considerations for use of anti-VEGF agents over PRP may include scenarios in which there is difficulty in performing PRP such as dense cataracts or vitreous hemorrhage, when PRP has failed in preventing PDR progression, and in patients with DME with PDR.[68]

As with DME, a potential drawback in the use of anti-VEGF therapy in the management of PDR is the increased number of visits and treatment compared with PRP.[68,69] Consequently, lack of adherence is a major concern. Of those allocated to the anti-VEGF group, approximately 30% of participants in the Protocol S trial and 9% of participants in the CLARITY trial were loss to follow-up.[63,65] A retrospective cohort study found that 22.1% of patients receiving anti-

VEGF therapy were loss to follow-up over a period of about 4 years, but statistically significantly more patients who received PRP were loss to follow-up (28.0%).[70]

Cost evaluations comparing PRP to anti-VEGF therapy have been conducted. One cost study used a Markov-style analysis and found PRP to be less expensive than intravitreal ranibizumab for PDR, taking into account both facility and non-facility settings.[71] In patients with PDR with concomitant vision-impairing DME, ranibizumab monotherapy may be a more cost-effective option than PRP. However, this cost benefit is lost in patients with PDR without baseline vision-impairing DME.[72]

Safety

In general, most clinical trials have reported a favorable safety profile for these agents. However, it must be noted that these studies often do not have adequate power to detect safety events, especially if rare. Conflicting results have been found in systematic reviews and meta-analyses. One systematic review and meta-analysis found an association between aflibercept or ranibizumab given monthly and potential increased risk for death, cerebrovascular accidents, and vascular death.[73] Another found that anti-VEGF agents do not increase the risk of systemic adverse events regardless of if treatment was given scheduled or as-needed.[74] Further data are needed to clarify the safety profile of these agents in patients with diabetes who already have increased cardiovascular risk.

Other adverse events to be aware of include endophthalmitis (incidence reported up to 1.6%), intraocular inflammation, intraocular pressure elevation (often transient and self-limiting), retinal detachment, and ocular hemorrhage.[75,76] Higher rates of intraocular inflammation and retinal vascular occlusion have been reported with brolucizumab compared with aflibercept (up to 5.3% vs. 1.1% and up to 1.6% vs. 0.5%, respectively, depending on brolucizumab dose and trial duration) in the KESTREL trial. In the KITE trial, the incidence of intraocular inflammation was 2.2% in the brolucizumab group and 1.7% in the aflibercept group; no difference in retinal vascular occlusion was observed between groups.[51,52] Conversely, cases of retinal vasculitis and or retinal vascular occlusion have not been reported with faricimab.[53]

CORTICOSTEROIDS

Inflammatory pathway activation is a proposed mechanism in DME. Therefore, medications such as corticosteroids that suppress pathways of inflammation are potential treatment options. Additionally, corticosteroids have been found to inhibit the expression of VEGFs in vascular smooth muscle cells and thus reduce blood vessel formation.[77]

DME

Data supporting the use of intravitreal corticosteroids is less promising than anti-VEGF agents. Superior efficacy and safety outcomes of intravitreal triamcinolone over focal or grid photocoagulation in patients with primarily DME (61%) and mild to moderately severe NPDR (61%) were not observed.[78]

Although there were benefits in visual acuity at 4 months in individuals receiving triamcinolone, those benefits were no longer present by 1 year. Additionally, by 2 years, patients receiving laser therapy showed improved visual acuity compared with patients receiving triamcinolone. Results regarding effects on retinal thickening paralleled the visual acuity results. In terms of safety, there was an increased percentage of patients with ocular hypertension and/or glaucoma and cataract surgery in the triamcinolone group compared with the laser therapy group. A follow-up study at 3 years showed similar results.[79]

Another study also found no benefit to the use of a corticosteroid compared with laser therapy. Study eyes with DME received prompt laser monotherapy, ranibizumab with prompt laser therapy, ranibizumab with deferred laser therapy, or triamcinolone with prompt laser therapy.[80,81] No difference was found in patients receiving the triamcinolone-laser therapy combination compared with laser monotherapy. Reduction in mean central subfield thickness was seen in all three medication-laser therapy combination groups compared with laser monotherapy at 1 year. However, benefits were lost in those patients receiving triamcinolone-laser therapy at 2 years with an increase in mean central subfield thickness from the 1- to 2-year visit. As with previous studies, intraocular pressure and cataract surgery were more frequent in patients receiving triamcinolone.

Intravitreal steroid injections require repeated administrations. Consequently, to reduce the need for repeated intravitreal injections, intravitreal corticosteroid implants have been developed and studied. Two steroids in three different implant products are available in the U.S.: dexamethasone (Ozurdex) and fluocinolone (Iluvien and Retisert). However, although studied in patients with DME, Retisert is not FDA approved for this indication.

Pooled results from an analysis of the dexamethasone intravitreal implant (Macular Edema: Assessment of Implantable Dexamethasone in Diabetes [MEAD] trial) found that a greater number of patients in the implant group had at least a ≥15-letter improvement in visual acuity and reduction in central retinal thickness than patients in the sham group.[82] Cataract-related adverse events in patients with phakic eyes were greater in those receiving the implant than in those receiving the sham.

A direct comparison of a corticosteroid implant with an anti-VEGF agent was examined in the Intravitreal Bevacizumab Versus Intravitreal Dexamethasone for Persistent Diabetic Macular Oedema (BEVORDEX) study.[83] This study compared dexamethasone implant with bevacizumab in patients with CIDME. Similar percentages of eyes achieved vision improvement by 10 or more letters with each group. Conversely, those eyes that received the dexamethasone implant achieved a greater reduction in mean central macular thickness. However, a greater number of eyes were associated with vision loss in the dexamethasone group secondary to cataract development. A greater number of injections were seen with the bevacizumab group. Of note, the benefits seen with reduction in mean central macular thickness with dexamethasone were lost at 24 months.[84]

Fluocinolone implants have been investigated in two studies. One study examined intravitreal implants releasing 0.2 µg/day or 0.5 µg/day of fluocinolone compared with sham injections in patients with persistent DME.[85] The two doses of fluocinolone each achieved greater percentages of patients who gained at least a

≥15–letter score compared with the sham group at 36 months (28.7% low dose, 27.8% high dose vs. 18.9% sham). A similar percentage was observed between the different doses. The incidence of cataracts and intraocular-related adverse events were higher in those patients receiving the steroid implant than the sham. Another study examined the Retisert implant delivering fluocinolone 0.59 mg.[86] Compared with standard of care, patients with persistent or recurrent DME randomized to receive the implant saw a greater improvement of visual acuity of at least three lines at 6 months and 2 years. This significance was lost at 3 years. Findings regarding retinal thickening at the center of the macula generally paralleled the above findings. Intraocular pressure and cataracts were greater in the implanted eyes.

With the introduction of anti-VEGF agents and concerns with safety, corticosteroids are rarely used first line, and when used, have been confined to select patient populations.[37] Frequent administrations and high cost of anti-VEGF agents may make sustained-release corticosteroid products attractive in comparison. However, the risk of adverse effects of corticosteroids often outweighs these benefits. Steroid therapy may be considered in patients who have conditions, such as recent cardiovascular events, in which the systemic adverse effects of anti-VEGF agents—although associations are limited—should be avoided; who have not responded to anti-VEGF therapy, especially in those with pseudophakic eyes; and post-vitrectomy patients with CIDME.[87]

RAS INHIBITORS

Good blood pressure control is central to preventing and arresting progression of diabetic retinopathy. However, data thus far supporting preferential selection of an antihypertensive agent have been inconclusive.

T1D

Three major controlled trials examined the effects of ACE inhibitors or ARBs in patients with T1D. The EUCLID trial examined the effects of lisinopril compared with placebo on retinopathy as a secondary endpoint. Patients had T1D (mean A1C of 7.1%), normotension (mean blood pressure of 123/81 mmHg), and primarily normoalbuminuria (85% of patients; median UAE rate of 7 µg/min).[88] Approximately 80% of patients had minimal NPDR or no retinopathy at baseline. Patients who received lisinopril had less progression of retinopathy by at least 1 level, by two or more grades, and to proliferative retinopathy compared with placebo. However, the study had limitations in terms of differences in baseline glycemia between the two groups and short follow-up (24 months).

Another trial (RASS) found similar benefits with an ACE inhibitor and an ARB.[89] When compared with placebo, both agents (enalapril and losartan) statistically significantly reduced the progression of retinopathy by two or more steps independent of changes in blood pressure. Patients had T1D (mean A1C of 8.5%), normotension (mean blood pressure of 120/70 mmHg), and normoalbuminuria (median UAE rate of 5.1 µg/min). At baseline, 74% of patients had minimal NPDR or no retinopathy. The retinopathy outcome was added a priori shortly after the study began.

Lastly, the DIRECT-Prevent 1 and DIRECT-Protect 1 studies examined the incidence and progression of retinopathy in patients with T1D, normotension, and normoalbuminuria on candesartan compared with placebo.[90] At baseline, those in the DIRECT-Prevent 1 trial had a mean A1C of 8.1%, mean blood pressure of 116/72 mmHg, and no retinopathy. Comparatively, those in the DIRECT-Protect 1 trial had a mean A1C of 8.5%, mean blood pressure of 117/74 mmHg, and a majority of patients had retinopathy at a level of 20 or 35 in the worst eye using the ETDRS scale (91%). With adjustment for blood pressure, candesartan statistically significantly reduced the incidence of retinopathy, defined as at least a three-step increase on the ETDRS scale. No significant difference was found in progression of diabetic retinopathy with the use of candesartan compared with placebo.

T2D

As with patients with T1D, the role of ACE inhibitors or ARBs in patients with T2D in preventing progression of diabetic retinopathy is conflicting. The BENEDICT trial was explored to determine the effects of trandolapril on diabetic retinopathy.[91] This was a prespecified secondary endpoint. Patients had T2D, normoalbuminuria, and hypertension or were on antihypertensive agents. A majority of patients did not have diabetic retinopathy (83.6%). They were randomized to trandolapril, verapamil, or combination therapy. In those individuals receiving trandolapril monotherapy or combination therapy, regression occurred more frequently compared with those receiving verapamil.

A similar study to the DIRECT-Protect 1 trial was conducted in patients with T2D (DIRECT-Protect 2).[92] In this study, patients with T2D (mean A1C of 8.2%), normotension or treated with antihypertensive agents (mean blood pressure of 123/76 mmHg in normotensive group, and 139/80 mmHg in the treated hypertensive group), and normoalbuminuria (mean UAE rate of 5.5 µg/min) were allocated to candesartan or placebo. Most patients had a retinopathy level of 20 or 35 in the worst eye based on the ETDRS scale (83%). No significant difference was found in progression of retinopathy. However, there was a statistically significant increase in risk of regression over the 4-year trial duration. It is unknown what a 5% difference between the two groups may mean clinically.

A retrospective cohort study using an insurance database in patients with T2D was conducted to investigate the risk of sight-threatening diabetic retinopathy (STDR) in patients receiving antihypertensive agents.[93] Interestingly, ACE inhibitors or ARBs and CCBs were associated with a significantly greater risk of developing STDR compared with β-blockers.

A systematic review and meta-analysis found beneficial effects of RAS inhibitors on reducing the risk of diabetic retinopathy and increasing the potential for regression of diabetic retinopathy, specifically in patients with normotension and T1D or T2D.[94] In patients with hypertension, RAS inhibitors were not associated with a difference in either outcome. When broken down by class, ACE inhibitors were found to decrease the risk of progression and increase the chance of regression, while ARBs were found to only increase the chance of regression.

Based on the literature above, it is difficult to ascertain the role of a specific class of antihypertensive agent in the treatment of diabetic retinopathy. Most evidence examining the effects of ACE inhibitors or ARBs is in patients with T1D or

T2D with normotension and normoalbuminuria. Patients with retinopathy often have concomitant nephropathy, in which RAS inhibitors have been shown to have a strong benefit in preventing progression.[6,69]

PPAR-α

The mechanism of action of a PPAR-α in the management of diabetic retinopathy is not fully elucidated. In addition to its lipid effects, fenofibrate has anti-inflammatory, antiangiogenic, antiapoptotic, and antioxidant effects that theoretically may be protective in diabetic retinopathy.[95]

The Fenofibrate Intervention and Event Lowering in Diabetes (FIELD) study was conducted in patients with T2D (mean A1C of 6.9%) to investigate coronary events.[96] However, retinopathy outcomes were examined as other endpoints. The mean blood pressure was 141/82 mmHg and mean LDL cholesterol was 119 mg/dL. Approximately 8% of patients had retinopathy at baseline. The fenofibrate group needed fewer laser treatments for retinopathy than the placebo group. A substudy of the FIELD trial examined patients without retinopathy at baseline.[97] Similarly, patients who received fenofibrate had a statistically significantly lower rate in needing laser treatment for diabetic retinopathy when compared with placebo. In patients with preexisting retinopathy, fewer experienced progression. No difference was seen in deterioration of visual acuity.

Diabetic retinopathy outcomes were examined in a substudy of the ACCORD trial.[18] In contrast with the FIELD study, patients in the ACCORD trial had a higher prevalence of preexisting diabetic retinopathy at baseline and a longer duration of diabetes. Regardless, the results of the study were consistent with those observed in the FIELD study. Patients in the fenofibrate group had a lower rate of retinopathy progression over the 4-year study period compared with the simvastatin group. No difference was seen in deterioration of visual acuity.

Due to limitations of its effects on cardiovascular outcomes, fenofibrate is often avoided as first-line therapy for the treatment of dyslipidemia. However, based on the above studies, considerations may be made for the use of fenofibrate in diabetic retinopathy progression.

ASPIRIN

Aspirin has been found to prevent leukocyte vascular occlusion and decrease production of inflammatory markers in diabetic retinopathy.[98] These mechanisms of action make it an attractive treatment option. However, clinical outcomes to support this hypothesis have not been well supported. In particular, the ETDRS study found that aspirin 650 mg daily had no effect on the progression of diabetic retinopathy or risk of vision loss.[99] Of note, aspirin also did not have an effect on the risk of vitreous hemorrhage among patients with PDR.[100] Therefore, although strong supporting evidence for the role of aspirin in the treatment of diabetic retinopathy is lacking, aspirin is safe to use in patients with diabetic retinopathy for its cardioprotective benefits.[69]

Table 26.2—Medications and Dosing

Medication	Typical dose(s)	Renal dose adjustment(s)	Hepatic dose adjustment(s)
Aflibercept (Eylea)*	2 mg once every 4 weeks for the first 5 injections, followed by 2 mg (0.05 mL) once every 8 weeks**	None	None
Bevacizumab (Avastin)	1.25 mg, may repeat every 4 weeks depending on response	None	None
Brolucizumab (Beovu)	6 mg once every 6 weeks for 5 doses, followed by 6 mg once every 8 to 12 weeks	None	None
Dexamethasone (Ozurdex)*	0.7-mg implant	None	None
Faricimab (Vabysmo)	6 mg once every 4 weeks for 6 doses, followed by 6 mg once every 4 to 16 weeks	None	None
Fluocinolone (Iluvien)*	0.19-mg implant	None	None
Fluocinolone (Retisert)	0.59-mg implant	None	None
Pegaptanib (Macugen)	0.3 mg once every 6 weeks	None	None
Ranibizumab (Lucentis)*	0.3 mg once a month	None	None
Triamcinolone (Triesence)	4 mg once	None	None

*FDA approved for diabetic macular edema **Some patients may require dosing every 4 weeks after the first 20 weeks. *Source*: refs. 38,78,86,114–121.

GLP-1 RAs

GLP-1 RAs are believed to exert neuroprotective effects that may be beneficial in the treatment of diabetic retinopathy beyond their effects on glycemic control.[101] Moreover, studies have shown the presence of GLP-1 receptors in human retinas, which helps support the idea that GLP-1 RAs may be useful in preventing or arresting retinal neurodegeneration.[101]

Currently, there is a lack of literature supporting the role of GLP-1 RAs in the treatment of diabetic retinopathy. When examined as secondary outcomes in major controlled trials examining primarily cardiovascular outcomes, effects of GLP-1 RAs were found to be neutral or even harmful. Specifically, the SUS-TAIN-6 trial observed that patients who received semaglutide had an increase in the progression of retinopathy compared with placebo.[102] Again, it must be emphasized that retinopathy was examined as a secondary outcome. Therefore, this finding must be taken into context and with caution. Analyses of other studies examining semaglutide did not have similar outcomes.[103,104] It is proposed that the worsening of retinopathy is associated with the speed and magnitude of improvement in glycemic control and not related to the medication itself.[105] More data are needed to define the role of this class of medication in the treatment of diabetic retinopathy.

COMBINATION THERAPY

Combination therapy may be a promising avenue for the treatment of diabetic retinopathy, particularly in cases not responding to initial therapy or with more severity. Currently, further studies are needed to solidify initial findings.

ANTI-VEGF + LASER THERAPY

The Ranibizumab Monotherapy or Combined with Laser Versus Laser Monotherapy for Diabetic Macular Edema (RESTORE) study found that ranibizumab combination therapy, in addition to ranibizumab monotherapy, was superior to laser treatment alone for DME. However, no differences in efficacy were found between the ranibizumab monotherapy or combination groups.[43] Similarly, patients receiving combination treatment with bevacizumab and macular photocoagulation did not experience better outcomes in terms of visual acuity or reduction in macular thickness than patients receiving monotherapy with bevacizumab.[106]

A potential role for combination therapy was alluded to in the Ranibizumab for Edema of the mAcula in Diabetes (READ-2) trial.[107] The study found that combined ranibizumab with macular laser photocoagulation may be beneficial in reducing the number of injections. Another role for combination therapy may be in PDR. A systematic review and meta-analysis found that anti-VEGF agents in patients with PDR may be used as an adjunct to PRP or pars plana vitrectomy.[108] Potential benefits of adjunctive use include improved visual activity and central retinal thickness, less intraoperative bleeding, decreased duration of surgery, and fewer retinal breaks.

CORTICOSTEROID + LASER THERAPY

Combination therapy with laser photocoagulation after 1 month was examined in the Primary Laser with Adjunctive Implantable Dexamethasone in DME (PLACID) trial.[109] Patients were allocated to dexamethasone implant or sham implant. Both groups received laser therapy at 1 month. Although no difference in percentage of patients who gained ≥10 letters in visual acuity at 12 months was found, the group who received the implant had significantly greater improvement at 1 month and 9 months. Cataract-related adverse events were more common in phakic study eyes that received the dexamethasone implant than the sham implant.

A few small studies have been conducted examining the combination of laser photocoagulation with intravitreal corticosteroids on diabetic retinopathy in patients primarily with PDR. These studies found improvement in visual acuity and central macular thickness with combination therapy compared with laser photocoagulation alone.[110,111]

ANTI-VEGF + CORTICOSTEROIDS

A phase 2 randomized clinical trial suggests that in patients with persistent DME, addition of a steroid may be harmful.[112] At 24 weeks, patients receiving ranibizumab and dexamethasone combination had a greater reduction in central subfield thickness compared with the ranibizumab monotherapy group. Of note, although no difference was found in mean visual acuity improvement, the study was not sufficiently powered to identify a difference. A higher proportion of patients developed a statistically significant increase in intraocular pressure in the combination group compared with the monotherapy group.

The efficacy of combination therapy with an anti-VEGF agent and steroid for the treatment of DME was analyzed in a meta-analysis.[113] The meta-analysis found that bevacizumab with intravitreal triamcinolone improved visual acuity at 3 months, but no difference was found at 6 months. Similarly, benefits of combination therapy were seen in central macular thickness at 3 months, but not at 6 months. Ocular hypertension ranged from 0 to 8.3% in the combination group, and there were no cases among the bevacizumab group. Results of the meta-analysis were limited by the short duration of the studies included.

MONOGRAPHS

Aflibercept (Eylea): https://dailymed.nlm.nih.gov/dailymed/drugInfo.cfm?setid=f96cfd69-da34-41ee-90a9-610a4655cd1c

Bevacizumab (Avastin): https://dailymed.nlm.nih.gov/dailymed/drugInfo.cfm?setid=939b5d1f-9fb2-4499-80ef-0607aa6b114e

Brolucizumab (Beovu): https://dailymed.nlm.nih.gov/dailymed/drugInfo.cfm?setid=5d1dc1fa-a2d3-46ed-9e9a-c1a036590d3d

Dexamethasone (Ozurdex): https://dailymed.nlm.nih.gov/dailymed/drugInfo.cfm?setid=4b204f44-6e8a-4d17-803c-268f0b04679f

Faricimab (Vabysmo): https://dailymed.nlm.nih.gov/dailymed/drugInfo.cfm?setid=04cc9ef7-c02a-4e92-a655-0062674e8487

Fluocinolone (Iluvien): https://dailymed.nlm.nih.gov/dailymed/drugInfo.cfm?setid=4400e471-7402-11df-93f2-0800200c9a66

Fluocinolone (Retisert): https://dailymed.nlm.nih.gov/dailymed/drugInfo.cfm?setid=1ab0f849-2a0d-47ce-ad05-768094da8cc9

Pegaptanib (Macugen): https://dailymed.nlm.nih.gov/dailymed/drugInfo.cfm?setid=45d03177-5d52-492c-b2e0-01afc7c8d2e0

Ranibizumab (Lucentis): https://dailymed.nlm.nih.gov/dailymed/drugInfo.cfm?setid=de4e66cc-ca05-4dc9-8262-e00e9b41c36d

Triamcinolone (Triesence): https://dailymed.nlm.nih.gov/dailymed/drugInfo.cfm?setid=3f045347-3e5e-4bbd-90f8-6c3100985ca5

REFERENCES

1. Solomon SD, Chew E, Duh EJ, et al. Diabetic retinopathy: a position statement by the American Diabetes Association. *Diabetes Care* 2017;40(3): 412–418

2. Yau JW, Rogers SL, Kawasaki R, et al. Global prevalence and major risk factors of diabetic retinopathy. *Diabetes Care* 2012;35(3):556–564

3. Xu J, Xu L, Wang YX, et al. Ten-year cumulative incidence of diabetic retinopathy. The Beijing Eye Study 2001/2011. *PLoS One* 2014;9(10):e111320

4. Jin P, Peng J, Zou H, et al. The 5-year onset and regression of diabetic retinopathy in Chinese type 2 diabetes patients. *PLoS One* 2014;9(11):e113359

5. Hammer SS, Busik JV. The role of dyslipidemia in diabetic retinopathy. *Vision Res* 2017;139:228–236

6. Lee MK, Han KD, Lee JH, et al. Normal-to-mildly increased albuminuria predicts the risk for diabetic retinopathy in patients with type 2 diabetes. *Sci Rep* 2017;7(1):11757

7. Klein R, Knudtson MD, Lee KE, et al. The Wisconsin Epidemiologic Study of Diabetic Retinopathy: XXII the twenty-five-year progression of retinopathy in persons with type 1 diabetes. *Ophthalmology* 2008;115(11):1859–1868

8. Klein R, Klein BE, Moss SE, et al. The Wisconsin epidemiologic study of diabetic retinopathy. II. Prevalence and risk of diabetic retinopathy when age at diagnosis is less than 30 years. *Arch Ophthalmol* 1984;102(4):520–526

9. Klein R, Klein BE, Moss SE, et al. The Wisconsin epidemiologic study of diabetic retinopathy. III. Prevalence and risk of diabetic retinopathy when age at diagnosis is 30 or more years. *Arch Ophthalmol* 1984;102(4):527–532

10. Wong TY, Cheung CM, Larsen M, et al. Diabetic retinopathy. *Nat Rev Dis Primers* 2016;2:16012

11. Romero-Aroca P, Baget-Bernaldiz M, Pareja-Rios A, et al. Diabetic macular edema pathophysiology: vasogenic versus inflammatory. *J Diabetes Res* 2016:2156273

12. Klein R, Klein BE, Moss SE, Cruickshanks KJ. The Wisconsin epidemiologic study of diabetic retinopathy. XIV. Ten-year incidence and progression of diabetic retinopathy. *Arch Ophthalmol* 1994;112(9):1217–1228

13. Klein R, Lee KE, Gangnon RE, Klein BE. The 25-year incidence of visual impairment in type 1 diabetes mellitus the Wisconsin epidemiologic study of diabetic retinopathy. *Ophthalmology* 2010;117(1):63–70

14. Klein R, Klein BE. Are individuals with diabetes seeing better? a long-term epidemiological perspective. *Diabetes* 2010;59(8):1853–1860

15. Nathan DM, Zinman B, Cleary PA, et al. Modern-day clinical course of type 1 diabetes mellitus after 30 years' duration: the diabetes control and

complications trial/epidemiology of diabetes interventions and complications and Pittsburgh epidemiology of diabetes complications experience (1983–2005). *Arch Intern Med* 2009;169(14):1307–1316

16. Nathan DM, Genuth S, Lachin J, et al. The effect of intensive treatment of diabetes on the development and progression of long-term complications in insulin-dependent diabetes mellitus. *N Engl J Med* 1993;329(14):977–986

17. UK Prospective Diabetes Study (UKPDS) Group. Intensive blood-glucose control with sulphonylureas or insulin compared with conventional treatment and risk of complications in patients with type 2 diabetes (UKPDS 33). *Lancet* 1998;352(9131):837–853

18. Chew EY, Ambrosius WT, Davis MD, et al. Effects of medical therapies on retinopathy progression in type 2 diabetes. *N Engl J Med* 2010;363(3):233–244

19. The Diabetes Control and Complications Trial Research Group. The relationship of glycemic exposure (HbA1c) to the risk of development and progression of retinopathy in the diabetes control and complications trial. *Diabetes* 1995;44(8):968–983

20. Lachin JM, Genuth S, Cleary P, et al. Retinopathy and nephropathy in patients with type 1 diabetes four years after a trial of intensive therapy. *N Engl J Med* 2000;342(6):381–389

21. Holman RR, Paul SK, Bethel MA, Matthews DR, Neil HA. 10-year follow-up of intensive glucose control in type 2 diabetes. *N Engl J Med* 2008;359(15):1577–1589

22. Patel A, MacMahon S, Chalmers J, et al. Intensive blood glucose control and vascular outcomes in patients with type 2 diabetes. *N Engl J Med* 2008;358(24):2560–2572

23. Hirsch IB, Brownlee M. Beyond hemoglobin A1c—need for additional markers of risk for diabetic microvascular complications. *JAMA* 2010;303(22):2291–2292

24. UK Prospective Diabetes Study Group. Tight blood pressure control and risk of macrovascular and microvascular complications in type 2 diabetes: UKPDS 38. *BMJ* 1998;317(7160):703–713

25. Ioannidou E, Tseriotis VS, Tziomalos K. Role of lipid-lowering agents in the management of diabetic retinopathy. *World J Diabetes* 2017;8(1):1–6

26. Modjtahedi BS, Bose N, Papakostas TD, et al. Lipids and diabetic retinopathy. *Semin Ophthalmol* 2016;31(1-2):10–18

27. Willis JR, Doan QV, Gleeson M, et al. Vision-related functional burden of diabetic retinopathy across severity levels in the United States. *JAMA Ophthalmol* 2017;135(9):926–932

28. Beck RW, Maguire MG, Bressler NM, et al. Visual acuity as an outcome measure in clinical trials of retinal diseases. *Ophthalmology* 2007;114(10): 1804–1809

29. Fortin P, Mintzes B, Innes M. A systematic review of intravitreal bevacizumab for the treatment of diabetic macular edema [Internet], 2012. Ottawa, Canadian Agency for Drugs and Technologies in Health. Available from https://www.ncbi.nlm.nih.gov/books/NBK169468/

30. Early Treatment Diabetic Retinopathy Study research group. Photocoagulation for diabetic macular edema. Early Treatment Diabetic Retinopathy Study report number 1. *Arch Ophthalmol* 1985;103(12):1796–1806

31. Nguyen QD, Brown DM, Marcus DM, et al. Ranibizumab for diabetic macular edema: results from 2 phase III randomized trials: RISE and RIDE. *Ophthalmology* 2012;119(4):789–801

32. The Diabetic Retinopathy Study Research Group. Preliminary report on effects of photocoagulation therapy. *Am J Ophthalmol* 1976;81(4):383–396

33. Evans JR, Michelessi M, Virgili G. Laser photocoagulation for proliferative diabetic retinopathy. *Cochrane Database Syst Rev* 2014(11):CD011234

34. Stefansson E. The therapeutic effects of retinal laser treatment and vitrectomy: a theory based on oxygen and vascular physiology. *Acta Ophthalmol Scand* 2001;79(5):435–440

35. Baker CW, Glassman AR, Beaulieu WT, et al. Effect of initial management with aflibercept vs laser photocoagulation vs observation on vision loss among patients with diabetic macular edema involving the center of the macula and good visual acuity: A randomized clinical trial. *JAMA* 2019;321(19):1880–1894

36. Busch C, Fraser-Bell S, Zur D, et al. Real-world outcomes of observation and treatment in diabetic macular edema with very good visual acuity: The OBTAIN study. *Acta Diabetol* 2019;56(7):777–784

37. Antonetti DA, Klein R, Gardner TW. Diabetic retinopathy. *N Engl J Med* 2012;366(13):1227–1239

38. Wells JA, Glassman AR, Ayala AR, et al. Aflibercept, bevacizumab, or ranibizumab for diabetic macular edema. *N Engl J Med* 2015;372(13):1193–1203

39. Simo R, Hernandez C. Intravitreous anti-VEGF for diabetic retinopathy: hopes and fears for a new therapeutic strategy. *Diabetologia* 2008;51(9): 1574–1580

40. MacDonald DA, Martin J, Muthusamy KK, et al. Aflibercept exhibits VEGF binding stoichiometry distinct from bevacizumab and does not support formation of immune-like complexes. *Angiogenesis* 2016;19(3):389–406

41. Kuo BL, Singh RP. Brolucizumab for the treatment of diabetic macular edema. *Curr Opin Ophthalmol* 2022;33(3):167–173

42. Joussen AM, Ricci F, Paris LP, et al. Angiopoietin/Tie2 signalling and its role in retinal and choroidal vascular diseases: a review of preclinical data. *Eye* (Lond) 2021;35(5):1305–1316

43. Mitchell P, Bandello F, Schmidt-Erfurth U, et al. The RESTORE study: ranibizumab monotherapy or combined with laser versus laser monotherapy for diabetic macular edema. *Ophthalmology* 2011;118(4):615–625

44. Ishibashi T, Li X, Koh A, et al. The REVEAL Study: Ranibizumab monotherapy or combined with laser versus laser monotherapy in Asian patients with diabetic macular edema. *Ophthalmology* 2015;122(7):1402–1415

45. Korobelnik JF, Do DV, Schmidt-Erfurth U, et al. Intravitreal aflibercept for diabetic macular edema. *Ophthalmology* 2014;121(11):2247–2254

46. Michaelides M, Kaines A, Hamilton RD, et al. A prospective randomized trial of intravitreal bevacizumab or laser therapy in the management of diabetic macular edema (BOLT study) 12-month data: report 2. *Ophthalmology* 2010;117(6):1078–1086.e2

47. Virgili G, Parravano M, Evans JR, et al. Anti-vascular endothelial growth factor for diabetic macular oedema: a network meta-analysis. *Cochrane Database Syst Rev* 2017;6:CD007419

48. Jampol LM, Glassman AR, Bressler NM, et al. Anti-vascular endothelial growth factor comparative effectiveness trial for diabetic macular edema: additional efficacy post hoc analyses of a randomized clinical trial. *JAMA Ophthalmol* 2016;134(12)

49. Bressler SB, Liu D, Glassman AR, et al. Change in diabetic retinopathy through 2 years: secondary analysis of a randomized clinical trial comparing aflibercept, bevacizumab, and ranibizumab. *JAMA Ophthalmol* 2017;135(6):558–568

50. Bressler NM, Beaulieu WT, Glassman AR, et al. Persistent macular thickening following intravitreous aflibercept, bevacizumab, or ranibizumab for central-involved diabetic macular edema with vision impairment: a secondary analysis of a randomized clinical trial. *JAMA Ophthalmol* 2018;136(3):257–269

51. Brown DM, Emanuelli A, Bandello F, et al. KESTREL and KITE: 52-week results from two phase III pivotal trials of brolucizumab for diabetic macular edema. *Am J Ophthalmol* 2022;238:157–172

52. Wykoff CC, Garweg JG, Regillo C, et al. Brolucizumab for treatment of diabetic macular edema (DME): 100-week results from the KESTREL and KITE studies [ARVO abstract 3849]. *Invest Ophthalmol Vis Sci* 2022;63(7):3849

53. Wykoff CC, Abreu F, Adamis AP, et al. Efficacy, durability, and safety of intravitreal faricimab with extended dosing up to every 16 weeks in patients with diabetic macular oedema (YOSEMITE and RHINE): two randomised, double-masked, phase 3 trials. *Lancet* 2022;399(10326):741–755

54. Ciulla TA, Pollack JS, Williams DF. Visual acuity outcomes and anti-VEGF therapy intensity in diabetic macular oedema: a real-world analysis of 28,658 patient eyes. *Br J Ophthalmol* 2021;105(2):216-221

55. Elman MJ, Ayala A, Bressler NM, et al. Intravitreal ranibizumab for diabetic macular edema with prompt versus deferred laser treatment: 5-year randomized trial results. *Ophthalmology* 2015;122(2):375–381

56. Schmidt-Erfurth U, Lang GE, Holz FG, et al. Three-year outcomes of individualized ranibizumab treatment in patients with diabetic macular edema: the RESTORE extension study. *Ophthalmology* 2014;121(5): 1045–1053

57. Wykoff CC, Abreu F, Adamis AP, et al. Efficacy, durability, and safety of intravitreal faricimab with extended dosing up to every 16 weeks in patients with diabetic macular oedema (YOSEMITE and RHINE): two randomised, double-masked, phase 3 trials. *Lancet* 2022;399(10326):741–755

58. Pershing S, Enns EA, Matesic B, et al. Cost-effectiveness of treatment of diabetic macular edema. *Ann Intern Med* 2014;160(1):18–29

59. Martin DF, Maguire MG. Treatment choice for diabetic macular edema. *N Engl J Med* 2015;372(13):1260–1261

60. Ross EL, Hutton DW, Stein JD, et al. Cost-effectiveness of aflibercept, bevacizumab, and ranibizumab for diabetic macular edema treatment: analysis from the diabetic retinopathy clinical research network comparative effectiveness trial. *JAMA Ophthalmol* 2016;134(8):888–896

61. Yannuzzi NA, Klufas MA, Quach L, et al. Evaluation of compounded bevacizumab prepared for intravitreal injection. *JAMA Ophthalmol* 2015;133(1):32–39

62. Maturi RK, Glassman AR, Josic K, et al. Effect of intravitreous anti-vascular endothelial growth factor vs sham treatment for prevention of vision-threatening complications of diabetic retinopathy: The Protocol W randomized clinical trial. *JAMA Ophthalmol* 2021;139(7):701–712

63. Gross JG, Glassman AR, Jampol LM, et al. Panretinal photocoagulation vs intravitreous ranibizumab for proliferative diabetic retinopathy: a randomized clinical trial. *JAMA* 2015;314(20):2137–2146

64. Gross JG, Glassman AR, Liu D, et al. Five-year outcomes of panretinal photocoagulation vs intravitreous ranibizumab for proliferative diabetic retinopathy: A randomized clinical trial. *JAMA Ophthalmol* 2018;136(10): 1138–1148

65. Sivaprasad S, Prevost AT, Vasconcelos JC, et al. Clinical efficacy of intravitreal aflibercept versus panretinal photocoagulation for best corrected visual acuity in patients with proliferative diabetic retinopathy at 52 weeks (CLARITY): a multicentre, single-blinded, randomised, controlled, phase 2b, non-inferiority trial. *Lancet* 2017;389(10085):2193–2203

66. Antoszyk AN, Glassman AR, Beaulieu WT, et al. Effect of intravitreous aflibercept vs vitrectomy with panretinal photocoagulation on visual acuity in patients with vitreous hemorrhage from proliferative diabetic retinopathy: a randomized clinical trial. *JAMA* 2020;324(23):2383–2395

67. Martinez-Zapata MJ, Marti-Carvajal AJ, Sola I, et al. Anti-vascular endothelial growth factor for proliferative diabetic retinopathy. *Cochrane Database Syst Rev* 2014;(11):CD008721

68. Osaadon P, Fagan XJ, Lifshitz T, Levy J. A review of anti-VEGF agents for proliferative diabetic retinopathy. *Eye* (Lond) 2014;28(5):510–520

69. American Diabetes Association; 12. Retinopathy, Neuropathy, and Foot Care. Standards of Care in Diabetes—2023. *Diabetes Care* 2023; 46(Suppl. 1):S203–S215

70. Obeid A, Gao X, Ali FS, et al. Loss to follow-up in patients with proliferative diabetic retinopathy after panretinal photocoagulation or intravitreal anti-VEGF injections. *Ophthalmology* 2018;125(9):1386–1392

71. Lin J, Chang JS, Smiddy WE. Cost evaluation of panretinal photocoagulation versus intravitreal ranibizumab for proliferative diabetic retinopathy. *Ophthalmology* 2016;123(9):1912–1918

72. Hutton DW, Stein JD, Glassman AR, et al. Five-year cost-effectiveness of intravitreous ranibizumab therapy vs panretinal photocoagulation for treating proliferative diabetic retinopathy: a secondary analysis of a randomized clinical trial. *JAMA Ophthalmol* 2019;137(12):1–9

73. Avery RL, Gordon GM. Systemic safety of prolonged monthly anti-vascular endothelial growth factor therapy for diabetic macular edema: a systematic review and meta-analysis. *JAMA Ophthalmol* 2016;134(1):21–29

74. Thulliez M, Angoulvant D, Pisella PJ, Bejan-Angoulvant T. Overview of systematic reviews and meta-analyses on systemic adverse events associated with intravitreal anti-vascular endothelial growth factor medication use. *JAMA Ophthalmol* 2018;136(5):557–566

75. Gupta A, Sun JK, Silva PS. Complications of intravitreous injections in patients with diabetes. *Semin Ophthalmol* 2018;33(1):42–50

76. Falavarjani KG, Nguyen QD. Adverse events and complications associated with intravitreal injection of anti-VEGF agents: a review of literature. *Eye* (Lond) 2013;27(7):787–794

77. Nauck M, Karakiulakis G, Perruchoud AP, et al. Corticosteroids inhibit the expression of the vascular endothelial growth factor gene in human vascular smooth muscle cells. *Eur J Pharmacol* 1998;341(2–3):309–315

78. Diabetic Retinopathy Clinical Research Network. A randomized trial comparing intravitreal triamcinolone acetonide and focal/grid photocoagulation for diabetic macular edema. *Ophthalmology* 2008;115(9):1447–1449, 1449.e1–10

79. Beck RW, Edwards AR, Aiello LP, et al. Three-year follow-up of a randomized trial comparing focal/grid photocoagulation and intravitreal triamcinolone for diabetic macular edema. *Arch Ophthalmol* 2009;127(3):245–251

80. Elman MJ, Aiello LP, Beck RW, et al. Randomized trial evaluating ranibizumab plus prompt or deferred laser or triamcinolone plus prompt laser for diabetic macular edema. *Ophthalmology* 2010;117(6):1064–1077.e1035

81. Elman MJ, Bressler NM, Qin H, et al. Expanded 2-year follow-up of ranibizumab plus prompt or deferred laser or triamcinolone plus prompt laser for diabetic macular edema. *Ophthalmology* 2011;118(4):609–614

82. Boyer DS, Yoon YH, Belfort R Jr., et al. Three-year, randomized, sham-controlled trial of dexamethasone intravitreal implant in patients with diabetic macular edema. *Ophthalmology* 2014;121(10):1904–1914

83. Gillies MC, Lim LL, Campain A, et al. A randomized clinical trial of intravitreal bevacizumab versus intravitreal dexamethasone for diabetic macular edema: the BEVORDEX study. *Ophthalmology* 2014;121(12):2473–2481

84. Fraser-Bell S, Lim LL, Campain A, et al. Bevacizumab or dexamethasone implants for DME: 2-year results (the BEVORDEX study). *Ophthalmology* 2016;123(6):1399–1401

85. Campochiaro PA, Brown DM, Pearson A, et al. Sustained delivery fluocinolone acetonide vitreous inserts provide benefit for at least 3 years in patients with diabetic macular edema. *Ophthalmology* 2012;119(10):2125–2132

86. Pearson PA, Comstock TL, Ip M, et al. Fluocinolone acetonide intravitreal implant for diabetic macular edema: a 3-year multicenter, randomized, controlled clinical trial. *Ophthalmology* 2011;118(8):1580–1587

87. Regillo CD, Callanan DG, Do DV, et al. Use of corticosteroids in the treatment of patients with diabetic macular edema who have a suboptimal response to anti-VEGF: recommendations of an expert panel. *Ophthalmic Surg Lasers Imaging Retina* 2017;48(4):291–301

88. Chaturvedi N, Sjolie AK, Stephenson JM, et al. Effect of lisinopril on progression of retinopathy in normotensive people with type 1 diabetes. The EUCLID Study Group. EURODIAB Controlled Trial of Lisinopril in Insulin-Dependent Diabetes Mellitus. *Lancet* 1998;351(9095):28–31

89. Mauer M, Zinman B, Gardiner R, et al. Renal and retinal effects of enalapril and losartan in type 1 diabetes. *N Engl J Med* 2009;361(1):40–51

90. Chaturvedi N, Porta M, Klein R, et al. Effect of candesartan on prevention (DIRECT-Prevent 1) and progression (DIRECT-Protect 1) of retinopathy in type 1 diabetes: randomised, placebo-controlled trials. *Lancet* 2008;372(9647):1394–1402

91. Ruggenenti P, Iliev I, Filipponi M, et al. Effect of trandolapril on regression of retinopathy in hypertensive patients with type 2 diabetes: a prespecified analysis of the benedict trial. *J Ophthalmol* 2010:106384

92. Sjolie AK, Klein R, Porta M, et al. Effect of candesartan on progression and regression of retinopathy in type 2 diabetes (DIRECT-Protect 2): a randomised placebo-controlled trial. *Lancet* 2008;372(9647):1385–1393

93. Lin JC, Lai MS. Antihypertensive drugs and diabetic retinopathy in patients with type 2 diabetes. *Ophthalmologica* 2016;235(2):87–96

94. Wang B, Wang F, Zhang Y, et al. Effects of RAS inhibitors on diabetic retinopathy: a systematic review and meta-analysis. *Lancet Diabetes Endocrinol* 2015;3(4):263–274

95. Noonan JE, Jenkins AJ, Ma JX, et al. An update on the molecular actions of fenofibrate and its clinical effects on diabetic retinopathy and other microvascular end points in patients with diabetes. *Diabetes* 2013;62(12):3968–3975

96. Keech A, Simes RJ, Barter P, et al. Effects of long-term fenofibrate therapy on cardiovascular events in 9795 people with type 2 diabetes mellitus (the FIELD study): randomised controlled trial. *Lancet* 2005;366(9500):1849–1861

97. Keech AC, Mitchell P, Summanen PA, et al. Effect of fenofibrate on the need for laser treatment for diabetic retinopathy (FIELD study): a randomised controlled trial. *Lancet* 2007;370(9600):1687–1697

98. Kohner EM. Aspirin for diabetic retinopathy. *BMJ* 2003;327(7423):1060–1061

99. Early Treatment Diabetic Retinopathy Study Research Group. Effects of aspirin treatment on diabetic retinopathy. ETDRS report number 8. *Ophthalmology* 1991;98(5 Suppl.):757–765

100. Chew EY, Klein ML, Murphy RP, et al. Effects of aspirin on vitreous/preretinal hemorrhage in patients with diabetes mellitus. Early Treatment Diabetic Retinopathy Study report no. 20. *Arch Ophthalmol* 1995;113(1):52–55

101. Hernandez C, Bogdanov P, Corraliza L, et al. Topical administration of GLP-1 receptor agonists prevents retinal neurodegeneration in experimental diabetes. *Diabetes* 2016;65(1):172–187

102. Marso SP, Bain SC, Consoli A, et al. Semaglutide and cardiovascular outcomes in patients with type 2 diabetes. *N Engl J Med* 2016;375(19):1834–1844

103. Vilsboll T, Bain SC, Leiter LA, et al. Semaglutide, reduction in glycated haemoglobin and the risk of diabetic retinopathy. *Diabetes Obes Metab* 2018;20(4):889–897

104. Pratley RE, Aroda VR, Lingvay I, et al. Semaglutide versus dulaglutide once weekly in patients with type 2 diabetes (SUSTAIN 7): a randomised, open-label, phase 3b trial. *Lancet Diabetes Endocrinol* 2018;6(4):275–286

105. Bethel MA, Diaz R, Castellana N, et al. HbA1c change and diabetic retinopathy during GLP-1 receptor agonist cardiovascular outcome trials: a meta-analysis and meta-regression. *Diabetes Care* 2021;44(1):290–296

106. Lee SJ, Kim ET, Moon YS. Intravitreal bevacizumab alone versus combined with macular photocoagulation in diabetic macular edema. *Korean J Ophthalmol* 2011;25(5):299–304

107. Nguyen QD, Shah SM, Khwaja AA, et al. Two-year outcomes of the ranibizumab for edema of the mAcula in diabetes (READ-2) study. *Ophthalmology* 2010;117(11):2146–2151

108. Simunovic MP, Maberley DA. Anti-vascular endothelial growth factor therapy for proflierative diabetic retinopathy: A systematic review and meta-analysis. *Retina* 2015;35(10):1931–1942

109. Callanan DG, Gupta S, Boyer DS, et al. Dexamethasone intravitreal implant in combination with laser photocoagulation for the treatment of diffuse diabetic macular edema. *Ophthalmology* 2013;120(9):1843–1851

110. Kang SW, Sa HS, Cho HY, Kim JI. Macular grid photocoagulation after intravitreal triamcinolone acetonide for diffuse diabetic macular edema. *Arch Ophthalmol* 2006;124(5):653–658

111. Maia OO Jr., Takahashi BS, Costa RA, et al. Combined laser and intravitreal triamcinolone for proliferative diabetic retinopathy and macular edema: one-year results of a randomized clinical trial. *Am J Ophthalmol* 2009;147(2):291–297.e292

112. Maturi RK, Glassman AR, Liu D, et al. Effect of adding dexamethasone to continued ranibizumab treatment in patients with persistent diabetic macular edema: a DRCR network phase 2 randomized clinical trial. *JAMA Ophthalmol* 2018;136(1):29–38

113. Jin E, Luo L, Bai Y, Zhao M. Comparative effectiveness of intravitreal bevacizumab with or without triamcinolone acetonide for treatment of diabetic macular edema. *Ann Pharmacother* 2015;49(4):387–397

114. Aflibercept (Eylea) injection, for intravitreal use [product information]. Tarrytown, NY, Regeneron Pharmaceuticals, May 2017

115. Rajendram R, Fraser-Bell S, Kaines A, et al. A 2-year prospective randomized controlled trial of intravitreal bevacizumab or laser therapy (BOLT) in the management of diabetic macular edema: 24-month data: report 3. *Arch Ophthalmol* 2012;130(8):972–979

116. Brolucizumab (Beovu) injection, for intravitreal use [product information]. East Hanover, NJ, Novartis Pharmaceuticals, December 2022

117. Dexamethasone (Ozurdex) implant, for intravitreal use [product information]. Madison, NJ, Allergan, May 2018

118. Faricimab (Vabysmo) injection, for intravitreal use [product information]. South San Francisco, CA, Genentech USA, Inc., January 2023

119. Fluocinolone (Iluvien) implant, for intravitreal use [product information]. Alpharetta, GA, Alimera Sciences, November 2016

120. Rinaldi M, Chiosi F, dell'Omo R, et al. Intravitreal pegaptanib sodium (Macugen) for treatment of diabetic macular oedema: a morphologic and functional study. *Br J Clin Pharmacol* 2012;74(6):940–946

121. Ranibuzumab (Lucentis) injection, for intravitreal use [product information]. South San Francisco, CA, Genentech USA, Inc., March 2018

Chapter 27
Medications for the Management of Depression

Megan Willson, PharmD, BCPS

INTRODUCTION

D
epression is one of the most common mental health disorders. The DSM-V
defines MDD as having five or more of the following symptoms during a
2-week period. These symptoms must include a depressed mood or loss of
interest or pleasure. Other symptoms are changes in weight, changes in sleep, agitation or slowing, lack of energy, worthlessness or guilt, decreased ability to con-
centrate, or recurrent thoughts of death.[1] Depression symptoms can range from
mild to severe and are truly different from just being sad. According to the Substance Abuse and Mental Health Services Administration (SAMHSA), 8.3% of the
of the U.S. adult population aged 18 years or older had a major depression episode
in 2021 with 5.7% having severe impairment as a result of their depression. The
prevalence of depression is highest in patients aged 18–25 years and reporting two
or more racial/ethnic backgrounds.[2] Risk factors for depression are both medical
and social. Some medical-related risk factors are biochemical, genetic, sleep disorders, and serious medical illness including diabetes. Social-related risk factors can
include abuse, gender, social support systems, and life events. Other factors to consider include substance use and abuse and certain medications.[3]

Serious chronic illnesses such as diabetes are known risk factors for MDD, but
MDD is also a risk factor for diabetes. Evidence also demonstrates additive effects
of comorbid MDD and diabetes to both morbidity and mortality. The bidirectional association has been observed in effect of treatment outcomes of both disease states.[4] Patients with diabetes have a 1.6 times greater risk of depression than
those without diabetes.[5] Another study showed that patients with newly diagnosed
diabetes were 30% more likely to have had an episode of depression in the past
3 years than individuals without diabetes.[4] A meta-analysis also demonstrated that
suicidal ideation and suicide attempts were increased in patients with depression
and diabetes.[6] Patients with T2D had a 24% increased risk of developing MDD.[4]
Mezuk and colleagues proposed the strongest correlation exists for MDD leading
to diabetes.[7]

The causal relationship between diabetes and depression is multifactorial.
General factors for depression impacting diabetes are antidepressant use, weight
gain, obesity, and lack of physical activity.[4,8] Further exploration of antidepressant
use has led to associations beyond the impact on weight gain or direct impact on
glycemic control. Higher doses of antidepressants used for longer periods of time
have led to increases in rates of diabetes. The factors associated with diabetes that

led to depression include emotional stress, metabolic syndrome, genetics, and obesity.[4,8,9]

Depression has a significant impact on both morbidity and mortality associated with diabetes as well, including worse glycemic control and insulin resistance, more micro- and macrovascular complications, as well as increased rates of mortality.[4,10,11] Research has demonstrated a relationship between diabetes outcomes and emotional stress and health-related quality of life.[12,13] Depression has been linked to poor self-care, diet, and medication adherence, which lead to decreased glycemic control. Patients with comorbid depression and diabetes treated with antidepressant medications are more likely to achieve good glycemic control than those not treated,[14] which indicates the strong need to recognize and treat depression in this population. The identification and treatment of the associated emotional distress is also important to address when treating the depression. Hyperglycemia and poor glycemic control are well-recognized contributing factors to macrovascular complications necessitating the management of co-morbid depression.

Due to the significant impact that treatment of depression can have on diabetes morbidity and mortality, this chapter will discuss the following major classes of antidepressants commonly used today: SSRIs; SNRIs; TCAs, atypical antidepressants, and serotonin modulators. A limited number of trials are focused on patients with diabetes, so most evidence is derived for treatment of depression in population-based studies.

Depression treatment follows some general rules or principles for treatment. Depression treatment begins with the acute phase, followed by the continuation phase, and concluded with the maintenance phase. The acute phase consists of initiation of pharmacotherapy, psychotherapy, or a combination of pharmacotherapy and psychotherapy or electroconvulsive therapy. Pharmacotherapy should be initiated at a low dose and titrated up to achieve symptom resolution while still maintaining a tolerable side-effect profile. If side effects occur, a reduction of dose can sometimes alleviate the symptoms. The acute phase should be continued for at least 6–12 weeks. Symptom relief can occur as early as 1–2 weeks but may take 4–6 weeks to show improvement with pharmacotherapy. A trial of 4–8 weeks at the maximal tolerated dose is adequate to determine if therapy is not effective. Full benefit with pharmacotherapy occurs at around 12 weeks. The continuation phase should continue for 4–9 months with the same therapy that induced remission of depression. The continuation phase should be used to prevent relapse. The maintenance phase should be used in patients with chronic depression, patients with three or more episodes of MDD, and those at high risk of relapse.[15] Pharmacotherapy initial treatment should be dictated by patient-specific considerations and anticipated side effects. First-line medications include SSRI and SNRI with atypical depressants and serotonin modulators as appropriate alternative medications.

Table 27.1—Goals of Therapy

- Remission of depression
- Preventing relapse of depression
- Avoiding adverse effects of pharmacotherapy
- Improving daily functioning

SSRIs

SSRIs are considered a first-line therapy, with or without combination psychotherapy, for the treatment of mild to moderate depression. This class is considered first line because of efficacy in clinical trials and overall tolerability. SSRIs used in combination with psychotherapy are also recommended as first line for severe forms of MDD. SSRIs can also be useful for the treatment of anxiety disorders.[15,16]

Class effects as well as individual medication characteristics must be considered when selecting an agent in the SSRI medication class. No medication in this class is considered superior to another. Also, no specific medication classes have been found to be superior to another class based on efficacy.[15] Each medication should be selected based on differences in side-effect profile and/or tolerability for the patient, dosing, or other drug characteristics. Most medications have a long elimination half-life allowing for once-daily dosing, except fluvoxamine, which should be taken twice daily.[17]

Although SSRIs are considered better tolerated than tricyclics or monoamine oxidase inhibitors, patients can still commonly experience side effects. Citalopram and escitalopram can cause a dose-related corrected QT (QTc) interval prolongation.[18,19] Paroxetine is more likely to cause sedation and upset stomach or nausea.[20] Sertraline is activating and has a high rate of diarrhea.[21] Fluoxetine is also considered to be activating.[22] Note also that paroxetine, fluvoxamine, and fluoxetine are metabolized by cytochrome enzymes, leading to drug interactions.[19,22] In a survey of approximately 400 patients, more than 50% complained of side effects during initial treatment with SSRIs. The three most commonly reported side effects were sexual dysfunction (17%), drowsiness (17%), and weight gain (12%).[23]

The side effect of weight gain is particularly troubling for patients with comorbid diabetes. Weight gain generally occurs over time with longer courses of therapy, which may be necessary with the treatment of depression. Differences are seen between individual medications in the class. In a trial comparing weight changes for fluoxetine, paroxetine, and sertraline, fluoxetine demonstrated a nonsignificant weight decrease, sertraline a nonsignificant weight increase, and paroxetine a significant weight gain.[24] One case-control study demonstrated that use of SSRIs not only increased weight but also increased the incidence of diabetes. High to moderate doses of SSRIs when used for longer than 2 years were associated with doubling of the risk of diabetes (incidence rate ratio 2.06, 95% CI 1.20–3.52). In reviewing individual medications, fluvoxamine and paroxetine had significantly positive incidence rate ratios influencing the overall weight gain associated with the SSRI medication class.[25]

SNRIs

SNRIs, like SSRIs, are considered first line for treatment of depression due to efficacy of treatment and tolerability of the medications. This class of medication may also be a good choice because of the benefit in chronic pain conditions like DPN. SNRIs are also approved to treat anxiety disorders.[15,16] The FDA has approved desvenlafaxine, duloxetine, milnacipran, levomilnacipran, and venlafaxine for the treatment of depression. Efficacy for treatment of depression is similar among the medications in this class.[15] Selection of a specific medication is dependent on side-effect profile, patient-specific symptoms, drug interactions, and other patient-specific factors.

The SNRI medications share some general characteristics but have unique profiles as well. SNRIs treat depression by blocking the reuptake of serotonin and norepinephrine. The effect on receptors is dose dependent. Venlafaxine blocks mostly serotonin at lower doses, but at doses of 225 mg and higher norepinephrine is affected.[26] Dosing in patients with severe renal and hepatic insufficiency may need to be reduced or avoided; however, medication doses should be titrated to the individualized patient effect. The most common side effects experienced were nausea and dizziness.[27–29] Elevations of blood pressure are seen with all medications except duloxetine.[27] Duloxetine demonstrated an initial decrease in weight of 0.4 kg compared to baseline in the first 12 weeks. At the end of the 34-week trial, however, patients receiving duloxetine had a weight increase of approximately 1 kg from baseline.[30] Levomilnacipran is weight neutral.[29] Abrupt discontinuation of medications in this class leads to decontamination syndrome, so these medications should be tapered to avoid withdrawal symptoms.[15] Sexual dysfunction can be problematic with this class of medications.[15]

TRICYCLIC ANTIDEPRESSANTS

Tricyclic and tetracyclic antidepressants are effective treatment for depression. These medications have also been shown to have similar efficacy to SSRIs and SNRIs; however, they are no longer used as a first-line treatment for depression. Medications in this class are considered equally efficacious. Due to significant side effects, this class of medication is used as second line or for resistant forms of depression. The tricyclics are also effective for the treatment of anxiety disorders, panic disorders, and neuropathy.[15]

Common medications used in this class are amitriptyline, imipramine, desipramine, and nortriptyline. The medications block reuptake of both serotonin and norepinephrine. Use-limiting side effects include cardiovascular effects such as arrhythmias and hypotension; anticholinergic effects such as constipation, dry eyes and mouth, sedation, and weight gain; and falls.[15] These medications also have varying degrees of affinity for histamine and muscarinic receptors, leading to the unwanted side-effect profile of weight gain, sedation, and other anticholinergic effects. Nortriptyline appears to have the least effect on histamine and muscarinic receptors and may be better tolerated. Most of these medications have therapeutic drug levels that may be monitored for efficacy or response and adherence to the medication. Some other adverse effects beyond the anticholinergic and antihistaminic effects are cardiac and lowering of the seizure threshold. Cardiac effects can include arrhythmias, heart block, sudden death, and orthostatic hypotension. These medications can also be fatal in cases of overdose.[15]

ATYPICAL ANTIDEPRESSANTS

The atypical antidepressants include bupropion and mirtazapine. These medications are different from other antidepressant medication classes due to different mechanisms of action. The mechanism of action of bupropion is not completely clear. It is classified as a dopamine and norepinephrine reuptake inhibitor with a majority of the effect on dopamine. It is generally used to treat MDD and seasonal affective disorder. The medication is also approved to assist in smoking cessation.[31] However, unlike other antidepressants, bupropion is not indicated in the treatment of anxiety. This medication may be considered when patients also need assistance in smoking cessation or have side effects with other antidepressants. The side-effect profile includes the potential for weight loss, anxiety, dry mouth, nausea, insomnia, and seizures. Sexual dysfunction is less with bupropion than with other antidepressants, so it may be considered a good alternative in patients who experience sexual dysfunction with other antidepressant classes.[31]

Mirtazapine is a tetracyclic compound with an unknown mechanism for its antidepressant properties. The antidepressant effects are thought to be through antagonism of central α-2 receptors, leading to increased central noradrenergic and serotonergic activity. It also has some antagonism to histamine receptors, peripheral α-1 adrenergic receptors, and muscarinic receptors.[32] Mirtazapine is similar in efficacy to SSRIs.[15] The adverse effects of mirtazapine include dry mouth, drowsiness, sedation, increased appetite, and weight gain.[32] Sedation is more prominent at lower doses and tends to go away at doses $\geq$30 mg per day.[33]

SEROTONIN MODULATORS

Serotonin modulators include trazodone, vilazodone, and vortioxetine. The serotonin modulators' effects are not completely understood but are thought to affect depression through inhibition of serotonin reuptake. The serotonin modulators have proven benefit in the treatment of depression compared to placebo.[34-36] Generally, trazodone is used more for its sedation effect than as a first-line therapy in the treatment of depression.[15] Common side effects for trazodone are sedation, dizziness, dry mouth, and nausea.[34] For vortioxetine, nausea and sexual dysfunction are the only adverse effects occurring in >10% of patients.[35] Patients taking vilazodone commonly experienced diarrhea, nausea, and headache.[36] Serotonin modulators go through hepatic metabolism, which can lead to drug interaction.[34-36]

Table 27.2—Dose and Dosage Adjustment for Commonly Used Medications

Drug	Initial dose (mg/day)	Usual dose (mg/day)	Dose adjustments
SSRIs			
Citalopram	20	20–40	Maximum dose of 20 mg daily in patients over age 60, hepatic impairment, or poor metabolizers of CYP2C19 or taking CYP2C19 inhibitors.
Escitalopram	10	10–20	Maximum dose of 10 mg daily in elderly and those with hepatic impairment. Use with caution in severe renal impairment. Doses up to 30 mg/day have been used in practice with additional benefit.
Fluoxetine	20	20–80	No renal adjustments. May require a reduced dose or frequency in hepatic dysfunction, elderly, or in patients with multiple comorbidities.
Paroxetine	20	20–50	Doses should not exceed 40 mg in elderly, debilitated, or severe renal or hepatic failure. Initial dose in this population should be 10 mg daily.
Sertraline	50	50–200	For mild hepatic impairment, the starting dose is 25 mg daily and the maximum dose is 100 mg daily. Avoid in moderate or severe hepatic impairment.
SNRIs			
Venlafaxine, immediate release	75	75–375	Reduce dose by 50% in patients with mild to moderate hepatic impairment. Reduce dose by 25% in with CrCl 10–70 mL/min.
Venlafaxine, extended release	37.5–75	75–225	Reduce dose by 50% in patients with mild to moderate hepatic impairment. Reduce dose by 25–50% in mild to moderate renal impairment and 50% for patients on hemodialysis or severe renal impairment.
Desvenlafaxine	50	50	Reduce dose for CrCl <30 mL/min to 25 mg per day or 50 mg every other day.
Duloxetine	20 twice daily	40–120	Not recommended for patients with CrCl <30 mL/min or patients with hepatic impairment. No additional benefits for doses greater than 60 mg/day.
Tricyclic Antidepressants			
Amitriptyline	25 three times daily	100–300	No renal or hepatic adjustments. Consider lower doses in elderly
Nortriptyline	25	25–150	No renal or hepatic adjustments.
Atypical Antidepressants			
Bupropion, immediate release	200	300–450	Moderate to severe hepatic impairment, 75 mg daily. Mild hepatic impairment or renal impairment, a dose and/or frequency reduction should be considered.
Bupropion, sustained release	150	300–400	Moderate to severe hepatic impairment, 100 mg daily or 150 mg every other day. Mild hepatic impairment or renal impairment, a dose and/or frequency reduction should be considered.

(continued)

Table 27.2 (continued)

Drug	Initial dose (mg/day)	Usual dose (mg/day)	Dose adjustments
Bupropion, extended release	150	300	Moderate to severe hepatic impairment, 150 mg every other day. Mild hepatic impairment or renal impairment, a dose and/or frequency reduction should be considered.
Mirtazapine	15	15–45	No renal or hepatic adjustments.
Serotonin Modulators			
Trazodone	150	150–600	No renal or hepatic adjustments.
Vilazodone	10	20–40	No renal or hepatic adjustments. Take with food
Vortioxetine	10	20	No renal or hepatic adjustments. Maximum recommended dose for poor metabolizers of CYP2D6 is 10 mg daily.

Source: refs. 17–22,27–29,31–32,34–36,38–44.

COMMON PRECAUTIONS

All medications can cause adverse reactions for patients. Some adverse events of concern for antidepressant agents are withdrawal syndrome with discontinuation of pharmacotherapy, an increased risk of suicidal thoughts or actions, and serotonin syndrome. Discontinuation syndrome can occur with most antidepressants, but is more common in agents with shorter half-lives. Some symptoms of discontinuation syndrome are similar to the flu, such as nausea, aches, chills, and some neurologic symptoms. Relapse of depression can occur with abrupt discontinuation. Serotonin syndrome is a rare condition that may occur as a result of too much serotonin in the body. This is more likely when using multiple medications that increase serotonin. Suicide and suicidal ideation are severe complications of depression. This is thought to be sometimes increased with the initiation of antidepressants, specifically in adolescents and young adults. Providers should assess patients for thoughts of suicide prior to initiation of therapy and monitor patients closely while on therapy.[15]

COMBINATION THERAPY

Achieving resolution of depressive symptoms is important to a patient's quality of life. Sometimes treatment with combination therapy is warranted to achieve remission. Combinations can often include addition of psychotherapy or the use of additional medications. Combination pharmacotherapy with psychotherapy should be considered as initial therapy for patients with severe depression or in hospitalized patients, and as augmentation to pharmacotherapy for patients not reaching remission on pharmacotherapy alone. Psychotherapy can come in many forms, such as family/marital, psychodynamic, group, problem-solving, interpersonal, and cognitive and behavioral therapies. Psychotherapies and pharmacotherapy have a synergistic benefit compared to either therapy alone. Pharmacotherapeutic combinations can also be used in individuals with incomplete response to single-agent therapy. Medications can be combined with another medication with a different mechanism of action.[15,16]

PHARMACOTHERAPY COMBINATIONS

When attempting combination or therapy augmentations, one should consider patient risk for side effects, comorbid conditions, and tolerability. Bupropion has shown synergistic effects when added to SSRI therapy, although caution should be used with the potential for drug-drug interactions. Also, mirtazapine has demonstrated beneficial effects when added to an SSRI or venlafaxine. Augmentation with second-generation antipsychotics can be used in patients who have depression with psychotic features but has also demonstrated benefit in patients who have incomplete response. The additional efficacy is not without risk. Increased weight gain, lipid alterations, as well as development of diabetes are significantly increased.[15] Symbyax is a combination of olanzapine and fluoxetine approved for bipolar 1 with depression.[37] Stimulant medications such as methylphenidate or modafinil have been used as add-on therapy to help with somnolence and fatigue.[15] Auvelity is a combination of dextromethorphan and bupropion. Dextromethorphan is an uncompetitive N-methyl D-aspartate (NMDA) receptor antagonist and sigma-1 receptor agonist. The mechanism for treatment of depression is unclear. The addition of dextromethorphan is felt to augment bupropion effects (package insert).

MONOGRAPHS

SSRI MEDICATIONS

Citalopram (Celexa): https://dailymed.nlm.nih.gov/dailymed/drugInfo.cfm?
setid=2632b547-2e13-447f-ac85-c774e437d6a8

Escitalopram (Lexapro): https://dailymed.nlm.nih.gov/dailymed/drugInfo.cfm?
setid=d5fbc8ce-bd41-4bd0-b413-0dea97e596c3

Fluoxetine (Prozac): https://dailymed.nlm.nih.gov/dailymed/drugInfo.cfm?
setid=9de65da4-73f8-4c88-8198-c92e63224ddb

Fluvoxamine (Luvox): https://dailymed.nlm.nih.gov/dailymed/drugInfo.cfm?
setid=6eeb14df-6fcf-a737-5359-5744eb4accea

Paroxetine (Paxil): https://dailymed.nlm.nih.gov/dailymed/drugInfo.cfm?
setid=89dd7e24-85fc-4152-89ea-47ec2b48a1ed

SNRI MEDICATIONS

Duloxetine (Cymbalta): https://dailymed.nlm.nih.gov/dailymed/drugInfo.
cfm?setid=2dde979d-b6f8-41d1-96fb-325c75ea3a74

Levomilnacipran (Fetzima): https://dailymed.nlm.nih.gov/dailymed/drugInfo.
cfm?setid=f371258d-91b3-4b6a-ac99-434a1964c3af

Venlafaxine (Effexor): https://dailymed.nlm.nih.gov/dailymed/drugInfo.cfm?setid=53c3e7ac-1852-4d70-d2b6-4fca819acf26

TRICYCLIC ANTIDEPRESSANTS

Amitriptyline (Elavil): https://dailymed.nlm.nih.gov/dailymed/drugInfo.cfm?setid=3d113e43-c694-427f-8b77-66be36a82374

Nortriptyline (Pamelor): https://dailymed.nlm.nih.gov/dailymed/drugInfo.cfm?setid=765d726b-fd4b-4ef7-afd7-9e7e9bf8cae6

ATYPICAL ANTIDEPRESSANTS

Bupropion (Wellbutrin XL): https://dailymed.nlm.nih.gov/dailymed/drugInfo.cfm?setid=60b270e4-29a4-474a-a2e9-e2c677bf59b5

Mirtazapine (Remeron): https://dailymed.nlm.nih.gov/dailymed/drugInfo.cfm?setid=9675333e-3064-c8cb-a4b4-6c74d9a82f17

SEROTONIN MODULATORS

Trazodone (Desyrel): https://dailymed.nlm.nih.gov/dailymed/drugInfo.cfm?setid=71961ab1-951d-1493-f76c-2ff25cca2a85

Vilazodone (Viibryd): https://dailymed.nlm.nih.gov/dailymed/drugInfo.cfm?setid=f917f30d-f2a7-43eb-836f-53eaa2a31cb0

Vortioxetine (Trintellix): https://dailymed.nlm.nih.gov/dailymed/drugInfo.cfm?setid=1a5b68e2-14d0-419d-9ec6-1ca97145e838

REFERENCES

1. American Psychiatric Association. *Diagnostic and Statistical Manual of Mental Disorders*. 5th ed., 2013

2. National Survey on Drug Use and Health. *2021 NSDUH Annual Reports*. Available from https://www.samhsa.gov/data/report/2021-nsduh-annual-national-report. Last updated January 2023. Accessed 6 March 2023

3. Healthline Editorial Team. Risk factors for depression [Internet]. Medically reviewed by Timothy J. Legg, 27 October 2016. Available from https://www.healthline.com/health/depression/risk-factors#1. Accessed 25 April 2018

4. Semenkovich K, Brown ME, Svrakic DM, Lustman PJ. Depression in type 2 diabetes mellitus: prevalence, impact and treatment. *Drugs* 2015;75: 577–587

5. Ali S, Stone MA, Peters JL, et al. The prevalence of co-morbid depression in adults with type 2 diabetes: a systematic review and meta-analysis. *Diabet Med* 2006;23(11):1165–1173

6. Elamoshy R, Bird Y, Thorpe L, Moraros J. Risk of depression and suicidality among diabetic patients: systematic review and meta-analysis. *J Clin Med* 2018;7:445

7. Mezuk B, Eaton WW, Albrecht S, Golden SH. Depression and type 2 diabetes over the lifespan. *Diabetes Care* 2008;31(12):2383–2390

8. Atasoy S, Johar H, Fang X, et al. Cumulative effect of depressed mood and obesity on type 2 diabetes incidence: findings from the MONICA/KORA cohort study. *J Psychosom Res* 2018;115:66–70

9. Xuan L, Zhao Z, Jia X, et al. Type 2 diabetes is causally associated with depression: a Mendelian randomization analysis. *Front Med* 2018;12(6):678–687. DOI:10.1007/s11684-018-0671-7. [Epub ahead of print]

10. Lustman PJ, Anderson RJ, Freedland KE, et al. Depression and poor glycemic control: a meta-analytic review of the literature. *Diabetes Care* 2000; 23(7):934–942

11. de Groot M, Anderson R, Freedland KE, et al. Association of depression and diabetes complications: a meta-analysis. *Psychosom Med* 2001;63(4):619–630

12. Burns RJ, Deschênes SS, Schmitz N. Cyclical relationship between depressive symptoms and diabetes distress in people with Type 2 diabetes mellitus: results from the Montreal Evaluation of Diabetes Treatment Cohort Study. *Diabetic Med* 2015;32:1272–1278

13. van Bastlaar KM, Pouwer F, Geelhoed-Duijvestijn PH, et al. Diabetes-specific emotional distress mediates the association between depressive symptoms and glycaemic control in Type 1 and Type 2 diabetes. *Diabet Med* 2010;27:798–803

14. Brieler JA, Lustman PJ, Scherrer JF, et al. Antidepressant medication use and glycaemic control in comorbid type 2 diabetes and depression. *Family Practice* 2016;33(1):30–36

15. American Psychiatric Association. *The Practice Guideline for the Treatment of Patients with Major Depressive Disorder.* 3rd ed, 2010. Available from https://www.psychiatry.org/psychiatrists/practice/clinical-practice-guidelines

16. American Psychological Association. *Clinical Practice Guideline for the Treatment of Depression Across Three Age Cohorts. Guideline Development Panel for the Treatment of Depressive Disorders.* 2019. Available from https://www.apa.org/depression-guideline

17. Fluvoxamine maleate [package insert]. Research Triangle Park, NC, Synthon Pharmaceuticals, Inc., 2007

18. Celexa (citalopram) [package insert]. Madison, NJ, Allergan USA, Inc., 2017

19. Lexapro (escitalopram oxalate) [package insert]. St. Louis, MO, Forest Pharmaceuticals, Inc., 2019

20. Paxil (paroxetine) [package insert]. Research Triangle Park, NC, GlaxoSmithKline, 2016

21. Zoloft (sertraline) [package insert]. New York, Roerig, 2018

22. Prozac (fluoxetine) [package insert]. Indianapolis, IN, Eli Lilly and Company, 2017

23. Hu XH, Bull SA, Hunkeler EM, et al. Incidence and duration of side effects and those rated as bothersome with selective serotonin reuptake inhibitor treatment for depression: patient report versus physician estimates. *J Clin Psychiatry* 2004;65:959–965

24. Fava M, Judge R, Hoog SL, et al. Fluoxetine versus sertraline and paroxetine in major depressive disorder: changes in weight with long-term treatment. *J Clin Psychiatry* 2000;61(11):863–867

25. Andersohn F, Schade R, Suissa S, Garbe E. Long-term use of antidepressants for depressive disorders and the risk of diabetes mellitus. *Am J Psychiatry* 2009;166:591–598

26. Debonnel G, Saint-André E, Hébert C, et al. Differential physiological effects of a low dose and high doses of venlafaxine in major depression. *Int J Neuropsychopharmacol* 2007;10(1):51–61

27. Cymbalta (duloxetine hydrochloride) [package insert]. Indianapolis, IN, Eli Lilly and Company, 2017

28. Effexor XR (venlafaxine hydrochloride) [package insert]. Philadelphia, PA, Wyeth Pharmaceuticals Inc., 2018

29. Fetizma (levomilnacipran) [package insert]. Irvine, CA, Allergan USA, Inc., 2017

30. Hudson JI, Wohlreich MM, Kajdasz DK, et al. Safety and tolerability of duloxetine in the treatment of major depressive disorder: analysis of pooled data from eight placebo-controlled clinical trials. *Hum Psychopharmacol* 2005;20:327–341

31. Wellbutrin XL (bupropion hydrochloride) [package insert]. Bridgewater, NJ, Valeant Pharmaceuticals North America LLC, 2017

32. Remeron (mirtazapine) [package insert]. Roseland, NJ, Organon USA Inc., 2018

33. Grasmäder K, Verwohlt PL, Kühn KU, et al. Relationship between mirtazapine dose, plasma concentration, response, and side effects in clinical practice. *Pharmacopsychiatry* 2005;38(3):113–117

34. Trazodone hydrochloride [package insert]. Weston, FL, Apotex Corp, 2017

35. Trintellix (vortioxetine hydrobromide) [package insert]. Deerfield, IL, Takeda Pharmaceuticals America, Inc., 2018

36. Viibryd (vilazodone hydrochloride) [package insert]. Madison, NJ, Allergan USA, Inc., 2018

37. Symbyax (olanzapine and fluoxetine hydrochloride) [package insert]. Indianapolis, IN, Eli Lilly and Company, 2018

38. Effexor (venlafaxine hydrochloride) [package insert]. Cranbury, NJ, Sun Pharmaceutical Industries, Inc., 2016

39. Pristiq (desvenlafaxine) [package insert]. Philadelphia, PA, Wyeth Pharmaceuticals Inc., 2018

40. Amitriptyline hydrochloride [package insert]. Chestnut Ridge, NY, Par Pharmaceuticals, 2017

41. Nortriptyline hydrochloride [package insert]. Greenville, NC, Mayne Pharma, 2016

42. Bupropion hydrochloride [package insert]. Weston, FL, Apotex Corp, 2017

43. Wellbutrin SR (bupropion hydrochloride) [package insert]. Research Triangle Park, NC, GlaxoSmithKline, 2017

44. Wade AG, Crawford GM, Yellowlees A. Efficacy, safety and tolerability of escitalopram in doses up to 50 mg in Major Depressive Disorder (MDD): an open-label, pilot study. *BMC Psychiatry* 2011;11:42. DOI:10.1186/1471-244X-11-42

Chapter 28
Medications for the Management of Hypoglycemia

Megan Giruzzi, PharmD, BCPS

Megan Giruzzi, PharmD, BCPS

INTRODUCTION

Hypoglycemia is a common complication of both T1D and T2D treatment that affects anywhere from 6 to 45% of the population.[1] Hypoglycemia is considered the major limiting factor for glycemic control in many patients with T1D or T2D.[2] Hypoglycemia has been defined in several different ways, and the definition has evolved over time. Despite the changes in the definition of hypoglycemia, the treatment recommendations and medication options for hypoglycemia have been consistent over the past decade.

Since the early 1930s, hypoglycemia has been defined as the presence of the Whipple triad. The Whipple triad consists of signs and symptoms of low blood glucose, low blood glucose levels, and the reversal of these signs and symptoms with administration or ingestion of glucose. In recent years there has been a growing concern regarding the incidence of hypoglycemic unawareness. Recent studies have observed hypoglycemia unawareness in 8–10% of patients with T1D and T2D.[3,4] With prolonged hypoglycemia, secondary to hypoglycemia unawareness, neurological complications such as behavioral changes, cognitive impairment, seizures, coma, and mortality are increased sixfold, affecting an estimated 4.9–9% of individuals.[5,6] This led the American Diabetes Association to redefine hypoglycemia and to create five classifications of it in 2013.[7] Most recently, the International Hypoglycemia Study Group redefined the classifications for hypoglycemia into three levels.[8] The first level is classified as the hypoglycemia alert value, where an SMBG or laboratory measurement of ≤70 mg/dL (3.9 mmol/L) is observed. Patients meeting this criterion can typically be treated with any form of fast-acting carbohydrate and should have their glycemic control regimen adjusted to prevent a future event. The second level is classified as clinically significant hypoglycemia, due to the risk for serious, potentially fatal consequences, where an SMBG or laboratory measurement is found to be <54 mg/dL (3.0 mmol/L). The third level is classified as severe hypoglycemia. For this classification, there is no specified glucose threshold; however, these patients will have hypoglycemia associated with severe cognitive impairment requiring assistance from another individual for recovery.[8] The second and third levels may require treatment with a parenteral formulation of dextrose or glucagon to reverse hypoglycemia and prevent complications. These three classifications were adapted by the American Diabetes Association in 2017 and are currently used to define and classify hypoglycemia within the *Standards of Care in Diabetes*.[2]

When an individual's blood glucose level begins to fall, multiple systems in the body are triggered to help resolve the hypoglycemic episode. The initial response of the body occurs when the blood glucose falls between 80 and 90 mg/dL. At this time, the pancreas begins to decrease the production of insulin and will begin to counterregulate by increasing glucagon production. The liver will quickly detect the increase in glucagon and respond by increasing both glycogenolysis and gluconeogenesis. In some patients, the glucagon production will be sufficient to resolve the hypoglycemic episode. In other patients, especially those whose glucose drops below 70 mg/dL, the adrenaline hormones will begin to play a key role to ensure the brain has a constant supply of glucose by limiting the use of glucose by nonessential tissues.[9-11]

The counterregulatory response is further carried out by the adrenal glands, which begin producing and releasing epinephrine. The epinephrine acts on certain body tissues, such as muscle, to decrease glucose use, as well as on the kidneys to decrease glucose clearance. Another counterregulatory response involves the peripheral nervous system, mediating an increase in acetylcholine. Acetylcholine and epinephrine then begin to trigger an autonomic response to alert the patient that their blood glucose is low. Lastly, cortisol and growth hormone are released and play a minor role in slowing the consumption of glucose by nonessential tissues to aid in the increase of blood glucose levels.[9-11]

During episodes of hypoglycemia, patients can experience a variety of symptoms that can be classified as either autonomic or neuroglycopenic. As previously mentioned, epinephrine and acetylcholine trigger the body's autonomic response. Typical symptoms of this response include tremors, diaphoresis, hunger, palpitations, anxiety, and sometimes pallor. It is important to note that medications such as β-blockers can mask the autonomic response, resulting in patients being unable to notice a hypoglycemic episode until the event progresses to the neuroglycopenic symptoms. Neuroglycopenic symptoms are caused by a lack of glucose in the CNS and are typically more distressing and severe. These symptoms include cognitive impairment, confusion, behavioral changes, anger, irritability, blurred vision, headaches, seizures, and loss of consciousness, leading to coma and even death.[11,12]

Acute hypoglycemia has been linked to a number of different consequences. In some cases, its effect can go beyond just the patient to affect others, especially if the episode is associated with a fall, motor vehicle accident, or other injury.[2] Hypoglycemia is associated with an increased risk for cardiovascular events, such as MI, stroke, and cardiovascular death. It has also been shown to cause QT prolongation and life-threatening ventricular arrhythmias.[13,14] Studies have found that patients with hypoglycemia are at an increased risk of developing dementia, both vascular and Alzheimer's disease. In adults, the degree of cognitive impairment has been associated with the frequency of severe hypoglycemia.[2,15] Patients with cognitive dysfunction may have difficulty identifying and treating low blood glucose levels; therefore, the risk of developing severe hypoglycemia may be greater. Lastly, numerous studies have documented the effect of hypoglycemia on quality of life. Patients with episodes of hypoglycemia report decreased overall health, mental health issues, and increased anxiety.

There are a number of factors that can contribute to hypoglycemia. The most common cause of hypoglycemia is antidiabetic medications. Antidiabetic oral medications with the highest risk of hypoglycemia include sulfonylureas and meglitinides. When used as monotherapy, they have been associated with an increased relative risk of 2–8; when used as part of a combination therapy, they are associated with a four- to eightfold increase in the frequency of hypoglycemic events.[16] Other oral medications that may be associated with a risk of hypoglycemia include aspirin, warfarin, allopurinol, and probenecid when used in combination with antidiabetic medications. When analyzing patients who are treated with insulin, the rates of hypoglycemia are greater than 15 times those of patients treated with oral medications. With several formulations of insulin on the market, there are profound variabilities in their pharmacokinetic and pharmacodynamic properties. Compared to longer-acting basal analogs such as insulin glargine and insulin detemir, NPH has been found to have a greater variability in its absorption profile and duration of action.[17] Furthermore, due to a lower variability profile, the basal analogs insulin detemir and insulin glargine are associated with a 31% risk reduction of nocturnal hypoglycemia and a 27% risk reduction of severe hypoglycemia in T1D and a 54% reduction in nocturnal hypoglycemia and 31% reduction in symptomatic hypoglycemia in T2D.[18,19] Other factors that contribute to hypoglycemia include alcohol ingestion, sudden reduction of corticosteroid dosing, hot weather, stress, acute illness (reduced oral intake and/or emesis), exercise, weight loss, acute kidney injury, chronic kidney disease, and hepatic disease. Elderly patients are at an increased risk of hypoglycemic events due to polypharmacy, cognitive impairment, and deteriorating renal function.

As mentioned previously, hypoglycemia unawareness is a growing concern. Hypoglycemia unawareness is defined as the asymptomatic onset of hypoglycemia. Patients will typically not recognize the autonomic warning symptoms and therefore are at an increased risk for morbidity and mortality. Studies have found that the increased risk of all-cause mortality remains for 4 years following a severe hypoglycemic event.[20] The major risk factors for hypoglycemia unawareness include duration of the disease, number of prior hypoglycemic events, frequent nocturnal hypoglycemia, aging, and more stringent glycemic control.[3] Major consequences of hypoglycemia unawareness include major macrovascular events, major microvascular events, venous thromboembolisms, severe arrhythmias, and cognitive dysfunction. Unfortunately, hypoglycemic unawareness can also lead to an increased risk of depression, missed days of work, and financial burdens.

HYPOGLYCEMIC PREVENTION

The prevention of hypoglycemic episodes is a critical component of diabetes management. The importance of SMBG should be stressed to patients at their initial diagnosis and reinforced longitudinally throughout management of their diabetes. In some patients, SMBG is not enough, and they will need CGM to detect hypoglycemia. Increasing evidence is emerging that CGM is a useful tool for decreasing the number of hypoglycemic episodes, specifically the time spent between 54 and 70 mg/dL in patients with T1D. One study with patients with T1D found that patients who were monitored with CGM for 28 days had a mean decrease in hypoglycemic events from 10.8 to 3.5.[21] Mixed data are published on the use of CGM in T2D. Some studies have shown an increase in the number of hypoglycemic events, due to the prevalence of hypoglycemic unawareness; others have shown no difference.[22] More studies are needed prior to recommending CGM for patients with T2D. Overall, CGM may be a useful tool to decrease the time spent in hypoglycemia. Patients must be educated to understand situations that increase their risk of hypoglycemia, including fasting for blood tests or procedures, delaying meals, during or after exercise, and while asleep. Additionally, patients should be counseled on the proper use of their antidiabetic agents, carbohydrate counting, and physical activity. Formal training programs have been developed to help increase awareness of hypoglycemia and to empower patients develop strategies to decrease hypoglycemia. Some of these programs include the Blood Glucose Awareness Training Program, Dose Adjusted for Normal Eating (DAFNE), and DAFNEplus. Education regarding these situations may not prevent all hypoglycemic episodes, but may increase a patient's self-awareness of their body's glucose demands in specific situations. All hypoglycemic events should be discussed and evaluated at every visit. The evaluation should include frequency of events, timing of events, current treatment regimen, and severity. Treatment regimens should be reevaluated if the patient is experiencing frequent or severe hypoglycemia. In certain situations of recurrent hypoglycemia, relaxing blood glucose targets for a couple of weeks may prevent unnecessary hypoglycemic episodes and reverse hypoglycemia unawareness. Specifically, patients who experience hypoglycemia unawareness, one level-three hypoglycemic event, or a number of unexplained level-two hypoglycemic events should have their glycemic targets adjusted to prevent hospitalizations, emergency department visits, and decrease their risk of mortality.[15,35]

TREATMENT OPTIONS

The backbone to hypoglycemic management is the consumption of pure glucose or fast-acting carbohydrates when a patient's glucose level falls below 70 mg/dL (3.9 mmol/L). Studies have found that either glucose or carbohydrates are effective; however, some data suggest that a hypoglycemic event will resolve faster with pure glucose. There are a number of fast-acting, oral glucose products that are readily available and easy to administer. Available glucose products include chewable tablets, oral gels, and liquids, which can be found at the local pharmacy (see Table 28.1). Although these products are readily available, they are not the only option. A patient can consume any type of fast-acting carbohydrate that is readily available, as long as the patient is conscious and demonstrates no difficulty in breathing or swallowing.

Patients being treated with medications that can cause hypoglycemia must be counseled on the appropriate amount of glucose to consume in order to raise their blood glucose quickly. In conscious individuals with a blood glucose <70 mg/dL (3.9 mmol/L), administration of 15–20 g of glucose is advised. Fifteen minutes after treatment, patients should recheck their blood glucose, and if they show continued hypoglycemia, the treatment should be repeated. This administration of 15 g of carbohydrates, followed by rechecking blood glucose levels in 15 min is

Table 28.1—Fast-Acting Glucose Products

Product (manufacturer)*	Carbohydrate amount	Dose
Liquids		
Dex4 (Perrigo)	15 g per bottle	1 bottle
TRUEplus Glucose Shot (Trividia Health)		
Gels		
Dex4 (Perrigo)	15 g per pouch	1 pouch
Glutose 15 (Perrigo)	15 g per tube	1 tube
Glutose 45 (Perrigo)	45 g per tube	1/3 of tube
Insta-Glucose (Valeant Pharmaceuticals)	24 g per tube	1 tube
Transcend (Transcend Foods)	15 g per pouch	1 pouch
TRUEplus Glucose Gel (Trividia Health)	15 g per pouch	1 pouch
Powder		
Elovate 15 (Diasan Corp)	15 g per packet	1 packet
Tablets		
Dex4 (Perrigo)	4 g per tablet	4 tablets, for 16 g carbohydrates
Glucolift (Jungell)		
Optimum (Magno-Humphries Labs)		
TRUEplus Glucose Tablets (Trividia Health)		
TRUEplus Soft Tabs (Trividia Health)		

*Store-brand glucose products contain the same amount of fast-acting glucose as the name-brand version and may serve as a cost-effective alternative.

often referred to as the "Rule of 15." Once a patient's SMBG returns to normal, they should consume a meal or snack to prevent the recurrence of hypoglycemia. This meal or snack should include a blend of carbohydrates, fats, and protein. Examples of snacks that a patient can consume include, but are not limited to, a peanut butter and jelly sandwich, cheese and crackers, or a granola bar. Patients should be advised to not overeat after these situations, as this may lead to a hyperglycemic state.

Education regarding hypoglycemia and management is important and should be revisited regularly with patients. All patients with diabetes should be counseled to carry a source of fast-acting glucose with them at all times. The "Rule of 15" further applies to the quantity of fast-acting candy sources such as M&Ms

and Skittles. It is recommended that a patient self-treat with 15 M&Ms or 15 Skittles during a hypoglycemic event.[20] Other options for fast-acting glucose sources that patients may use other than oral glucose products include 4 ounces of regular fruit juice or regular soda (not diet); 2 tablespoons of raisins; 1 tablespoon of corn syrup, table sugar, or honey; 8 ounces of nonfat or 1% milk; hard candy or jellybeans (see package for number to consume); or a spoonful of commercial cake frosting. All of these sources will rapidly raise blood glucose levels. Patients experiencing hypoglycemia should initially avoid ingesting high-fat or protein-based foods or drinks. Both protein and fats will impact and slow the absorption of glucose into the system, prolonging the acute hypoglycemic episode.

All patients that experience a hypoglycemic episode should continue to regularly monitor their glucose throughout the remainder of the day, while resuming a regular eating schedule. A patient should also contact their physician and discuss the hypoglycemic episode and determine whether adjustment with their treatment regimen is needed.

GLUCAGON

If a patient is unable to self-administer oral glucose products due to swallowing difficulties or unconsciousness, another option that may be used is glucagon. Glucagon is produced by the α-cells in the pancreas and is released when the concentration of glucose in the blood falls between 80 and 90 mg/dL. When released, it works to raise blood glucose levels and prevent or reverse hypoglycemia. When the body is not able to produce enough glucagon, other systems in the body respond to alert patients to the hypoglycemic event. Unfortunately, some patients will lose consciousness before being able to adequately treat the event. In these situations, exogenous glucagon is available as a hypoglycemic antidote and may be administered for the management of hypoglycemia. Therefore, glucagon should be prescribed for all individuals at increased risk of clinically significant hypoglycemia. This includes, but is not limited to, all T1D patients, children with diabetes, and any patient who has experienced a hypoglycemic event of <54 mg/dL (3.0 mmol/L).

When released and/or administered, glucagon triggers adenylate cyclase in the liver to stimulate the conversion of AMP to cAMP. The increase in cAMP leads to a degradation of stored glycogen to rapid-acting glucose. This process is known as glycogenolysis, resulting in return to a euglycemic state rapidly, reversing hypoglycemia. In order for this mechanism to be effective at increasing blood glucose levels, there must be a preexisting hepatic glycogen store for breakdown. Patients at risk of having depleted glycogen stores include geriatric patients, patients with low body weight, and chronic alcoholics. These patients have been found to have a reduced response or no response to glucagon. In situations where glycogen stores are depleted, other methods of raising blood glucose must be employed, including the administration of intravenous dextrose.

Table 28.2—Glucagon Prescribing Information for Treatment of Hypoglycemia

Medication	Available formulations	Dosage
Glucagon	Kit and solution for reconstitution	IM, IV, Subcutaneous, Intranasal: Dose may be repeated in 15 min as needed
	Dry powder (white nasal powder)	Adults & Pediatrics >44 lbs (20 kg): 1 mg by injection
	Single-dose pre-filled HypoPen autoinjector	Pediatrics <44 lbs (20 kg): 0.5 mg or dose equivalent to 20–30 µg/kg
	Single-dose pre-filled syringe	If a patient fails to respond to glucagon injection, IV dextrose must be given
		Intranasal: administer 3 mg (one actuation) into single nostril
		Pre-filled autoinjector and syringe: >45 kg: 1-mg dose <45 kg: 0.5-mg dose

IM, intramuscular; IV, intravenous.

Glucagon, when used for the emergent treatment of hypoglycemia, is administered parenterally via an intravenous, intramuscular, or subcutaneous injection. For adults and pediatrics weighing more than 44 lbs (20 kg), administration of a 1 mg dose is appropriate. In patients weighing less than 44 lbs (20 kg), a 0.5 mg dose or a dose equivalent to 20–30 µg/kg, not exceeding 1 mg, would be appropriate (see Table 28.2). Prior to administration, glucagon kits will need to be reconstituted. Patients and family members should be counseled on how to reconstitute the solution and to not inject the solution unless the solution is clear and a waterlike consistency. The glucagon injection should be administered in the patient's buttock, arm, or thigh. The patient should then be turned on their side, due to the risk of vomiting. Following administration of glucagon, immediately call 911. A clinical response and return to consciousness should occur within 15 min of administration. If there is a delayed response, administration of an additional dose of glucagon is appropriate. Replacement with intravenous 50% dextrose solution may be preferred in these situations to ensure that an adequate glucose response is achieved. After consciousness is obtained, patients should ingest carbohydrates to prevent hypoglycemic recurrence and assist in the replenishment of glucose to replace glycogen stores in the liver. Patients should consume a fast-acting carbohydrate, followed by a long-acting carbohydrate that can be combined with some protein and small amounts of fat as mentioned previously. In December 2020, the FDA approved the first generic glucagon for injection, a 1 mg/vial packaged in an emergency kit.[31] The emergency kit is approved for the treatment of severe hypoglycemia and as a diagnostic aid in radiologic examinations of the stomach and intestinal tract.[31]

Recently, intranasal glucagon has made its way back into clinical trials as a potential alternative for injectable glucagon. It was first studied more than 20 years ago; however, none of those studies led to the FDA approval of a nonparenteral glucagon preparation.[23] Many challenges have been reported with the reconstitution of injectable glucagon, such as opening the package, removing the needle sheath, mixing the ingredients, bending the needle, and time to reconstitution (ranging from 2.5–3 min on average).[24,25] Intranasal glucagon has the ability to overcome most of these obstacles since there is no need for reconstitution because of its dry powder formulation. When evaluating intranasal glucagon's efficacy, it has been found to be noninferior to injectable glucagon; however, in studies, the time to resolution of a hypoglycemic event when blood glucose is <50 mg/dL was 16 min with intranasal glucagon versus 13 min with injectable glucagon.[23,25] Although statistically there was a 3 min difference, when taking into account the time to reconstitute the injectable glucagon, both formulations work in about the same amount of time; therefore, there is no clinical difference. On July 24, 2019, the FDA approved Baqsimi, the first intranasal formulation of glucagon. Baqsimi was approved for severe hypoglycemia for adults and children over the age of 4 years. The recommended dose of Baqsimi is 3 mg administered via intranasal device into one nostril. Patients, caregivers, and family members should be counseled to insert the tip of the device into one nostril and to press the device plunger all the way until the green line is no longer showing. Once the dose has been administered, immediately call 911. If an additional dose is needed, a new Baqsimi device will be needed, since each device contains only one dose of glucagon. If there has been no response after 15 minutes, an additional 3 mg dose may be administered while waiting for emergency medical services.[27]

Furthermore, research has been ongoing for a glucagon solution formulation that does not require reconstitution. On September 10, 2019, the FDA approved Gvoke, a liquid-stable form of glucagon that is available as an autoinjectable, prefilled syringe, as a rescue treatment for severe hyoglycemia. In clinical trials, Gvoke has been proven to be noninferior to the reconstituted injectable glucagon. One study performed in 81 adult patients with T1D, found that the time from administration of glucagon for plasma glucose to increase by ≥ 20 mg/dL from baseline was 11.36 minutes in the Gvoke group compared with 8.02 minutes in the reconstituted injectable glucagon group.[28,29] The study also looked at the time from administration of glucagon to complete resolution of 4 autonomic symptoms of hypoglycemia: sweating, tremor, palpitations, and feeling of nervousness. Resolution of symptoms on average took 13.8 minutes in the Gvoke group compared with 12 minutes in the reconstituted glucagon group.[28,29] Although resolution of symptoms and time to effect took slightly longer with the Gvoke group, when taking into account the time to reconstitute glucagon, there is no difference. In fact, Gvoke may be preferred due to the anxiety that is accompanied with reconstituting glucagon for subcutaneous administration. For adult and pediatric patients weighing more than 45 kg, administration of a 1 mg dose is appropriate. In patients weighing less than 45 kg, a 0.5 mg dose is recommended.[30] Family members and caregivers should be counseled on how to use the prefilled pen. Prior to administration, visual inspection is required to ensure the solution appears clear and colorless (a pale yellow is okay) and is free of particles. If the solution is discolored or contains particles, it should not be used. After visually inspecting the solution, remove the needle cap and inject the solution into the lower abdomen, outer thigh, or outer upper arm at a 90 degree angle. The autoinjector should be held against the skin for at least 5 seconds, to ensure full administration of the glucagon dose. The patient should then be turned on their side, due to the risk of vomiting, and 911 should be called. If the patient has not responded after 15 minutes, an additional dose may be administered while waiting for emergency medical services. If an additional dose is needed, a new Gvoke prefilled syringe will be needed, since each syringe contains only one dose of glucagon. Although this is currently a novel solution, there is an additional liquid-stable glucagon analog formulation in the works by Adocia.

Glucagon is a well-tolerated medication, with nausea and vomiting being the most common side effect associated with its injectable formulation. This effect may be compounded by the body's natural hypoglycemic response. In clinical trials, the common adverse effects associated with intranasal glucagon include nasal irritation, ocular irritation, head or facial discomfort, and some nausea and vomiting. Glucagon has positive inotropic and chronotropic effects; therefore, patients with underlying cardiovascular conditions such as arrhythmias and hypertension should be monitored closely following administration. Monitoring parameters should include blood pressure, blood glucose, ECG, heart rate, and mentation. Glucagon carries contraindications for administration in patients with known hypersensitivity, pheochromocytoma, insulinoma, and glucagonoma.

In terms of special populations, glucagon is relatively safe in pregnancy. Although exact effects are unknown due to limited data available, there is no concern for teratogenicity and the effects of prolonged hypoglycemia outweigh the risk of harm. It is unknown whether this medication is excreted in human milk; therefore, caution should be exercised in nursing women. There are no dosing adjustments required for patients with renal or hepatic impairment.

There is not an extensive list of drug interactions for concern; however, the use of glucagon in combination with vitamin K antagonists such as warfarin may enhance the bleeding risk. This interaction is noted with much larger doses of glucagon than are used in hypoglycemic management. Nonetheless, patients at a high risk for bleeding should be monitored for fluctuations in INR and signs/symptoms of bleeding.

DASIGLUCAGON

Dasiglucagon is the next-generation glucagon and is the first glucagon product to be provided in a ready-to-use, aqueous formulation. Dasiglucagon is unique in that it has seven amino acid substitutions to increase the physical and chemical stability in aqueous media, eliminating the need for reconstitution before injection. In a phase 3, randomized trial of patients with T1D, patients received 150% of their usual basal rate with a target blood glucose of 55 mg/dL. Patients then received dasiglucagon, placebo, or glucagon.[32] Median time to plasma glucose recovery was 10 minutes with dasiglucagon vs. 12 minutes with glucagon. The safety profiles of both dasiglucagon and glucagon were consistent with the known adverse effects of glucagon treatment, with the most common drug-related adverse events of nausea, vomiting, and headache comparable between treatment groups.[32] Similar efficacy and safety results were obtained in a similar study with children and adolescents,[33] showing that dasiglucagon is an acceptable alternative to glucagon during a severe hypoglycemic event.

The FDA approved dasiglucagon (Zegalogue) on March 22, 2021, for the treatment of severe hypoglycemia for pediatric and adult patients with diabetes age 6 years and older. Dasiglucagon is available as an autoinjectable, 0.6 mg/0.6 mL single-dose prefilled syringe.[34] A patient or caregiver should inject the solution into the lower abdomen, buttock, thigh, or upper arm. Once the dose has been given, immediately call 911. If there is no response after 15 minutes, an additional dose of dasiglucagon can be given; however, a new device will be needed, since each device contains only one dose of dasiglucagon. Dasiglucagon is generally well tolerated, with nausea, vomiting, and headache being the most common encountered adverse reactions. Patients may also experience injection site pain and diarrhea. Contraindications are similar to glucagon, including pheochromocytoma and insulinoma. Lastly, dasiglucagon is only effective if patients have sufficient hepatic glycogen present. If patients are in a state of starvation, have adrenal insufficiency, or chronic hypoglycemia, dasiglucagon may be ineffective at increasing blood glucose to adequate levels to overcome the hypoglycemic event.

In terms of special populations, dasiglucagon has not been studied in pregnant patients; therefore, little is known about its risk of miscarriage and major birth defects. However, it is important to keep in mind that untreated hypoglycemia can cause complications and be fatal. There is also no information on dasiglucagon's presence in human milk. Dasiglucagon is a peptide and would be expected to be broken down to its constituent amino acids in the infant's digestive tract and is therefore unlikely to cause harm to an exposed infant.

There is not an extensive list of drug interactions for concern. The use of dasiglucagon like glucagon in combination with vitamin K antagonists such as warfarin may enhance the bleeding risk. When used in patients taking β-blockers, it may have a transient increase in pulse and blood pressure. Lastly, when given to patients who are also taking indomethacin, dasiglucagon may lose its ability to raise blood glucose.

SUMMARY

Hypoglycemia is a commonly encountered complication of glycemic control. It affects a patient's quality of life and can be an economic burden. It is important to properly educate patients to be able to recognize the early signs and symptoms of hypoglycemia and appropriately manage their hypoglycemic event with fast-acting carbohydrates or injectable glucagon. Furthermore, patients should be counseled to follow up with their provider after a hypoglycemic event to have their glycemic regimen adjusted as necessary to prevent future events.

MONOGRAPH

Glucagon kit: https://dailymed.nlm.nih.gov/dailymed/drugInfo.cfm?setid=f09feb8e-6651-4708-a811-bb5264712059

Gvoke (glucagon prefilled syringe): https://dailymed.nlm.nih.gov/dailymed/drugInfo.cfm?setid=92385737-dbad-98c5-e053-2995a90a2805

Baqsimi (glucagon nasal powder): https://dailymed.nlm.nih.gov/dailymed/drugInfo.cfm?setid=3fdb4e92-2e19-487d-9f14-99871e9fd15a

Zegalogue (dasiglucagon injection, solution): https://dailymed.nlm.nih.gov/dailymed/drugInfo.cfm?setid=c6c32b47-c47c-4a7f-8d4d-23578f663217

REFERENCES

1. Edridge CL, Dunkley AJ, Bodicoar DH, et al. Prevalence and incidence of hypoglycaemia in 532,542 people with type 2 diabetes on oral therapies and insulin: a systematic review and meta-analysis of population based studies. *PLoS One* 2015;10(6):e0126427

2. American Diabetes Association. 6. Glycemic targets: Standards of Medical Care in Diabetes—2022. *Diabetes Care* 2023;45(Suppl. 1):S83–S96

3. Czyzewska K, Czerniawska E, Szadkowska A. Prevalence of hypoglycemia unawareness in patients with type 1 diabetes. *Pediatr Diabet* 2012;13 (Suppl. 17):77

4. Schopman JE, Geddes J, Frier BM. Prevalence of impaired awareness of hypoglycaemia and frequency of hypoglycaemia in insulin-treated type 2 diabetes. *Diabetes Res Clin Pract* 2010;87:64–68

5. Marrett E, Radican L, Davies MJ, Zhang Q. Assessment of severity and frequency of self-reported hypoglycemia on quality of life in patients with type 2 diabetes treated with oral antihyperglycemic agents: a survey study. *BMC Res Notes* 2011;4:251

6. Martin-Timon I, Canizon-Gomez FJ. Mechanisms of hypoglycemia unawareness and implications in diabetic patients. *World J Diabetes* 2015;6(7):912–926

7. Seaquist ER, Anderson J, Childs B, et al. Hypoglycemia and diabetes: a report of a work group of the American Diabetes Association and the Endocrine Society. *Diabetes Care* 2013;36:1384–1395

8. International Hypoglycaemia Study Group. Glucose concentrations of less than 3.0 mmol/L (54 mg/dL) should be reported in clinical trials: a joint position statement of the American Diabetes Association and the European Association for the Study of Diabetes. *Diabetes Care* 2017;40:155–157

9. Briscoe VJ, Davis SN. Hypoglycemia in type 1 and type 2 diabetes: physiology, pathophysiology, and management. *Clin Diabetes* 2006;24:115–121

10. Cryer PE, Davis SN, Shamoon H. Hypoglycemia in diabetes. *Diabetes Care* 2003;26:1902–1912

11. Kenny C. When hypoglycemia is not obvious: diagnosing and treating under-recognized and undisclosed hypoglycemia. *Prim Care Diabetes* 2014;8:3–11

12. White JR. The contribution of medications to hypoglycemia unawareness. *Diabetes Spectrum* 2007;20(2):77–80

13. Frier BM. Hypoglycemia in diabetes mellitus: epidemiology and clinical implications. *Nat Rev Endocrinol* 2014;10:711–722

14. Zoungas S, Patel A, Chalmers J, et al. Severe hypoglycemia and risks of vascular events and death. *N Engl J Med* 2010;363:1410–1418

15. Punthakee Z, Miller ME, Launer LI, et al. ACCORD Group of Investigators: ACCORD-MIND Investigators. Poor cognitive function and risk of severe hypoglycemia in type 2 diabetes: post hoc epidemiologic analysis of the ACCORD trial. *Diabetes Care* 2012;35:787–793

16. Phung OJ, Scholle JM, Talwar M, Coleman CI. Effect of noninsulin antidiabetic drugs added to metformin therapy on glycemic control, weight gain, and hypoglycemia in type 2 diabetes. *JAMA* 2010;303:1410–1418

17. Vora J, Heise T. Variability of glucose-lowering effect as a limiting factor in optimizing basal insulin therapy: a review. *Diabetes Obes Metab* 2013;15:701–712

18. Monami M, Marchionni N, Mannucci E. Long-acting insulin analogues verses NPH human insulin in type 1 diabetes. A meta-analysis. *Diabetes Obes Metab* 2009;11;372–378

19. Monami M, Marchionni N, Mannucci E. Long-acting insulin analogues verses NPH human insulin in type 2 diabetes: a meta-analysis. *Diabetes Res Clin Pract* 2008;81:184–189

20. Morales J, Schneider D. Hypoglycemia. *Am J Med* 2014;127(10 Suppl.):S17–S24

21. Heinemann L, Freckmann G, Ehrmann D, et al. Real-time continuous glucose monitoring in adults with type 1 diabetes and impaired hypoglycaemia awareness or severe hypoglycaemia treated with multiple daily insulin injections (HypoDE): A multicentre, randomised controlled trial. *Lancet* 2018;391:1367–377

22. Beck RW, Riddlesworth TD, Ruedy K, et al. Continuous glucose monitoring versus usual care in patients with type 2 diabetes receiving multiple daily insulin injections: A randomized trial. *Ann Intern Med* 2017;167:365–374

23. Rickels MR, Ruedy KJ, Foster CN, et al. Intranasal glucagon for treatment of insulin-induced hypoglycemia in adults with type 1 diabetes: a randomized crossover noninferiority study. *Diabetes Care* 2016;39(2):264–270

24. Pontiroli AE. Intranasal glucagon: a promising approach for treatment of severe hypoglycemia. *J Diabetes Sci Technol* 2015;9(1):38–43

25. Yale JF, Dulede H, Egeth M, et al. Faster use and fewer failures with needle-free nasal glucagon versus injectable glucagon in severe hypoglycemia rescue: a simulation study. *Diabetes Technol Ther* 2017;19(7):423–432

26. Boido A, Ceriani V, Pontiroli AE. Glucagon for hypoglycemic episodes in insulin-treated diabetic patients: a systematic review and meta-analysis with a comparison of glucagon with dextrose and of different glucagon formulations. *Acta Diabetol* 2015;52(2):405–412

27. Baqsimi [package insert]. Indianapolis, IN, Eli Lilly and Company, 2019

28. G-Pen Compared to Lilly Glucagon for Hypoglycemia Rescue in Adults with Type 1 Diabetes. In: ClinicalTrials.gov [Internet]. Available from https://clinicaltrials.gov/ct2/show/NCT03439072

29. Xeris Pharmaceuticals, Inc. Annual Report Pursuant to Section 13 or 15 of the Securities Exchange Act of 1934, 6 March 2019. Available from https://www.xerispharma.com/images/xeris-annual-report-2018.pdf

30. Gvoke [package insert]. Chicago, IL, Xeris Pharmaceuticals, Inc., 2019

31. U.S. Food & Drug Administration. FDA approves first generic of drug used to treat severe hypoglycemia. Available from https://www.fda.gov/news-events/press-announcements/fda-approves-first-generic-drug-used-treat-severe-hypoglycemia. Accessed 4 February 2021

32. Pieber TR, Aronson R, Hovelmann E, et al. Dasiglucagon—A next-generation glucagon analog for rapid and effective treatment of severe hypoglycemia: results of phase 3 randomized double-blind clinical trial. *Diabetes Care* 2021;44(6):1361–1367

33. Batterlina T, Tehranchi R, Bailey T, et al. Dasiglucagon, a next-generation ready-to-use glucagon analog, for treatment of severe hypoglycemia in children and adolescents with type 1 diabetes: Results of a phase 3, randomized controlled trial. *Pediatr Diabetes* 2021;22(5):734–741

34. Zegalogue [package insert]. Søborg, Denmark, Zealand Pharma A/S, 2021

35. Zoungas S, Patel A, Chalmers J, et al.; ADVANCE Collaborative Group. Severe hypoglycemia and risks of vascular events and death. *N Engl J Med* 2010;363:1410–1418

Chapter 29
Medications for the Management of Obesity

Nicholas R. Giruzzi, PharmD, BCPS

INTRODUCTION

O besity is a chronic medical condition that is the result of a long-term mismatch in energy balance, in which daily energy intake exceeds daily energy use.[1] The daily energy balance is affected by multiple factors including metabolic rate, appetite, diet, and physical activity.[1] Obesity is associated with many health risks, including hypertension, hyperlipidemia, T2D, CHD, stroke, gallbladder disease, osteoarthritis, sleep apnea, respiratory problems, and some cancers.[2] Obesity has also been associated with an increased risk of all-cause and cardiovascular mortality. The 1998 overweight and obesity clinical guidelines[3] defined overweight as a BMI of 25–29.9 kg/m^2 and obesity as a BMI of ≥30 kg/m^2. According to reports from the CDC, more than one-third (36.5%) of U.S. adults have obesity.[4] In 2008, the estimated medical cost of obesity in the U.S. was $147 billion.[4] The average medical costs were $1,429 more in those who were obese than those with a normal weight.[4]

As confirmed by multiple studies, there is strong evidence showing that weight management can delay or even prevent the progression from prediabetes to T2D and may be beneficial in the treatment.[5] Evidence-based research strongly suggests that medical nutrition therapy provided by a registered dietitian who is experienced in the management of diabetes is clinically effective.[6] Outcomes from randomized controlled nutrition therapy studies have documented decreases in A1C of approximately 1% in patients with newly diagnosed T1D, 2% in patients with newly diagnosed T2D, and 1% in patients with a long-standing history of T2D (average duration of 4 years).[6]

Weight loss can be attained with lifestyle modifications and programs that help the patient achieve a daily energy deficit,[5] and maintaining this over the long term is done by maintaining a neutral energy deficit. There are many benefits associated with weight loss, including decreased A1C, lipid levels, and blood pressure, that may be seen with as little as 5% weight loss.[7] However, a sustained weight loss over the long term of ≥7% is the optimal scenario. Many different diets have been studied, such as those restricting certain foods (high fat or high carbohydrate), which creates the necessary energy deficit that leads to weight loss.[5] Healthcare professionals play an important role not only in educating patients about dietary changes but also in providing ongoing support and encouragement for these patients.

Although diet and exercise are the backbone of therapy for weight management, those interventions alone may not be sufficient to achieve weight loss goals.

This circumstance is when pharmacological therapies should be considered. The FDA defines the indication for obesity pharmacotherapy as a BMI >30 kg/m^2 or a BMI >27 kg/m^2 with at least one obesity-associated comorbid condition.[8] This means a very large percentage of the U.S. adult population meets the criteria for pharmacological weight management therapy. The goals of weight management therapy include the prevention of further weight gain, reduction of body weight, and maintaining weight loss over the long term.[9,10]

PHARMACOLOGICAL MANAGEMENT OF OBESITY

PHENTERMINE

Phentermine (Lomaira; Adipex-P) is classified as a CNS stimulant and anorexiant. Phentermine has FDA approval as a short-term weight management agent in appropriate patients, but it is often prescribed off-label for long-term use.[11] Phentermine is a federally controlled (C-IV) medication. A meta-analysis[7] of six randomized, controlled trials of phentermine lasting 2–24 weeks reported patients on phentermine 15–30 mg/day lost an average of 3.6 kg more than patients receiving placebo, with a mean total weight loss of 6.3 kg.

Pharmacology

Mechanism of Action

Phentermine is a sympathomimetic amine. Its mechanism in reducing appetite is secondary to its CNS effects: phentermine stimulates the hypothalamus to release norepinephrine, which leads to a reduction in hunger and signals fat cells to break down stored fat, resulting in weight loss.[12,13]

Pharmacokinetics

Phentermine is available as both capsules and tablets, with the onset of action varying depending on the timing of administration and meals. Phentermine is well absorbed, with maximal plasma concentrations reached within 3–4 h. Less than 20% of the dose is protein-bound, and phentermine is minimally metabolized by the liver. Between 62 and 85% of the drug is excreted unchanged in the urine, with an elimination half-life of approximately 20 h.[12,13]

Treatment Advantages and Disadvantages

Clinical use of phentermine should be limited to short-term weight management in appropriate patients.[9,12,13] Phentermine is an effective adjunct to diet, exercise, and behavioral modification for producing weight loss compared to placebo. A clinical downside of phentermine use is that it should only be used for short-term management (<12 weeks), and typically patients will experience some weight regain after discontinuation, which can be discouraging.[12,13]

Therapeutic Considerations

Warnings and Precautions

Phentermine use is contraindicated in patients with a history of CVD, within 14 days of MAOI use, and in those with hyperthyroidism. Phentermine can also cause CNS depression, and use is associated with primary pulmonary hypertension (PPH), for which patients usually present initially with dyspnea. Treatment should be discontinued in patients who develop new and unexplained symptoms of dyspnea. Phentermine has also been associated with direct cardio-toxic effects, including HF and valvular heart disease; its use should be cautioned in patients with a history of these diseases. Patients with a history of substance abuse, agitation, hyperthyroidism, glaucoma, or recent (within 14 days) use of MAOI therapy should also avoid the use of phentermine.[12,13]

Special Populations

Phentermine is an FDA pregnancy category X medication. The use of phentermine is contraindicated during pregnancy due to lack of potential benefit and possible fetal harm. It is unknown whether phentermine is excreted in human milk; however, other amphetamines are present in human milk, and the risk/benefit of using phentermine should be considered prior to use. Safety and efficacy in children under the age of 18 years have not been evaluated, so use in this population should be avoided. Caution is warranted in patients with kidney disease. A dose reduction is recommended in patients with severe kidney disease (eGFR 15–29 mL/min/1.73 m^2), limiting the dose to 15 mg daily. Use in patients with an eGFR <15 mL/min/1.73 m^2, including hemodialysis, has not been studied and should be avoided.[12,13]

Adverse Effects and Monitoring

All patients using phentermine should be monitored for PPH, valvular heart disease, CNS side effects, and withdrawal effects including weight gain. Common adverse effects associated with phentermine use include dry mouth, dizziness, headache, insomnia, and restlessness.[9,12,13]

Drug Interactions

Concomitant use with MAOIs is contraindicated, and should only be initiated after a minimum of 14 days following discontinuation of MAOI use. All patients under consideration for phentermine therapy should be checked for potential drug interactions. See Table 29.1 for more drug interaction information.[12,13]

Dosage and Administration

Dosage and administration of phentermine varies depending on the product formulation. Lomaira comes as a tablet and should be dosed at 8 mg by mouth three times daily approximately 30 min prior to a meal. Adipex-P comes as a tablet or capsule and should be dosed at 15–37.5 mg/day in one dose or two divided doses. It should be dosed before a meal or 1–2 h after a meal. Dosing for both formulations should be maintained at the lowest effective doses. Administration of either formulation should be avoided in the late evening to prevent insomnia, due to its amphetamine-like characteristics. See Table 29.2 or refer to the full prescribing information for more dosing guidance.[12,13]

ORLISTAT

Orlistat is the only noncentrally acting medication with FDA approval for obesity management. Orlistat should be used in conjunction with a reduced-calorie diet in adults with either an initial BMI of ≥30 kg/m^2 or an initial BMI of ≥27 kg/m^2 and at least one weight-related comorbid condition.[14] Orlistat is a gastric and pancreatic lipase inhibitor, available as both a prescription (Xenical) and

Table 29.1 — Drug Interactions for Weight Loss–Management Agents

Substance	Interaction
Phentermine (Lomaira; Adipex-P)	
Acebrophylline	May enhance stimulatory effect of CNS stimulants; Risk X: Avoid combination
Alcohol (Ethyl)	May enhance the adverse/toxic effect of phentermine; Risk C: Monitor
Alkalinizing Agents	May decrease the excretion of amphetamines; Risk D: Consider modification
Ammonium Chloride	May decrease the serum concentration of amphetamines, likely due to enhanced excretion of amphetamines in urine; Risk C: Monitor
Antacids	May decrease the excretion of amphetamines; Risk C: Monitor
Antihistamines	May diminish the sedative effect of antihistamines; Risk C: Monitor
Antihypertensive Agents	May diminish the antihypertensive effects; Risk C: Monitor
Antipsychotic Agents	May diminish stimulatory effect of amphetamines; Risk C: Monitor
Ascorbic Acid	May decrease serum concentration of amphetamines; Risk C: Monitor
Atomoxetine	May enhance hypertensive and tachycardic effect of sympathomimetic; Risk C: Monitor
Bupropion	May enhance neuroexcitatory and/or seizure potentiating effects; Risk C: Monitor
Cannabinoid-Containing Products	May enhance tachycardic effect of sympathomimetic; Risk C: Monitor
Carbonic Anhydrase Inhibitors	May decrease excretion of amphetamines; Risk C: Monitor
Cocaine (Topical)	May enhance hypertensive effects; Risk D: Consider Modification
CYP2D6 Inhibitors	May increase serum concentration of amphetamines; Risk C: Monitor
Ethosuximide	Amphetamines may diminish the therapeutic effect of ethosuximide; Risk C: Monitor
Linezolid	May enhance the hypertensive effect of sympathomimetics; Risk D: Consider Modification
Lithium	May diminish stimulatory effect of amphetamines; Risk C: Monitor
Methenamine	May decrease the serum concentration of amphetamines; Risk C: Monitor
MAOIs	May enhance hypertensive effect; at least 14 days should elapse between discontinuation of an MAOI and initiation of treatment with bupropion; Risk X: Avoid Combination
Multivitamins	May decrease the serum concentration of amphetamines; Risk C: Monitor
Opioid Analgesics	Amphetamines may enhance the analgesic effect of opioid analgesics; Risk C: Monitor
Phenobarbital	Amphetamines may decrease the serum concentration of phenobarbital; Risk C: Monitor

(continued)

Table 29.1 (continued)

Substance	Interaction
Phenytoin	Amphetamines may decrease the serum concentration of phenytoin; Risk C: Monitor
Seizure Threshold–lowering Drugs	Extreme caution with concomitant use; Risk C: Monitor
Tricyclic Antidepressants	May enhance stimulatory effect of amphetamines and may also potentiate the cardiovascular effects of amphetamines; Risk C: Monitor
Urinary Acidifying Agents	May decrease serum concentration of amphetamines; Risk C: Monitor
Orlistat (Xenical, Alli)	
Amiodarone	A reduction in serum concentration of amiodarone with coadministration; Risk C: Monitor
Anticonvulsants	Convulsions have been reported in patients taking orlistat with antiepileptic drugs; Exceptions: fosphenytoin, pentobarbital, thiopental; Risk C: Monitor
Antiretroviral Drugs	Loss of virological control has been reported in HIV-infected patients. Patients should be monitored frequently for changes in HIV RNA levels; Drugs include: atazanavir, ritonavir, tenofovir disoproxil fumarate, emtricitabine and combinations; Risk C: Monitor
Cyclosporine	Reductions in cyclosporine plasma levels were observed. Administer orlistat at least 3 h before or after cyclosporine and monitor for decreased serum concentrations even with dose separation; Risk D: Consider Modification
Fat-Soluble Multivitamins	Coadministration may decrease efficacy and absorption of vitamins; therefore, separation of orlistat by 2–4 h is advised; Risk D: Consider Modification
Levothyroxine	Concomitant use may result in decreased levothyroxine levels
Paricalcitol	Decreased serum concentration with coadministration; when combination must be used, consider administering paricalcitol at least 1 h before or 4–6 h after the administration of orlistat; Risk D: Consider Modification
Propafenone	Coadministration may decrease serum concentrations; Risk C: Monitor
Vitamin D Analogs	Coadministration may decrease serum concentration of vitamin D analogs by inhibiting absorption; Risk D: Consider Modification
Warfarin	Concomitant use may result in an enhanced anticoagulant effect; Risk C: Monitor
Liraglutide (Saxenda)	
α-Lipoic Acid	May enhance hypoglycemic effect of antidiabetic agents; Risk C: Monitor
Androgens	May enhance the hypoglycemic effect of blood glucose–lowering agents; Risk C: Monitor
Guanethidine	May enhance the hypoglycemic effects of antidiabetic agents; Risk C: Monitor
Hypoglycemia-Associated Agents	Antidiabetic agents used in combination (oral and noninsulin injectables) may enhance the hypoglycemic effect; Risk C: Monitor
Insulins	May enhance hypoglycemic effects of insulins; Risk D: Consider Modification

(continued)

Table 29.1 (continued)

Substance	Interaction
MAOIs	May enhance the hypoglycemic effects; Risk C: Monitor
Pegvisomant	May enhance the hypoglycemic effects of blood glucose–lowering agents; Risk C: Monitor
Prothionamide	May enhance the hypoglycemic effects of blood glucose–lowering agents; Risk C: Monitor
Quinolones	Quinolones may diminish the therapeutic effect of blood glucose–lowering agents; Risk C: Monitor
Salicylates	May enhance the hypoglycemic effect of blood glucose–lowering agents; Risk C: Monitor
Selective Serotonin Reuptake Inhibitors	May enhance the hypoglycemic effect of blood glucose–lowering agents; Risk C: Monitor
Sulfonylureas	May enhance the hypoglycemic effects of sulfonylureas; Risk D: Consider Modification
Thiazide and Thiazide-like Diuretics	May diminish the therapeutic effect of antidiabetic agents; Risk C: Monitor
Semaglutide	
Alpha-lipoic acid	May enhance hypoglycemic effect of antidiabetic agents; Risk C: Monitor
Androgens	May enhance hypoglycemic effect of blood glucose lowering agents; Risk C: Monitor
Direct Acting Antivirals	May enhance hypoglycemic effect of antidiabetic agents; Risk C: Monitor
Furosemide	May diminish therapeutic effect of semaglutide, while semaglutide may increase concentration of furosemide; Risk C: Monitor
GLP-1 Agonists	May enhance adverse/toxic effects of GLP-1 agonists; Risk X: Avoid
Hypoglycemic Associated Agents	May dimmish or enhance the therapeutic effect; Risk C: Monitor
Insulins	May enhance hypoglycemic effect of insulins; Risk D: consider modification
MAOIs	May enhance hypoglycemic effects; Risk C: Monitor
Pegvisomant	May enhance the hypoglycemic effect of Agents with Blood Glucose Lowering Effects; Risk C: Monitor
Prothionamide	May enhance the hypoglycemic effect of Agents with Blood Glucose Lowering Effects; Risk C: Monitor
Quinolones	Quinolones may diminish the therapeutic effect of blood glucose-lowering agents; Risk C: Monitor
Salicylates	May enhance the hypoglycemic effect of Agents with Blood Glucose Lowering Effects; Risk C: Monitor
SSRIs	May enhance the hypoglycemic effect of Agents with Blood Glucose Lowering Effects; Risk C: Monitor
Sulfonylureas	GLP-1 agonists may enhance the hypoglycemic effect of sulfonylureas; Risk D: consider modification
Thiazide and Thiazide-like Diuretics	May diminish the therapeutic effect of antidiabetic agents; Risk C: Monitor

(continued)

Table 29.1 (continued)

Substance	Interaction
Tirzepatide	
Alpha-lipoic acid	May enhance hypoglycemic effect of antidiabetic agents; Risk C: Monitor
Androgens	May enhance hypoglycemic effect of blood glucose lowering agents; Risk C: Monitor
Beta-Blockers	May enhance or diminish the hypoglycemic effect of antidiabetic agents: Rick C: Monitor
Bortezomib	May enhance or diminish therapeutic effect of antidiabetic agents: Risk C: Monitor
Direct Acting Antivirals	May enhance hypoglycemic effect of antidiabetic agents; Risk C: Monitor
Etilefrine	May dimmish the therapeutic effect of antidiabetic agents. Risk C: Monitor
Hormonal Contraceptives	May decrease blood concentrations of hormonal contraceptives; patients should switch to a non-oral hormonal contraceptive method, or add a barrier method to contraception, for 4 weeks after initiation and each dose escalation. Risk D: Consider therapy modification
Hypoglycemic Associated Agents	May dimmish or enhance the therapeutic effect; Risk C: Monitor
Insulins	May enhance hypoglycemic effect of insulins; consider insulin dose reduction when used in combination. Risk D: Consider therapy modification
Liraglutide	May enhance adverse/toxic effect of GLP-1 agonists. Risk X: Avoid combination
Quinolones	May enhance hypoglycemic effect or diminish therapeutic effect of blood glucose lowering agents, Risk C: Monitor
Semaglutide	May enhance adverse/toxic effect of GLP-1 agonists. Risk X: Avoid combination
Sincalide	Drugs that affect gallbladder function may dimmish therapeutic effect of sincalide; patients should consider discontinuing drugs that may affect gallbladder motility prior to using sincalide to stimulate gallbladder contraction. Risk D: Consider therapy modification
Sulfonylureas	GLP-1 agonists may enhance the hypoglycemic effect of sulfonylureas; Risk D: consider modification
Thiazide and Thiazide-like Diu-retics	May diminish the therapeutic effect of antidiabetic agents; Risk C: Monitor
Phentermine/Topiramate (Qsymia)	
Please see Phentermine section for specific interactions related to that component	
Antiepileptic Medications	Concomitant administration of phenytoin or carbamazepine with topiramate in patients with epilepsy decreased plasma concentrations of topiramate by 48% and 40%, respectively

Concomitant administration of valproic acid and topiramate has been associated with hyperammonemia with and without encephalopathy. The combination has also been associated with hypothermia |
| Carbonic Anhydrase Inhibitors | Concomitant use may increase the severity of metabolic acidosis and may also increase the risk of kidney stone formation |

(continued)

Table 29.1 (continued)

Substance	Interaction
CNS Depressants including Alcohol	Concomitant use with alcohol or CNS depressants may potentiate CNS depression such as dizziness or cognitive adverse reactions or other centrally mediated effects of these agents
MAOIs	Phentermine use within 14 days of MAOIs is contraindicated due to risk of hypertensive crisis
Non-Potassium Sparing Diuretics	Concomitant use may potentiate potassium-wasting action of the diuretics, monitor for hypokalemia
Oral Contraceptives	Qsymia decreased the exposure of ethinyl estradiol by 16% and increased exposure to norethindrone by 22%. Increased risk of pregnancy is not anticipated; however, irregular bleeding (spotting) may occur more frequently due to both the increased exposure to progestin and lower exposure to estrogen
Naltrexone/Bupropion Extended Release (Contrave)	
CYP2B6 Inducers	May reduce the efficacy by reducing bupropion exposure
CYP2B6 Inhibitors	Drugs such as ticlopidine or clopidogrel can increase concentrations of bupropion exposure, leading to increased adverse reactions
CYP2D6 Substrates	Bupropion inhibits CYP2D6 and can increase concentrations of drugs metabolized by CYP2D6, leading to increased adverse reactions
Dopaminergic Drugs	CNS toxicity can occur when used concomitantly with Contrave
Drug-Laboratory Test Interactions	Contrave can cause false-positive urine test results for amphetamines
MAOI	Increased risk of hypertensive reactions can occur when used concomitantly
Seizure Threshold–lowering Drugs	Extreme caution with concomitant use
Cellulose and Citric Acid Hydrogel (Plenity)	
Metformin	Cellulose and citric acid hydrogel mimics the effects of food on metformin pharmacokinetics

NMS, Neuroleptic Malignant Syndrome.

Table 29.2—Prescribing Information for Weight Loss–Management Agents

Generic (brand)	Ingredient/strength	Dosage*
Phentermine (Lomaira)	Tablet, 8 mg	Adults ■ 8 mg by mouth three times daily. Individualize to achieve adequate response with lowest effective dose.
Phentermine (Adipex-P)	Tablet, 37.5 mg Capsule: ■ 15 mg ■ 30 mg ■ 37.5 mg	Adults ■ 15–37.5 mg/day in one dose or two divided doses. Individualize to achieve adequate response with lowest effective dose
Orlistat (Xenical) Orlistat (Alli)	Capsule, 120 mg Capsule, 60 mg	Adults ■ Rx: Recommended dosing is 120 mg by mouth three times per day with each meal containing fat ■ OTC: 60 mg by mouth three times daily with each main meal containing fat (maximum: 180 mg/day)
Liraglutide (Saxenda)	Subcutaneous Pen, 6 mg/mL, 3 mL	Adults and children >12 years: Daily Dose ■ Week 1: 0.6 mg ■ Week 2: 1.2 mg ■ Week 3: 1.8 mg ■ Week 4: 2.4 mg ■ Week 5: 3 mg (target dose)
Semaglutide (Wegovy)	Subcutaneous Pen: ■ 0.25 mg/0.5 mL ■ 0.5 mg/0.5 mL ■ 1 mg/0.5 mL ■ 1.7 mg/0.75 mL ■ 2.4 mg/0.75 mL	Adults and children >12 years ■ Week 1–4: 0.25 mg weekly ■ Week 5–8: 0.5 mg weekly ■ Week 9–12: 1 mg weekly ■ Week 13–16: 1.7 mg weekly ■ Week 17 onward: 2.4 mg weekly
Tirzepatide	Subcutaneous Pen: ■ 2.5 mg/0.5 mL ■ 5 mg/0.5 mL ■ 7.5 mg/0.5 mL ■ 10 mg/0.5 mL ■ 12.5 mg/0.5 mL ■ 15 mg/0.5 mL	Adults ■ Week 1-4: 2.5 mg weekly ■ Week 5-8: 5 mg weekly ■ Week 9-12: 7.5 mg weekly ■ Week 13-16: 10 mg weekly ■ Week 17-20: 12.5 mg weekly ■ Week 21-24: 15 mg weekly
Phentermine/Topiramate (Qsymia)	Extended-release Capsules: ■ 3.75/23 mg ■ 7.5/46 mg ■ 11.25/69 mg ■ 15/92 mg	Adults: ■ Take once daily in morning to prevent insomnia ■ Recommended: 3.75/23 mg daily for 14 days; increase to 7.5/46 mg daily ■ Discontinue or dose escalation if 3% weight loss not achieved after 12 weeks ■ Discontinue is 5% weight loss not achieved on maximum dose of 15/92 mg/day

(continued)

Table 29.2 (continued)

Generic (brand)	Ingredient/strength	Dosage*
Naltrexone/Bupropion Extended Release (Contrave)	Tablet, 8/90 mg	Adults: Morning/Evening Dose ■ Week 1: 1 tablet (8/90 mg)/None ■ Week 2: 1 tablet (8/90 mg)/1 tablet (8/90 mg) ■ Week 3: 2 tablets (16/180 mg)/1 tablet (8/90 mg) ■ Week 4: 2 tablets (16/180 mg)/2 tablets (16/180 mg) Moderate to Severe Renal Impairment ■ 1 tablet twice daily Hepatic Impairment ■ Maximum dose of 1 tablet daily
Cellulose and Citric Acid Hydrogel (Plenity)	Capsule, 0.75-g/capsule	Adults: 1. Swallow 3 capsules (2.25 g) with water 2. After taking capsules, drink 2 additional glasses of water (8 fl oz/250 mL each) 3. Wait 20–30 minutes to begin meal

*All therapies are adjunct to a reduced-calorie diet and increased physical activity.

over the counter (Alli) at half the strength.[14] The Xenical in the Prevention of Diabetes in Obese Subjects (XENDOS) trial was conducted to assess the efficacy of orlistat in preventing T2D in obese patients.[15] The study demonstrated that orlistat plus behavioral counseling led to meaningful weight loss through 4 years of therapy, with twice as much weight loss compared to the placebo.[15] Those in the orlistat group lost 10.6 kg at 1 year and maintained a loss of 5.8 kg at 4 years, compared to 6.2 kg and 3.0 kg, respectively, in the placebo group.[15] In patients with T2D, those treated with orlistat experienced a reduction in body weight more than the placebo.[16]

Pharmacology

Mechanism of Action

Orlistat is a reversible inhibitor of gastrointestinal and pancreatic lipases. It works by exerting its therapeutic activity in the lumen of the stomach and small intestine by forming a covalent bond with the active serine residue site of gastric and pancreatic lipase. The inactivated enzymes are thus unavailable to hydrolyze dietary fat, in the form of triglycerides, into absorbable free fatty acids and monoglycerides. The undigested triglycerides are not absorbed, and the resulting caloric deficit leads to weight loss.[14]

Pharmacokinetics

Systemic exposure to orlistat is minimal and >99% bound to lipoproteins and albumin. The onset of action is between 24 and 48 h, with a duration of action between 48 and 72 h. Orlistat has an elimination half-life of 1–2 h. Approximately 97% of the drug is excreted in the feces, 83% unchanged.[14]

Therapeutic Considerations

Warnings and Precautions

Orlistat is contraindicated in pregnancy, chronic malabsorption syndrome, cholestasis, and known hypersensitivity. There have been postmarketing reports indicating severe liver injury, so patients should be closely monitored. There have also been reports of increased urinary oxalate, resulting in acute renal disease. As such, renal function should be monitored. Substantial weight loss has been associated with an increase in the risk of cholelithiasis.[14]

Special Populations

Orlistat is contraindicated in pregnancy and is listed as an FDA pregnancy category X medication. Caution should be exercised in nursing mothers since secretion in human milk is unknown. Safety for use in patients below the age of 12 years and patients over the age of 65 years has not been established.[14]

Adverse Effects and Monitoring

Orlistat is associated with a variety of side effects mainly resulting from its mechanism of action in the gastrointestinal tract. Common adverse effects (≥5% incidence and at least twice that of placebo) associated with the use of orlistat include oily spotting, flatus with discharge, fecal urgency, fatty/oily stool, oily evacuation, increased defecation, and fecal incontinence. Patients should have their BMI, diet (calorie and fat intake), thyroid function, liver function, and renal function monitored throughout their duration of medication therapy.[14]

Drug Interactions

The use of orlistat is associated with interactions with cyclosporine, fat-soluble vitamin supplements, levothyroxine, anticoagulants, amiodarone, antiepileptic, and antiretroviral therapy. Orlistat can decrease the absorption of these medications, altering their efficacy.[14] See Table 29.1 for more drug interaction information.

Dosage and Administration

The recommended dosage depends on the formulation. Dosing for prescription orlistat (Xenical) is 120 mg by mouth three times daily with each main meal containing fat. The dose may be given during or up to 1 h after the meal and may be omitted if the meal is occasionally missed or contains no fat. Dosing for the OTC formulation of orlistat (Alli) is 60 mg by mouth three times daily with each main meal containing fat, up to a maximum of 180 mg per day. Patients on orlistat should be maintained on a nutritionally balanced, reduced-calorie diet that contains approximately 30% of calories from fat. The manufacturer does not have any dosing recommendations for hepatic or renal impairment.[14] See Table 29.2 or refer to the full prescribing information for further guidelines.

LIRAGLUTIDE

Liraglutide (Saxenda), a GLP-1 RA, was approved by the FDA in 2016 for chronic weight management. Liraglutide is also marketed under the brand name Victoza, which is FDA approved for the management of T2D, but at a lower dosage (max of 1.8 mg/day). Liraglutide (Saxenda) is also approved for chronic weight management among pediatric patients ages 12 and older. As part of the Satiety and Clinical Adiposity—Liraglutide Evidence in Nondiabetic and Diabetic Individuals (SCALE) program, there were three trials with a primary outcome of weight loss.[17,18] The SCALE Maintenance trial treated nondiabetic patients with liraglutide or placebo following a 12-week, low-calorie-diet run-in period in which they achieved ≥5% weight loss. After 1 year, liraglutide-treated patients achieved significantly greater weight loss than those treated with the placebo (6.2% vs. 0.2%, $P < 0.0001$). Significantly more patients in the SCALE Maintenance trial lost ≥5% of body weight in the treatment group after randomization than in the placebo group.[18]

The SCALE Obesity and Prediabetes trial was a 2-year extension of the SCALE Maintenance trial. The goal of the 2-year extension was to evaluate the proportion of overweight and obese individuals with prediabetes who progressed to a diagnosis of T2D. At 160 weeks, 26 (2%) participants treated with liraglutide versus 46 (6%) participants in the placebo group were diagnosed with T2D. These results indicate that liraglutide may reduce the risk of developing diabetes in obese patients with prediabetes.[19]

The SCALE Diabetes trial was designed to investigate efficacy and safety of liraglutide (3.0 mg and 1.8 mg) versus placebo for weight management in overweight or obese adults with T2D.[20] A ≥5% weight loss occurred in 54.3% and 40.4% of patients treated with liraglutide 3.0 mg and 1.8 mg, respectively, compared with 21.4% of patients treated with placebo. A ≥10% weight loss occurred in 25.2% and 15.9% of patients treated with liraglutide 3.0 mg and 1.8 mg, respectively, compared with 6.7% of patients treated with placebo. These results indicate that liraglutide, in conjunction with lifestyle changes, is more effective than placebo at reducing weight.[20] In December 2020, the FDA approved liraglutide (Saxenda) for chronic weight management in patients 12 years and older who are obese, defined by cut-offs that correspond to a BMI of 30 kg/m² for adults, and who weigh more than 60 kg (132 lbs).[21] A 56-week, double-blind, placebo-controlled study among 251 patients aged 12 to 17 years was complete.[22] The primary end point of the trial was change in BMI at week 56. The study split the participants into liraglutide (n=125) and placebo (n=126), with liraglutide showing superior to the placebo with regard to the change from baseline in BMI standard deviation at week 56 (-0.22 [95% CI -0.37 to -0.08] $P = 0.02$). The study also demonstrated greater percentages of patients achieving both a 5% and 10% weight loss in the liraglutide group compared with the placebo. Adverse effects were similar to those in the adult trials.[22]

Pharmacology

Mechanism of Action

Liraglutide is a long-acting analog of human GLP-1, an incretin hormone. Like other GLP-1 RAs, liraglutide has multiple mechanisms of action, including increasing glucose-dependent insulin secretion, decreasing inappropriate glucagon secretion, increasing β-cell growth and replication, and slowing gastric emptying. GLP-1 RAs also act centrally on neurons in the hypothalamus, leading to a satiety-inducing effect that is believed to be the most relevant to its role in weight loss.[21]

Pharmacokinetics

Following the subcutaneous administration of liraglutide, maximum concentrations are achieved between 8 and 12 h after dosing. Exposure to the drug increased proportionally in the dose range of 0.6–3 mg. Liraglutide is extensively bound to plasma proteins (>98%). The elimination half-life of liraglutide is approximately 13 h, making it suitable for once-daily administration.[23]

Therapeutic Considerations

Warnings and Precautions

Liraglutide is contraindicated in patients who are pregnant and those with a personal or family history of medullary thyroid carcinoma or multiple endocrine neoplasia type 2. Use of liraglutide has also been associated with thyroid C-cell tumors, acute pancreatitis, gallbladder disease, serious hypoglycemia with the use of additional secretagogue agents, heart rate increase, and renal impairment. Caution should be used in patients with a history of any of these conditions.[23]

Special Populations

Liraglutide (Saxenda) is contraindicated in pregnancy. There is no available data on the presence of liraglutide in human milk, the effects on a breast-fed infant, or on milk production. There is limited experience with liraglutide in patients with renal impairment; however, there have been postmarketing reports of acute renal failure and worsening of chronic renal failure with liraglutide use. Caution should be used in those with hepatic impairment, although data are limited. Liraglutide slows gastric emptying, so use should be cautioned in patients with a history of gastroparesis.[23]

Adverse Effects and Monitoring

Common adverse effects associated with the use of liraglutide include nausea (39%), hypoglycemia (monotherapy 16%), diarrhea (21%), constipation (19%), vomiting (16%), headache (14%), decreased appetite (10%), dyspepsia (10%), fatigue (8%), dizziness (7%), abdominal pain (5%), and increased lipases (5%). Monitoring while using liraglutide includes blood glucose, renal function, signs or symptoms of pancreatitis and gallbladder disease, triglycerides, and body weight at 16 weeks.[23]

Drug Interactions

As stated previously, liraglutide causes delays in gastric emptying; thus, use may impact the absorption of all concomitantly administered oral medications. In clinical trials, liraglutide did not affect the absorption of orally administered medications to a clinically relevant degree. Due to the effect liraglutide has on lowering blood glucose levels, the administration with additional diabetes medications dramatically increases the risk of hypoglycemia compared with monotherapy (in T2D, combination therapy with sulfonylurea: 44%; monotherapy: 16%; nondiabetic: 2–3%).[23] See Table 29.1 for more drug interaction information.

Dosage and Administration

Liraglutide (Saxenda) is a subcutaneously administered medication. The recommended target dose for chronic weight management is 3 mg daily. This recommended target dose should be attained by a titration schedule. Patients should start with 0.6 mg/day at baseline and increase daily dose by 0.6 mg every week as tolerated. Patients should adhere to the dosing escalation recommendations until achieving the 3-mg dosage. If patients do not tolerate an increased dose during dose escalation, consider delaying the escalation by an additional week and rechallenge. The slow titration helps to minimize side effects, especially those related to the gastrointestinal tract. Clinical judgment should be used when determining whether to continue the medication in patients unable to tolerate the 3-mg per day dose. If patients are experiencing a benefit from a lower dose, it may be reasonable to maintain the maximum tolerated dose; however, liraglutide doses of <3 mg have not been FDA approved for weight management. The FDA recommends evaluation of weight loss after 16 weeks of therapy. Clinical trials assessing weight loss have shown that patients who lose ≥4% of baseline weight during this 16-week time frame will likely continue to lose weight, while those who lose <4% of baseline weight are unlikely to lose significantly more weight with therapy continued beyond 16 weeks. There are no dosing adjustments necessary in patients with renal or hepatic impairment, although caution is advised.[23] See Table 29.2 or refer to the full prescribing information for further guidelines.

SEMAGLUTIDE

On June 4, 2021, the FDA approved Wegovy (semaglutide) injection (2.4 mg once weekly) for chronic weight management in adults with obesity or overweight with at least one weight-related condition (such as high blood pressure, T2D, or high cholesterol), for use in addition to a reduced-calorie diet and physical activity.[24] The safety and efficacy of semaglutide for weight management were studied in four 68-week trials, referred to as the STEP (Semaglutide Treatment Effect in People with obesity) program. On January 3, 2023, the FDA approved Wegovy (semaglutide) for treating obesity in pediatric patients aged 12 years and older.

The STEP 1 trial is a double-blind trial that enrolled 1,961 adults with obesity or overweight with coexisting conditions who did not have diabetes, and randomly assigned them in a 2:1 ratio to receive treatment with once-weekly subcutaneous semaglutide (2.4 mg dose) or placebo, plus lifestyle interventions for 68 weeks.[25] The primary end points were percentage change in body weight and weight reduction of at least 5%.[25] The results showed that from baseline to week 68, the mean change in body weight was –14.9% (–15.3 kg) in the treatment group compared with –2.4% (–2.6 kg) in the placebo group ($P < 0.001$).[25] There were more participants in the semaglutide group than in the placebo group who achieved weight reductions of 5% or more (1,047 [86.4%] vs. 182 [31.5%]), 10% or more (838 [69.1%] vs. 69 [12%]), and 15% or more (612 [50.5%] vs. 28 [4.9%]) at 68 weeks ($P < 0.001$ for all three).[25] Nausea and diarrhea were the most common adverse events with semaglutide. This STEP 1 trial demonstrated 2.4 mg of semaglutide once weekly plus lifestyle intervention was associated with sustained, clinically significant reductions in body weight.[25]

The STEP 2 trial is a randomized, double-blind, double-dummy, placebo-controlled, multicenter superiority study that enrolled adults with a BMI of at least 27 kg/m² and glycated hemoglobin 7–10% who had been diagnosed with diabetes at least 180 days prior to screening.[26] Patients were randomly assigned (1:1:1) to subcutaneous semaglutide 2.4 mg, semaglutide 1 mg, or visually matching placebo once a week for 68 weeks, plus lifestyle interventions.[26] The primary endpoints were similar to the STEP 1 trial, assessed by intention to treat for 2.4 mg semaglutide vs. placebo. The mean change in body weight from baseline to week 68 was –9.6% (2.4 mg semaglutide) vs. -3.4% (placebo) ($P < 0.001$),[26] and more patients on semaglutide 2.4 mg achieved weight reductions of at least 5%

(267 [68.8%] vs. 107 [28.5%]) (*P* < 0.001).[26] There were more frequent adverse events associated with semaglutide 2.4 mg (87.6%) and 1 mg (81.8%) than the placebo (76.9%).[26] The study results demonstrated in patients with overweight or obesity, with T2D, semaglutide 2.4 mg once weekly achieved superior weight loss compared with placebo.[26]

The STEP 3 trial is a randomized, double-blind, parallel-group, 68-week study that looked to compare the effects of once-weekly semaglutide 2.4 mg vs. placebo for weight management as an adjunct to intensive behavioral therapy in overweight and obese adults without diabetes.[27] There were 611 patients randomized (2:1) to semaglutide 2.4 mg or placebo, both combined with low-calorie diet for the first 8 weeks and intensive behavioral therapy, in the form of 30 counseling visits during 68 weeks,[27] to observe two primary end points of change in body weight and loss of 5% or more in body weight. At week 68, the estimated mean body weight change from baseline was –16% for semaglutide compared with –5.7% for placebo (*P* < 0.001),[27] with more patients treated with semaglutide losing at least 5% of baseline body weight (86.6% vs. 47.6%, *P* < 0.001).[27] Gastrointestinal side effects were more frequent with semaglutide compared with the placebo (82.8% vs. 63.2%). Similar with STEP 1 and STEP 2 trials, in overweight or obese adults, once-weekly subcutaneous semaglutide, as an adjust to intensive behavioral therapy and an initial low-calorie diet, results in significantly greater weight loss during 68 weeks than the placebo.[27]

Finally, the STEP 4 trial looked at comparing the effect of continuing or withdrawing treatment with semaglutide on weight loss maintenance in overweight or obese adults in a randomized, double-blind withdrawal study. The primary end point was percent change in body weight from week 20 to week 68.[28] There were 902 participants at baseline that received once-weekly subcutaneous semaglutide during the run-in phase, and after 20 weeks (16 weeks dose escalation; 4 weeks maintenance dose), patients who reached 2.4 mg/week semaglutide dose were randomized (2:1) to 48 weeks of continued semaglutide maintenance or switched to placebo, plus lifestyle interventions in both groups.[28] In the group that continued semaglutide, mean body weight change from week 20 to 68 was –7.9% compared with +6.9% with the switch to placebo (–14.8 percentage point difference; *P* < 0.001).[28] Like previous trials, gastrointestinal events were reported in 49.1% of participants who continued semaglutide vs. 26.1% with placebo. This study demonstrates that continued use of semaglutide results in further weight loss, while discontinuation of treatment may result in weight gain.[28]

Pharmacology

Mechanism of Action

Semaglutide acts as a GLP-1 receptor agonist that selectively binds to and activates the GLP-1 receptor, the target for native GLP-1, which is a physiologic regulator of appetite and caloric intake. Semaglutide increases glucose-dependent insulin secretion, decreases inappropriate glucagon secretion, slows gastric emptying, and also acts in the areas of the brain involved in appetite regulation and caloric intake.[29]

Pharmacokinetics

Following subcutaneous administration of semaglutide, maximum concentrations are achieved in 1–3 days after dosing. The steady-state exposure increased proportionally with doses to 2.4 mg once-weekly. Semaglutide is extensively bound to plasma albumin (>99%), which results in decreased renal clearance. The elimination half-life of semaglutide injection is approximately 1 week, meaning that it will be present for 5–7 weeks in circulation after the last dose of 2.4 mg.[29]

Therapeutic Considerations

Warnings and Precautions

Semaglutide is contraindicated in patients with a personal or family history of medullary thyroid carcinoma or multiple endocrine neoplasia syndrome type 2. Use of semaglutide has been associated acute pancreatitis, gallbladder disease, increased heart rate, psychiatric effects, and renal impairment. Caution should be used in patients with a history of any of these conditions.[29]

Special Populations

Based on animal reproduction studies, there may be potential risks to the fetus from exposure to semaglutide during pregnancy, and weight loss offers no benefit to the pregnant patient and may cause fetal harm. There are no data on the presence of semaglutide or its metabolites in human milk, the infant, or on milk production. Safety and efficacy of semaglutide for weight loss have not been established in pediatric patients. No dose adjustment is recommended for renal or hepatic impairment but caution is advised.[29]

Adverse Effects and Monitoring

Common adverse effects associated with the use of semaglutide include nausea (44%), diarrhea (30%), vomiting (24%), constipation (24%), abdominal pain (20%), headache (14%), fatigue (11%), dyspepsia (9%), dizziness (8%), abdominal distension (7%), eructation (7%), hypoglycemia (6%), flatulence (6%), and gastroenteritis (6%).[29]

Monitoring while using semaglutide includes blood glucose, heart rate, body weight, renal function, signs/symptoms of pancreatitis, triglycerides, signs/symptoms of gallbladder disease and behavioral changes.[29]

Drug Interactions

Semaglutide subcutaneous injection delays gastric emptying; thus, use may impact the absorption of all concomitantly administered oral medications. In clinical trials, semaglutide did not affect the absorption of orally administered medications, but monitoring is suggested. See Table 29.1 for more drug interaction information.[29]

Dosage and Administration

Semaglutide (Wegovy) is a subcutaneously administered medication. The recommended target dose for chronic weight management is 2.4 mg once weekly for both pediatrics and adults. This recommended target dose should be attained by the recommended dose titration schedule. Patients should begin with 0.25 mg once weekly injection on weeks 1–4, doubling the dose to 0.5 mg once weekly weeks 5–8, and again to 1 mg weekly in weeks 9–12. For weeks 13–16 patients should inject a 1.7 mg dose weekly and at week 17 that dose is increased to the target 2.4 mg once weekly injection. If patients do not tolerate a dose escalation, consider delaying the escalation for another 4 weeks at the previous tolerated dose. If patients cannot tolerate 2.4 mg dose, it is recommended to discontinue medication; however, clinical judgement should be used when determining whether to continue or discontinue a medication. If patients are experiencing benefits from a lower dose, it may be reasonable to maintain the maximum tolerated dose; however, doses of <2.4 mg once weekly have not been FDA approved for weight management.[29]

TIRZEPATIDE

Tirzepatide (Mounjaro), a novel glucose-dependent insulinotropic polypeptide (GIP)/GLP-1 RA, was approved by the FDA in May 2022 for the treatment of T2D. Although not currently approved for weight loss, clinical trials for the treatment of T2D showed promising weight loss, and you may start seeing off-label use in practice. Due to these finding, the FDA granted Fast Track designation for the investigation of tirzepatide for the treatment of adults with obesity, or overweight with weight-related comorbidities.[30] The SURMOUNT clinical trial program is currently in process, and we have results from the SURMOUNT-1 clinical trial and are awaiting the final results of SURMOUNT-2/3 trials in 2023.

The SURMOUNT-1 evaluated the efficacy and safety of tirzepatide in adults with obesity or overweight who did not have diabetes.[31] Adults 18 years of age and older, with a BMI of 30 or more or a BMI of 27 or more and at least one weight-related complication, with the exception of diabetes, were enrolled in this trial.[31] Participants were randomly assigned in a 1:1:1:1 ratio to receive tirzepatide at a dose of 5 mg, 10 mg, 15 mg, or a placebo, administered subcutaneously once weekly for 72 weeks as an adjunct to lifestyle intervention.[31] The mean change in weight at week 72 was –15% (95% CI –15.9 to –14.9) with a 5 mg weekly dose of tirzepatide, –19.5% (95% CI –20.4 to –18.5) with the 10 mg dose, and –20.9% (95% CI –21.8 to –19.9) with a 15 mg dose.[31] The change in weight at week 72 for the placebo was –3.1% (95% CI –4.3 to –1.9).[31] All three tirzepatide doses were superior to placebo.[31] At week 72, more participants had reductions in body weight of 10% or more, 15% or more, and 20% or more from baseline than participants in the placebo ($P < 0.001$).[31] Between 78.9% and 81.9% of participants in the tirzepatide groups reported at least one adverse event as compared with 72% of those in the placebo group, with the most frequent reported events being gastrointestinal.[31]

Pharmacology

Mechanism of Action
Tirzepatide is a GIP/GLP-1 RA that increases glucose-dependent insulin secretion, decreases inappropriate glucagon secretion, and slows gastric emptying.[32] In a glucose-dependent manner, tirzepatide enhances insulin secretion in the first and second phases, and reduces glucagon levels.[32]

Pharmacokinetics
Following subcutaneous administration, maximum concentrations are achieved between 8 and 72 hours.[32] Tirzepatide has an elimination half-life of 5 days, enabling once-weekly dosing.[32] This drug is highly bound to plasma albumin (99%) and metabolites are excreted in the urine and feces.[32]

Therapeutic Considerations

Warnings and Precautions

Tirzepatide is contraindicated in patients with a personal or family history of medullary thyroid carcinoma or in patients with Multiple Endocrine Neoplasia syndrome type 2. Use of tirzepatide has also been associated with thyroid C-cell tumors, acute pancreatitis, acute gallbladder disease, serious hypoglycemia with the use of additional secretagogue agents, and renal impairment. Caution should be used in patients with a history of any of these conditions.[32]

Special Populations

Tirzepatide has insufficient data for its use in pregnant women. Animal studies have shown there may be risks to the fetus, so use is not recommended. There is no data on the presence of tirzepatide in animal or human milk, the effects on the breastfed infant, or the effects on milk production. No dose adjustments with tirzepatide are recommended in patients with renal impairment or hepatic impairment as no change in pharmacokinetics was observed.

Adverse Effects and Monitoring

Common adverse effects associated with the use of tirzepatide include diarrhea (11%), increased serum amylase (33%), increased serum lipase (31%), and nausea (12%). Other considerations include sinus tachycardia (5%), abdominal pain (5%), dyspepsia (5%), constipation (6%), and vomiting (5%).[32] Monitoring while using tirzepatide includes blood glucose, GI adverse reactions, kidney function, signs and symptoms of pancreatitis and gallbladder disease, and worsening diabetic retinopathy.[32]

Drug Interactions

Tirzepatide delays gastric emptying, and therefore has the potential to alter absorption of orally administered medications. Patients using oral hormonal contraceptives should be advised to switch to a non-oral contraceptive method or add a barrier method of contraception for 4 weeks after initiation and for 4 weeks after each dose escalation.[32] Due to tirzepatide's effect on lowering blood glucose levels, co-administration with additional diabetes medications can increase the risk of hypoglycemia, specifically with insulin secretagogues or insulin.[32] See Table 29.1 for more drug interaction information.

Dosage and Administration

Tirzepatide is a subcutaneous injection that is not currently approved for weight loss, although it is being studied at 5 mg, 10 mg, and 15 mg dosages. Once clinical trials are complete and finalized data is submitted and approved by the FDA, comments will be provided on specific weight loss dosing.

COMBINATION PRODUCTS

PHENTERMINE-TOPIRAMATE EXTENDED RELEASE (ER)

Phentermine/topiramate ER is a combination product that was approved by the FDA in 2012 for weight management under the brand name Qsymia.[33] This medication is classified as a schedule IV controlled substance.[30] The EQUIP trial provided an evaluation of the safety and efficacy of phentermine-topiramate ER (3.75/23 mg and 15/92 mg) versus placebo on weight loss and metabolic improvements when added to a reduced-calorie diet.[34] Patients lost an average 5.1% (3.75/23 mg dose), 10.9% (15/92 mg dose), and 1.6% (placebo) of their baseline body weight. The percentage of patients achieving weight loss of ≥5% was significantly more in the treatment groups versus the placebo.[34]

The CONQUER clinical trial was a 56-week phase 3 trial designed to assess the efficacy and safety of two doses of phentermine plus topiramate ER as an adjunct to diet and lifestyle modification for weight loss and metabolic risk reduction in individuals who were overweight and obese, with two or more risk factors. Patients were assigned to placebo, once-daily phentermine 7.5/46 mg, or once-daily phentermine 15/92 mg. At 56 weeks, weight losses of 1.4 kg, 8.1 kg, and 10.2 kg were recorded in the placebo, 7.5/46-mg, and 15/92-mg groups, respectively. Patients achieving at least 5% weight loss were 21%, 62%, and 70% in the placebo, 7.5/46-mg, and 15/92-mg groups, respectively. This study concluded that the combination of phentermine and topiramate may be a valuable treatment for obesity in comparison to the placebo.[35]

The SEQUEL randomized clinical trial was a 52-week extension study in eligible patients that completed the CONQUER study and complied with treatment. The objective of this study was to evaluate the long-term efficacy and safety of phentermine/topiramate ER combination in overweight and obese subjects. After the 52-week extension (week 108), the phentermine/topiramate ER combination was associated with significant, sustained weight loss, indicating that this is a potentially effective option for the sustained treatment of obesity.[36]

Pharmacology

Mechanism of Action

Phentermine, as discussed previously, is a sympathomimetic amine with a mechanism of reducing appetite secondary to the CNS effects, which include the stimulation of the hypothalamus to release norepinephrine leading to a reduction in hunger and signaling fat cells to break down stored fat, resulting in weight loss.[33]

The mechanism of topiramate on chronic weight management is not fully understood, although it may be due to its effects on both appetite suppression and satiety enhancement, induced by a combination of pharmacologic effects.[33]

Pharmacokinetics

High-fat meals do not affect the pharmacokinetic profiles of either medication in combination. Phentermine is approximately 17.5% bound to plasma proteins, while topiramate is 15–41% protein-bound. Phentermine is primarily metabolized by CYP3A4 with a mean terminal half-life of approximately 20 h. Topiramate does not show extensive hepatic or renal metabolism, with about 70% of the dose existing as unchanged metabolites. Minor amounts are metabolized in the liver via hydroxylation, hydrolysis, and glucuronidation. Topiramate has a mean terminal half-life of approximately 65 h.[33]

Therapeutic Considerations

Warnings and Precautions

The use of phentermine/topiramate ER is contraindicated during pregnancy due to an increased risk of oral clefts (cleft lip and/or palate). Its use is also associated with an increased heart rate, suicidal behavior and ideation, acute myopia and secondary angle closure glaucoma, mood and sleeping disorders, cognitive impairment, and elevations in creatinine and metabolic acidosis. Patients should be advised against abrupt discontinuation of phentermine/topiramate as it can precipitate seizure activity due to the topiramate component.[33]

Special Populations

Phentermine/topiramate ER is contraindicated in pregnancy and is listed as an FDA category X medication. Because topiramate is a known teratogen (cleft lip and/or palate), pregnancy should be ruled out prior to initiating phentermine/topiramate ER, and women of childbearing age should be advised to use contraception and to have monthly pregnancy testing during use. Topiramate and amphetamine derivatives such as phentermine are excreted into human milk; therefore, its use should be avoided in breast-feeding. In patients with renal impairment (CrCl <50 mL/min) and those with moderate hepatic impairment, dosing should not exceed 7.5/46 mg once daily.[33]

Adverse Effects and Monitoring

Common adverse effects (≥5% incidence and at least 1.5 times placebo) that are associated with the use of phentermine/topiramate ER include paresthesia, dizziness, dysgeusia, insomnia, constipation, and dry mouth. Patients on phentermine/topiramate ER should have their blood chemistries—including bicarbonate, creatinine, potassium, and glucose—monitored at baseline and periodically throughout treatment. Monthly pregnancy testing is recommended for female patients while using this medication. Patients should also monitor their weight. If after 12 weeks on the recommended 7.5/46-mg daily dosing a 3% weight loss has not been achieved, the medication should be discontinued or escalated to the next dose of 11.25/69 mg daily.[33]

Drug Interactions

Phentermine/topiramate ER has many potential drug interactions, including with MAOIs, oral contraceptives, CNS depressants such as alcohol, non-potassium sparing diuretics, antiepileptics, and carbonic anhydrase inhibitors.[33] See Table 29.1 for more detailed drug interaction information.

Dosage and Administration

Patients should be advised to take phentermine/topiramate ER by mouth, once daily in the morning with or without food. Treatment should be initiated with the 3.75/23-mg tablet for 14 days and then should be increased to the 7.5/46-mg tablet, the recommended target dose. If a 3% weight loss is not achieved in 12 weeks, the dose may be escalated to 11.25/69 mg daily for 14 days followed by 15/92 mg once daily. If at this time a 5% weight loss is not achieved after an additional 12 weeks on the 15/92-mg dose, the medication should be discontinued. In patients with a CrCl <50 mL/min or moderate hepatic impairment, dosing should not exceed 7.5/46-mg once daily. In patients who have been stabilized, the dose should gradually be decreased if discontinuation is desired. Patients should be advised to take the dose every other day for at least 1 week prior to discontinuation to avoid precipitating a seizure. See Table 29.2 or refer to the full prescribing information for further guidelines.[33]

NALTREXONE-BUPROPION SR

Naltrexone-bupropion SR is another combination product marketed for weight management under the brand name Contrave. This medication is an anorexiant agent approved for weight management. Naltrexone-bupropion SR is not approved for use in the treatment of major depressive disorder or other psychiatric disorders.[34] Several randomized trials have shown weight loss and improvements in obesity-related comorbid conditions, including a trial of naltrexone-bupropion SR in patients with obesity and T2D.[38] Those treated with the medication for 1 year lost 5.9% of initial body weight and had an A1C reduction of 0.6% compared to 2.2% weight loss and 0.1% A1C reduction with the placebo.[38]

Pharmacology

Mechanism of Action

Naltrexone-bupropion SR has two components: naltrexone, an opioid receptor antagonist, and bupropion, a relatively weak inhibitor of the neuronal reuptake of dopamine and norepinephrine. The exact neurochemical effects of naltrexone-bupropion leading to weight loss are not fully understood. Studies suggest that naltrexone and bupropion have effects on two separate areas of the brain involved in the regulation of food intake. Those areas are located in the hypothalamus, which is the appetite regulatory center, and the mesolimbic dopamine circuit, which is also known as the reward center. Besides decreasing appetite, the combination also decreases cravings for high-calorie, pleasurable foods.[37]

Pharmacokinetics

Following oral administration, the time to peak concentration is 2 h for naltrexone and 3 h for bupropion. When taken with a high-fat meal, the food effect increased the AUC and C_{max} for naltrexone and bupropion. Thus, naltrexone-bupropion SR should not be taken with a high-fat meal, as it may increase the systemic exposure of the active ingredients. Naltrexone is not metabolized by cytochrome P450 enzymes, while bupropion inhibits CYP2D6 and is metabolized by CYP2B6. Bupropion is metabolized into three active metabolites (erythrohydrobupropion, threohydrobupropion, and hydroxybupropion), which have longer elimination half-lives. Following oral administration of naltrexone-bupropion SR, the mean elimination half-life was approximately 5 h for naltrexone and 21 h for bupropion.[37]

Therapeutic Considerations

Warnings and Precautions

This medication contains bupropion, thus patients with major depressive disorder may experience worsening of their depression and/or suicidal ideation. However, in clinical trials with naltrexone-bupropion SR, no suicides or attempts were reported. Patients should be appropriately counseled about this risk. Bupropion may cause seizures, so use is cautioned in patients with a history of seizures. Due to the naltrexone component, patients using opioid medications are at risk for an opioid overdose and/or opioid withdrawal, and use of this medication is contraindicated. Naltrexone-bupropion SR may increase blood pressure, and therefore is contraindicated in patients with uncontrolled hypertension.[37]

Special Populations

Naltrexone-bupropion SR is contraindicated in pregnancy and carries an FDA category X label, because weight loss therapy is not recommended in pregnant women, and there have been inconsistent reports of adverse fetal events such as cardiovascular malformations following maternal use of bupropion. The constituents and metabolites of this combination are known to be secreted in human milk; therefore, use in nursing mothers is not recommended. A pooled analysis of naltrexone-bupropion SR suggests no clinically meaningful differences in patients based on sex and race. Although this medication has not been specifically studied in patients with hepatic failure, the individual components have. Patients with hepatic impairment should have the dose reduced to a maximum dose of 8/90 mg twice daily (50% reduction). Similarly, in patients with renal impairment, the dose should be reduced, and its use is not recommended in those with ESRD. Naltrexone-bupropion should be used with caution in elderly patients due to a greater risk of drug accumulation when used chronically, precipitating adverse drug reactions.[37]

Adverse Effects and Monitoring

Common adverse effects (≥10% incidence) that are associated with the use of naltrexone-bupropion include nausea, constipation, headache, vomiting, insomnia, dry mouth, and diarrhea. Patients, especially those with a psychiatric disorder, should also be monitored for changes in mood. Patients should be monitored for weight loss.[37]

Drug Interactions

The use of naltrexone-bupropion should be cautioned with medications that can lower the seizure threshold, as well as other dopaminergic drugs (e.g., levodopa and amantadine), as this can lead to CNS toxicity. Bupropion is a CYP2D6 inhibitor; therefore, this medication can increase exposure to CYP2D6 substrates. See Table 29.1 for more drug interaction information.[37]

Dosage and Administration

When initiating this medication, patients should be started on a low dose and then titrate the dose every week until a maximum dosage of two tablets in the morning and two tablets in the evening is established. This phased titration greatly improves the tolerability of this medication. Although the weekly dose escalation was forced in clinical trials regardless of tolerability, patients who continue to experience side effects may benefit from a slower dose titration over several months. If a patient has not lost at least 5% of their baseline body weight after 12 weeks at the target dose of two tablets (16/180 mg) twice daily, therapy should be discontinued. In clinical trials, naltrexone-bupropion SR was administered with meals, but high-fat meals should be avoided.[37] Similar to liraglutide, early weight loss of ≥5% at 16 weeks predicted better long-term weight loss with naltrexone-bupropion at 1 year compared to those with <5% weight loss.[39] In patients with moderate or severe renal impairment, the maximum recommended dose is one tablet (8/90 mg) twice daily, and its use is not recommended for those with ESRD.[32] In patients with hepatic impairment, the maximum dosage is one tablet (8/90 mg) daily. Caution should be exercised in elderly patients due to a greater risk of accumulation leading to adverse drug reactions.[37] See Table 29.2 or refer to full prescribing information for further guidelines.

CELLULOSE AND CITRIC ACID HYDROGEL

Cellulose and citric acid hydrogel is a novel nonsystemic, superabsorbent hydrogel developed for the treatment of overweight or obesity.[38] This new cellulose and citric acid hydrogel was approved by the FDA under the brand name Plenity in April 2019. The cellulose and citric acid hydrogel is considered a medical device because it achieves its primary intended purpose through mechanical modes of action.[40]

The Gelesis Loss of Weight (GLOW) study provided an assessment of the safety and efficacy of this device in patients with overweight and obesity, with and without T2D. GLOW was a 24-week multicenter, randomized, double-blind, placebo-controlled study. For 24 weeks, patients self-administered 3 capsules containing either 2.25 g of cellulose and citric acid hydrogel or the placebo with 500 mL of water 20–30 minutes prior to lunch and dinner in conjunction with a hypocaloric diet of 300 kcal/day below their calculated energy requirement. Patients were also instructed to perform daily moderate-intensity exercise (for example, 30 minutes of walking per day) and maintain their smoking habits during the study. Patients lost an average of 6.4% (treatment group) and 4.4% (placebo) of their baseline body weight at 24 weeks. Significantly more patients in the treatment group achieved >5% weight loss versus placebo (59% vs. 42%), and 27% of patients in the treatment group lost >10% of their body weight versus 15% in the placebo. The most common adverse effect in each group was gastrointestinal (GI) related and only when grouping all of the GI side effects together was there a significant difference between the groups.[40]

The Gelesis Loss of Weight 24-week Extension (GLOW-EX) evaluated the effectiveness over a 48-week exposure, while also assessing the weight loss benefit of adding the treatment after patients had successful weight loss with lifestyle modifications (placebo) over the initial 24 weeks. GLOW-EX offered the last 52 patients completing the GLOW study who had lost >3% body weight from baseline an opportunity to participate in his open-label extension; 39 patients (21 from treatment and 18 from placebo) were enrolled. The patients treated in the GLOW study achieved a mean of 7.1% (SD 2.8%) weight loss at the time of enrollment compared with 7.1% (SD 4.1%) among those originally in the placebo group. Continuing the treatment resulted in a mean 7.6% (SD 5.1%) weight loss at 48 weeks, showing maintenance of weight loss at 48 weeks. The addition of the treatment to patients initially in the placebo group resulted in a mean of 9.4% (SD 6.4%) weight loss at 48 weeks.[40] The safety results in GLOW-EX were consistent with the GLOW safety results.

Patients with diabetes and an A1C of <8.5% were included as participants in the study. In the GLOW study there were 32 patients in the treatment group and 36 patients in the placebo group with prediabetes (FPG >100 mg/dL and <126 mg/dL) or drug-naïve T2D (FPG >126 mg/dL) based on two consecutive FPG measurements at visits 1 and 233. The mean percentage change in body weight from baseline to 24 weeks was –8.1% (SD 6.5%) and –5.6% (SD 4.9%) for the treatment and placebo groups, respectively. More patients with prediabetes and drug-naïve T2D achieved >7.5% (53%) and >10% (44%) reduction in weight compared with 25% and 14%, respectively, for the placebo.[40]

Device Characteristics

Indications for Use

Plenity is indicated to aid in weight management in overweight and obese adults with a body mass index (BMI) of 25–40 kg/m², when used in conjunction with diet and exercise.[41]

Mechanism of Action

Two naturally derived building blocks, modified cellulose cross-linked with citric acid create a three-dimensional matrix. Each capsule contains thousands of superabsorbent hydrogel particles, and when consumed orally with a meal, the capsules disintegrate in the stomach and release the particles. When fully hydrated, the individual nonclustering particles occupy about a quarter of average stomach volume. The gel particles mix with ingested foods, creating a larger volume with higher elasticity and viscosity in the stomach and small intestine, promoting satiety and fullness.[41]

Pharmacodynamics and Pharmacokinetics

Plenity is not systemically absorbed and is considered a medical device due to its mechanical modes of action. Onset of action is seen with satiety, occurring 20–30 minutes after ingestion.[41]

Considerations

Warnings and Precautions

The use of Penity is contraindicated in pregnancy due to the importance of moderate weight gain being required for positive fetal outcomes. Patients who experience severe abdominal pain or diarrhea should discontinue use and contact their medical provider. Use should be avoided in patients with esophageal anatomic anomalies, suspected strictures, and complications from prior GI surgery that may affect mobility and transit.[41]

Special Populations

Plenity is contraindicated in pregnancy. Since it is not systemically absorbed, there are no dose adjustments necessary in patients with renal or hepatic impairment.[41]

Adverse Effects and Monitoring

Common adverse effects that are associated with the use of Plenity that were greater than placebo include all GI-related adverse events combined, of which 98% were classified as mild or moderate. Adverse effects that were seen in patients on Plenity that were equivalent to the placebo include abdominal distention and pain, bloating, constipation, cramping, diarrhea, flatulence, vomiting and gastro-esophageal reflux disease (GERD). Patients and providers should monitor BMI, weight, and blood glucose in patients with diabetes while on Plenity.[41]

Drug Interactions

In a pharmacokinetic study looking at the effect on metformin of cellulose and citric acid as a single dose under feeding conditions resulted in no change to the pharmacokinetic parameters of metformin. Under fasting conditions, the cellulose and citric acid hydrogel decreased the metformin AUC and C_{max}. The study suggests that cellulose and citric acid mimics the effects of food on metformin pharmacokinetics. Other drug interactions have not been identified. Packaging indicates that all medications should be taken during the morning while in a fasting state or at bedtime; however, if a patient must take a dose with food, all medications should be taken after the meal has started. The risk of drug interactions may outweigh the benefit of using cellulose and citric acid hydrogel, especially with medications that have narrow therapeutic windows.[41] See Table 29.1 for drug interaction information.

Dosage and Administration

Patients should be advised to take cellulose and citric acid hydrogel with water twice a day, 20–30 minutes before lunch and dinner. Each dose includes 3 capsules provided in a single blister pack. After taking the capsules, patients should be advised to drink 2 additional glasses of water (8 fl oz or 250 mL) each. See Table 29.2 or refer to the full prescribing information for further guidelines.[41]

SUMMARY

Obesity is a chronic medical condition that results from a long-term mismatch in energy balance and affects almost 40% of U.S. adults. There are many health risks that are associated with obesity, including T2D, cardiovascular effects, osteoarthritis, respiratory problems, and even some cancers. These risks can be decreased by implementing an appropriate, personalized weight loss regimen. The regimen should include lifestyle modifications to diet and exercise and may include the use of pharmacotherapy. Decreasing the health risks associated with obesity will have long-term benefits that may also include a decreased financial burden. Goals of therapy are preventing further weight gain, an eventual weight loss, and maintaining this lower weight over the long term. There are many agents that can be used as adjunct therapy to diet and exercise. Selection ultimately comes down to patient-specific factors, and the cost and benefit seen with these medications.

MONOGRAPHS

Liraglutide (Saxenda): https://dailymed.nlm.nih.gov/dailymed/drugInfo.cfm?setid=3946d389-0926-4f77-a708-0acb8153b143

Naltrexone/Bupropion ER (Contrave): https://dailymed.nlm.nih.gov/dailymed/drugInfo.cfm?setid=ed2da3a6-0614-4bea-8e82-962cbaae6428

Orlistat (Xenical; Alli): https://dailymed.nlm.nih.gov/dailymed/drugInfo.cfm?setid=5bbdc95b-82a1-4ba5-8185-6504ff68cc06

Phentermine (Lomaira; Adipex-P): https://dailymed.nlm.nih.gov/dailymed/drugInfo.cfm?setid=737eef3b-9a6b-4ab3-a25c-49d84d2a0197

Phentermine/Topiramate (Qsymia): https://dailymed.nlm.nih.gov/dailymed/drugInfo.cfm?setid=40dd5602-53da-45ac-bb4b-15789aba40f9

Semaglutide oral tablet (Rybelsus): https://dailymed.nlm.nih.gov/dailymed/drugInfo.cfm?setid=27f15fac-7d98-4114-a2ec-92494a91da98

Semaglutide injection (Ozempic): https://dailymed.nlm.nih.gov/dailymed/drugInfo.cfm?setid=adec4fd2-6858-4c99-91d4-531f5f2a2d79

Semaglutide injection (Wegovy): https://dailymed.nlm.nih.gov/dailymed/drugInfo.cfm?setid=ee06186f-2aa3-4990-a760-757579d8f77b

REFERENCES

1. Delaet D, Schauer D. Obesity in adults. *Clin Evid Handbook* 2010;216–217

2. American College of Cardiology/American Heart Association Task Force on Practice Guidelines, Obesity Expert Panel, 2013. Expert Panel Report: Guidelines (2013) for the management of overweight and obesity in adults. *Obes* (Silver Spring) 2014;22(Suppl. 2):S41–S410. DOI:10.1002/oby.20660

3. National Institutes of Health. Clinical guidelines on the identification, evaluation, and treatment of overweight and obesity in adults—the evidence report. *Obes Res* 1998(6 Suppl. 2):51S–209S

4. Centers for Disease Control and Prevention. Adult Obesity Facts [Internet], 29 August 2017. Available from https://www.cdc.gov/obesity/data/adult.html. Accessed 25 April 2020

5. American Diabetes Association. 7. Obesity management for the treatment of type 2 diabetes: Standards of Medical Care in Diabetes—2018. *Diabetes Care* 2018;41(Suppl. 1):S65–S72

6. Pastors JC, Warshaw H, Daly A, et al. The evidence for the effectiveness of medical nutrition therapy in diabetes management. *Diabetes Care* 2002; 25(3):608–613

7. Franz MJ, Boucher JL, Rutten-Ramos S, VanWormer JJ. Lifestyle weight-loss intervention outcomes in overweight and obese adults with type 2 diabetes: a systematic review and meta-analysis of randomized clinical trials. *J Acad Nutr Diet* 2015;115:1447–1463

8. Kahan S, Fujioka K. Obesity pharmacotherapy in patients with type 2 diabetes. *Diabetes Spectrum* 2017;30(4):250–257

9. World Health Organization (WHO). Fact sheet: obesity and overweight. [article online], 2017. Available from http://www.who.int/en/news-room/fact-sheets/detail/obesity-and-overweight. Accessed 25 April 2018

10. Jensen MD, Ryan DH, Apovian CM, et al. 2013 AHA/ACC/TOS guideline for the management of overweight and obesity in adults: a report of the American College of Cardiology/American Heart Association Task Force on Practice Guidelines and the Obesity Society. *J Am Coll Cardiol* 2014;63:2985–3023

11. Patel D. Pharmacotherapy for the management of obesity. *Metabolism* 2015;64:1376–1385

12. Adipex-P (phentermine) [package insert]. Horsham, PA, Teva Select Brands, March 2017. Available from https://dailymed.nlm.nih.gov/dailymed/drug Info.cfm?setid=f5b2f9d8-2226-476e-9caf-9d41e6891c46

13. Lomaira (phentermine) [package insert]. Newtown, PA, KVK-Tech, September 2016. Available from https://dailymed.nlm.nih.gov/dailymed/drug Info.cfm?setid=cde9fb09-e5af-434d-8874-e4f9f974d893

14. Xenical (orlistat) [package insert]. South San Francisco, CA, Genentech USA Inc., December 2017. Available from https://dailymed.nlm.nih.gov/ dailymed/drugInfo.cfm?setid=5bbdc95b-82a1-4ba5-8185-6504ff68cc06

15. Torgerson JS, Hauptman J, Boldrin MN, Sjostrom L. XENical in the prevention of diabetes in obese subjects (XENDOS) study: a randomized study of orlistat as an adjunct to lifestyle changes for the prevention of type 2 diabetes in obese patients. *Diabetes Care* 2004;27:155–161

16. Rucker D, Padwal R, Li SK, et al. Long term pharmacotherapy for obesity and overweight: updated meta-analysis. *BMJ* 2007;335:1194–1199

17. Fujioka K, O'Neil PM, Davies M, et al. Early weight loss with liraglutide 3.0 mg predicts 1-year weight loss and is associated with improvements in clinical markers. *Obes* 2016;24:2278–2288

18. Wadden TA, Hollander P, Klein S, et al. Weight maintenance and additional weight loss with liraglutide after low-calorie-diet-induced weight loss: the SCALE maintenance randomized study. *Int J Obes* 2013;37:1443–1451

19. Le Roux CW, Astrup A, Fujioka K, et al. 3 years of liraglutide versus placebo for type 2 diabetes risk reduction and weight management in individuals with prediabetes: a randomized, double-blind trial. *Lancet* 2017;380:1399–1409

20. Davies MJ, Bergenstal R, Bode B, et al. Efficacy of liraglutide for weight loss among patients with type 2 diabetes: the SCALE diabetes randomized clinical trial. *JAMA* 2015;314(7):687–699

21. U.S. Food & Drug Administration. FDA approves weight management drug for patients aged 12 and older. 4 December 2020. Available from www. fda.gov/drugs/drug-safety-and-availability/fda-approves-weight -management-drug-patients-aged-12-and-older

22. Kelly AS, Auerbach P, Barrientos-Perez M, et al. A randomized, controlled trial of liraglutide for adolescents with obesity. *N Engl J Med* 2020; 382:2117–2128. DOI:10.1056/NEJMoa1916038.

23. Saxenda (liraglutide) [package insert]. Plainsboro, NJ, Novo Nordisk Inc., May 2017. Available from https://dailymed.nlm.nih.gov/dailymed/drug Info.cfm?setid=3946d389-0926-4f77-a708-0acb8153b143

24. U.S. Food & Drug Administration. FDA approves new drug treatment for chronic weight management, first since 2014. June 2021. Available from https://www.fda.gov/news-events/press-announcements/fda-approves-new-drug-treatment-chronic-weight-management-first-2014

25. Wilding JP, Batterham RL, Calanna S, et al. Once-weekly semaglutide in adults with overweight or obesity. *NEJM* 2021;384(11):989–1002. DOI:10.1056/NEJMoa2032183.

26. Davies M, Faerch L, Jeppesen OK, et al. Semaglutide 2.4 mg once a week in adults with overweight or obesity, and type 2 diabetes (STEP 2): a randomized, double-blind, double-dummy, placebo-controlled, phase 3 trial. *Lancet* 2021;397:971–984

27. Wadden TA, Bailey TS, Billings LK, et al. Effect of subcutaneous semaglutide vs placebo as an adjunct to intensive behavioral therapy on body weight in adults with overweight or obesity: The STEP 3 randomized clinical trial. *JAMA* 2021;325(14):1403–1413. DOI:10.1001/jama.2021.1831

28. Rubino D, Abrahamsson N, Davies M, et al. Effect of continued subcutaneous semaglutide vs placebo on weight loss maintenance in adults with overweight or obesity: the STEP 4 randomized clinical trial. *JAMA* 2021; 325(14):1414–1425. DOI:10.1001/jama.2021.3224

29. Wegovy (semaglutide) [package insert]. Plainsboro, NJ, Novo Nordisk Inc., June 2021. Available from https://dailymed.nlm.nih.gov/dailymed/drugInfo.cfm?setid=ee06186f-2aa3-4990-a760-757579d8f77b

30. [Lilly] Lilly Investors. Lilly receives U.S. FDA Fast Track designation for tirzepatide for the treatment of adults with obesity, or overweight with weight-related comorbidities, 6 October 2022. Available from https://investor.lilly.com/news-releases/news-release-details/lilly-receives-us-fda-fast-track-designation-tirzepatide

31. [SUR-1} Jastreboff A, Aronne L, Ahmed N, et al. Tirzepatide once weekly for the treatment of obesity. *N Engl J Med* 2022; 387:205-16. DOI: 10.1056/NEJMoa2206038

32. Mounjaro (tirzepatide) [package insert]. Indianapolis, IN. Lilly USA, LLC., September 2022. Available from https://dailymed.nlm.nih.gov/dailymed/drugInfo.cfm?setid=d2d7da5d-ad07-4228-955f-cf7e355c8cc0

33. Qsymia (phentermine/topiramate) [package insert]. Campbell, CA, Vivus Inc., June 2017. Available from https://dailymed.nlm.nih.gov/dailymed/drugInfo.cfm?setid=40dd5602-53da-45ac-bb4b-15789aba40f9

34. Allison DB, Gadde KM, Garvey WT, et al. Controlled-release phentermine/topiramate in severely obese adults: a randomized controlled trial (EQUIP). *Obes* 2012;20:330–342

35. Gaddle KM, Allison DB, Ryan DH, et al. Effects of low-dose, controlled-release, phentermine plus topiramate combination on weight and associated comorbidities in overweight and obese adults (CONQUER): a randomized, placebo-controlled, phase 3 trial. *Lancet* 2011;377(9774):1341–1352

36. Garvey WT, Ryan DH, Look M, et al. Two-year sustained weight loss and metabolic benefits with controlled-release phentermine/topiramate in

obese and overweight adults (SEQUEL): a randomized, placebo-controlled, phase 3 extension study. *Am J Clin Nutr* 2012;95:297–308

37. Contrave (naltrexone/bupropion) [package insert]. Deerfield, IL, Takeda Pharmaceuticals America, Inc., September 2014. Available from https://dailymed.nlm.nih.gov/dailymed/drugInfo.cfm?setid=ed2da3a6-0614-4bea-8e82-962cbaae6428

38. Hollander P, Gupta AK, Plodkowski RA, et al. Effects of naltrexone sustained-release/bupropion sustained-release combination therapy on body weight and glycemic parameters in overweight and obese patients with type 2 diabetes. *Diabetes Care* 2013;36:4022–4029

39. Fukioka K, Plodkowski R, O'Neil PM, et al. The relationship between early weight loss and weight loss at one year with naltrexone ER/bupropion ER combination therapy. *Int J Obes* 2016;40:1369–1375

40. Greenway FL, Aronne, LJ, Raben A, et al. A randomized, double-blind, placebo-controlled study of Gelesis100: A novel nonsystemic oral hydrogel for weight loss. *Obesity* 2019;27(2):205–216

41. Plenity [instructions for use]. Boston, MA, Gelesis, Inc., 2019

Chapter 30
Immunizations and Diabetes

Kimberly C. McKeirnan, PharmD, BCACP
Nicole M. Rodin, PharmD, MBA

INTRODUCTION

Complications from vaccine-preventable diseases lead to hospitalization and sometimes death. The CDC considers T1D and T2D to be high-risk health conditions that can result in serious and long-term health consequences due to illness from vaccine-preventable diseases.[1] Patients with T1D or T2D are at higher risk for serious complications from contracting these diseases, even when diabetes is well managed. Patients with diabetes are at an increased risk of glycemic fluctuations, increased risk of hepatitis B infection, and even an increased risk of death by vaccine-preventable diseases.[1] This chapter will provide an overview of available vaccines, recommendations specifically for people with diabetes, and information about available vaccine resources.

VACCINATION SCHEDULES

Vaccination schedules are available from the CDC as a guide for which vaccines are needed and recommended timing of administration. Vaccination schedules developed for healthcare providers are available categorized by patient age (birth to 18 years, 19 years and older) and also by medical condition.[2] Patient-friendly schedules are also available categorized by age for infants and children, preteens and teens, and adults.[2] Catch-up schedules are available for patients who need immunizations that were recommended at younger ages.

The Advisory Committee on Immunization Practices (ACIP) also has useful vaccination resources for specific medical conditions. Figure 30.1 displays an informational table called Vaccinations for Adults with Diabetes.[3] This resource lists common adult vaccinations along with recommendations on the need for vaccines indicated specifically for patients with diabetes. The CDC also has helpful condition-specific patient infographics explaining the importance of being vaccinated and which vaccines are recommended. The diabetes infographic is shown in Figure 30.2.[4]

VACCINES

The CDC vaccination schedules provide a foundation for the vaccines that everyone should receive. However, additional recommendations are provided for peo-

Vaccinations for Adults with Diabetes

The table below shows which vaccinations you should have to protect your health if you have diabetes. Make sure you and your healthcare provider keep your vaccinations up to date.

Vaccine	Do you need it?
COVID-19	**Yes!** All adults are recommended to get a primary series of COVID-19 vaccine plus booster doses when eligible
Hepatitis A (HepA)	**Maybe.** You need this vaccine if you have a specific risk factor for hepatitis A* or simply want to be protected from this disease. The vaccine is usually given in 2 doses, 6–18 months apart.
Hepatitis B (HepB)	**Yes!** All adults younger than 60 are recommended to complete a 2- or 3-dose series of hepatitis B vaccine, depending on the brand. If you are 60 or older, you or your healthcare provider may decide you should be vaccinated because people with diabetes are at increased risk for hepatitis B.
Hib (*Haemophilus influenzae* type b)	**Maybe.** Some adults with certain high-risk conditions,* for example, lack of a functioning spleen, need vaccination with Hib. Talk to your healthcare provider to find out if you need this vaccine.
Human papilloma-virus (HPV)	**Yes!** You should get this vaccine if you are 26 years or younger. Adults age 27 through 45 may also be vaccinated against HPV after a discussion with their healthcare provider. The vaccine is usually given in 2 or 3 doses (depending on the age at which the first dose was given) over a 6-month period.
Influenza (Flu)	**Yes!** You need to be vaccinated against influenza every fall (or even as late as winter or spring) for your protection and for the protection of others around you.
Measles, mumps, rubella (MMR)	**Maybe.** You need at least 1 dose of MMR vaccine if you were born in 1957 or later. You may also need a second dose.* People with weakened immune systems should not get MMR vaccine.
Meningococcal ACWY (MenACWY)	**Maybe.** You may need MenACWY vaccine if you have one of several health conditions,* for example, if you do not have a functioning spleen, and also boosters if your risk is ongoing. You need MenACWY if you are age 21 or younger and a first-year college student living in a residence hall and you either have never been vaccinated or were vaccinated before age 16.
Meningococcal B (MenB)	**Maybe.** You may need MenB if you have one of several health conditions,* for example, if you do not have a functioning spleen, and also boosters if your risk is ongoing. You may also consider getting the MenB vaccine if you are age 23 or younger (even if you don't have a high-risk medical condition) after a discussion with your healthcare provider.
Pneumococcal (PPSV23; PCV15, PCV20)	**Yes!** Adults with diabetes need to get either PCV20 alone, or PCV15 followed 1 year later by PPSV23. If you have previously received either PCV13 and/or PPSV23, your healthcare provider can determine what additional doses you may need.
Tetanus, diph-theria, whooping cough (pertussis) (Tdap, Td)	**Yes!** If you have not received a dose of Tdap during your lifetime, you need to get a Tdap shot now. After that, you need a Tdap or Td booster dose every 10 years. Consult your healthcare provider if you haven't had at least 3 tetanus- and diphtheria-toxoid containing shots sometime in your life or if you have a deep or dirty wound.
Varicella (Chickenpox)	**Maybe.** If you have never had chickenpox, never were vaccinated, or were vaccinated but only received 1 dose, talk to your healthcare provider to find out if you need this vaccine.*
Zoster (shingles)	**Yes!** If you are 19 or older and have a weakened immune system or are 50 or older, you should get a 2-dose series of the Shingrix brand of shingles vaccine, even if you were already vaccinated with Zostavax.

* Consult your healthcare provider to determine your level of risk for infection and your need for this vaccine.

Are you planning to travel outside the United States? Visit the Centers for Disease Control and Prevention's (CDC) website at wwwnc.cdc.gov/travel/destinations/list for travel information, or consult a travel clinic.

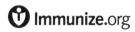 **Immunize**.org   FOR PROFESSIONALS www.immunize.org / FOR THE PUBLIC www.vaccineinformation.org

www.immunize.org/catg.d/p4043.pdf • Item #P4043 (6/22)

Figure 30.1—ACIP Table Vaccinations for Adults with Diabetes.[3]

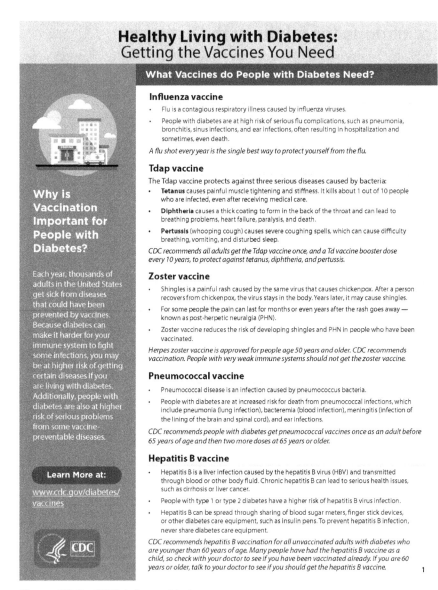

Healthy Living with Diabetes:
Getting the Vaccines You Need

What Vaccines do People with Diabetes Need?

Why is Vaccination Important for People with Diabetes?

Each year, thousands of adults in the United States get sick from diseases that could have been prevented by vaccines. Because diabetes can make it harder for your immune system to fight some infections, you may be at higher risk of getting certain diseases if you are living with diabetes. Additionally, people with diabetes are also at higher risk of serious problems from some vaccine-preventable diseases.

Learn More at:

www.cdc.gov/diabetes/vaccines

CDC

Influenza vaccine

- Flu is a contagious respiratory illness caused by influenza viruses.
- People with diabetes are at high risk of serious flu complications, such as pneumonia, bronchitis, sinus infections, and ear infections, often resulting in hospitalization and sometimes, even death.

A flu shot every year is the single best way to protect yourself from the flu.

Tdap vaccine

The Tdap vaccine protects against three serious diseases caused by bacteria:

- **Tetanus** causes painful muscle tightening and stiffness. It kills about 1 out of 10 people who are infected, even after receiving medical care.
- **Diphtheria** causes a thick coating to form in the back of the throat and can lead to breathing problems, heart failure, paralysis, and death.
- **Pertussis** (whooping cough) causes severe coughing spells, which can cause difficulty breathing, vomiting, and disturbed sleep.

CDC recommends all adults get the Tdap vaccine once, and a Td vaccine booster dose every 10 years, to protect against tetanus, diphtheria, and pertussis.

Zoster vaccine

- Shingles is a painful rash caused by the same virus that causes chickenpox. After a person recovers from chickenpox, the virus stays in the body. Years later, it may cause shingles.
- For some people the pain can last for months or even years after the rash goes away — known as post-herpetic neuralgia (PHN).
- Zoster vaccine reduces the risk of developing shingles and PHN in people who have been vaccinated.

Herpes zoster vaccine is approved for people age 50 years and older. CDC recommends vaccination. People with very weak immune systems should not get the zoster vaccine.

Pneumococcal vaccine

- Pneumococcal disease is an infection caused by pneumococcus bacteria.
- People with diabetes are at increased risk for death from pneumococcal infections, which include pneumonia (lung infection), bacteremia (blood infection), meningitis (infection of the lining of the brain and spinal cord), and ear infections.

CDC recommends people with diabetes get pneumococcal vaccines once as an adult before 65 years of age and then two more doses at 65 years or older.

Hepatitis B vaccine

- Hepatitis B is a liver infection caused by the hepatitis B virus (HBV) and transmitted through blood or other body fluid. Chronic hepatitis B can lead to serious health issues, such as cirrhosis or liver cancer.
- People with type 1 or type 2 diabetes have a higher risk of hepatitis B virus infection.
- Hepatitis B can be spread through sharing of blood sugar meters, finger stick devices, or other diabetes care equipment, such as insulin pens. To prevent hepatitis B infection, never share diabetes care equipment.

CDC recommends hepatitis B vaccination for all unvaccinated adults with diabetes who are younger than 60 years of age. Many people have had the hepatitis B vaccine as a child, so check with your doctor to see if you have been vaccinated already. If you are 60 years or older, talk to your doctor to see if you should get the hepatitis B vaccine.

1

Figure 30.2—CDC Infographic.[4]

ple with specific medical conditions. For patients with diabetes, the CDC specifically recommends vaccination against influenza, hepatitis B, pneumococcal diseases, herpes zoster (shingles), and the combination vaccine for tetanus, diphtheria, and pertussis.

INFLUENZA

Influenza is a respiratory illness affecting the nose, throat, and lungs caused by infection with the influenza virus. Complications from influenza can lead to pneumonia, bronchitis, sinus infections, and ear infections in all people, but it can also cause blood glucose fluctuations in those with diabetes. Acute illness may cause hyperglycemia, but dietary inconsistency due to the general malaise and feeling not well during the course of illness can also lead to hypoglycemia in patients taking antihyperglycemic agents. Many influenza medications contain high levels of sugar. It is good practice to recommend increasing the frequency of blood glucose testing during this time. Annual influenza vaccinations are recommended by the CDC and are FDA approved for people with diabetes.[5] The available influenza vaccines comprise four influenza viruses, also known as quadrivalent influenza vaccines, that researchers believe will be most common in the upcoming influenza season. Influenza vaccine is generally administered intramuscularly in one dose.[5] For patients over the age of 65 years, the ACIP preferentially recommends a quadrivalent high-dose influenza vaccine, a quadrivalent recombinant influenza vaccine, or a quadrivalent adjuvanted inactivated influenza vaccine. If none of these are available then any other age-appropriate influenza vaccine may be used.[5] The influenza vaccine has been shown to reduce the risk of getting sick with the flu, as well as to reduce the risk of having a serious outcome if infected, such as a stay in the hospital.[5]

HEPATITIS B

Hepatitis B is a vaccine-preventable liver infection caused by the hepatitis B virus (HBV), which is transmitted by bodily fluid. People with diabetes have higher rates of hepatitis B, because outbreaks associated with blood glucose monitoring procedures have occurred.[6] There is approximately a 60% increase in prevalence in patients with diabetes for contracting HBV and up to a twofold increase in acquiring the virus.[7] In most people, hepatitis B is an acute illness, but in patients with reduced immune function, hepatitis B can become a chronic infection leading to cirrhosis, cancer, liver failure, or death.[6] The hepatitis B vaccine is available as a two- or three-dose series of intramuscular injections, although one hepatitis B vaccine has an FDA-approved four-dose accelerated schedule.

PNEUMOCOCCAL DISEASE

Infection with pneumococcal bacteria can lead to meningitis, pneumonia, and bacteremia. There are currently three different pneumococcal vaccines recommended by the CDC for routine administration to adults: the 15-valent pneumococcal conjugate vaccine (PCV15), the 20-valent pneumococcal conjugate vaccine (PCV20), and the pneumococcal polysaccharide vaccine (PPSV23).[8] For all people ages 65 years and older who have never received a pneumococcal conjugate vaccine, the ACIP recommends administering either PCV15 or PCV20. If PCV15 is administered, it should be followed by a dose of PPSV23. If PCV20 is used, no additional vaccination is necessary unless other risk factor exist.

Vaccination against pneumococcal diseases is also recommended for people with an increased risk for infection, including patients with diabetes, even when under the age of 65 years. People ages 18 to 64 who have not previously received a pneumococcal vaccination and have certain underlying medical conditions or other risk factors should receive one dose of either PCV15 or PCV20.[8] Similar to the recommendations for older adults, if PCV15 is administered, it should be followed by a dose of PPSV23 1 year later.[2] All three pneumococcal vaccines are administered individually as a one-dose intramuscular or subcutaneous injection. Doses of PCV15 and PPSV23 should ideally be given 1 year apart, although a minimum dosing interval of 8 weeks can be considered for adults with immuno-compromising conditions.[2] If the patient has previously been vaccinated with PPSV23 before the age of 65 years, they should receive the PCV15 or PCV20 vaccine at age 65 years, at least 1 year after their last pneumococcal vaccine.[8]

HERPES ZOSTER

Herpes zoster, also known as shingles, is caused by the chickenpox virus in the form of reactivating the varicella zoster virus, which remains dormant in the nervous system after infection. Shingles presents as a painful rash that develops on one side of the body. The rash usually resolves in 2–4 weeks, but some patients have complications, such as postherpetic neuralgia (PHN), which can cause pain lasting for years. The CDC recommends all people over the age of 50 years receive a recombinant zoster vaccine. The newer recombinant zoster vaccine is a two-dose series and was FDA approved in 2017. A previous zoster vaccine, zoster vaccine live, was used in the U.S. until November 2020, but is no longer available or recommended. Even people who were previously vaccinated with zoster vaccine live should receive the full schedule of the new recombinant vaccine in order to more adequately prevent shingles and the complications caused by the disease.[9]

TETANUS, DIPHTHERIA, PERTUSSIS

Tetanus is a vaccine-preventable infection that is caused by Clostridium tetani bacteria. Tetanus primarily presents as painful muscle contractions in the jaw, also known as "lockjaw." Tetanus itself is not spread among humans. The Clostridium tetani bacteria spreads through mediums such as soil, dust, or manure. Pertussis is also known as whooping cough. This is a respiratory disease that is caused by the Bordetella pertussis bacteria. It is known for the violent, uncontrollable coughing associated with the disease that often makes it hard to breathe.[10] Protection against these infections is offered in a variety of combination products. For patients who are younger than 7 years of age, diphtheria and tetanus (DT) and diphtheria, tetanus, and pertussis (DTaP) combinations are offered. For patients who are 7 years of age or older, the same combinations of diphtheria and tetanus (Td) and diphtheria, tetanus, and pertussis (Tdap) exist with differing doses of the diphtheria component. According to the CDC, this is to be used as a booster that should be updated every 10 years in diabetic patients.[11]

COVID-19

Infection of SARS-CoV-2, the strain of coronavirus responsible for the coronavirus pandemic (COVID-19), has a wide variety of presentations that can differ based on variant. COVID-19 is transmitted in airborne particles and has a high rate of transferability. The most common path of transmission occurs through close contact (with 6 feet). Upon infection, signs and symptoms can vary but are most seen through fever, chills, cough, shortness of breath and difficulty beathing, fatigue and loss of smell and taste.[12] The clinical presentation of COVID-19 in patients with diabetes can precipitate complications such as DKA, hyperosmolar hyperglycemic state (HHS), and severe insulin resistance.[13] Additionally, patients with diabetes are at a higher risk for developing more serious complications from COVID-19 infection. This risk is compounded in patients with diabetes who also have multiple comorbidities and are older adults. Severe illness may result in hospitalization, intubation, and may be fatal.[14]

The COVID-19 vaccination series with a booster vaccination are recommended for patients with T1D and T2D due to the increased risk and vulnerability of severe illness with COVID-19 in both patient populations.[15] COVID-19 vaccines from Pfizer-BioNTech and Moderna, for which the FDA provided emergency use authorization (EUA) in December 2020, use novel mRNA technology. This vaccine type injects mRNA intramuscularly, which is translated to create proteins that the body should recognize to be similar to the SARS-CoV-2 virus. By recognizing this similar protein, the body mounts an immune response, which leads to the creation of antibodies that are able to initiate immune defenses when the SARS-CoV-2 proteins are encountered again. A COVID-19 vaccine from Janssen, for which the FDA provided EUA in February 2021, utilizes viral vector technology. A viral vector uses a modified version of a dead virus to introduce the pathogen to the cells. This aids in creating antibodies that are able to initiate immune defenses when the virus is present. A third type of COVID-19 vaccine, the protein subunit vaccine Novavax, received EUA in 2022. Novavax vaccine contains spike protein pieces of the SARS-CoV-2 virus along with an adjuvant, which improves the immune response to the spike protein. The mRNA, viral vector, and protein subunit vaccines have been proven to be safe and effective for decreasing rates of transmission and avoiding severe illness.[16]

CONCLUSION

T1D and T2D increase risk for complications from vaccine-preventable diseases even when the diabetes is well managed. The CDC recommends that patients with diabetes be up to date with the flu vaccine and the tetanus, diphtheria, pertussis vaccine, and for these patients to maintain an altered schedule when receiving the pneumococcal series, the hepatitis B series, and protection against herpes zoster.[1,2] Following these recommended schedules and reducing complications from vaccine-preventable diseases will lead to lower hospitalization rates and fewer deaths for patients with diabetes.

REFERENCES

1. Centers for Disease Control and Prevention (CDC). Diabetes type 1 and type 2 and adult vaccination [Internet], 2 May 2016. Updated 1 November 2016. Available from https://www.cdc.gov/vaccines/adults/rec-vac/health-conditions/diabetes.html. Accessed 17 February 2023

2. CDC. Information for adult patients: 2018 recommended immunizations for adults: by age [Internet]. Available from https://www.cdc.gov/vaccines/schedules/hcp/imz/adult.html. Accessed 17 February 2023

3. Immunization Action Coalition. Vaccinations for adults with diabetes [Internet], June 2018. Available from http://www.immunize.org/catg.d/p4043.pdf. Accessed 17 February 2023

4. CDC. Healthy living with diabetes: getting the vaccines you need [Internet], May 2018. Available from https://www.cdc.gov/vaccines/adults/rec-vac/health-conditions/diabetes/infographic/images/global/footer/diabates_en.pdf. Accessed 17 February 2023

5. Grohskopf LA, Blanton LH, Ferdinands JM, et al. Prevention and Control of Seasonal Influenza with Vaccines: Recommendations of the Advisory Committee on Immunization Practices - United States, 2022–23 Influenza Season. MMWR Recomm Rep. 2022;71(1):1–28. Published 2022 August 26

6. CDC. Viral hepatitis [Internet], 12 October 2021. Available from https://www.cdc.gov/hepatitis/hbv/index.htm. Accessed 17 February 2023

7. Hepbtalk. Hepatitis B precautions for people living with diabetes [Internet], 20 March 2018. Hepatitis B Foundation and Baruch S. Blumberg Institute. Available from www.hepb.org/blog/hepatitis-b-precautions-people-living-diabetes/. Accessed 17 February 2023

8. CDC. Pneumococcal vaccine recommendations [Internet], 13 February 2023. Available from https://www.cdc.gov/vaccines/vpd/pneumo/hcp/recommendations.html. Accessed 17 February 2023

9. CDC. Shingles (herpes zoster) [Internet], 3 February 2022. Available from https://www.cdc.gov/shingles/index.html. Accessed 17 February 2023

10. CDC. Epidemiology and prevention of vaccine-preventable diseases. The Pink Book [Internet]. Available from https://www.cdc.gov/vaccines/pubs/pinkbook/downloads/pert.pdf

11. CDC. Tetanus [Internet], 16 September 2022. Available from hhttps://www.cdc.gov/vaccines/vpd/tetanus/index.html. Accessed 17 February 2023

12. CDC. Symptoms of COVID-19 [Internet], 22 December 2020. Updated 26 Octover 2022. Available from https://www.cdc.gov/coronavirus/2019-ncov/symptoms-testing/symptoms.html. Accessed 17 February 2023

13. Kim NY, Ha E, Moon JS, Lee YH, Choi EY. Acute hyperglycemic crises with coronavirus disease-19: case reports. *Diabetes Metab J* 2020;44(2):349

14. Guo W, Li M, Dong Y, et al. Diabetes is a risk factor for the progression and prognosis of COVID-19. *Diabetes Metab Res Rev* 2020;https://onlinelibrary.wiley.com/doi/full/10.1002/dmrr.3319

15. Powers AC, Aronoff DM, Eckel RH. COVID-19 vaccine prioritisation for type 1 and type 2 diabetes. *Lancet Diabetes Endocrinol.* 18 January 2021. Available from https://www.thelancet.com/journals/landia/article/PIIS2213-8587(21)00017-6/fulltext

16. CDC. Overview of COVID-19 vaccines [Internet], 1 November 2022. Available from: https://www.cdc.gov/coronavirus/2019-ncov/vaccines/different-vaccines/overview-COVID-19-vaccines.html. Accessed 21 February 2023

Index

Note: Page numbers followed by *f* refer to figures. Page numbers followed by *t* refer to tables. Page numbers in **bold** indicate an in-depth discussion of the topic.

A

A1C
α-glucosidase inhibitors, 85, 190, 192–193
biguanides, 80, 95
bile acid sequestrant, 250–252, 417
cardiovascular outcome trials, 296*t*, 298*t*, 305*t*
chronic kidney disease, 345
combination therapy, 65–66
diabetic retinopathy, 517, 524
dopamine-2 receptor agonist, 261
DPP-4 inhibitors, 86, 198, 200, 208
gastroparesis, 474
glinides, 84, 162–163, 168
GLP-1 RAs, 88–89, 219, 220, 223, 227–228, 232
glucose lowering medications, 60*f*
glycemic recommendation, 17
injectable therapy, 61*f*, 82*f*
insulin therapy, 1–4, 40, 42, 43*f*, 50, 89
metformin, 81
niacin, 415*t*
noninsulin treatment, 9
obesity, 565
pramlintide, 238–240, 241*t*, 242
SGLT2 inhibitors, 87, 176, 180
sulfonylureas, 84, 145, 147–148
thiazolidinediones, 86, 125–128, 140

type 1 diabetes, 9
type 2 diabetes, 56–57, 60*f*
abdominal pain, 193, 245, 255, 415*t*
abemaciclib, 113
abuse, 540. *See also* substance use/abuse
AC2993 Diabetes Management for Improving Glucose Outcomes (AMIGO) trial, 218*t*
acarbose, 62*t*, 85, 190–196
ACE inhibitors. *See* angiotensin-converting-enzyme (ACE) inhibitors
acebrophylline, 568*t*
acellular matrix tissue, 377, 378, 379*t*
acetylcholine, 553
acid-reducing medications, 429
ACIP Table Vaccinations for Adults with Diabetes, 595*f*
acromegaly, 260
Action for Health in Diabetes (Look AHEAD) trial, 300
Action in Diabetes and Vascular Disease: Preterax and Diamicron Modified Release Controlled Evaluation (ADVANCE) trial, 148, 271, 274*t*, 517
Action in Diabetes and Vascular Disease: Preterax and Diamicron MR Controlled Evaluation-Blood Pressure (ADVANCE BP) trial, 272
Action to Control Cardiovascular Risk in Diabetes blood pressure

CPSIA information can be obtained
at www.ICGtesting.com
Printed in the USA
JSHW010735270723
45478JS00002B/3